HKPropel >> Accessing your HKPropel digital product is easy!

T0260481

If it's your first time using HKPropel:

1. Visit HKPropel.HumanKinetics.com.
2. Click the "New user? Register here" link on the opening screen to register for an account and rede your one-time-use access code.
3. Follow the onscreen prompts to create your HKPropel account. Use a **valid email address** as your username to ensure you receive important system updates and to help us find your account if you ever need assistance.
4. Enter the access code exactly as shown below, including hyphens. You will not need to re-enter this access code on subsequent visits, and this access code cannot be redeemed by any other user.
5. After your first visit, simply log in to HKPropel.HumanKinetics.com to access your digital product.

If you already have an HKPropel account:

1. Visit HKPropel.HumanKinetics.com and log in with your username (email address) and password.
2. Once you are logged in, click the arrow next to your name in the top right corner and then click **My Account**.
3. Under the "Add Access Code" heading, enter the access code exactly as shown below, including hyphens, and click the **Add** button.
4. Once your code is redeemed, navigate to your Library on the Dashboard to access your digital content.

> **Product: Athletic Training and Therapy HKPropel Access**
>
> **Access code: 53ZW-JD3R-SZQI-Z51G**

NOTE TO STUDENTS: If your instructor uses HKPropel to assign work to your class, you will need to enter a class enrollment token in HKPropel on the **My Account** page. This token will be provided **by your instructor at no cost to you**, but it is required **in addition** to the unique access code that is printed above.

Helpful tips:

You may reset your password from the log in screen at any time if you forget it.

Your license to this digital product will expire **1 year** after the date you redeem the access code. You can check the expiration dates of all your HKPropel products at any time in **My Account**.

If you purchased a used book, you may purchase a new access code by visiting US.HumanKinetics.com and searching for "Athletic Training and Therapy HKPropel Access."

For assistance, contact us via email at HKPropelCustSer@hkusa.com.   02-2021

Athletic Training and Therapy

FOUNDATIONS OF BEHAVIOR AND PRACTICE

Leamor Kahanov, EdD, ATC, LAT
SUNY Oneonta

Ellen K. Payne, PhD, LAT, ATC, EMT
Moravian College

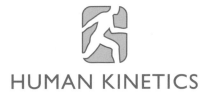

HUMAN KINETICS

Library of Congress Cataloging-in-Publication Data

Names: Kahanov, Leamor, 1969- author. | Payne, Ellen K., 1978- author.
Title: Athletic training and therapy : foundations of behavior and practice
 / Leamor Kahanov, Ellen K. Payne.
Description: First edition. | Champaign, IL : Human Kinetics, Inc., 2022. |
 Includes bibliographical references and index.
Identifiers: LCCN 2020034380 (print) | LCCN 2020034381 (ebook) | ISBN
 9781492560586 (paperback) | ISBN 9781492596523 (epub) | ISBN
 9781492560593 (pdf)
Subjects: LCSH: Sports medicine. | Sports injuries--Treatment.
Classification: LCC RC1210 .K32 2021 (print) | LCC RC1210 (ebook) | DDC
 617.1/027--dc23
LC record available at https://lccn.loc.gov/2020034380
LC ebook record available at https://lccn.loc.gov/2020034381

ISBN: 978-1-4925-6058-6 (print)
ISBN: 978-1-4925-6366-2 (loose-leaf)

Copyright © 2022 by Leamor Kahanov and Ellen K. Payne

Human Kinetics supports copyright. Copyright fuels scientific and artistic endeavor, encourages authors to create new works, and promotes free speech. Thank you for buying an authorized edition of this work and for complying with copyright laws by not reproducing, scanning, or distributing any part of it in any form without written permission from the publisher. You are supporting authors and allowing Human Kinetics to continue to publish works that increase the knowledge, enhance the performance, and improve the lives of people all over the world.

The online learning content that accompanies this product is delivered on HK*Propel*, HKPropel.HumanKinetics.com. You agree that you will not use HK*Propel* if you do not accept the site's Privacy Policy and Terms and Conditions, which detail approved uses of the online content.

To report suspected copyright infringement of content published by Human Kinetics, contact us at **permissions@hkusa.com**. To request permission to legally reuse content published by Human Kinetics, please refer to the information at **https://US.HumanKinetics.com/pages/permissions-information**.

The web addresses cited in this text were current as of September 2020, unless otherwise noted.

Senior Acquisitions Editor: Joshua J. Stone; **Acquisitions Editor:** Jolynn Gower; **Developmental and Managing Editor:** Amanda S. Ewing; **Copyeditor:** Joy Hoppenot; **Proofreader:** Pamela S. Johnson; **Indexer:** Rebecca L. McCorkle; **Permissions Manager:** Dalene Reeder; **Senior Graphic Designer:** Nancy Rasmus; **Cover Designer:** Keri Evans; **Cover Design Specialist:** Susan Rothermel Allen; **Photograph (cover):** Sciepro/Science Photo Library/Getty Images; **Photographs (interior):** Marco Calderon Photography, Inc./ © Human Kinetics, unless otherwise noted; **Photo Asset Manager:** Laura Fitch; **Photo Production Specialist:** Amy M. Rose; **Photo Production Manager:** Jason Allen; **Senior Art Manager:** Kelly Hendren; **Illustrations:** © Human Kinetics, unless otherwise noted; **Printer:** Walsworth

We thank Moravian College in Bethlehem, Pennsylvania, for assistance in providing the location for the photo shoot for this book.

Printed in the United States of America   10   9   8   7   6   5   4   3   2   1

The paper in this book was manufactured using responsible forestry methods.

Human Kinetics
1607 N. Market Street
Champaign, IL 61820
USA

United States and International
Website: **US.HumanKinetics.com**
Email: info@hkusa.com
Phone: 1-800-747-4457

Canada
Website: **Canada.HumanKinetics.com**
Email: info@hkcanada.com

E7214 (paperback) /
E7288 (loose-leaf)

Tell us what you think!
Human Kinetics would love to hear what we
can do to improve the customer experience.
Use this QR code to take our brief survey.

This textbook is dedicated to Josh Stone, who started us along this journey.

CONTENTS

PART I   Foundation of Professional Practice

PART III   Immediate and Emergency Care

PART IV   Injury and Illness Evaluation

PREFACE

Athletic Training and Therapy: Foundations of Behavior and Practice is written for entry-level graduate students of athletic training. The text is intended for students who have a foundational understanding of health and exercise sciences from their undergraduate education, including coursework in biology, anatomy, physiology, wellness, nutrition, exercise physiology, biomechanics, and statistics. The primary goal of the text is to deliver the following:

- A broad competency-based educational foundation for entry-level graduate students in athletic training
- An introductory foundation of athletic training and health care behaviors and professional practice
- An evidence-based underpinning of athletic training and health care behaviors and practices
- The foundational information necessary for a professional athletic training program
- A succinct and concise presentation of critical information that engages the contemporary student as a member of the interprofessional health care team

Organization

The textbook helps students incorporate concepts of evidence-based medicine, cultural competence, interprofessional practice, prevention, health promotion, acute care, therapeutic interventions and rehabilitation basics, and administrative management into a global health care context of assessing and managing injuries and illnesses. Contemporary concepts in athletic training are presented to orient students toward an expanding scope of professional knowledge. Cultural competence, special populations, epidemiology, and emerging therapeutic interventions are a few of the subjects unique to the current textbook.

- Part I presents information essential to managing professional practice in athletic training. Specifically, the chapters provide key information in health care administration from the athletic trainer's lens, including gaining cultural competence to address diversity in patient care. The chapters also address maintaining professional

currency and practice through an understanding of research and ethical obligations. The concepts in part I are integrated throughout the textbook to provide a comprehensive understanding of the scope of the athletic training profession, the use of evidence-based practice, health care promotion, cultural competence, and management and administration.

- Part II focuses on the athletic trainer's role in injury and illness prevention, including important concepts for athletic training students who are beginning educational programs and their first clinical rotations. It includes introductory information on blood-borne pathogens, preparticipation examinations (PPE), weather monitoring, hydration, taping and bracing, and fitting of fitness and protective equipment.
- Part III of the textbook presents entry-level information on emergency planning and acute care procedures. It also discusses emergent injury and illness assessment, placing the important components of assessment in the context of a holistic view of emergency planning and immediate care.
- Part IV addresses aspects of common injuries and illnesses and the evaluation and referral process for nonemergent conditions. In addition to the essentials of evaluation and diagnosis, this section provides an understanding of the patient, including life span, special populations, and psychosocial aspects of health care. This section provides information on a range of illnesses and types of evaluation used to address the increasing diversity that athletic trainers encounter in client populations and work settings. Unique to this section is information regarding medical imaging, an expanding responsibility for athletic trainers.
- Part V presents therapeutic interventions, a principle component of an athletic trainer's practice. It provides a comprehensive overview of therapeutic and medical interventions for athletic trainers, including therapeutic modalities and exercises, pharmacology, and casting procedures. It also provides information that orients students to emerging practices.

Together, the chapters in this textbook introduce athletic training students to health care concepts and professional practices in their field to help develop a comprehensive knowledge base that supports interprofessional engagement for serving a diverse population.

Strategic Alliance Coverage

The authors focus on identifying and integrating foundational information of the athletic training behaviors and professional practices required for training programs accredited by the Commission on Accreditation of Athletic Training Education (CAATE). Each chapter includes a listing of the CAATE standards addressed in that chapter. The CAATE standards are an essential component of the Strategic Alliance (NATA, BOC, and CAATE) that informs the athletic training profession on essential knowledge and skills.

The material in this textbook is consistent with the domains of athletic training clinical practice as defined by the National Athletic Trainers' Association Executive Council for Education (NATA-ECE) and the seventh edition of the Board of Certification (BOC) Practice Analysis. The text also adheres to the BOC Standards of Practice.

The text highlights current concepts, expanding professional settings, and the need to enhance team-based care. This book emphasizes the foundational knowledge students will need to obtain national certification by successfully completing the BOC examination.

Key Features

The text is unique in its attention to changing instructional methods and its aim to engage adult students with an integration of digital and traditional classroom content. The authors focus on presenting comprehensive foundational information in a succinct and graphic-rich environment.

In addition, the textbook includes the following to aid student understanding:

- Learning objectives clearly and succinctly present the goals of each chapter to help students focus their reading and studying, both now and when they are preparing for the BOC examination.

- Glossary terms are identified in bold print throughout the text.
- A graphic-rich presentation of key concepts and foundational information augments the text.
- The Clinical Bottom Line section that closes each chapter summarizes key concepts.
- Evidence-Based Athletic Training sidebars highlight research (e.g., position statements, systematic literature reviews, high-level RCTs) to connect research findings with the concepts presented in each chapter.
- Foundational Skills sidebars provide directions for common skills for entry-level athletic trainers.

Instructor Resources in HKPropel

A variety of instructor resources are available online within the instructor pack in *HKPropel*:

- *Presentation package.* More than 700 PowerPoint slides cover the key concepts of each chapter, including select art, photos, and tables.
- *Image bank.* Most of the art, photos, and tables from the text are provided as individual files for use in PowerPoints, student handouts, and so on.
- *Instructor guide.* The instructor guide includes a sample syllabus and chapter-specific files that include the chapter objectives, a chapter summary, lecture outline, ideas for student activities, and answers to the case studies.
- *Test package.* More than 650 questions are provided that instructors can use to make their own tests and quizzes.

Instructor ancillaries are free to adopting instructors, including an ebook version of the text that allows instructors to add highlights, annotations, and bookmarks. Please contact your Sales Manager for details about how to access instructor resources in *HKPropel*.

NATA Practice Domains

1. Injury and illness prevention and wellness
2. Examination, assessment, and diagnosis
3. Immediate and emergency care
4. Therapeutic intervention
5. Health care administration and professional responsibility

Reprinted from www.nata.org/about/athletic-training/obtain-certification.

Student Resources in HK*Propel*

Students have access to a variety of online resources in HK*Propel*:

- *Case studies:* Two case studies per chapter let students demonstrate critical thinking and decision-making skills to improve patient outcomes.
- *Foundational skills check sheets:* These check sheets can be used to ensure students follow the correct steps for select foundational skills.
- *Foundational skills videos:* These videos demonstrate a variety of skills such as conducting culturally competent patient interactions, administering fitness and wellness tests, properly fitting equipment, correctly applying taping procedures, accurately taking vital signs, and properly completing therapeutic modalities.
- *Flash cards:* Students can test themselves on the glossary terms used in each chapter.

BOC Standards of Practice

Preamble

The primary purpose of the Practice Standards is to establish essential duties and obligations imposed by virtue of holding the ATC credential. Compliance with the Practice Standards is mandatory.

The BOC does not express an opinion on the competence or warrant job performance of credential holders; however, every Athletic Trainer and applicant must agree to comply with the Practice Standards at all times.

Standard 1: Direction

The Athletic Trainer renders service or treatment under the direction of, or in collaboration with a physician, in accordance with their training and state's statutes, rules and regulations.

Standard 2: Prevention

The Athletic Trainer implements measures to prevent and/or mitigate injury, illness and long term disability.

Standard 3: Immediate Care

The Athletic Trainer provides care procedures used in acute and/or emergency situations, independent of setting.

Standard 4: Examination, Assessment and Diagnosis

The Athletic Trainer utilizes patient history and appropriate physical examination procedures to determine the patient's impairments, diagnosis, level of function and disposition.

Standard 5: Therapeutic Intervention

The Athletic Trainer determines appropriate treatment, rehabilitation and/or reconditioning strategies. Intervention program objectives include long and short-term goals and an appraisal of those which the patient can realistically be expected to achieve from the program. Appropriate patient-centered outcomes assessments are utilized to document the efficacy of interventions.

Standard 6: Program Discontinuation

The Athletic Trainer may recommend discontinuation of the intervention program at such time the patient has received optimal benefit of the program. A final assessment of the patients' status is included in the discharge note.

Standard 7: Organization and Administration

The Athletic Trainer documents all procedures and services in accordance with local, state and federal laws, rules and guidelines.

Reprinted by permission from BOC, *BOC Standards of Professional Practice*, Version 3.3. https://bocatc.org/public-protection/standards-discipline/standards-discipline/standards-of-professional-practice.

- *Quizzes:* Instructors may assign short quizzes to complete within HK*Propel* to demonstrate student mastery of each chapter's content.

Here is a listing of the videos and check sheets provided in HK*Propel:*

Foundational Skills Videos

Chapter 4
Culturally incompetent patient interaction
Culturally competent patient interaction

Chapter 7
Exam glove removal

Chapter 9
30-second chair stand test
Handgrip dynamometer
Standing long jump
Vertical jump test
YMCA bench press test

Chapter 11
Football helmet fitting
Football shoulder pad fitting

Chapter 12
Application of a compression
Closed basketweave for the ankle
Kinesiology taping for the lower leg
Figure-eight shoulder spica
Wrist hyperflexion or hyperextension
Taping for a sprained thumb
Buddy taping for finger sprain

Chapter 14
Pulse assessment
Respiration rate assessment
Blood pressure assessment
Capillary refill

Chapter 21
Ultrasound application
Ultrasound application under water
Closed kinetic chain exercise
Open kinetic chain exercise
Balance training

Foundational Skills Check Sheets

Chapter 2
Writing a PICO question
Completing critical appraisal steps

Chapter 5
Writing SOAP notes

Chapter 7
Removing protective gloves
Handwashing

Chapter 8
Completing an ergonomic assessment

Chapter 9
Measuring height
Measuring resting heart rate
Measuring shoulder flexibility with the back scratch test

Chapter 11
Fitting a standard football helmet
Fitting football shoulder pads
Removing a face mask and helmet
Removing traditional shoulder pads

Chapter 12
Ankle taping
Hip spica wrap for flexor strain
Hip spica wrap for adductor strain
Shoulder spica wrap
Wrist hyperextension taping
Buddy taping
Crutch fitting
Cane fitting
Crutch walking

Chapter 13
Calling 911

Chapter 14
Assessing rectal temperature
Assessing blood pressure
Assessing capillary refill
Assessing blood glucose level
Applying a tourniquet
Applying a cervical collar
Administering an epinephrine autoinjector

Chapter 16
Completing the evaluation process

Chapter 19
Applying goal-setting principles

Chapter 23
Administering medication
Using a meter-dosed inhaler

CAATE STANDARDS

The following Commission of Accreditation of Athletic Training Education (CAATE) 2020 standards are covered in this text:

Standard 39: The coordinator of clinical education is a core faculty member whose primary appointment is to the athletic training program and who has responsibility to direct clinical education. The coordinator of clinical education's experience and qualifications include the following:

- Contemporary expertise in athletic training
- Certification and good standing with the Board of Certification
- Possession of a current state athletic training credential and good standing with the state regulatory agency in the state in which the program is housed (in states with regulation)
- Previous clinical practice in athletic training

Annotation: The title of this individual is determined by the institution, and the position should be consistent with the responsibilities of others at the institution who have similar roles. This individual is not the same person as the program director.

Standard 40: The coordinator of clinical education is responsible for oversight of the clinical education portion of the program. This includes the following responsibilities:

- Oversight of student clinical progression
- Student assignment to athletic training clinical experiences and supplemental clinical experiences
- Clinical site evaluation
- Student evaluation
- Regular communication with preceptors
- Professional development of preceptors
- Preceptor selection and evaluation

Annotation: Communication with the preceptors includes familiarizing them with the program framework. Professional development of preceptors is specific to development of their role as preceptor.

Standard 45: Preceptors are health care providers whose experience and qualifications include the following:

- Licensure as a health care provider, credentialed by the state in which they practice (where regulated)
- BOC certification in good standing and state credential (in states with regulation) for preceptors who are solely credentialed as athletic trainers
- Planned and ongoing education for their role as a preceptor
- Contemporary expertise

Annotation: Preceptor education is designed to promote an effective learning environment and may vary based on the educational expectations of the experiences. The program must have a plan for ongoing preceptor training.

Standard 50: The program has administrative and technical support staff to meet its expected program outcomes and professional education, scholarship, and service goals.

Standard 55: Students must gain foundational knowledge in statistics, research design, epidemiology, pathophysiology, biomechanics and pathomechanics, exercise physiology, nutrition, human anatomy, pharmacology, public health, and health care delivery and payor systems.

- Annotation: Foundational knowledge areas can be incorporated as prerequisite coursework, as a component of the professional program, or both.

Standard 56: Advocate for the health needs of clients, patients, communities, and populations.

- Annotation: Advocacy encompasses activities that promote health and access to health care for individuals, communities, and the larger public.

Standard 57: Identify health care delivery strategies that account for health literacy and a variety of social determinants of health.

Standard 58: Incorporate patient education and self-care programs to engage patients and their families and friends to participate in their care and recovery.

Standard 59: Communicate effectively and appropriately with clients/patients, family members, coaches, administrators, other health care professionals, consumers, payors, policy makers, and others.

Standard 60: Use the International Classification of Functioning, Disability, and Health (ICF) as a framework for delivery of patient care and communication about patient care.

Standard 61: Practice in collaboration with other health care and wellness professionals.

Standard 62: Provide athletic training services in a manner that uses the best evidence to inform practice.

- Annotation: Evidence-based practice includes using best research evidence, clinical expertise, and patient values and circumstances to connect didactic content taught in the classroom to clinical decision making.

Standard 63: Use systems of quality assurance and quality improvement to enhance client/patient care.

Standard 65: Practice in a manner that is congruent with the ethical standards of the profession.

Standard 66: Practice health care in a manner that is compliant with the BOC Standards of Professional Practice and applicable institutional/organizational, local, state, and federal laws, regulations, rules, and guidelines. Applicable laws and regulations include (but are not limited to) the following:

- Requirements for physician direction and collaboration
- Mandatory reporting obligations
- Health Insurance Portability and Accountability Act (HIPAA)
- Family Education Rights and Privacy Act (FERPA)
- Universal Precautions/OSHA Bloodborne Pathogen Standards
- Regulations pertaining to over-the-counter and prescription medications

Standard 67: Self-assess professional competence and create professional development plans according to personal and professional goals and requirements.

Standard 68: Advocate for the profession.

- Annotation: Advocacy for the profession takes many shapes. Examples include educating the general public, public sector, and private sector; participating in the legislative process; and promoting the need for athletic trainers.

Standard 69: Develop a care plan for each patient. The care plan includes (but is not limited to) the following:

- Assessment of the patient on an ongoing basis and adjustment of care accordingly

- Collection, analysis, and use of patient-reported and clinician-rated outcome measures to improve patient care
- Consideration of the patient's goals and level of function in treatment decisions
- Discharge of the patient when goals are met or the patient is no longer making progress
- Referral when warranted

Standard 70: Evaluate and manage patients with acute conditions, including triaging conditions that are life threatening or otherwise emergent. These include (but are not limited to) the following conditions:

- Cardiac compromise (including emergency cardiac care, supplemental oxygen, suction, adjunct airways, nitroglycerin, and low-dose aspirin)
- Respiratory compromise (including use of pulse oximetry, adjunct airways, supplemental oxygen, spirometry, meter-dosed inhalers, nebulizers, and bronchodilators)
- Conditions related to the environment: lightning, cold, heat (including use of rectal thermometry)
- Cervical spine compromise
- Traumatic brain injury
- Internal and external hemorrhage (including use of a tourniquet and hemostatic agents)
- Fractures and dislocations (including reduction of dislocation)
- Anaphylaxis (including administering epinephrine using automated injection device)
- Exertional sickling, rhabdomyolysis, and hyponatremia
- Diabetes (including use of glucometer, administering glucagon, insulin)
- Drug overdose (including administration of rescue medications such as naloxone)
- Wounds (including care and closure)
- Testicular injury
- Other musculoskeletal injuries

Standard 71: Perform an examination to formulate a diagnosis and plan of care for patients with health conditions commonly seen in athletic training practice. This exam includes the following:

- Obtaining a medical history from the patient or other individual
- Identifying comorbidities and patients with complex medical conditions

- Assessing function (including gait)
- Selecting and using tests and measures that assess the following, as relevant to the patient's clinical presentation:
  - Cardiovascular system (including auscultation)
  - Endocrine system
  - Eyes, ears, nose, throat, mouth, and teeth
  - Gastrointestinal system
  - Genitourinary system
  - Integumentary system
  - Mental status
  - Musculoskeletal system
  - Neurological system
  - Pain level
  - Reproductive system
  - Respiratory system (including auscultation)
  - Specific functional tasks
- Evaluating all results to determine a plan of care, including referral to the appropriate provider when indicated

Standard 72: Perform or obtain the necessary and appropriate diagnostic or laboratory tests—including (but not limited to) imaging, blood work, urinalysis, and electrocardiogram- –to facilitate diagnosis, referral, and treatment planning.

Standard 73: Select and incorporate interventions (for pre-op patients, post-op patients, and patients with nonsurgical conditions) that align with the care plan. Interventions include (but are not limited to) the following:

- Therapeutic and corrective exercise
- Joint mobilization and manipulation
- Soft tissue techniques
- Movement training (including gait training)
- Motor control/proprioceptive activities
- Task-specific functional training
- Therapeutic modalities
- Home care management
- Cardiovascular training

Standard 74: Educate patients regarding appropriate pharmacological agents for the management of their condition, including indications, contraindications, dosing, interactions, and adverse reactions.

Standard 75: Administer medications or other therapeutic agents by the appropriate route of administration upon the order of a physician or other provider with legal prescribing authority.

Standard 77: Identify, refer, and give support to patients with behavioral health conditions. Work with other health care professionals to monitor these patients' treatment, compliance, progress, and readiness to participate. These behavioral health conditions include (but are not limited to) the following:

- Suicidal ideation
- Depression
- Anxiety disorder
- Psychosis
- Mania
- Eating disorders
- Attention deficit disorders

Standard 78: Select, fabricate, and/or customize prophylactic, assistive, and restrictive devices, materials, and techniques for incorporation into the plan of care, including the following:

- Durable medical equipment
- Orthotic devices
- Taping, splinting, protective padding, and casting

Standard 79: Develop and implement strategies to mitigate the risk for long-term health conditions across the lifespan. These include (but are not limited to) the following conditions:

- Adrenal diseases
- Cardiovascular disease
- Diabetes
- Neurocognitive disease
- Obesity
- Osteoarthritis

Standard 80: Develop, implement, and assess the effectiveness of programs to reduce injury risk.

Standard 81: Plan and implement a comprehensive preparticipation examination process to affect health outcomes.

Standard 82: Develop, implement, and supervise comprehensive programs to maximize sport performance that are safe and specific to the client's activity.

Standard 83: Educate and make recommendations to clients/patients on fluids and nutrients to ingest prior to activity, during activity, and during recovery for a variety of activities and environmental conditions.

Standard 85: Monitor and evaluate environmental conditions to make appropriate recommendations to start, stop, or modify activity in order to prevent environmental illness or injury.

Standard 87: Select and use biometrics and physiological monitoring systems and translate the data into effective preventive measures, clinical interventions, and performance enhancement.

Standard 88: Perform administrative duties related to the management of physical, human, and financial resources in the delivery of health care services. These include (but are not limited to) the following duties:

- Strategic planning and assessment
- Managing a physical facility that is compliant with current standards and regulations
- Managing budgetary and fiscal processes
- Identifying and mitigating sources of risk to the individual, the organization, and the community
- Navigating multipayor insurance systems and classifications
- Implementing a model of delivery (for example, value-based care model)

Standard 91: Develop, implement, and revise policies and procedures to guide the daily operation of athletic training services.

- Annotation: Examples of daily operation policies include pharmaceutical management, physician referrals, and inventory management.

Standard 92: Develop, implement, and revise policies that pertain to prevention, preparedness, and response to medical emergencies and other critical incidents.

Reprinted in part by permission of the Commission of Accreditation of Athletic Training Education (CAATE), *2020 Standards for Professional Masters Programs.* https://caate.net/wp-content/uploads/2018/09/2020-Standards-for-Professional-Programs-copyedited-clean.pdf.

ACKNOWLEDGMENTS

For their love and support during the writing process, Mitch, Noam, and Yonah have my unending love and gratitude.

—Leamor

This project would not have been possible without the guidance of my mentors throughout my career and the love and support of Woody Brownell. Thank you!

—Ellen

We wish to thank the contributing authors, models, and most importantly Amanda Ewing for all their help in making Josh Stone's vision come to life.

—Leamor and Ellen

Foundation of Professional Practice

Part I of this text focuses on the formative information that students need for professional practice. The foundation for athletic training practice is a historical understanding of the profession and its responsibilities and knowledge of how to manage and interpret research, the management and administration of athletic training, and cultural literacy. Understanding the underpinnings of the profession and practice is critical to the provision of patient-centered care and continued professional growth.

Chapter 1 discusses the history of athletic training, certification and education requirements, and the foundational behaviors for professional practice. Unique to this text is an extensive section on interprofessional education and the health care team. Chapter 2 provides an overview of evidence-based practice and the research principles important for interpreting the literature to help students understand the whys of current practice and advance as professional knowledge grows and changes over time. Because athletic trainers work in diverse settings and have a large role on health care teams, chapters 3 and 4 seek to help students understand population health and engage with a range of different patients. Chapters 3 and 4 are unique to most introductory athletic training texts in that they address the relationship between athletic training and public health and the cultural competency needed for a patient-centered approach to working with a diverse population. They discuss population health, injury surveillance, and social determinants of health as they relate to athletic training. Lastly, chapters 5 and 6 provide essential information for the management and administration of health care in athletic training settings, including policy and best practices that are grounded in health care ethics.

CHAPTER 1
Athletic Training and the Health Care Team

Leamor Kahanov, EdD, ATC, LAT

CAATE STANDARDS

The following CAATE 2020 standards are covered in this chapter:

Standard 59

Standard 61

Standard 65

Standard 66

Standard 68

CHAPTER OBJECTIVES

After reading this chapter, you will be able to do the following:

- Describe athletic training history and the current route to certification

- Understand foundational behaviors of professional practice

- Identify interprofessional practice as a component of patient-centered care

- Identify members of the athletic training health care team and the role athletic trainers play with the team

- Summarize professional ethics in athletic training

Athletic training is a health care profession recognized for specific skills and knowledge. The formal education process for professional membership began in 1950 with the creation of the **National Athletic Trainers' Association (NATA)**.[1,2] At the time, the NATA facilitated the education process and advocated for the profession and its vision. The education process for athletic trainers has evolved from an apprenticeship or internship model to a nationally recognized formal curriculum, and the profession has expanded to include a broader range of places of employment and **competencies**.[1,2] Today, approximately 25,000 people in the United States are employed as athletic trainers and approximately 45,000 members of the NATA identify as athletic trainers.

According to the NATA, **athletic trainers** (ATs) are

> health care professionals who render service or treatment, under the direction of or in collaboration with a physician, in accordance with their education and training and the states' statutes, rules and regulations. As a part of the health care team, services provided by ATs include injury and illness prevention, wellness promotion and education, emergent care, examination and clinical diagnosis, therapeutic intervention, and rehabilitation of injuries and medical conditions.[3]

Athletic trainers work as interprofessional team members in a variety of settings:[4,6]

- Clinics
- Hospitals
- Physicians' offices
- Health and fitness clubs
- Sport or performance-enhancement clinics
- Centers for professional and Olympic sports
- Centers for amateur, recreational, and youth sports
- Colleges and universities
- Junior or community colleges
- Secondary schools
- Industrial or occupational settings
- Corporate settings
- Centers for performing arts
- Workplaces for members of the military, law enforcement, and government

The scope of practice for athletic trainers is regulated by their state's practice act, regardless of the practice setting. As of January 2021, the ATC credential and the BOC requirements are recognized by 49 states plus the District of Columbia for eligibility and/or regulation of the practice of athletic trainers.

Becoming an Athletic Trainer

To become an athletic trainer, you must go through a formal education process and pass a national certification examination. Each state regulates additional requirements for professional practice after national certification. One avenue for entry-level professional practice exists. The **Commission on Accreditation of Athletic Training Education (CAATE)** ensures that athletic training curriculum covers the appropriate skills, knowledge, and behaviors based on professional standards. Students who complete a CAATE-accredited athletic training program at the bachelor's and master's levels are eligible for the national certification examination, which is facilitated and

monitored by the **Board of Certification (BOC)**. Starting in 2022, entry-level education will be available only at the master's level. Someone who successfully completes the BOC examination is called a certified athletic trainer (ATC). ATCs must maintain a level of competence to retain certification.

Professional Education (Entry-Level Education)

Professional education for athletic training occurs at the graduate level. A multitude of undergraduate majors and courses may serve as the precursor for graduate education in athletic training.

CAATE-accredited master's programs use a standards-based approach that includes both didactic (classroom) and clinical (hands-on employment setting) experiences. Programs follow a medical-based education model. Athletic training education prepares students to provide comprehensive patient care in five domains of clinical practice. Students must receive formal instruction in the core competencies, which include the following subjects:[1-5]

Core Competencies

- Patient-centered care
  - Care plan
  - Examination, diagnosis, and intervention
- Interprofessional practice and interprofessional education
- Evidence-based practice

Quality Improvement

- Health care informatics
- Professionalism
- Patient or client care
- Prevention, health promotion, and wellness
- Health care administration

Practice Domains of Athletic Training

BOC-certified athletic trainers are educated, trained, and evaluated in five major practice domains:[3-5]

1. Injury and illness prevention and wellness promotion
2. Examination, assessment, and diagnosis
3. Immediate emergency care
4. Therapeutic intervention
5. Health care administration and professional responsibility

Continuing Education

Continuing education requirements promote competence, development of current knowledge and skills, and enhancement of professional skills and judgment. These activities must focus on increasing athletic trainers' knowledge, skills, and abilities.

Professional practice information is continually changing based on new evidence, so you must keep up with current knowledge to ensure patient safety and appropriate clinical practice. Certified athletic trainers are required to provide the BOC with evidence of their continuing education. The BOC website lists the many avenues available for continuing education. Because these opportunities are ever changing, you should routinely check the BOC website for approved continuing education opportunities. According to the CAATE and the NATA, continuing education requirements are meant to ensure that ATs continue to do the following:[1-5]

- Stay on the cutting edge in the field of athletic training
- Obtain current information for professional development
- Explore new knowledge in specific content areas
- Master new skills and techniques
- Expand approaches to effective athletic training
- Further develop professional judgment
- Conduct professional practice in an ethical and appropriate manner

Postprofessional Education

Postprofessional education in athletic training can occur through doctoral education or a residency program. Several universities grant a clinical doctorate in athletic training specific to research, skills, advocacy, and practice.

Postprofessional residency programs are accredited by the CAATE to provide additional education in specialized areas of professional practice. These planned programs of study provide both clinical and didactic education. The following specialties are CAATE-approved areas of residency:[1,5]

- Prevention and wellness
- Urgent and emergent care
- Primary care
- Orthopedics
- Rehabilitation
- Behavioral health
- Pediatrics
- Performance enhancement

Interprofessional Approach to Health Care Delivery

As part of patient care, athletic trainers interface with a multitude of different professionals depending on their employment setting and the type of patients they serve. For example, an athletic trainer in an inpatient hospital setting may interact with phlebotomists, physical therapists, occupational therapists, speech pathologists, physicians, and social workers. Likewise, an athletic trainer at the secondary-school level may coordinate care with school counselors, school nurses, and coaches. The more efficient and transparent the care coordination, the better the patient outcomes.[5,6]

Since the current health care environment is increasingly reliant on team-based care for improving patient outcomes, you must integrate interprofessional care into your practice.[5-7,8,12-14] A team approach is optimal for ensuring high-quality health care and fostering **patient-centered care**. A well-functioning health care team improves the patient's experience and outcomes.[6]

Interprofessional collaboration may also reduce medical errors and enhance job satisfaction and retention.[5-8] Efficient interprofessional teams may contribute to health care reform in the United States.[10,11] Athletic trainers are a critical component of health care teams for active people. They often act as the hub of care, particularly in employment settings where they interact with patients daily or several times a week.[6]

In 2009, six national associations representing higher education in allopathic and osteopathic medicine, dentistry, nursing, pharmacy, and public health formed the Interprofessional Educational Collaborative (IPEC) to promote and encourage interprofessional learning experiences. The IPEC established common core competencies for interprofessional collaborative practice to help guide curricula development across the health professions. The IPEC's four core competency domains are as follows:[15,16]

FOUNDATIONAL SKILL

Interprofessional Education and Practice

The most widely accepted definition of **interprofessional practice (IPP)**, or interprofessional education (IPE), is when "two or more professions learn with, about and from each other to enable effective collaboration and improve health outcomes."[8,15,16]

FOUNDATIONAL SKILL

Core Competencies for Interprofessional Collaborative Practice

The following are the core competencies for Interprofessional Collaborative Practice:[15,16]

Competency 1: Values/Ethics for Interprofessional Practice
Work with individuals of other professions to maintain a climate of mutual respect and shared values.

Competency 2: Roles and Responsibilities
Use the knowledge of one's own role and those of other professions to appropriately assess and address the health care needs of patients and to promote and advance the health of populations.

Competency 3: Interprofessional Communication
Communicate with patients, families, communities, and professionals in health and other fields in a responsive and responsible manner that supports a team approach to the promotion and maintenance of health and the prevention and treatment of disease.

Competency 4: Teams and Teamwork
Apply relationship-building values and the principles of team dynamics to perform effectively in different team roles to plan, deliver, and evaluate patient/population centered care and population health programs and policies that are safe, timely, efficient, effective, and equitable.

1. Values and ethics for interprofessional practice
2. Roles and responsibilities
3. Interprofessional communication
4. Teams and teamwork

Athletic Trainers as Members of Health Care Teams

In patient-centered care, a cohesive team of health care providers collaborates to focus on patient needs. Depend-ing on the situation, the athletic trainer may be the leader of the team or a team member delivering a specialized component of the care. Athletic trainers may work with a host of professionals in medicine, health care, and institutional environments. Table 1.1 lists common and additional members of the **health care team**. To ensure patient privacy while enhancing and augmenting patient care, health care professionals discuss relevant medical information only with appropriate members of the team.

FOUNDATIONAL SKILL

Essentials for Members of the Health Care Team

Members of health care teams must do the following preparatory work:

- Make sure all patient information is accessible to medical team members.
- Make all contact information for medical specialists readily available in the office and the patient chart.
- Identify the team leader for the purpose of discharge and team coordination.
- Develop a routine team discussion for coordinating patient care.
- If team leader, when the team identifies that discharge from care is appropriate, promptly provide written communication to the team.
- If team member, maintain appropriate follow-up and patient care until receiving written notification of discharge from care from the team leader.

TABLE 1.1   Members of the Health Care Team in Athletic Training

Team member	Team relationship
Common members	
Dentist	Provides emergency care of dental injuries Fits and potentially manufactures mouth guards Conducts preseason dental examinations when appropriate
Nurse	Assists with care outside of the scope of sports medicine management and injuries (registered nurse) Diagnoses and manages common illnesses and diseases and prescribes medications (nurse practitioner)
Nutritionist	Provides nutrition and eating programs and plans to assist active populations
Occupational therapist	Works with patients with physical, developmental, or emotional challenges to improve daily living and working environments Assists in work environments to facilitate the development of accommodations to enhance function
Osetopathic physician	Doctor of osteopathic medicine (DO) Fully licensed physicians Practice in all medical specialties, but primary care and orthopedics are a focus Receive special training in the musculoskeletal system Provide patients with holistic care by combining medical knowledge and training with the latest advances in medical technology
Physical therapist	Augments rehabilitative programs for injured people
Physician	Allopathic physicians, or MDs Practice in every specialty area Treat symptoms and diseases using drugs, radiation, or surgery Perform various responsibilities related to the maintenance of health, including both acute care and prevention Also called conventional medicine, mainstream medicine, and Western medicine
Physician assistant	Assumes many of the responsibilities a physician conducts, such as diagnosing and managing illnesses and diseases and prescribing medication
Podiatrist (DPM)	Manages foot issues Performs foot surgery Constructs orthotic devices
Additional members	

Biomechanist	Exercise physiologist	Member of school health services
Chiropractor	Massage therapist	Social worker
Emergency medical technician or paramedic	Orthodontist	Sports psychologist
Equipment personnel	Referee	Strength and conditioning specialist

Athletic Training History

The origins of athletic training are traced back to ancient Greek and Roman civilizations, where coaches and trainers helped athletes reach top performance. In modern times, athletic training came into existence in 1881 when James Robinson was hired to assist the Harvard University football team with conditioning (see figure 1.1). The first known educational resource in the field was the book *Athletic Training*, written by Dr. Bilik in 1916,[20] which later was called *The Trainers Bible*. Ten years after authoring the book, Dr. Bilik began teaching summer workshops for athletic trainers "based on sound, logical, physiological, scientific facts."[20] Next, the legendary Cramer brothers began giving traveling workshops after their experience working with the U.S. Olympic team in 1932.[20] Some early athletic trainers learned skills through these different workshops, but most just learned the trade by doing it. At the beginning, apprenticeship was the only route to becoming an athletic trainer, and this method of learning still influences the profession today.

In 1938, the National Athletic Trainers' Association (NATA) was founded to support athletic trainers, but it ended in 1944 due to World War II. In 1950, athletic trainers reorganized and founded a new version of the NATA in Kansas City with 101 members; this form of

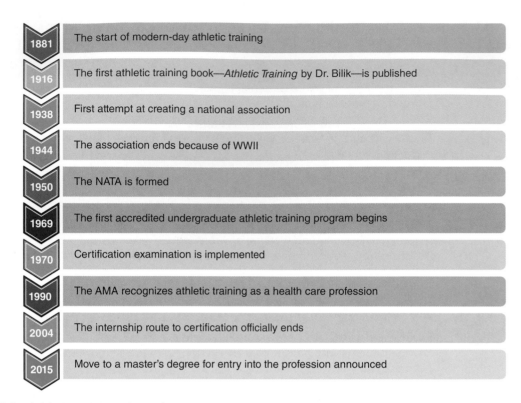

FIGURE 1.1 Athletic training chronology.

Primary Professional Organizations Relevant to Athletic Training

- *American Academy of Family Physicians (AAFP):* promotes standards for family medicine physicians
- *American Academy of Pediatrics, Committee:* promotes education of pediatric physicians on the medical needs of children in sport
- *American College of Sports Medicine (ACSM):* promotes education and research in areas of sports medicine for health and wellness professionals
- *American Orthopaedic Society for Sports Medicine (AOSSM):* promotes wellness and fitness in sport and research and development of safe and effective medicine
- *American Physical Therapy Association (APTA), Sports Physical Therapy Section:* supports a forum for professionals associated with physical therapy to discuss treatment and education of people who participate in sport
- *International Federation of Sports Medicine (FIMS):* promotes the study of sports medicine in over 100 countries
- *National Academy of Sports Medicine (NASM):* supports education for professionals in sports medicine in order to enhance the lives of people in sport
- *National Athletic Trainers' Association (NATA):* promotes standards for athletic trainers
- *National Strength and Conditioning Association (NSCA):* promotes the field of strength and conditioning
- *NCAA Committee on Competitive Safeguards and Medical Aspects of Sports (NCAA):* promotes innovative education and solutions to enhance results in sport

the organization continues today.[21] Part of the recurring discussion among the men of the NATA at that time was how to strengthen the profession and gain recognition within the health care community.[20]

In 1956, the NATA formed a committee to address the educational requirements of athletic trainers.[21] In 1959, the first athletic training curriculum began in higher education institutions and focused on the care and treatment of athletic injuries and teaching high school.[1,14] The first undergraduate athletic training education programs began in 1969 at Mankato State University, Indiana State University, Lamar University, and the University of New Mexico.[1,14] Indiana State University was also the first school to allow women to enroll in their program. In 1970, the first certification examination for people wanting to be recognized as certified athletic trainers was developed and implemented by the NATA.[21] The evolution of the certification examination parallels the changes in athletic training curriculum to this day. In 1989, the NATA and the certification body, the NATA's Board of Certification (NATABOC), split into two organizations.

In 1990, the AMA officially recognized the profession of athletic training. In 1993, the AMA's Committee on Allied Health Education and Accreditation (CAHEA) developed requirements for educating entry-level athletic trainers, which led to the process of accrediting academic programs. When CAHEA disintegrated, accreditation moved to the Commission on Accreditation of Allied Health Education Programs (CAAHEP). In 1997, a major change to athletic training education occurred when the Board of Certification (BOC) eliminated the internship route to certification.[21] Prior to this ruling, an athletic training student was eligible to sit for the national certification examination through one of two routes: the internship route or the curriculum route. The curriculum route required students to complete coursework and practicum hours through a nationally accredited athletic training program. The last year a student from the internship route could sit for the certification examination was 2004.[21] The elimination of the internship route helped standardize athletic training education and align it with programs from other allied health care disciplines.[9]

In 2006, the Joint Review Committee on Educational Programs in Athletic Training (JRC-AT), now known as the Commission on Accreditation of Athletic Training Education (CAATE), became the accrediting agency for athletic training education.[8,17,20-22] In 2015, the CAATE announced that the entry-level master's program would move to being the only route to certification for athletic trainers. This would allow for a transition from bachelor's programs to entry-level master's programs by 2022. In 2019, the CAATE accredited the first school outside of the United States, Universidad Camilo José Cela (UCJC) in Madrid, Spain.

Professional Ethics

Athletic trainers must practice **professional ethics** at all times to ensure that they maintain and employ the highest standards of integrity, conduct, and care.[6,15-17] In 1993, the NATA developed a code of ethics to ensure appropriate professional behavior among athletic trainers.[6,18,19] The NATA Code of Ethics was reaffirmed in 2005 and again in 2018. The Code of Ethics has four principles:

1. Members shall practice with compassion, respecting the rights, well-being, and dignity of others.

2. Members shall comply with the laws and regulations governing the practice of athletic training, National Athletic Trainers' Association (NATA) membership standards, and the NATA code of ethics.

3. Members shall maintain and promote high standards in their provision of services.

4. Members shall not engage in conduct that could be construed as a conflict of interest, reflects negatively on the athletic training profession, or jeopardizes a patient's health and well-being.

Athletic trainers should read the Code of Ethics, which includes more detailed information under each of the four principles. Athletic trainers who act in an unethical manner or breach the Code of Ethics may have their professional certification (BOC) suspended or revoked. Additional health care regulations are identified in chapter 5.

CLINICAL BOTTOM LINE

- Athletic training is a health care profession, recognized by the American Medical Association, for clinicians who specialize in working with the active population.

- Employment opportunities for athletic training range from outpatient and inpatient rehabilitation positions to sales jobs. Athletic trainers have vast opportunities for affecting the health care outcomes of active people.

- In patient-centered care, athletic trainers must work closely with other health care professionals to ensure patient safety and optimal outcomes. Athletic trainers are integral participants in interprofessional collaborative teams. The members of a health care team vary depending on the athletic trainer's employment setting.

- Athletic training has a rich history tracing back to the late 1800s. The profession has transitioned from caring solely for athletes to working with active people in various settings.

- Athletic training education began as an apprenticeship model and transitioned to a college- or university-based curriculum that meets accreditation requirements. Students who complete an entry-level education in athletic training may take the national certification examination, which allows them to practice the profession.

- The Code of Ethics for athletic trainers is affirmed by the National Athletic Trainers' Association (NATA). Athletic trainers who fail to uphold standards of professional ethics are subject to suspension or loss of certification.

 Go to HK*Propel* to complete the activities and case studies for this chapter.

CHAPTER 2

Evidence-Based Practice and Basic Research Principles

Leamor Kahanov, EdD, ATC, LAT

CAATE STANDARDS

The following CAATE 2020 standard is covered in this chapter:

Standard 55

CHAPTER OBJECTIVES

After reading this chapter, you will be able to do the following:

- Define *evidence-based practice*
- Outline foundational research methods
- Describe various types of research
- Understand the use of research in clinical decision making and reasoning
- Apply ethical considerations in research practices

Athletic trainers are required to make clinical decisions based on the best scholarly evidence available combined with their clinical expertise and critical analysis of the patient's needs and values. This component of practice is known as critical reasoning.[1]

Athletic trainers are obligated to provide optimal care for patients. Synthesizing the research to determine best practices is essential to achieving that outcome. This chapter provides a foundational understanding of the role of evidence-based research in athletic training, as well as research terminology and models. Athletic trainers interested in evidence-based practice and research principles should investigate the information in each section further.

Definition of Evidence-Based Practice

Evidence-based practice means using the current and best evidence available in research to make clinical decisions that serve patients and achieve optimal outcomes.[2-12] Evidence-based practice is highly linked to research principles. You will need to understand the types of research and how research is conducted in order to evaluate research and best apply it when making a diagnosis, providing treatment, and rehabilitating patients.[2-12]

Evidence-based practice is best applied when the appropriate evidence is coupled with patient experiences and clinical expertise, also known as the three pillars of evidence (figure 2.1).[2-12] Ultimately, application of evidence-based practice results in patient-centered practice, where an informed patient is part of the treatment or rehabilitation decision-making process.

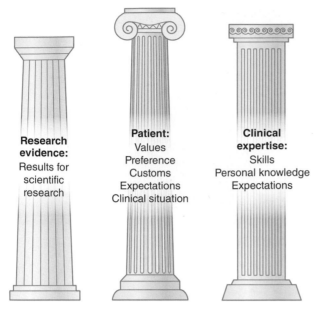

FIGURE 2.1   Three pillars of evidence.

Research is a vital component of improving patient care. Benefits of evidence-based practice include the following:[2-12]

- Increased levels of patient satisfaction
- Reduced harm
- Individualized care
- Enhanced treatment, therapy, diagnostic procedures, and preventive measures
- Better outcomes
- Lower-cost options for the patient

Research Design and Levels of Evidence

Research is an organized method for finding answers to questions. In athletic training, and medicine in general, research helps practitioners manage patient injuries, illness, and issues. Knowledge garnered from research may be assimilated into clinical practice based on the research evidence.

Research design is a blueprint for the collection, measurement, and analysis of data. It outlines a framework for the plan of investigation. Appropriate selection of a research design can aid a researcher choosing a methodology that best addresses research questions. Inappropriate selection of research design may result in incongruent outcomes that do not address or answer the research question. Table 2.1 outlines how to select a research design based on the research question.

The level of research evidence is based on the quality of the research design, validity, and applicability to patient care (table 2.2). The levels or grades of the evidence or research help athletic trainers make critical care decisions grounded in the strength of the research. Level I research provides the strongest evidence (figure 2.2). All levels of research are essential in providing an array of knowledge.[13]

Qualitative and Quantitative Research

Research and the collection of evidence are separated into two major categories: qualitative and quantitative. The data collection methods of quantitative and qualitative research are significantly different, leading to different types of outcome data.

- **Qualitative** research is primarily used to gain an understanding of opinions, motivations, phenomena, and situations that may not be quantifiable through numbers.[14-26]
- **Quantitative** research is used to quantify the problem through numerical data or data that can be transformed into usable statistics.[14,15,27]

Defining Evidence-Based Practice

Evidence-based practice is the application of the following:

- Research that may prove or disprove an accepted method, treatment, therapy, diagnostic procedure, or preventive measure
- Research that demonstrates new methods of care that are more accurate or effective or less harmful

Evidence-based practice should not:

- Serve as a blueprint for diagnosis, treatment, or therapy in health care
- Guarantee that research is available to answer clinical questions
- Be used in isolation without incorporating clinical skills and the patient

TABLE 2.1   **Clinical Questions and Suggested Research Design**

Research design	Definition	Clinical question answered	Example of question
Meta-analysis	A subset of systematic reviews that combine qualitative and quantitative study data into a single conclusion with greater statistical power	All clinical questions	Do people with fewer cases of CA-MRSA follow a different disinfection procedure than other people?
Systematic review	Document that provides a comprehensive review of all relevant studies on a particular clinical question	All clinical questions	Does regularly disinfecting prevent CA-MRSA infections compared to nonuse of disinfectants?
Practice guideline	Statement produced by a panel of experts outlining current best practices informed by extensive review of the literature. Typically used by governments or professional associations.	All clinical questions	What is best way to prevent CA-MRSA?
Randomized controlled trial	Design that randomly assigns participants into an experimental group or control group to assess the variable studied	Quality improvement Diagnosis Prevention **Etiology** Therapy	Does a specific disinfectant affect the contraction of CA-MRSA?
Cohort study	Design where one or more samples (called cohorts) are followed prospectively to determine disease or injury outcomes	Therapy Etiology Diagnosis Prevention	Does the use of a specific disinfectant decrease the incidence of CA-MRSA in high school wrestlers?
Case-control study (also known as retrospective studies)	Study design that compares patients with disease, injury, or a certain outcome with patients who do not have the medical issue	Therapy Etiology Prevention Prognosis	What are the effects of disinfectant use in high school wrestlers diagnosed with CA-MRSA?
Case report	Design that describes and interprets one individual case that is typically unique, followed over a long period of time	Therapy Prevention Prognosis	Is there any connection between agoraphobia and recurring CA-MRSA infections in an otherwise healthy person?

TABLE 2.2   **Levels of Evidence**

Level of evidence	Description	Practical application in athletic training and clinical practice guidelines
Level I	Systematic review or meta-analysis of randomized controlled trials (RCTs) Clinical practice guidelines predicated on systematic reviews of RCTs Three or more RCTs of good quality with similar results	• Prognosis • Differential diagnosis • Treatment/therapy • Prevention • Economic decisions of care

> continued

Table 2.2 >*continued*

Level of evidence	Description	Practical application in athletic training and clinical practice guidelines
Level II	A minimum of one well-designed RCT	• Quality improvement • Differential diagnosis • Prevention • Treatment/therapy
Level III	Well-designed controlled trails without randomization (i.e., **quasi-experimental**)	
Level IV	Well-designed case-control or cohort studies	• Therapy • Prevention • Prognosis
Level V	Systematic review of descriptive and qualitative studies (metasynthesis)	• Quality improvement • Impetus for future research • Unique clinical practice issues, treatment/therapy • Social and psychological intervention
Level VI	A single or number of integrated studies that are descriptive or qualitative in nature	
Level VII	Opinion of authorities or reports of expert committees	• Differential diagnosis • Prevention • Treatment/therapy

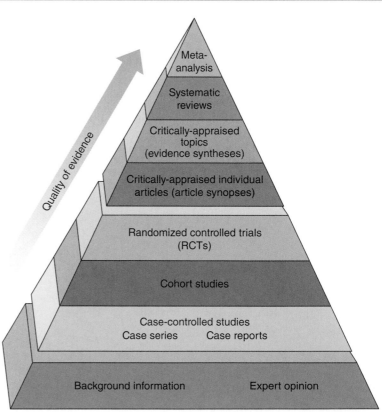

Quality of evidence

Meta-analysis

Systematic reviews

Critically-appraised topics (evidence syntheses)

Critically-appraised individual articles (article synopses)

Randomized controlled trials (RCTs)

Cohort studies

Case-controlled studies
Case series   Case reports

Background information   Expert opinion

FIGURE 2.2   Quality of evidence pyramid.

Qualitative Research

Qualitative is a non-numerical type of social science research based on words, feelings, emotions, sounds, and other unqualifiable elements of data (table 2.3).[14-26] Qualitative research is generally exploratory, seeking to identify and interpret social life or events of a targeted population or person. Qualitative research can be used to assess opinions, motivations, and culture that can be practically applied to inform practitioners of the context of injury or illness and unique events or happenings in medicine and to address social and psychological issues associated with patients.[14-26]

Quantitative Research

Quantitative research is a numerical representation of information about a specific phenomenon. Quantitative

TABLE 2.3   **Common Qualitative Methods**

Qualitative method	Definition	Focus	Data collection	Sample size	Example	Practical application
Ethnography	Researcher immerses himself with the participants to understand the culture, motivations, and goals of the group	Culture or context	Interviews and observations	1 (may have group or organization study)	Researcher positions himself as a nursing home patient to understand the environment	May help practitioners better understand the environment to make appropriate changes to improve patient satisfaction
Narrative	Description through written or spoken words or visual representation of people	Individual experience	Individual stories and documentation	1 or 2	Explore how people proceed through cancer diagnosis and treatment	May help practitioners render better care Increase understanding of patients' psyche
Phenomenological	Direct investigation of a person or group's experience or a particular phenomenon	Individual or group experience	Interviews	5-25	Investigate the athletic trainer's experience in professional sports	May assist in improving a work environment
Grounded theory	Inductive process of identifying constructs to create a theory	Development of theory from observations and documentation	Interviews	20-60 or until consistent theme emerges (data saturation)	Explore compliance of postoperative ACL surgery patients	Help athletic trainers communicate the importance of compliance to patients by learning reasons for noncompliance, as understood by research themes
Case study	Investigation of a contemporary phenomenon or unique real-life issue, disease, or injury	Experiences of a person, organization, or event	Interviews, observations, and documentation	1 (may have group or organization study)	Investigate a unique case of cuboid syndrome	Inform practitioners on a unique injury diagnosis and potential treatment

research methods provide descriptions, examine relationships, and determine cause-and-effect relationships. Quantifying a program with numerical data helps athletic trainers identify patterns and causation in a range of populations, from small to large, that can inform their clinical practice. There are four major types of quantitative research (table 2.4).

Critical Appraisal of the Literature

Critical appraisal of the literature is a process of systematically analyzing research to assess its trustworthiness, value, and relevance before using it to inform clinical practice decisions.[28] Research that lacks quality

TABLE 2.4 **Major Types of Quantitative Research**

Design	Definition	Level of evidence	Example	Practical application
Descriptive research	Systematic collection of information through description. The researcher typically does not have a hypothesis but provides information about a phenomenon.	Level IV	People with acute 2nd degree ankle sprains were surveyed and observed to determine when they self-determined to remove crutches.	Application of an improved timeline for crutch use with 2nd degree ankle sprains based on patients' perceived symptoms
Correlational research	Determination regarding the relationship between two or more variables	Level IV (case-controlled or cohort study) Level V (systematic review) Level VI (qualitative)	Patients with acute 2nd degree ankle sprains were assessed to determine when they began full weight-bearing and the length of time to return to activities of daily living.	Application of an improved timeline for crutch use with 2nd degree ankle sprains
Causal-comparative (quasi-experimental)	Cause-and-effect relationship Similar to experimental design but lacks randomization of groups	Level IV (case-controlled or cohort study) Level V (systematic review) Level VI (qualitative)	People in assisted living were tested for ankle strength. Researchers followed up 1 year later to see who had sustained 2nd degree ankle sprains to determine if preinjury weakness correlated with increased ankle sprains.	Potential measures for strength to prevent ankle sprains in the elderly
Experimental research (true experiment)	Cause-and-effect relationship whereby subjects are randomly assigned to groups to assess outcomes between a control group and experimental group with a researcher-manipulated variable	Level II (randomized control trial)	People with acute 2nd degree ankle sprains were randomly grouped into a control group and a group given acetaminophen as part of the treatment regime to determine efficacy and timeline for returning to activities of daily living.	Potential inclusion or exclusion of the use of acetaminophen with 2nd degree ankle sprains in improving the timeline of return to activities of daily living

(for example, is biased or has misleading results) may allow for false conclusions that misdirect clinical practice, potentially harming patients. Multiple appraisal

methods and tools have been articulated and developed in the literature,[29] but the basis of all models require the following process:

FOUNDATIONAL SKILL

Critical Appraisal Steps

The following outlines how to complete a critical appraisal:[30-35]

1. *Abstract*
   * Do the findings match the related question?
   * Are there reasons to doubt the findings without reading the whole article?
   * Do you want to know more after reading the abstract?

2. *Introduction and discussion*
   * Do these sections help you identify the key concepts, goals, subjects, and themes of the research?
   * Do these sections directly relate to answering the research question?

3. *Methodology*
   * Does the methodology provide a step-by-step description of the study process?
   * Where and on whom was the study conducted?
   * Does the study use **primary** or **secondary data**?
   * How was the data collected?
   * Is the data trustworthy?
   * Does the study adequately control for different groups (when appropriate)?
   * Are the statistical methods appropriate?
   * Is the sample large enough to produce significant results?
   * Are the measures well established prior to study development?
   * Do the measures accurately reflect the study's research question?

4. *Results*
   * Are the results consistent with the tables and figures provided?
   * Are the results consistent with the data derived from the statistical methods?
   * Are the data appropriately articulated?
   * Are the data consistent with the research question asked?

5. *Discussion*
   * How do the results compare or contrast with previous research?
   * Is the appraisal of the contrasting or comparative research reliable and trustworthy?
   * Are interpretations of the results consistent with the data or actual findings?
   * Do the discussion and abstract sections match?
   * Are limitations of the study discussed?

6. *Conclusion*
   * Does the conclusion address the research inquiry?
   * Does the conclusion match the data and discussion?

7. *Other criteria*
   * Are the results applicable to my population?
   * Is the research timely and relevant?

1. Assess if the research methodology is appropriate for the research question.
2. Scrutinize the data collection and process.
3. Determine if the findings presented are consistent with the data analysis.
4. Draw a conclusion as to whether the literature is trustworthy and valuable enough to make clinical decisions.

Role of Evidence in the Clinical Decision-Making Process

Athletic trainers must combine evidence-based practice with their clinical experience and the uniqueness of each patient's case to achieve successful outcomes.[4,7,8,10,36] This section presents a nonexhaustive representation of several models to provide context for evidence-based practice.

Stepwise models, called **disablement models**, provide a structure for assessing patient health status that accounts for the person and environment. Disablement models describe the effect of injury or disease on patient function, which shifts the focus from the disease or injury to the patient.

Understanding disablement models allows athletic trainers to ask more pointed questions during patient history and evaluation, direct specific diagnostic tests, and evaluate the known literature to create a patient-centered treatment plan.[8,37-39] The two most notable disablement models used by health care providers are the Nagi model and World Health Organization (WHO) ICF model.

The Nagi model (figure 2.3)[8,37-42] was the impetus for the WHO's International Classification of Functioning, Disability and Health (ICF).[33,34] The ICF disablement model (figure 2.4) is used to assess and track the effect of health conditions on activity.[8,37-39] The Nagi and ICF models use the injury or disease pathology and a description of the end result of impairments and functional limitations. Disablement models can be used to determine treatment plans and desired outcomes for the patient.[37-39]

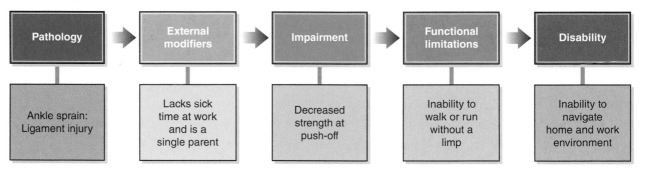

FIGURE 2.3 Nagi model.

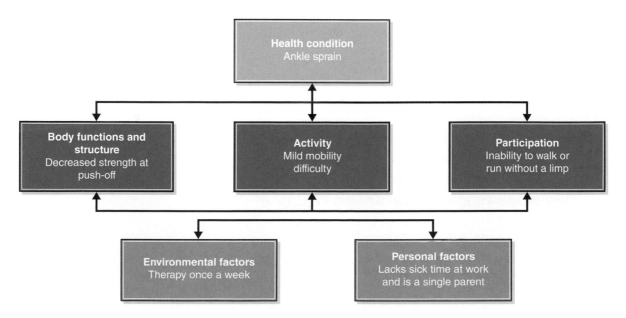

FIGURE 2.4 World Health Organization's ICF disablement model.

An additional model or strategy for assessing the usefulness of including research in clinical decision making is the PICO framework.[43,44] PICO stands for patient, intervention, comparison, and outcome.[2,10,11,45-48]

P: patient; the focus of the research

I: intervention; methods used to address the question

C: comparison (optional)

O: outcome; benefits of the clinical intervention

Use of the PICO framework narrows the focus to improve the specificity and clarity of the identified clinical problems. A PICO disablement model provides a guide for clinical decisions to better select research during the literature pre-search reference interviews, which leads to more precise search results.[2,10,49]

Applying Evidence-Based Practice

Applying research to practice through an evidence-based process requires critical analysis of the literature.[2,6,10,28,30,46,49,50] Multiple processes have been identified that vary in language and number of steps, as identified in previous sections.[2,6,29-31,47] However, regardless of the model used, there are unifying processes for evaluating the research and determining its applicability to clinical practice:

- Identify a concern or question to solve a patient or practice concern or issue.
- Evaluate and assimilate the literature to determine if the evidence is valid and valuable.
- Apply the assimilated literature to change clinical practice.
- Evaluate the outcomes and usefulness of the change in clinical practice.

Although each evidence-based process model has unifying components, the transition to using the clinical decision with individual patients must follow key components that are consistent among practitioners.

Making clinical decisions should be based on the following:[30]

- Use the highest level of evidence possible (level I or II).
- Understand that evidence-based decision making may involve less evidence from higher on the pyramid.
- Know that evidence may not exist for your clinical question or problem.
- Move down the pyramid as needed when evidence doesn't exist to make the best possible decision for the patient.

Understanding Diagnostic Tests

In your role, you must make clinical decisions based on diagnostic tests and their ability to determine or exclude injury and disease. You must also be able to predict or estimate the likelihood that a patient will have an injury or disease from the outcome of a test. You will need to understand the sensitivity, specificity, predictive value, and likelihood ratio of diagnostic tests in order to appropriately evaluate and diagnose patient conditions (figure 2.5).[45,51-56]

- *Sensitivity.* **Sensitivity** is the proportion of patients with an injury or disease that have a positive test or result. The higher the sensitivity, the more correctly the test has identified patients with that injury or disease.
- *Specificity.* **Specificity** is the proportion of patients *without* the injury or disease who have a negative result. The higher the specificity, the more correctly the test has identified patients without the injury or disease.
- *Positive predictive value.* The **positive predictive value (PPV)** is the proportion of patients with a positive diagnostic test who actually have the injury or disease. PPV = true positive (true positive + false positive).

EVIDENCE-BASED ATHLETIC TRAINING

Five Steps of Evidence-Based Practice

The five steps of evidence-based practice are as follows:[2,10,49]

1. Determine the clinical problem and ask an answerable question.
2. Identify the best evidence for answering the question.
3. Critically appraise the evidence gathered to determine its usefulness.
4. Apply results to clinical practice, identifying potential changes to practice.
5. Assess outcome changes to practice.

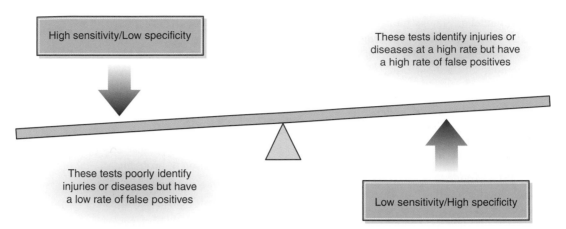

FIGURE 2.5 Specificity and sensitivity.

- *Negative predictive value.* The **negative predictive value (NPV)** is the proportion of patients with a negative diagnostic test who do not have the injury or disease. NPV = true negative (true negative + false positive).
- *Likelihood ratio.* The **likelihood ratio** indicates how many times a patient with an injury or disease will have a certain diagnostic result compared to the same result in patients without the injury or disease. Likelihood ratio for positive test = probability of patient with disease having a positive test/probability of patient without disease having a positive test.

Usefulness of Sensitivity and Specificity

Sensitivity and specificity are components of diagnostic testing and medical diagnosis that are both needed to convey important information regarding the usefulness of testing to reach a correct diagnosis. Diagnostically, test sensitivity relates to the ability to correctly identify the injury or illness, whereas specificity relates to the ability to correctly identify individuals who do not have an injury or illness.[53,57]

- The purpose of a diagnostic test is to determine the probability or likelihood of a correct diagnosis.
- Sensitivity and specificity are not practical for estimating the probability of injury or disease.
- Predictive values provide a measure of a diagnostic test's performance outcomes.

FOUNDATIONAL SKILL

Using the Data to Interpret Diagnostic Tests

- SNout: high sensitivity, negative result, rule out. A diagnostic test with 80% sensitivity will identify 80% of the patients with an injury or disease and miss 20% of patients with the injury or illness.
- SPin: high specificity, rule in. A diagnostic test with 80% specificity will identify 80% of patients with the disease and 20% without the injury or disease.
- A positive predictive value of 20% means that if the test result was positive, the patient has a 20% chance of having the injury or disease.
- A negative predictive value of 20% means that if a test result was negative, the patient has an 80% chance of having the injury or disease.

Research Ethics and Institutional Review Board

Research ethics focuses on the standards and conduct of researchers in the development, design, data collection, and dissemination of research.[58-60] Adhering to ethical conduct in research promotes trust in the outcomes, particularly when using them to inform practices in patient diagnosis, prevention, treatment, therapy, and responsibility to the public. A code of professional conduct also allows researchers to collaborate with the knowledge that their cohorts are behaving with like accountability, respect, and fairness.

The norms of professional conduct that inform researchers of acceptable and unacceptable behavior may be interpreted differently based on culture, background, and experiences. Therefore, to explicitly define accepted professional conduct in research, the United States mandates the review and monitoring of research with human subjects through an institutional review board (IRB).

General ethical principles include the following:[61-63]

- *Autonomy.* Research should afford people the right to determine their participation. Participants should also have an understanding of what is being requested of them in the research study. The informed consent process is the key to protecting individual autonomy.

- *Beneficence.* The researcher is obligated to ensure that participation in research maximizes benefits for participants and society. She must also minimize harm to participants. Sound research design is the key to ensuring minimal risk and maximum benefit.

- *Deception.* Deception of research participants jeopardizes informed consent and may cause harm. Deception may also erode public and individual trust in researchers.

- *Justice.* The duty of the researcher is to select participants equitably by avoiding members of vulnerable populations who may be coerced (i.e., minors, prisoners, people with mental challenges).

Consent from participants ensures an understanding of the research activities and upholds their right to decline participation or components of participation. Consent for participation should include the following:[61-63]

- *Disclosure.* Potential participants must be apprised of the nature of the study, purpose activities, benefits, foreseeable risks, stress, discomforts, compensation, their rights if injured, confidentiality, and anonymity. Research disclosures to participants should include a clear statement of the procedures or activities in the study. Participants must also understand that participating in a medical study is not the same as receiving clinical treatment.

- *Understanding.* Researchers must provide the opportunity for potential participants to ask questions and obtain answers regarding the study. The informed consent form should be clearly written in layman's terms, avoiding technical jargon.

- *Voluntariness.* A participant's consent to participate in research must be voluntary and free of any coercion or promise of benefits due to participation.

- *Competence.* The participant must be competent to give consent. Children, people with altered mental status and other members of vulnerable populations, such as people who have diseases or need emergency care, may not provide consent.

- *Consent.* Potential participants in research must provide authorization of consent to participate, preferably in writing.

- *Exculpatory language.* Informed consent forms cannot include exculpatory language that waives any legal rights of the participant or releases the investigator or sponsor from liability for negligence.

Researchers should uphold the principles of conducting and reporting information, which include the following:[58,60]

- *Honesty.* Reporting data honestly may reduce inaccurate application. Falsification or misrepresentation of data may deceive colleagues and the public.

- *Objectivity.* Minimizing, avoiding, and disclosing bias that may affect research outcomes is imperative to making critical decision on research validity and transferability.

- *Integrity.* Sincere application of action and agreements creates the consistency that is valued in research.

- *Carefulness.* Concerted effort to minimize errors and negligence in data collection, design, correspondences, and global research activities adds validity to the outcomes and increases the assurance that data applications will benefit patients.

The application of research ethics is overseen by an institutional review board (IRB). An IRB defines research ethics to minimize personal interpretation of appropriate behavior with human subjects. The IRB is an independent committee tasked with approving, monitoring, and reviewing biomedical and behavioral research that involves human subjects. The committee is charged with assessing research protocols, ethics, and methods to preserve the rights and welfare of human participants in a research study. Based on an analysis of the research study, the IRB makes formal decisions regarding whether the study should be conducted or completed.

Institutional review boards have the following characteristics:[64-66]

- Mandated in the United States and regulated by these bodies:
  - Food and Drug Administration (FDA)
  - Department of Health and Human Services (specifically the Office for Human Research Protections)

- Housed by medical, governmental, and educational institutions but are independent from those institutions
- Should be consulted to determine the level of review
  - Exempt: benign risk to subjects
  - Expedited: minimal risk to subjects
  - Full board: greater than minimal risk to subjects

An assumption of ethical research as governed by IRBs allows trust in the data and outcomes for evidence-based applications to practice. Athletic trainers should thoroughly understand research processes and ethical standards prior to conducting research.

CLINICAL BOTTOM LINE

- Application of the best research in clinical practice, defined as evidence-based practice, is based on combining three pillars of evidence:
  - Research evidence, which includes the results for scientific research
  - Patient values, preferences, and customs; expectations; and the clinical situation
  - Clinical expertise, including the practitioner's skills, personal knowledge, and expectations
- Qualitative and quantitative are the two overarching types of research that can inform clinical practice. Qualitative research is a non-numerical approach that focuses on opinions, motivations, phenomena, cultures, and environments. Quantitative research is a numerical assessment of problems or issues through data.
- The disablement model shifts the focus from the disease or injury to the patient by creating a stepwise approach to influencing clinical decision making. The stepwise approach includes the health, structure, activity level, participation, environmental factors, and personal factors to assist the patient or practitioner in making decisions that will affect the patient's disease or injury.
- Sensitivity and specificity provide practitioners with information to best use diagnostic testing.
  - SNout, sensitivity to rule out, is a high sensitivity test. A negative result indicates that the practitioner should rule out the disease or injury. A diagnostic test with 80% sensitivity will identify 80% of the patients with an injury or disease and miss 20% of patients with the injury or illness.
  - SPin, specificity to rule in, is a high specificity test. A positive result indicates that the practitioner should rule in the disease or injury. A diagnostic test with 80% specificity will identify 20% of patients with the disease and 80% without the injury or disease.
- Ethical research inspires public trust in research through honesty, objectivity, integrity, and carefulness. To ensure ethical research practices, institutional review boards (IRB) safeguard the use of human subjects. Research studies that include humans as a component of inquiry are required to obtain permission and oversight from an IRB.

 Go to HK*Propel* to complete the activities and case studies for this chapter.

Go to HK*Propel* to download foundational skill check sheets for (1) writing a PICO question and (2) completing critical appraisal steps.

CHAPTER 3

Public Health and Athletic Training

Samuel Johnson, PhD, ATC, CSCS

CAATE STANDARDS

The following CAATE 2020 standards are covered in this chapter:

Standard 55

Standard 57

Standard 80

CHAPTER OBJECTIVES

After reading this chapter, you will be able to do the following:

- Compare a public health approach and a medical approach to improving health

- Describe the intersection of athletic training and public health

- Describe the sequence of prevention as it relates to the injuries and illnesses athletic trainers encounter

- Define *injury surveillance*

- Explain key issues related to injury surveillance

- Describe how athletic trainers identify risk factors and mechanisms of injury

- Differentiate *primary, secondary,* and *tertiary prevention*

- Define *health disparity* and *health equity*

- Describe the social determinants of health

- Differentiate between prevention program efficacy and effectiveness

- Describe the social-ecological model

- Explain how prevention program effectiveness is evaluated

Athletic trainers, like other health care providers, aim to improve the health of the people they care for. To achieve this, you will need an understanding of what is considered **health**. According to the World Health Organization, "health is a state of complete physical, mental and social well-being and not merely the absence of disease or infirmity."[1] Patient-centered, culturally competent health care encompasses the whole person and considers the environment in which the patient lives, works, and plays. By improving the health of patients, the health of the broader population will increase as well. This is the public health approach, and this chapter identifies the foundational principles of public health needed to accomplish this.

Defining Public Health

Public health is defined in many ways, but its primary function is to promote the health of populations. In order to accomplish this, public health professionals work to prevent injuries, illnesses, and diseases from occurring or recurring. This is done in multiple ways:

- Assessing the health status of a population

- Educating and empowering communities regarding health

- Developing policies to protect patients' health

- Linking patients with medical services

- Evaluating the effectiveness of prevention programs

Due to the breadth of the field, public health professionals use an interdisciplinary approach when trying to improve health. The Centers for Disease Control and Prevention (CDC), the leading public health agency in the United States, defines 10 essential functions of public health:[2]

1. Monitor health status to identify and solve community health problems

2. Diagnose and investigate health problems and health hazards in the community

3. Inform, educate, and empower people about health issues

4. Mobilize community partnerships and action to identify and solve health problems

5. Develop policies and plans that support individual and community health efforts

6. Enforce laws and regulations that protect health and ensure safety

7. Link people to needed personal health services and assure the provision of health care when otherwise unavailable

8. Assure a competent public and personal health care workforce

9. Evaluate effectiveness, accessibility, and quality of personal and population-based health services

10. Research for new insights and innovative solutions to health problems

The core functions of public health are assessment, policy development, and assurance. Within each of the functions are individual services that public health provides (figure 3.1).

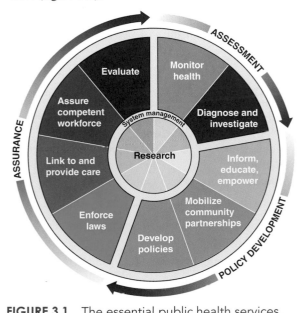

FIGURE 3.1 The essential public health services.

Reprinted from Centers for Disease Control and Prevention, *10 Essential Public Health Services*, (2020). https://www.cdc.gov/publichealthgateway/publichealthservices/essentialhealthservices.html.

Public health and medicine approach the challenge of health and medical care from distinct, complementary perspectives.[3] The focus of most medical professionals is caring for the patient. Although prevention is an important aspect of this goal, it often does not happen as effectively as desired because patients typically do not seek care until after the condition has occurred. This delay in accessing care hampers the ability of the medical professional to promote strategies that may prevent the condition. Public health focuses on improving the health of populations by focusing on prevention. Table 3.1 provides some examples of the perspectives of both disciplines. Each approach has unique values. In order to maximize health, both approaches are needed.[4]

Intersection of Athletic Training and Public Health

Athletic trainers are health care professionals who provide care for physically active people. Historically, athletic trainers worked with athletes on sports teams. However, as the profession has grown, so have the settings athletic trainers work in. For example, athletic trainers now work in the performing arts, public safety, the military, and industry, just to name a few settings. Part of the reason for this is the wide-ranging education athletic trainers receive, specifically within the five domains of athletic training:[5]

1. Injury and illness prevention and wellness promotion

2. Examination, assessment, and diagnosis

3. Immediate and emergency care

4. Therapeutic intervention

5. Health care administration and professional responsibility

Athletic trainers are well aligned with the medical approach, particularly as it relates to providing care to patients who are active. In most jurisdictions, athletic trainers are required to work in collaboration with or under the supervision of a physician; thus, they naturally become advocates for interprofessional practice.

Unlike many other medical professionals, athletic trainers typically provide services beyond the confines of a traditional medical clinic. Athletic trainers are often on site where the patients are, such as at a school, fire station, or warehouse. This means patients can seek care from the athletic trainer at the location of their activity or work, allowing for immediate care for injuries and illnesses. When needed, the athletic trainer refers the patient to other professionals.

The athletic trainer's availability on site at the school or workplace also gives her the opportunity to develop and implement injury and illness prevention programs.

TABLE 3.1   Perspectives of Public Health and Medicine

Medicine	Public health
Primary focus on individual patients	Primary focus on the population
Personal service ethic, conditioned by the awareness of social responsibilities	Public service ethic, tempered by individual concerns
Emphasis on diagnosis, treatment, and care for the whole patient	Emphasis on prevention and health promotion for the whole community
Medical paradigm places predominant emphasis on medical care	Public health paradigm employs a spectrum of interventions aimed at the environment, human behavior and lifestyle, and medical care
Well-established profession with sharp public image	Multiple professional identities with diffuse public image
Uniform system for certifying specialists beyond professional medical degrees	Variable certification of specialists beyond professional public health degrees
Lines of specialization organized, for example, by the following: • Organ system (cardiology, neurology) • Patient group (obstetrics, pediatrics) • Etiology and pathophysiology (oncology, infectious disease) • Technical skill (radiology, surgery)	Lines of specialization organized, for example, by the following: • Analytic method (epidemiology, toxicology) • Setting and population (occupational health, international health) • Substantive health problem (environmental health, nutrition)
Biologic sciences central, stimulated by the needs of patients; move between laboratory and bedside	Biologic sciences central, stimulated by major threats to health of populations; move between laboratory and field
Numeric sciences increasing in prominence, although still a relatively minor part of training	Numeric sciences an essential feature of analysis and training
Social sciences tend to be an elective part of medical education.	Social sciences are an integral part of public health education.

Adapted by permission from H.V. Fineberg, "Public Health and Medicine Where: The Twain Shall Meet," *American Journal of Preventitive Medicine* 41, 4 Suppl 3 (2011): S149-151.

In fact, athletic trainers working in high schools report that preventive services are the primary reason patients seek their services, accounting for nearly 50% of all services provided.[6]

Additionally, in many settings, the athletic trainer is responsible for the health of an entire group or population. From a public health perspective, a population is not just based on a geographic area. Here are just a few examples of populations athletic trainers serve:

• All the athletes on a sports team
• All the dancers in a ballet company
• All the student-athletes in a school
• All the firefighters in a fire department or district
• All the employees in a distribution warehouse
• All the soldiers in a battalion

Because athletic trainers work at both the patient and population levels, additional opportunities exist for more effective prevention. As this chapter later discusses,

health and healthy choices are influenced by many factors. Although athletic trainers cannot directly influence all of these, they have the opportunity to affect many of them. Their wide-ranging education and training allow athletic trainers to provide both initial and follow-up care and referral as needed. By engaging the patient and other stakeholders, such as coaches, school or work administrators, teammates, coworkers, family members, and other health care professionals, the athletic trainer is well suited to promote the health of the population.

The relationship between caring for an individual patient and also an entire population is somewhat unique for a health care provider. This highlights the intersection of athletic training and public health. At its core, public health emphasizes "prevention over treatment, populations over individuals, and engagement at multiple levels."[7] The role of the athletic trainer aligns with public health and medical approaches because athletic training encompasses both prevention and treatment and the health of both the patient and the population. Athletic trainers also engage stakeholders on multiple levels. This intersection between athletic training and public health appears to be a natural fit, but in order to be successful, you need to be acquainted with the public health approach to prevention.

Sequence of Prevention

One of the domains of athletic training is injury and illness prevention. As an athletic trainer, you will be well positioned to provide preventive services due to the fact you will often work with people before an injury occurs. For example, nearly half of the services that athletic trainers in high schools provided were preventive.[6] Yet, this may be an underestimate due to the fact that many of the preventive services the athletic trainer performs— such as assessing environmental conditions for safety, developing emergency action plans, and providing injury screening—are typically undocumented.

Since prevention is a key component of practicing athletic training and improving health, you should understand how to develop and implement preventive interventions. One of the most influential approaches to sports injury prevention was introduced in 1992 by van Mechelen and colleagues.[8] The four-step sequence of prevention was based on other prevention models used in public health. Although the focus of the 1992 review was on sports injury, you can apply the concepts to injury and illness prevention in any athletic training setting. Here are the four steps:

1. Establish the extent of the problem
2. Establish the etiology and the mechanism of injury
3. Develop and introduce preventive interventions
4. Evaluate the intervention

Establishing the Extent of the Problem

The first step of injury and illness prevention is determining the problem. This is done primarily by assessing the frequency of the injury (e.g., the prevalence or incidence) and the consequences of injury (e.g., severity, burden).[8] In other words, how many injuries are there and how bad are they?

Injury Surveillance

One approach to determining the extent of the problem is to track the frequency and duration of injuries and illnesses that occur in a specific population. This is most commonly done through **surveillance**, which is the systematic and ongoing collection, analysis, and dissemination of data in order to prevent and control injuries and illnesses.[9-11] Surveillance has been called the cornerstone of public health practice[9,12] due to the fact that the data from injury surveillance systems are the foundation of evidence-based decisions for preventing injuries and illnesses.[12]

Surveillance is rooted in the public health field of **epidemiology**, which is "the study of the distribution and determinants of health-related states or events (including disease), and the application of this study to the control of diseases and other health problems."[13] Although epidemiologists use injury surveillance to establish the extent of the problem, it is just one tool used to study the causes of injuries and illnesses. This chapter focuses only on key foundational issues related to injury surveillance in athletic training.

Clinicians can perform injury surveillance by tracking the number of injuries and illnesses the people they provide care for suffer and how long the injuries persist. For example, an athletic trainer in the industrial setting may want to know how many people suffered low back injuries over a certain period of time. As an athletic trainer, you can do this in several ways. You could record all the low back injuries during the time of interest. Alternatively, you could use existing health records to ascertain this information. As the use of electronic health records for injury documentation has increased, it has become easier to tally the number of injuries that have occurred. Although using health records for injury surveillance has become easier, it is important to understand that health records and injury surveillance are not the same.

The goal of injury surveillance is to establish the extent of the problem with the goal of eventually reaching a preventive solution. However, certain conditions are relatively rare, and it may take a long time to reach the critical threshold needed to determine a problem exists and develop an intervention. For example, an athletic trainer providing services to a basketball team may be concerned about noncontact anterior cruciate ligament (ACL) injuries and wish to track the frequency of these injuries on the team. However, with only around 15 athletes on a basketball team, it would likely take multiple playing seasons before enough ACL injuries occurred for the athletic trainer to make any evidence-based decisions on the extent of the injury. Because of this, it is common to combine data from multiple clinicians at multiple sites to create an injury surveillance system. Currently, most of the injury surveillance systems that athletic trainers use and provide injury data to are specific to sports (table 3.2). However, as athletic trainers expand their services to new settings and are able to combine patient records from large health care organizations to create big data sources, it is likely that new surveillance systems will be available to inform athletic training practice in the future.

TABLE 3.2 **Examples of Sports Injury Surveillance Systems**

Name of system	Scope	Responsible organization	Source of data	Dates
National Collegiate Athletic Association (NCAA) Injury Surveillance Program (ISP)	Injury and exposure data of a subset of NCAA intercollegiate athletes	NCAA	Athletic trainers	1982 to present
National Center for Catastrophic Sport Injury Research (NCCSIR)	Severe sports-related injuries and illnesses for organized sports at all levels	Based at the University of North Carolina at Chapel Hill	Athletic trainers, coaches, school administrators, parents, and athletes	All sports: 1982 to present Football: 1968 to present
National High School Sports-Related Injury Surveillance System	Monitors injuries among high school athletes in selected sports	Colorado School of Public Health	Athletic trainers using the High School Reporting Information Online (High School RIO) system	2005 to present
High School National Athletic Treatment, Injury, and Outcomes Network (High School NATION)	Injury, treatment, and patient-reported outcomes of public high school athletes	The Datalys Center	Athletic trainers	2011 to present

When multiple athletic trainers collect data for a combined surveillance system, it is critical that the data be collected consistently. Therefore, injury surveillance systems have specific parameters for recording the injury information, including what is considered an injury, how the injury is classified, and how the cumulative injuries are reported.

Injury Definition Although a health record should record all patient encounters, injury surveillance systems often focus on certain injuries and illnesses. Different surveillance systems employ different definitions of injury,

and only those injuries that meet that system's definition are recorded. For example, some systems record only injuries and illnesses that occurred as a direct result of the activity. Others record only time-loss injuries and illnesses, such as injuries that result in missing at least one day of activity. Clinicians reviewing data from injury surveillance systems need to understand the definitions used in the system in order to make informed decisions. For example, if only time-loss injuries were reported, that may not reflect the burden placed on the athletic trainer to treat non-time-loss injuries.

EVIDENCE-BASED ATHLETIC TRAINING

Injury Surveillance Program

Injury surveillance is an important tool for determining the extent of the injuries and illnesses affecting a population. Data from injury surveillance systems can help athletic trainers determine which conditions are problematic, focus prevention efforts, and monitor the effects of implemented prevention programs. Prevention can take many forms, including changes in policies, such as laws, regulations, or rules. The National Collegiate Athletic Association (NCAA) is the governing body of many college athletics programs and determines the rules for the sports under its jurisdiction. Additionally, the NCAA has an injury surveillance program (ISP). An article that reviewed the ISP's methods reported multiple examples of rules changes where the ISP data were used.[14] For example, analysis of concussions in hockey led to rules changes and emphasis in officiating on reducing hitting from behind and contact to the head. Rules changes in women's lacrosse required eye protection to minimize the risk of catastrophic eye injury. More recently, there have been changes to kickoff rules in football in an effort to reduce injuries during these plays. It apparent that data from injury surveillance systems can have wide-ranging effects on health and safety.

Injury Classification Since the goal of surveillance systems is to combine injury and illness data from multiple clinicians at multiple sites, everyone providing data needs to record it the same way to allow the injuries to be grouped accurately. To assist the clinician with this, injury surveillance systems often use a specific classification system.

One of the classification systems most commonly used throughout medicine is the International Classification of Diseases (ICD) system. This classification system is based on a clinician's diagnosis of the condition. The ICD classification system is a built-in feature of many electronic health record systems due to its role in reimbursement for services. Because of its availability in the health records system, athletic trainers may use it to classify injuries when performing injury surveillance. However, this classification system is so broad, its use is uncommon in the injury surveillance systems used by athletic trainers.[15]

A number of different coding systems specific to sports injuries exist, and the Orchard Sports Injury and Illness Classification System is one of the most common. This system, currently on its 13th version, is based on a system where injuries are coded with a three-dimensional lettering system and illnesses with a two-dimensional system.[15] Specifically, the first letter for the injury code is based on the body part (e.g., K = knee, S = shoulder), the second letter on the tissue type (e.g., L = ligament, T = tissue), and the third letter on the pathology type. For illnesses, the organ system or region are the first letters, with "M" signifying medical conditions, (e.g., MN = neurological, MG = gastrointestinal) and the remaining letters indicating the etiology or pathology (e.g., A = allergy, I = infection). Table 3.3 presents examples of codes from the system.

The advantage of a system like this is that all knee injuries could be queried by examining all injuries that start with the letter K. If all injuries to the tendons around the knee are of interest, then all injuries starting with KT could be tallied. If frequency of a specific condition, such as patellar tendinopathy, was of interest, the specific KTP2 code could be examined. The specificity of conditions relating to sports medicine and the fact that the coding system is open source and freely available have made the Orchard system one of the most common injury classification systems used by sports injury surveillance systems.

Measuring the Frequency of Injuries and Illnesses

To determine the extent of injuries and illnesses, it is essential to understand how many people are affected by them. At its simplest level, injury surveillance is counting the number of conditions that occur. Although this may suffice if you want to determine the extent of the problem for your team or worksite, it is insufficient if you want to compare to other groups or data from existing injury surveillance systems.[16] Suppose that you want to compare injuries between two different worksites, but one site has more employees. Or that you want to compare injuries between two teams, but one team has a longer season. In both of those examples, you could not use injury counts alone to accurately compare the different groups. Therefore, the injury count data needs to consider aspects of the population to allow you to generalize the results.

Accounting for these differences is accomplished by determining the proportion of people in the population of interest who have or develop the condition. This is done by calculating the **prevalence**, which is a measure of how many people have the condition at any given time, and the **incidence**, which is a measure of how often new cases of the condition occur[16] (see table 3.4). Both prevalence and incidence can give you important information about the extent of the problem and, in some cases, the risk of the activity, but is one better? It depends on what you want to know. It has been suggested that it is more appropriate to use incidence for acute conditions and prevalence for overuse conditions.[16]

Although the incidence of an injury or illness can be calculated as the proportion of the population at risk

TABLE 3.3 Examples of Knee Injury Codes from the Orchard Sports Injury and Illness Classification System

Injury	Code
MCL injury	KL3
Grade 1 MCL sprain	KLV
Grade 2 MCL sprain	KLW
Grade 3 MCL sprain (complete rupture)	KLM
Patellar tendon injury	KTP
Patellar tendinopathy	KT2
Patellar tendon rupture	KT1

TABLE 3.4 **Prevalence and Incidence**

	Prevalence	Incidence
Calculation	$\dfrac{\text{Number of existing cases}}{\text{Total population at risk}}$	$\dfrac{\text{Number of new cases over a specific time}}{\text{Total population at risk}}$
Example	$\dfrac{\text{6 swimmers with rotator cuff tendinopathy at the start of the season}}{\text{30 swimmers on the team}}$ = 20% prevalence of rotator cuff tendinopathy on the team at the halfway point of the season	$\dfrac{\text{3 swimmers develop rotator cuff tendinopathy over course of the season}}{\text{30 swimmers on the team}}$ = 10% incidence of rotator cuff tendinopathy over the course of the season
	$\dfrac{\text{10 wildland firefighters have strep throat at day 12 of deployment}}{\text{800 firefighters at the fire camp}}$ = 1.25% prevalence of strep throat in firefighters living at fire camp	$\dfrac{\text{20 wildland firefighters develop strep throat over 21-day deployment}}{\text{800 firefighters at the fire camp}}$ = 2.5% incidence of strep throat during a 21-day fire deployment

that develops the condition over a specific time, there is often interest in calculating the incidence as a function of time at risk. The time at risk is termed an **exposure** and is used as the denominator in the incidence calculation.

For example, many existing sports injury surveillance systems define an exposure as participating in one practice or one competition. That is, the time at risk of sustaining an injury is one practice or one competition.

TABLE 3.5 **Exposure Level Descriptions**

Exposure level	Time at risk	Incidence calculation	Example	Advantages	Disadvantages
Season or year	1 athlete participating in 1 season is an exposure of 1 athlete-season. 1 worker working over the course of 1 year is an exposure	Number of new cases per season or number of new cases per year	3.6 concussions per player-seasons	Easy to collect	The length of the season is not the same for all sports or teams so the time at risk is not equal. For example, one team makes playoffs so the players have a longer season and have a greater time at risk.
Actual number of days or events participated in	1 practice is an exposure. 1 day at work is an exposure	Number of new cases per days of participation	1.3 concussions per 1,000 practice exposures	More detailed than the athlete-season or year method	Not all practices and competitions are the same length. For example, a 2-hr practice is considered one exposure, just as one 30-min practice is counted as one exposure. The time at risk is different for these practices, but the exposure calculation indicates they are the same.
Actual time at risk	A 2-hr practice is 2 hr at risk or 2 hr of exposure. An 8-hr work shift is 8 hr of exposure	Number of new cases per actual time spent at risk	4.7 concussions per 1,000 player hours	More detailed measure of time at risk	Resource intensive to collect. Some sports competitions do not have a defined length of time (e.g., baseball), so this level of exposure is likely unmeaningful.

Recording and Reporting Epidemiological Data

Incidence is the calculated rate of how often an injury occurs and is often expressed relative to the time the person is at risk. This might be reported at 0.9 hamstring injuries per 1,000 hours of exposure (time at risk) or 0.28 hamstring injuries per player season.[16] These injury rates, although informative, may be difficult for the practitioner or patient to fully understand in terms of the risk of participation. Therefore, the International Olympic Committee consensus statement Methods for Recording and Reporting of Epidemiological Data on Injury and Illness in Sport 2020 suggests converting the data into a statistic that the end user can understand.[16] For example, if there are 0.28 hamstring injuries per player per season and there are 25 players on the team, this could be calculated to a total of 7 hamstring injuries per team per season.[16] This is a quantity that is easier to understand. The consensus statement concludes that sharing understandable statistics may increase the likelihood of practitioners and athletes participating in a prevention program to reduce hamstring injuries.

Table 3.5 provides examples of different exposure levels along with some advantages and disadvantages of using those time periods as the denominator. The choice of exposure level can influence the results, so the choice is an important consideration when attempting to measure or interpret incidence data.

Measuring the Consequences of Injuries and Illnesses

Although understanding the frequency and ultimately the risk of injury or illness is essential, it is also important to learn the effect or consequences of the condition on both the patient and the population. This has been termed the burden of the condition and has been quantified in public health using measures such as financial cost, mortality, and morbidity.[16] Similar to determining the frequency of the injury, there are multiple ways to assess the severity of injuries.

Athletic trainers provide care for life-threatening conditions, such as sudden cardiac arrest, heat stroke, or hypovolemic shock. Due to the risk of death, these types of the conditions would be considered the most severe. Therefore, even though the incidence of these conditions is small, athletic trainers need to be prepared to act to prevent death by developing emergency action plans, ensuring life-saving equipment is available, and practicing the plan, among other things.

Other injuries that athletic trainers provide care for can lead to permanent damage or chronic disease. For example, people who suffer anterior cruciate ligament (ACL) injuries are more likely to have osteoarthritis of that knee joint later in life.[17] Although not life-threatening, chronic disease increases risk for other health conditions and reduces quality of life. Due to the risk of long-term health consequences, these conditions are the focus of prevention programs, such as those that reduce the risk of ACL injury.

Severity can also be measured by the duration of the condition. Using this method, the longer someone suffers from the condition, the more severe it is considered. For the injured person, this means a longer period of time in pain or discomfort, time potentially lost from activity (e.g., sport, work), and psychosocial effects.[18] For workers, injuries with a longer duration result in loss of productivity and potentially profits for the employer. Finally, clinicians may be affected because the longer the duration of the injury, the more treatments will have to be performed. More treatments mean a greater resource cost in time and money.

Similar to measuring incidence and prevalence, the choice of how to measure severity should be based on the goals of the prevention program. The goal may be a reduction in time-loss injuries, a decrease in insurance claims from a preventable injury, a lessening of the number of treatments the athletic trainer has to deliver, or a combination of these, among other goals. Unfortunately, there is no one-size-fits-all approach to determining severity.

Severity is just one part of determining the extent of the problem. You must also consider the frequency of the injury, as measured through the incidence or prevalence. Focusing on one or the other—severity or frequency—in isolation may not provide the full picture of the extent of the problem.[19] This can be challenging for the athletic trainer because establishing the extent of the problem requires a multifaceted approach. Injury surveillance is an important aspect, but it should not be seen as an end in itself. Instead, it should be used as a crucial tool to inform the subsequent steps of preventing injury and illness and promoting health.[10,20]

Establishing the Etiology and the Mechanism of Injury

Injury surveillance can help determine the magnitude of the problem (e.g., risk, severity). However, it does not necessarily provide information about what caused the injury. To do this, you will need the **etiology**, or the cause of injury, and the mechanism of injury. Without these two elements, you will not be able to develop and implement a preventive program.[20]

Risk Factors

Risk is the probability of an adverse event or consequence, in this case, an injury or illness. In other words, the greater the probability of injury, the greater the risk. Certain activities carry more risk than others and are thus considered riskier to participate in.

Certain factors increase the risk for injury or illness and are termed **risk factors**. Risk factors are often divided into intrinsic (individual characteristics) and extrinsic (external or environmental characteristics):

Intrinsic Risk Factors

- Sex
- Fitness level
- Strength
- Range of motion
- Psychological characteristics
- Previous history of injury

Extrinsic Risk Factors

- Environmental conditions
- Equipment
- Playing surface conditions

The risk factors associated with a specific injury or illness will dictate the prevention strategies you employ. For example, excessive pronation is a risk factor for several lower-extremity injuries, so you may prescribe strengthening exercises or an orthotic to help prevent injury. Likewise, you will monitor weather conditions when there is a risk of lightning in the area and notify participants that it is unsafe to be outside. Both are examples of factors that increase the risk of injury and how the athletic trainer performs actions to mitigate the risk.

Although the distinction between intrinsic and extrinsic risk factors is important, it is also essential to recognize the difference between modifiable and non-modifiable risk factors.[21] If a risk factor is nonmodifiable, there is nothing you can do to reduce the risk associated with that factor. Focus on risk factors that are modifiable when designing injury prevention programs.

For example, young (13- to 24-year-old) female athletes are at the greatest risk for suffering noncontact ACL injuries.[22] Yet both age and sex are considered nonmodifiable risk factors. However, certain movement patterns have also been associated with increased risk of noncontact ACL injuries.[22] Since movement patterns are potentially modifiable, you may want to implement a multicomponent prevention program to alter the athlete's technique to reduce the risk of an ACL injury.[22]

Understanding the difference between intrinsic and extrinsic risk factors and modifiable and nonmodifiable risk factors is important when developing a prevention strategy. Several other issues related to risk factors are important to understand. Sports injuries are typically the result of the interaction of multiple risk factors, not a single risk factor.[23,24] Just because someone has an intrinsic risk factor for a condition or is exposed to extrinsic risk factors associated with a specific condition does not mean he will suffer the injury or acquire the illness.

Determinants of Health

Health differences exist among members of a population. Understanding why these differences exist will help you work with patients to achieve their health goals.

For example, people with lower education or incomes, of specific races or ethnic backgrounds, and from certain environments are disproportionately affected by chronic disease.[25,26] These are examples of what are considered **health disparities**. Health differences and health disparities are not necessarily the same.[27] Just because certain activities or experiences result in a higher rate of injury, such as more shoulder injuries in throwing athletes than runners, does not mean it is a health disparity. Although health differences may be important for an athletic trainer to address, health disparities relate specifically to how certain groups have fewer advantages when it comes to health and health care.[27] In short, the burden of disease is not distributed equitably across the population.[28] A goal of public health is eliminating health disparities by promoting **health equity**, which means all people have the opportunity to attain the highest level of health.

To eliminate health disparities and health inequities, it is important to understand what actually determines health. These factors are called the determinants of health[29] and fall under the following broad categories:

- Biology and genetics, such as age, sex, ethnicity, and family history
- Individual behavior, such as diet, amount of physical activity, and substance abuse
- Health services, such as having access to quality health care
- Social factors, such as the environments where people live, work, and play
- Policy, such as laws and regulations

Powerful, complex relationships exist between these determinants.[26] Further, evidence is mounting that the social determinants play a very large role in determining health, but most of the resources in health care are directed at the other determinants, mainly medical services.[25] Social determinants include many aspects of the environments people live in and experience. One approach has been to organize these aspects into five different areas that serve as the underlying factors of the social determinants of health (figure 3.2):[29]

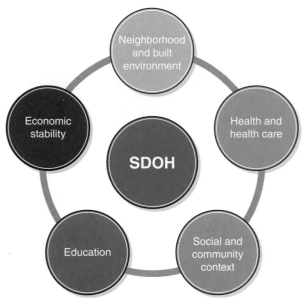

FIGURE 3.2 The five areas underlying the social determinants of health (SDOH).

Reprinted from HealthyPeople.gov. https://www.healthypeople.gov/2020/topics-objectives/topic/social-determinants-of-health.

1. Economic stability: food or housing insecurity
2. Education: access to and level of education
3. Social and community context: level of engagement in the community; any discrimination experienced
4. Health and health care: access to health care and health literacy
5. Neighborhood and built environment: environmental conditions, access to healthy foods, exposure to crime and violence, quality of housing

You may be asking yourself what role athletic trainers have in addressing the health inequities. How can an athletic trainer make a difference in addressing the social determinants of health? Aren't these factors beyond the control of any one person?

First, consider that health begins in homes, schools, workplaces, neighborhoods, and communities.[4,29] Unlike most other health care professionals, athletic trainers often work in schools or workplaces, which allows them to interact with people within their social and physical environments. Athletic trainers also often interact with the families and friends of the people they provide services to, which can have a significant influence. Because athletic trainers serve on site, their patients have greater access to care and do not have to leave the school or workplace to seek treatment, which can affect education and economic stability, respectively.

Athletic trainers also commonly provide services to and care for people who belong to groups or populations

EVIDENCE-BASED ATHLETIC TRAINING

Social Determinants of Health

Asthma is a respiratory condition that affects people across the life span and is the most common chronic disease affecting children in the United States.[31] Uncontrolled asthma leads to costly emergency department visits, hospitalizations, missed school or work days, and decreased quality of life.[31] Asthma disproportionately affects those with low socioeconomic status, and the prevalence is greater in some minority populations. For example, African American and Hispanic children are more likely to visit the emergency departments due to asthma compared to non-Hispanic white children.[32] A person's biology does not fully explain why she develops asthma and has better or worse asthma outcomes. It has long been known that social factors also play a significant role.[33] These factors, known as social determinants of health, include exposure to allergens, second-hand smoke, and pests and rodents in the home; environmental pollutants in the neighborhood of the house or school; or work environments that are unsafe or expose the person to toxins.[33] Despite their significant influence on health, these factors are rarely addressed in a typical health care setting. Therefore, an approach that addresses these health disparities is needed. One approach is to use population health principles to influence factors outside of a traditional health clinic, specifically in the home, school, and work environments.[32] Athletic trainers are trained in the management of asthma. Since they often provide care where people work, go to school, and play, they are well positioned to understand and help address the social determinants related to asthma.

that have suffered health disparities and health inequities. For example, athletic trainers work with adolescents from the LGBTQ+ community, who have greater incidence of anxiety, depression, and suicide than their heterosexual peers.[30] Additionally, athletic trainers may work with people from lower socioeconomic backgrounds who have greater health inequities than patients who are more socially and economically advantaged. As such, you must establish the cause of the conditions you are attempting to prevent for your patients before developing and implementing a prevention program.

Developing and Introducing Preventive Interventions

The next step in the sequence of prevention is introducing prevention measures.[8] In some cases, this is straightforward because the prevention strategy already exists. For example, if you want to prevent noncontact ACL injuries, your next step may be to implement a lower-extremity injury prevention program. However, in many cases, the prevention program has yet to be developed.

Due to this and other reasons (discussed in the next section), Finch proposed a modification to the sequence of prevention. She called this the Translating Research into Injury Prevention Practice (TRIPP) framework.[20] As table 3.6 shows, the first change modified stage 3 of the sequence of prevention model to focus on identifying potential solutions and then developing the preventive measures.

The process of identifying potential solutions involves using information gathered in the first two stages: What is the problem and what is causing the problem? Doing this helps ensure that the program addresses the actual problem and is evidence based.

Due to the varied nature of the injuries and illnesses you will encounter throughout your career as an athletic trainer, it is beyond the scope of this chapter to describe in detail specific prevention programs that you may choose to introduce. Instead, this chapter focuses on concepts to consider when developing the program.

Preventive efforts can occur at different stages of the progression of the condition, and each stage serves a critical role in promoting the health of the population.

- *Primary prevention.* This step involves intervening before the injury or illness occurs. For example, you might implement an injury prevention program to prevent lower-extremity musculoskeletal injuries.
- *Secondary prevention.* Here, you will identify the injury or illness at the earliest stages and develop strategies to lessen the effect. For example, you might ensure that an automated external defibrillator is used as quickly as possible following a patient's unexplained collapse.
- *Tertiary prevention.* Managing the injury or illness after it occurs slows the progression and helps patients manage their health as much as possible despite the injury or illness. For example, you may help a patient manage her diabetes by providing resources and information on proper management.

The goal is to implement the preventive intervention before health is affected. In public health, this is called working upstream. Ideally, the further upstream that the intervention can be implemented, the more likely it is that the intervention will be successful. However, many health problems require a combination of primary, secondary, and tertiary prevention strategies. You should determine what stage or stages the prevention program is targeting and develop a program based on that.

TABLE 3.6 Comparison of Two Prevention Models

Model stage	Sequence of prevention model[8]	Translating Research into Injury Prevention Practice (TRIPP) framework[20]
1	Establish the extent of the injury problem.	Conduct injury surveillance.
2	Establish the etiology and mechanism of injury.	Establish etiology and mechanism of injury.
3	Introduce the preventive measures.	Identify potential solutions and develop preventive measures.
4	Assess the effectiveness of the prevention measure by repeating stage 1.	Evaluate the preventive measure under ideal conditions.
5	_____	Describe the intervention context to inform implementation strategies.
6	_____	Evaluate the effectiveness of the preventive measures in the implementation context.

Adapted from van Mechelen, Hlobil, and Kemper (1992); Finch (2006).

Stages of Prevention

Athletic trainers are well positioned to help prevent injuries and illnesses because they often provide care where the patient works or plays. This access can allow the athletic trainer to do the following:

- Intervene before an injury or illness occurs
- Intervene at the earliest stages of the condition to lessen the effects
- Assist a patient in managing a condition in an effort to maintain health despite having the injury or illness

A public health approach identifies these different stages as primary, secondary, and tertiary prevention. For example, you may implement a shoulder strengthening program for your patients to prevent a rotator cuff injury from occurring in the first place (primary prevention). You may recognize the signs and symptoms of a rotator cuff tendinopathy early and begin treatment and rehabilitation before the patient suffers a rotator cuff tear (secondary prevention). In the cases where the rotator cuff is torn and the patient is not a candidate for surgery, you may provide treatment and rehabilitation to help the patient manage the injury in order to maintain activity. The goal is to use primary prevention as much as possible, but it is impossible to prevent *all* conditions from occurring. You should leverage the unique role you have with your patients to promote prevention at all stages.

Regardless of the stage of prevention that is being targeted, it is important that you work to engage key stakeholders when identifying potential solutions. This is discussed in more detail in the next section on introducing the prevention program. Understanding the stakeholders' perspective from the beginning of the process will likely aid in the success of the program.

Evaluating the Intervention

The final stage of the sequence of prevention is to evaluate the effectiveness of the preventive intervention. The need to evaluate the program to ensure it works may seem obvious; however, this step is often incomplete.

In the original sequence of prevention model, evaluating for effectiveness was done by repeating stage 1, establishing the extent of the problem.[8] In other words, by conducting injury surveillance or research studies on frequency and severity, the effectiveness of the intervention could be determined. Again, this seems like a straightforward approach. However, several factors should be considered when determining effectiveness.

The TRIPP framework proposed that the sequence of prevention model should be expanded by three additional steps:[20]

1. Introducing and testing the intervention under ideal conditions
2. Understanding the real-world contexts
3. Evaluating the intervention in real-world situations

This is particularly important for interventions that have just been developed because, ideally, existing programs that you might choose to use would have already progressed through the three stages. Unfortunately, that is not always the case.

Evaluating the Intervention Under Ideal Conditions

According to the TRIPP model, after development of the preventive measure, you should assess the program under ideal conditions.[20] What are ideal conditions? Generally, this means that the program was carried out under highly controlled conditions. This could include in laboratory settings, in small groups, or in tightly controlled studies. Typically, the people receiving the intervention are given resources, such as equipment, reminders, or incentives to complete the program, that will likely be unavailable when the prevention program is performed under real-world conditions.

Trials tested under ideal conditions are termed efficacy trials.[34] When a prevention program has been shown to work under ideal conditions, it is considered **efficacious**. If the program is found not to be efficacious, you should return to the previous step and consider other potential solutions. On the other hand, if the program is efficacious, you may move on to the next step.

Describe the Intervention Context

In order for a prevention program to be successful, the people who would benefit from the intervention need to use it. Unfortunately, many prevention programs that have shown to be efficacious are not being adopted and implemented. Therefore, before translating an efficacious program into practice, you need to understand the context of the real world.

Understanding the Barriers and Facilitators   When gaining an understanding of the real-world context for a program, knowing the factors that may be hindering its use may lead to insights. On the other hand, realizing why some people are using the program or what would help others use the program is also valuable information.

Barriers are factors that hinder people from adopting or implementing the prevention program. There are many reasons why prevention programs are not being used, and it is unlikely that one approach can address all barriers. Table 3.7 provides some common barriers to using injury prevention programs. You should work to engage people who might benefit from the program to understand their perspective and then consider strategies for encouraging success of the program.

The factors that aid in the use of the prevention program are called facilitators. One approach to determining the facilitators is developing solutions to the barriers, which would ideally aid in the uptake of the program. Although this is an important step, you should also engage with the stakeholders to determine other facilitators. You might ask people who have already adopted the program what helped them to begin using the program and those who are not yet using the program what would help them try it. Although numerous barriers probably exist, there are likely many facilitators as well. Engaging the stakeholders is key.

Social-Ecological Model   Another important aspect of understanding the real-world context is to learn what drives someone's behavior and what might help him

change the behavior for the positive. In this case, what causes someone to decide to use a prevention program? One approach that has been used in health promotion is the social-ecological model (figure 3.3 and table 3.8), which suggests that behavior is determined by the following:[35]

- Intrapersonal factors
- Interpersonal processes
- Institutional factors
- Community factors
- Public policy

At each level, different approaches are used to change individual behavior. However, behavior is affected and

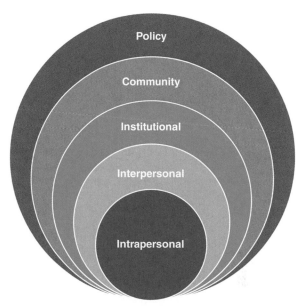

FIGURE 3.3   Five levels of the social-ecological model.

TABLE 3.7   **Examples of Barriers to Prevention Program Use and Potential Solutions**

Potential barrier	Potential solution
Lack of knowledge of the problem or the prevention strategy	Education on the risks and benefits of the preventive strategy
Patients' perception that the condition is unlikely to affect them	Education on the risks and engagement to understand the patients' perceptions
Perception that what is already being done is enough to prevent the injury	Engagement with the patients to understand what is currently being done and if it is likely to be successful
Lack of time to complete the prevention program	Work with patients to determine ways to deliver the prevention program considering the time constraints
Lack of resources (e.g., personnel, money, equipment)	Work with patients to determine ways to deliver the prevention program in ways that are less resource intensive or find resources to help implement the program

TABLE 3.8 **Details of the Social-Ecological Model**

Factor	Definition	Examples	Approach to change behavior
Intrapersonal	Individual characteristics that influence behavior	Knowledge Attitudes Self-efficacy	Changing someone's knowledge, attitudes, and beliefs
Interpersonal	Interpersonal processes and groups providing identity and support	Family, friends, and peers Teammates and coaches Coworkers and supervisors	Engaging people close to the patient to promote a change in behavior, such as family members and friends
Institutional or organizational	Social institutions with organizational characteristics and rules and regulations for operation	School for interscholastic sports Company in terms of employees Other social groups such as churches or clubs	Changing the organization's culture to promote health and safety
Community	Relationships between organizations, institutions, and networks within defined boundaries	Geographic boundaries such as neighborhood, town, state, and region Relationships between organizations Social networks	Understanding the community norms and then developing interventions that take those norms into consideration
Policy	Local, state, and national laws, policies, and regulations	Laws (local, state, federal) Governing body policies and regulations (such as NCAA or NFHS for sports or OSHA for workplace safety)	Developing policies that promote health and safety

shaped by multiple levels, and it ultimately shapes and affects each of the levels as well.

The social-ecological model is a multifaceted framework that you can use to guide behavior change and ultimately promote prevention efforts. Efforts may target the individual level or peers or other social networks. Others may involve creating policies at the institutional level or advocating for new laws. When attempting to understand the context of the real world to introduce a prevention program, you must look beyond the patient and consider other factors that may influence her choices.

Taken together, understanding this context provides information about how to translate the program into practice in the real world.[20] It also allows for ideas on how to target or market the program to those who may use it.[20]

Evaluate the Intervention in the Real World

After understanding the real-world context, you should disseminate the program to the target population. When a program has been shown to work under real-world conditions, it is considered effective.[34] **Effectiveness** is the goal of any prevention program because that means it works in the real world. Assessing for effectiveness is the last stage of both the sequence of prevention model and the TRIPP framework.

How is effectiveness assessed? Ideally, there would be a reduction in the negative outcome that is trying to be prevented. In other words, the problem that was identified in stages 1 and 2 of the sequence of prevention has been reduced or eliminated. For example, a lower-extremity injury prevention program would be considered effective if it is used by athletes in the real world and it demonstrates a reduction in lower-extremity injuries. This can be accomplished through injury surveillance.

One of the challenges with assessing the outcomes is that some happen infrequently. For example, some catastrophic injuries are very rare, and the outcome of interest may not always be captured by the surveillance system. This is discussed previously in terms of why the surveillance system needs to be sufficiently large to capture a critical threshold of the injuries in order to make informed conclusions. However, even large systems may

EVIDENCE-BASED ATHLETIC TRAINING

Prevention of Anterior Cruciate Ligament Injury

Anterior cruciate ligament (ACL) injury can be devasting to patients and put them at risk for osteoarthritis, a debilitating chronic health condition. Therefore, athletic trainers should attempt to prevent ACL injuries, particularly those that occur without direct contact. The National Athletic Trainers' Association position statement Prevention of Anterior Cruciate Ligament Injury reports that multicomponent training programs that provide feedback on technique and include at least three of the common exercise categories (i.e., strength, plyometrics, agility, balance, and flexibility) have grade A evidence to reduce the risk (1) of noncontact ACL injuries in girls aged 12 to 18 and (2) of other noncontact and indirect-contact knee injuries in active people.[22] Despite the strong evidence that these programs should be part of clinical practice, several studies found that only around 20% of youth soccer coaches reported performing a structured knee injury prevention training program.[36,37] This is an example of a prevention program that works under ideal conditions (i.e., efficacious) not adopted and implemented in real-world settings (i.e., effective). To increase the effectiveness of these prevention programs, athletic trainers need to better understand the barriers and facilitators to using these programs.

be insufficient. In those cases, other approaches may be used. For example, an assessment of how many people are using the prevention program could be determined. Although this is not a direct assessment of effectiveness, it provides some information until enough data are available to determine effectiveness.

A broader view is that the goal of both medicine and public health is to improve the health of individual people and the greater population. Therefore, it may be appropriate to assess health through measures of quality of life and function. These are often referred to as patient-centered outcomes since the focus is on patients' perception of

their health and function. Athletic trainers are using these assessments more often in clinical practice.

Regardless of the approach, assessing effectiveness is an important stage of injury and illness prevention to ensure that the prevention program is working. Unfortunately, this stage is often incomplete. The sequence of prevention is a continual process. It does not end once the program has been developed and introduced. Instead, it builds on itself with the goal of creating better and more effective prevention strategies, ultimately resulting in improved health for the individual patient and the population.

CLINICAL BOTTOM LINE

- Athletic trainers in many settings serve a unique role by providing services at both the patient and population levels. In addition, athletic trainers are well suited to provide preventive care to those they work with. These facts highlight the intersection of athletic training and public health.
- When establishing the risk of participating in certain activities, athletic trainers should consider both the frequency and consequences of injuries and illnesses.
- Health is more than just the absence of disease and is the result of more than just a person's biology. Instead, where he lives, works, attends school, and plays all have a role in his health and, as a result, that of the community as a whole.
- Before introducing an injury- or illness-prevention program, the athletic trainer should engage stakeholders at multiple levels to determine what they perceive as critical barriers and facilitators to the prevention program's success.
- To maximize the influence athletic trainers can have on the health of the patients and populations they work with, they must implement effective prevention programs. Using the concepts of injury and illness prevention, rooted in the public health approach, will increase their chances of success. The more upstream their approaches and the more contextual factors they consider, the greater the health benefits to their patients.

 Go to HK*Propel* to complete the activities and case studies for this chapter.

CHAPTER 4

Cultural Literacy in Patient-Centered Care

Marsha Grant-Ford, ATC, PhD
Leamor Kahanov, EdD, ATC, LAT

CAATE STANDARDS

The following CAATE 2020 standards are covered in this chapter:

Standard 56

Standard 57

Standard 65

CHAPTER OBJECTIVES

After reading this chapter, you will be able to do the following:

- Understand the definition of patient-centered care

- Define cultural literacy or competence

- Apply considerations for cultural literacy in patient-centered care

- Apply ethical considerations and advocacy for cultural literacy in clinical decisions

Athletic trainers are obligated to provide optimal care for patients; this includes being sensitive to differences. This chapter provides a foundation for understanding the role of the provider in improving patient outcomes through cultural literacy and sensitivity to the biases that affect health care. The first principle of the NATA's code of ethics directs members to respect the rights, welfare, and dignity of all.[1] The purpose of this chapter is to provide the foundational knowledge to improve patient outcomes and communication. Educational programs coordinate programs that help students understand personal values, identities, and biases; explore culturally sensitive and professionally appropriate attitudes, beliefs, and values; and learn professional socialization in clinical education. Ideally, the clinical education experience provides opportunities to learn delivery of appropriate, sensitive, and specific patient-centered care.[2-5]

Additionally, the CAATE core competencies direct professionals to advocate for the health needs of clients, patients, communities, and populations and communicate effectively and appropriately. Ultimately, a successful educational program would move the athletic training student along the continuum from a passive to more active advocacy role, providing care that is respectful of the patient's values and beliefs, mitigates health disparities in athletic medicine, and improves patient outcomes. This includes understanding specifically how age, religion or spirituality, socioeconomic status, race and ethnicity, gender and sexual identity, ability, and the many permutations of these identities form the benchmark against which athletic trainers evaluate others and how patients will evaluate them and interpret their language and behavior.[2-5] It is only when health care professionals understand the historical experiences and perspectives of less privileged groups that they can grow in self-awareness, which enables them to substantively improve their patients' experience.[6]

Patient-Centered Care Definition

In 2001, the Institute of Medicine endorsed a change in their focus from a paternalistic philosophy of care to patient-centered care.[7] Paternalistic care established physicians as the authority, with the right to make autocratic decisions for the patient. **Patient-centered care (PCC)** is an approach to therapeutic interactions with patients that delivers the care in a responsive and respectful way. Clinicians who espouse PCC are charged with the following:[7]

- Knowing their patients' preferences and values
- Engaging them in discussion and decisions regarding their pathology and treatment plan
- Executing therapeutic interventions consistent with the patient's needs and choices

There is persuasive evidence that PCC improves patient outcomes in a variety of settings.[8]

Empathy, or the ability to understand a patient's perspective, is required in the provision of PCC.[8] Demonstration of empathy and compassion are NATA professional behaviors. Researchers have established that empathy positively influences a clinician's ability to reduce prejudice, discern social determinants and inequities in health care, build a relationship with the patient, and improve patient outcomes by increasing their compliance with therapeutic interventions.[8,9] Educators can use a variety of teaching strategies to develop and maintain empathy; people can become less empathetic if this value is not supported in didactic and clinical education.

Person-First Language

The effectiveness of patient care can be negatively or positively affected by the words that health care clinicians choose. Patients need to feel that they, and not their injury or illness, are the most important part of their relationship with their clinician. Person-first language emphasizes the person rather than the diagnosis (see table 4.1 for examples). It eliminates references to a person's disability when it is not pertinent to the discussion. It also does not refer to people who do not have a condition as "normal," which implies that people with a disability are not normal. Avoid the words "abnormal" or "deformed," which suggest that a person has not met an ideal of perfection, as well as metaphors that are descriptors or insults for disabilities (table 4.2).

TABLE 4.1 **Examples of Person-First Language**

Don't say	Do say
Learning disabled student-athletes often have a history of multiple ACEs.	Student-athletes with learning disabilities often have a history of multiple ACEs.
Chris is confined to a wheelchair and is a tennis player.	Chris is a para-tennis athlete.
Specific medical documentation must be provided by ADHD athletes in the event that a medical exemption for positive drug screen is necessary.	Athletes with ADHD must provide specific medical documentation in the event that a medical exemption for positive drug screen is necessary.
The athlete has bilateral stumps below the knee.	The athlete has a bilateral below-the-knee amputation.
I provide clinical coverage for special ed students practicing for Special Olympics.	I provide clinical coverage for students with cognitive impairments who are practicing for Special Olympics.

ACE = adverse childhood experiences; ADHD = attention-deficient/hyperactivity disorder.

TABLE 4.2 **Insulting Terms**

Terms	Category of impairment
Retard, schizo, special ed, psycho, spaz, insane	Cognitive or intellectual
Deaf and dumb, deaf mute, hearing challenged	Sensory
Fit	Neurological
Crippled, crip, deformed, spaz, lame, dwarf, midget	Physical

Identity-Based Language

- The Deaf community values the Platinum Rule as opposed to the Golden Rule. The Platinum Rule says to "treat others as they want to be treated."

- The Deaf community and, to a smaller extent, the Autistic community, prefer identity-based language to denote that their social interactions and communication style are different rather than negative.

- When using identity-based language, which is implicit in the person-first shift in academia and scholarly journal style guides, avoid use of the word "disability."[10]

- The International Paralympic Committee directs clinicians to avoid the terms "disabled athlete" and "athlete with a disability." The respectful terminology is "athlete with an impairment," "para-athlete," or "adaptive sport athlete."[11]

There are many impairments and impairment combinations. Memorizing an expansive list of preferred terms would be challenging for clinicians who do not work with these populations regularly. When in doubt, ask the client how he wants to be addressed.

Group Identities

Our identity contributes to how we see ourselves and how others treat us. The words that people use to categorize themselves are important because they provide insights into the complicated history, values, and behaviors they identify with. Since patients do not leave their cultural identities outside the athletic training facility, clinicians must be aware of those things that affect their patients' thoughts, behaviors, experiences, the clinical relationship, and the therapeutic intervention designed to meet their needs.[12]

The goal of this section is not to provide a list of terms to memorize, but rather to help you understand how the power differentials between groups came to be, how inequities are created and perpetuated, how the patient's world may differ from the world the athletic trainer has been conditioned to see, and the athletic trainer's responsibility in navigating all these differences. When clinicians do not give groups and clients the autonomy to determine their labels, patient care and results are significantly affected.[10,13]

Racial and Ethnic Identity Group Names

Capitalizing racial identity group names validates and empowers the group members. Black and White are very broad skin color descriptions for people of many ethnicities and from many countries of origin. In the United States, *Black* refers to people who are descendants of North American slaves with sub-Saharan ancestry.

Immigrants from African nations like Nigeria or Ghana and Caribbean immigrants have different ethnic identities from African Americans, yet they also consider themselves Black. This chapter also capitalizes the term *White* to be respectful of the group identities the term represents and to be consistent in sentence construction. It is used for anyone who indicates "White" on research demographic intake forms, often people of European ancestry (e.g., Italian American, Danish American, Australian American).

Ethnicity delineates a group of people with a distinct shared ancestry and cultural identity. It is often inappropriately used as a euphemism for race. The ethnic group or groups that people identify with may be either a minority or a majority in their country of residence. Commonly, but not always, members of ethnic groups share geography, language, communication style, religion, and ritual. Members of minority ethnic groups may share an experience of **marginalization** within the dominant culture. According to its demographic data, the NATA has members from many Asian ethnic groups (Japanese, Chinese, Filipino), European (often White) ethnic groups (Spanish, Dutch, Lithuanian, Scottish), Hispanic ethnic groups (Puerto Rican, Cuban, Brazilian, Columbian), Native American/Pacific Islanders (Inupiat, Tongan, Sioux, Navajo), and Black groups.[118] The designation *Black* (rather than *Hispanic*) is intended to categorize American people who are descendants of enslaved people.

Ethnicity at times depends on the social setting. People with a South American, Caribbean, or Central American heritage may not perfectly fit into the simplified categories identified in this chapter. Brazilians are thought of by some people as Hispanic, although their language is Portuguese. A Chinese American teenager raised in a Chinese family in the United States would typically identify as Chinese. When visiting Hong Kong, however, she may report that she feels more American.

Ethnicity also determines how patients define health or injury, express pain, and seek help; as a result of health disparities, ethnicity also affects patient outcomes. When clinicians make assumptions about a patient based on a rote list of ethnic characteristics, patient interactions can easily be compromised.

People of Color

"People of color" is a phrase used to describe the collective experience of people who do not identify as White. When writing or speaking about something that affects African Americans, Alaska Natives and Pacific Islanders, Asian Americans, Latina/o/x people, and Native Americans similarly, it is appropriate to use "people of color." It is not appropriate, however, to use "people of color" when referring specifically to African Americans; here, the preferred term is *Black*.

Hispanic and Latino

Much like people with ancestry from the continent of Africa, people with ancestry from Spanish- and Portuguese-speaking countries prefer to identify themselves according to their family's country of origin—for example, Mexican, Dominican, or Columbian. The term selected for government use and medical documentation is *Hispanic*. This phrase is not without controversy, though; there have been historical objections in some areas of the United States, and it homogenizes more than 20 ethnic groups, some of which do not speak Spanish. The label widely used in lieu of *Hispanic* is *Latino*.

The two terms are often distinguished by using *Hispanic* when referring to a person whose ancestry is from a Spanish-speaking country or culture and *Latino* when referring to people from Latin America. Through this lens, a Brazilian or Haitian basketball player would be considered Latino but not Hispanic. Because Spanish is a gendered language, its speakers commonly use the terms *Latino* (male), *Latina* (female), and *Latino* (group of males and females).[14,15]

The gender-neutral term *Latinx* has recently started to be used. It was created for those who identify as gender fluid and as a challenge to the masculine focus of the term *Latino*.[14,15] Another option is to use *Latina/o/x*. This chapter will reference *Latina/o/x* when research suggests that discrimination or disparity is grounded in the intersection of Latin American ancestry and language.[14,18-20]

Sexual Identity

When speaking about sexual identity, use the terms "identity" or "sexual orientation." The term "sexual preference," which was often used in the past, is considered disrespectful because it implies that sexual attraction is a voluntary choice.

Family Structure

The concept of family has varying meanings, both culturally and legally. Athletic trainers must be mindful of respecting clients with different family structures. This may involve families that are single parent, two parents, of the same sex or gender, or with parents and guardians with various sexual identities. A child's legal guardians may be from her extended biological family, such as aunts, uncles, and grandparents. In traditional settings, you may also work with children in the foster care system who are being raised by people who are not biologically or socially related to them. Strive to use inclusionary language in your oral and written communication and instructions to prevent barriers to care and compliance. Make sure you are clear about relationships when talking with patients and clients and use respectful salutations and references. You might ask the following questions: Who do you live with? Is (parent/guardian's) last name the same as yours? How does (parent/guardian) prefer to be addressed? Is it possible for (parent/guardian) to receive a call from me at work?

Salutations

Salutations are important and set the tone for the relationship. Their use in different cultures is influenced by **power distance**, which refers to the level of comfort

---

EVIDENCE-BASED ATHLETIC TRAINING

Health Care Inequities in Practice Settings

One goal of athletic trainers is to eliminate health care inequities in their practice. As such, you should avoid ambiguity about the social minorities you refer to. Approximately 53% of student-athletes in the high school setting are people of color. NCAA demographic data indicate that 33%, 38%, and 25% (in Divisions I, II, and III, respectively) of student-athletes are ethnic minorities.[16] In the general population, about 40% of people identify as racial or ethnic minorities.[17] As of December 2019, about 20% of certified athletic trainers identified as ethnic minorities.[16] These data demonstrate that athletic trainers will interact with many patients who do not look like them. See chapter 3 for additional information on health disparities.

group members have with power, influence, and wealth inequalities. There are two extremes of power distance: high and low. Country cultures with a high power distance include Mexico, India, and Saudi Arabia. Countries with low power distance include the United Kingdom and Israel. A student-athlete from Mexico (high power distance) may defer to his parents with regard to whether the ACL injury will be rehabilitated or surgically reconstructed; when addressing his parents, use the Mr./Mrs. or Senor/Senora salutation. The Quaker religion, also called the Society of Friends, is a group that values low power distance. Titles that reinforce sexist, classist, or racist ideals are avoided; students in Quaker schools call adults and teachers by their first names.[21]

Culture, Ethnicity, and Personal Core Values

Our personal core values are influenced by our family units, social groups, education, religion, and culture. Everyone has cultural identities, and one's attitudes, beliefs, and actions within that culture are grounded in these personal core values. The behaviors (conscious and unconscious), knowledge, beliefs, style of dress, language, manners, protocol, rituals, morals, and attitudes of a social group distinguish culture as a social construct.

Culture is learned and passed down; it is also adaptive across time.

Robust research regarding attributes of patients, such as race, cultural background, and gender, has been developed to guide clinical interactions. The foundation for meaningful relationships with patients is self-awareness, or an understanding of how the athletic trainer's own attitudes and beliefs can affect patients. Athletic trainers should manage their own behaviors to create an inclusive clinical setting.[1,7,22]

Livermore[21] has expanded the concept of culture developed by previous researchers to distinguish between different cultures based on group preferences in several categories of dimensions of culture. Table 4.3 presents the cultural identities most applicable to health care behaviors, compliance, and communication.

Pain Management

Pain management is a foundational component of therapeutic intervention where you must consider the patient's culture. Male and female patients respond differently to pain.[24-26] There are two cultural coping styles: emotive or stoic. The difference is not in whether the pain is experienced but how pain is expressed. **Emotive** people are demonstrative in expressing their emotions.[27] **Stoicism** means not showing emotion after painful or

TABLE 4.3 Categories of Dimensions of Culture and Health Behaviors

Cultural dimension	Influence on health behaviors and communication
Individualist vs. collectivist	Decision making
Low vs. high power distance	Views on authority
Low vs. high uncertainty avoidance	Planning for the future
Cooperative vs. competitive	Clinical expectations and compliance
Punctuality vs. relationships	Time orientation
Direct vs. indirect communication	Explicit vs. implicit communication style
Neutral expressiveness vs. affective	Emotional expression for pain and communication
Tight vs. loose social norms	Strength of conformity to societal norms

Adapted by permission from D.A. Livermore, *Leading With Cultural Intelligence: The Real Secret to Success*, (New York, NY: Amacom, 2015), 93-98.

Cultural Influence on Pain Presentation

Stoic Cultures	Emotive Cultures
Asian	Polish
English	French
Dutch	Spanish
Finnish	Italian
	Some African American subcultures
	Latin American

pleasurable experiences. (See sidebar for examples of the intersection of culture and pain expression.) People who identify strongly with ethnic groups are more likely to ascribe to the cultural influences of that group. Culturally influenced responses can be altered or negated by other influences, such as acculturation, personality, or socioeconomic status. [25,28-30]

Religious values also influence expression of pain and pain management. [27,29,31,33] A patient who practices Buddhism may believe that pain is a consequence for negative behavior in a past or present life; refusal of pain medication is a way to repay that debt. [31] In some African American cultures, pain is seen as God's will; therefore, members may delay seeking treatment. [32] A patient who espouses traditional Irish cultural values may view a painful experience as an opportunity to prove his spiritual worthiness. [31]

The cultural value described in the preceding examples is expressiveness; the categories are affective versus neutral. In stoic cultures, control of feelings and emotions are important signs of respect and dignity. Members of these groups prefer to stick to the point and "keep a stiff upper lip." Therefore, their facial expressions are not likely to reveal what they are thinking or feeling. Examples are the United Kingdom, Germany, the Netherlands, Finland, and most Asian countries. Japanese culture is often considered to be one of the most neutral world countries. Saving face is a hallmark of Asian cultures; at all costs, dignity cannot be compromised, especially in the presence of others. Even public praise is avoided. In contrast, people from emotive cultures are expressive communicators, using an array of facial expressions and frequent gesturing. When they are excited, their verbal expression can be loud. This value varies within some country cultures and socioeconomic groups. [21]

Language

Language is another central aspect of culture. If athletic trainers use words without a thorough understanding of their nuances in different cultures, the potential for miscommunication is high. [11] English words used to describe certain types of pain that are diagnostic red flags for health care professionals may not have meaning to patients who describe pain from the reference point of the ethnic cultural descriptors that they are most familiar with. The imagery and numerical symbols used on analog pain scales can easily be misinterpreted by someone using another cultural frame of reference. [34] The possibility of making a diagnostic error or having a patient perceive mistreatment contributes to inequities in therapeutic outcomes. [28]

Written materials should also be examined through the lens of reading level proficiency. Many institutional review boards recommend that investigators aim for between a 6th and 8th grade reading level when writing consent forms. The following national standards are of special note to athletic trainers in traditional settings because these requirements ensure that they are receiving accurate information and relayed correct information to the patient and guardian (in the case of a minor). [35]

- Standard 5 requires a translator to assist people with limited English proficiency and sensory impairment.
- Standard 7 specifies that untrained people and minors should not be used as translators.

When educational translators are not available and athletic trainers are managing emergent situations without professional translation expertise, the potential for legal liability is high. The best defense against malpractice is to document the steps taken to provide the standard of care. [36]

Race

Race is a social construct and a societal category that is not grounded in biology. Racial classification systems used in the United States are not applicable to people in other countries, and systems in use in any given country may not be valid across countries. The U.S. Census divides people into racial categories based primarily on superficial, visible physical characteristics (predominantly skin color) that vary between and within countries and across time. For practitioners, it is important to understand that less than 6 human genes determine skin color. In contrast, blood type is a potential medical classifier with more gene variability. Because there is no biological or genetic basis for most relationships between disease and race, the Centers for Disease Control and Prevention advise paying minimal attention to race when determining matters of public health. Yet, knowledge on this topic is important for athletic trainers in order to understand a patient's outlook and provide effective care.

Geography is a better indicator than race for identifying inclination toward disease or illness. For example, sickle cell disease has been characterized as a Black disease, but it most often appears in certain countries, including some from sub-Saharan Africa, but also Greece (particularly Orchomenos), Italy, Turkey, India, and some Central and South American countries. [37-39] A clinician who is aware that sickle cell status is a geographical rather than racial genetic anomaly with endless parental permutations can provide more focused patient care. Clinical focus on culture and ethnicity rather than race helps athletic trainers provide patient-centered care. [37-40]

For athletic trainers working in traditional settings, the identities that are important to explicitly address may vary. For example, the effects of marginalization and privilege of a patient with an acute ankle sprain are salient as opposed to sexual identity. Clinicians must be mindful that some patients might not want certain therapeutic interventions because of their religious or spiritual beliefs.[41]

The danger of making assumptions and prejudging cultural or ethnic groups is marginalization (table 4.4). The cultural bias associated with marginalization is ethnocentrism. Someone grounded in an ethnocentric philosophy views his culture as superior. Ethnocentrism is incongruent with holistic clinical practices.[41]

Intersectionality

All identities, including race, vary along a continuum. Everyone has multiple identities that intersect and create their distinct life experiences. The overlapping of two or more identities is called **intersectionality**. This intersectionality creates unique experiences for a person based on the various interactions that occur with the dominant group in the United States. A person's particular intersectionality is based in part on the number of combinations of their identities and the environment in which their experiences take place. People experience discrimination differently depending on their overlapping identities. Intersectionality becomes more complex when one of the variables is race. The same person can simultaneously experience both privilege and oppression.

In the management of athletic injury, the dominant group varies depending on the social group. For example, for someone with a disability, the dominant group is people without disabilities. For someone who identifies with the female gender, the dominant group is males. For someone who identifies as Asian, the dominant group in the United States is White people. If the athletic trainer's cultural identities are considered as well, the permutation of relationship variables is astronomical. Athletic trainers will need understanding and insight on these topics to achieve optimal patient relationships and outcomes and ultimately provide patient-centered care.

Race and Patient-Centered Care

Athletic trainers work with people with a huge range of realities and experiences. They should be mindful that in the medical culture, White privilege is in full effect. This chapter defines racism as power plus privilege. Racism and all the other isms differ, because regardless of gender, socioeconomic level, ability, or age, White people have a more privileged status in the United States.

Professional Culture and Core Values

Athletic training students may not be aware of the additional identity they take on by participating in the medical culture. The medical field is a culture with specific professional core values (table 4.5). Because athletic

TABLE 4.4 Marginalized Identities in the United States

Classification	Identity
Gender	Women, transgender people, nonbinary people
Sexual identity	Lesbian, gay, and bisexual people
Socioeconomic class	People in poverty
Age	Youth and elders
Race and ethnicity	African American, Black, Asian and Asian American, Latina/o/x and Latin American, Native American/Indian, and biracial/multiracial people
Ability	People with mental or physical disabilities
Religion or spirituality	People who practice Buddhism, Islam, Mormonism, or Judaism

TABLE 4.5 Professional Core Values in the Medical Field

Medical cultural attribute	Example beliefs and behaviors among medical professionals
Profession-specific ethics and values	Hippocratic Oath NATA Code of Ethics
Disease epidemiology	"Pathogens cause disease." "Medications cure disease."
Ego-driven	Patients and subordinates may experience medical professionals as rude, arrogant, or intimidating. Medical professionals discourage questions, hide their human side, and must not show weakness or indecisiveness.

> continued

Table 4.5   >*continued*

Medical cultural attribute	Example beliefs and behaviors among medical professionals
Guiding ethical principle	Accede to The Ethic of Reciprocity (The Golden Rule of Medicine)
Dress code	The white coat is equated with someone deserving of respect and its length signifies the level of expertise. Athletic trainers often wear khaki-colored pants and polo shirt.
Distinctive lexicon	The field uses a language system of medical abbreviations based on Latin (NPO), acronyms (ADLs), words that have lost their beginnings (e.g., [arthro]*scope*, [spine] *board*), words that have lost their endings (e.g., *consult*[ation], *prep*[are]), words that have lost both the beginning and ending (e.g., [pre]*script*[ion]), and slang terms that are euphemisms for offensive terminology (e.g., *gatekeeper*).
Core values	*Nursing:* caring, integrity, diversity, excellence *Physical therapy:* accountability, altruism, compassion, excellence, integrity, professional duty, social responsibility *Athletic training:* respect, caring, social responsibility, accountability, excellence, integrity *Medicine:* well-being, equity and justice, excellence, professionalism, leadership, compassion, inclusion

TABLE 4.6   Actions and Core Values

Core value	Sample behavior examples
Respect	Assure that patients feel that clinicians listen to and validate their concerns. Make a concerted effort to learn about patients' cultures and beliefs. Include patients in decision making.
Caring	Commit to effective communication with respect to all variables. Advocate for patient needs. Be attentive to achieving the greatest outcome for patients. Acknowledge biases and eradicate their influence in patient interactions.
Social responsibility	Encourage cultural humility in all aspects of life. Provide community leadership and promote volunteerism. Advocate for social and institutional policy that affects the well-being of patients.
Accountability	Be attentive to patient needs. Accept and acknowledge consequences for behaviors. Continually seek to improve the quality of care delivered. Pursue and respond to performance feedback.
Excellence	Consistently use multiple evidence sources in clinical decision making. Demonstrate exemplary knowledge and skill.
Integrity	Adhere to the highest standards of practice within the profession (Code of Ethics, IRB). Prudently and sensitively use power, including abstaining from use of privilege. Use core values to resolve conflict and solve problems. Confront bias and harassment regardless of the source. Practice in accordance with one's limitations.

trainers are educated in the medical model, this adds another layer to their own particular cultural and ethnic intersectionality. To mitigate prejudging and provide patient-centered care, be aware that you will view your patients though a very specific lens.

The National Athletic Trainers' Association has not yet explicitly delineated professional core values; however, the moral compass for professional behaviors in athletic training has been set with the NATA Code of Ethics.[1] The American Physical Therapy Association (APTA) has delineated some sample behaviors that indicate the congruence of actions with core values. Table 4.6 identifies core values shared by both the NATA and APTA.

Stereotypes

A **stereotype** is a belief about the characteristics of a social group; it is a preconceived generalization.[42] Societal stereotypes are pervasive and unavoidable. People form stereotypes over the course of their lives from their observations and personal experiences and direct and indirect interactions with family, friends, educators, and the media. The genesis of stereotypes is believed to be grounded in group dynamic theory.[42,43] People have a need to belong to a group and to classify themselves (in-group) and others (out-group) into social groups. Members of the same in-group are naturally inclined to view one other as having positive attributes. Conversely, either consciously or unconsciously, people categorize members of out-groups as generic or homologous, and they may associate negative qualities with the groups.[44,45] This rudimentary intergroup categorization can be considered to be a simple form of prejudice.[45]

Stereotypes can be consciously acknowledged or unconsciously accepted. Members of groups that are not particularly susceptible to social oppression often view stereotypes as harmless generalizations.[43,45,46]

Throughout U.S. history, the oppressive treatment of racial minority groups (including laws against interracial marriage, appropriation of homelands, forced migration, internment, and slavery) is inextricably linked with the genesis and perpetuation of negative stereotypes. Conscious or unconscious acceptance of negative stereotypes ignores individual and cultural variation among people. Negative stereotypes are particularly dangerous because they serve as the justification for unjust treatment in the United States.[43,46] Stereotypes can be triggered quickly in high-prejudiced and low-prejudiced people because racial designations can be processed in microseconds. The effect of negative stereotypes can be mitigated in motivated people.[42,43] Stereotypes are the basis for implicit and explicit bias.[43,45]

Implicit and Explicit Biases

Biases are based on stereotypes. *Everyone has biases.* Simply knowing about group stereotypes can trigger information-processing distortions. Conscious thoughts and actions are called explicit bias. **Implicit bias** is the result of unconscious judgment and behavior toward members of a social group. Interactions with stereotyped groups are influenced primarily by the person's implicit biases, which can include both verbal and nonverbal behaviors.[42] Acting on stereotypes can be routed around conscious thought.[42] Implicit bias resulting from repeated reinforcement of social stereotypes has been detected in children as young as 3 years old. Despite the tendency for people to become more egalitarian as they age with respect to their explicit biases based on age, gender, and race, implicit biases do not change.[42]

Unconscious biases, which are rooted in stereotyping, affect clinical decision making. Biases regarding race, which exist in all of us, are influenced by systemic racism and the narratives that play out within our highly racialized society. Clinicians tend to default to stereotyping when they are under a heavy cognitive load. Athletic trainers, especially in the traditional setting, routinely have low clinician-to-patient ratios and experience daily cognitive loads that extend for most of the academic year.[49]

Everyone has implicit bias, even the members of social groups that are most often discriminated against.[50,51] The effect of bias is compounded further by privilege and power, which are unfairly allocated by society according to any combination of group identities, including mental health, body size, stigmatized disease status, socioeconomic status, gender and sexual identity, skin color, able-bodiedness, country of origin, English fluency, religion or spirituality, geography, or age. Implicit biases similar to levels identified in the general population have been found in physicians and health care providers.[42,52] Implicit bias has a negative effect on clinician relationships with patients.[53]

EVIDENCE-BASED ATHLETIC TRAINING

Implicit Bias Measurement

Check your implicit bias. Implicit bias is commonly measured with the Implicit Association Test (IAT) available online from Harvard University's Project Implicit website.[47] The IAT bypasses conscious awareness by comparing the speed at which people associate the words "good" and "bad" with certain images (similar to the cognitive concussion testing procedures familiar to athletic training students). The degree of bias correlates with the magnitude of the speed difference in keystrokes.[42] Like all people, health care professionals have unconscious biases that may not be congruent with their conscious values and behaviors. Knowing about your biases and addressing them can improve your patient-centered care.[48]

Prejudice and Discrimination

Prejudice and discrimination are based on stereotypes and implicit biases.[45] Everyone has prejudices as a result of in-group preferences.[43] Prejudices are pervasive, negative attitudes (thoughts) toward a person or group. The negative effects of prejudice can be mitigated in people who have eternalized egalitarian values; however, this process is more challenging than simply moderating stereotypical beliefs. Discrimination is negative behavior or action toward members of a group.[45] When a power or status differential exists between groups, the marginalized people are subject to prejudice and discrimination from the dominant group. Patients who are members of marginalized groups are predisposed to experiencing prejudice and discrimination in the health care system and from individual clinicians.[22] Prejudice and discrimination negatively affect patient outcomes and cause depression and anxiety, somatic symptoms, toxic stress, negative coping behaviors, and chronic disease.[53]

Isms

Considering the isms (e.g., racism, sexism, agism) moves the conversation from preconceived judgments (thoughts) to the unjust treatment or oppression (both individual and institutional) of patients in less powerful groups. Unjust oppressive treatment supported by policies and laws creates a power imbalance between sociocultural groups. Powerful groups are inclined to maintain social disparities; this tendency is fueled by the habit to stereotype, which leads to discrimination.[43,54,55] Although people in less powerful groups also stereotype members of powerful groups, their biases are not considered an ism in the same way because of the difference in resources to affect societal change between the two groups.[43] The equation "power + prejudice = racism" is frequently used in sociological literature to describe this dynamic as it applies to race.[43,54] This equation can be applied to the other cultural groups with a caveat.

Oppression refers to unjust treatment with regard to status. When applied to patients under medical care, this partly explains the perpetuation of health disparities in patient interactions, treatment decisions, treatment compliance, and health outcomes.[42,50,53] Medical mistreatment and health disparities do not occur in a vacuum; the stage for injustice has been set by history and the norms of U.S. society at large.

History and Politics in Power and Privilege

History is often the genesis of power and privilege, which vary by country, culture, and religion. Here are some examples of power and privilege in American history.

- Chinese immigrants were long prevented from becoming citizens because in 1882, members of Congress passed the Chinese Exclusion Act. Historically, most of the elected U.S. representatives have been members of the socioeconomic elite, Protestant Christians, heterosexual, able-bodied, European American men.
- During World War II, Japanese Americans were imprisoned by the executive order of President Roosevelt. In 1988, reparations were offered to all surviving victims.
- Jim Crow laws were enacted by state and local legislators to enforce segregation in the southern United States.
- Despite religious tolerance being a central tenet of America's founding fathers, several religious groups have experienced discrimination. People who practice Judaism and Islam continue to experience discrimination, prejudice, and assault.[56]
- People with lower socioeconomic status are not protected. Examples of class-based oppression are inequalities in education access, minimum wage laws, and limited low-income housing.

Although they are not always motivated by altruism, groups with power have made concessions that benefited oppressed groups. Power distribution results from the actions of the dominant group through media, education, and institutional policies and practices.[57] Here are some examples.

- Some women received the right to vote in 1920 because the group in power (White men) supported the 19th amendment to the Constitution of the United States.
- Rights for disabled people were granted in 1990 when, after decades of struggle and advocacy, the group in power (nondisabled representatives of the electorate) supported the Americans with Disabilities Act.
- Native Americans were granted civil rights in 1968 when Congress passed the Indian Civil Rights Act.

Privilege

Privilege is unearned social and cultural advantages or entitlements that are awarded to a majority group based on the qualities valued by the dominant culture. It benefits the dominant group and marginalizes minority groups (table 4.7). Someone can be both privileged by virtue

TABLE 4.7   **Groups With Privilege in the United States**

Majority group identity	Majority groups with privilege in the United States	Example of majority group privilege
Gender	Cisgender men	I can choose my gender on a standardized form. I don't need to constantly remind people of my name or my pronouns. I can walk alone at night without fear of being harmed. I can decide whether to have children without anyone questioning my masculinity. I can generally work or walk down a street without fear of sexual harassment. I am paid equitably for my work. I am not judged as emotional when I am passionate about an issue. My expertise in my field is not questioned.
Sexual identity	Heterosexual people	School may evoke a "one parent rule" for school activities so as not to offend or have to address different family units by encountering same sex parents on school grounds. I will not be fired because of my sexual identity.
Socioeconomic class	Upper-class people	I have never gone to bed hungry. I can afford medical and mental health care in my chosen facility and in the case of a medical emergency. I haven't ever had to avoid seeking medical attention due to economic reasons. I don't worry about how medical emergencies will affect my spending. I can use variants of language like slang without having my intelligence or integrity questioned. I can seek a full-time unpaid internship without worrying that it will affect my finances.
Age	Young adult and middle-aged people	My age is not a punch line for jokes. People do not automatically assume I am slow, dim-witted, or closed-minded. I don't need to lie about my age due to fear of negative perceptions or comments. People do not express that I am too old to be driving, competing in organized sport, going to the gym, or wearing certain clothing styles.
Race and ethnicity	White and biracial or multiracial people with fairer skin tones	During my health profession education, I never struggled to find professors and academic role models who shared my race. My ability as a health professional is not judged by my accent. I don't fear being stopped, delayed, unjustly detained, inappropriately touched, injured, or killed by the police because of my race.
Ability	People who are temporarily able-bodied	The source of my daily mobility is not touched, manipulated, or leaned on by strangers. People do not perpetually try to help me. People will not have low expectations of me as a result of my disability.
Religion and spirituality	Christians	The religious scripture on which I swear an oath in a legal setting is that of my faith. I can expect to have time off to celebrate religious holidays. When I turn on the TV, I see people of my religion or culture represented in a positive way.

of membership in a majority group and oppressed as a result of membership in a minority group.[58,59] The concept of privilege is not meant to suggest that someone has not struggled or is not conscientious. Nor is privilege a reflection on one's character or integrity. It is not uncommon for privileged people to be unaware of or disregard their privilege; many are also unaware that privilege has been a long-standing component of marginalization of minority groups.[41] Identity, marginalization, and privilege affect the lives of people on a daily basis.[41] Privilege and oppression change over time and with respect to one's experience and the context.[6]

Microaggressions

Microaggressions are a form of discrimination in which verbal, nonverbal, intentional, unintentional, or environmental insults are made to or about marginalized societal groups (table 4.8).[57] Microaggressions were first described in 1970 as racial transgressions directed

TABLE 4.8   Examples of Microaggressions

	Gender	SES	Race	Ethnicity	Age	Sexual orientation	Religion/spirituality	Ability
Endorsing stereotypes	Humor and jokes Having abilities questioned	"The working poor are poor but happy." These are people embedded in a social structure that is complex.[70]	Crossing to the other side of the street when a Black man approaches (i.e., assuming he is a violent threat)	"You speak such good English." (i.e., assuming someone is foreign born) "I'm an alien in my own land."	Dismissive jokes about older people (e.g., bad at technology, looking good for your age)	"Don't act so gay" (i.e., assumption is that everyone who identifies as gay acts the same)[81]	Moving when a Muslim woman wearing hijab sits next to you in a lecture hall (i.e., assumption is that Muslim people are a violent threat)[57]	Assuming that people with disabilities are not capable
Assuming homogeneity	"Why haven't you had children?"	People from lower socioeconomic groups have more mental illness. (i.e., assuming that all who identify as low SES are the same)[70]	Saying Happy Kwanza to a Black student	Saying Happy Chinese New Year to a student who is Korean[57]	Using the term "the elderly" to suggest that everyone in a certain age demographic thinks the same way	"You are not like those gay people." (i.e., all people who identify as gay are the same)	"Can I pray for you?" (i.e., my God and your God are the same)	"You don't look like you have a disability."
Pathologizing	"He will grow out of it." (i.e., being transgender is not normal and needs to be fixed)	Responding "That's crazy" when someone shares an aspect of their reality with regard to low SES status	Asking a Black woman "Why do you have to be so loud?"	Pathologizing a cultural or communication style: "Just calm down."	___	"Being gay is just a phase." (i.e., Homosexuality is something to be fixed)[81]	T-shirt that says "Recovering Catholic" (i.e., Catholicism is a disease)[57]	"When will you get a cochlear implant?" (i.e., deafness is something to be fixed; people with disabilities are broken)

	Gender	SES	Race	Ethnicity	Age	Sexual orientation	Religion/ spirituality	Ability
Disparaging	Heterosexist, sexist, and transphobic language: "slut" (vs "player"), "chick," "bitch," "sweetie," "honey," "young lady," "sissy"	"Those people" (i.e., people experiencing low SES status should be viewed as a social other out of society's mainstream)[71]	Racial slur[71] "Indian giver" "That's so White of you."	"You people" "I Jewed him down."	"Old geezer," "old bag" Patronizing language: "sweetie," "honey," "dear"	Hateful slurs[81]	Using "God" in profanity (i.e., the central tenet of your spirituality is only a profane expletive)[57]	Using slurs (e.g., "crip") or baby talk Ignoring the person Using dismissing language (e.g., "she suffers from")
Invalidating	Telling people that they are exaggerating about their reality (e.g., number of catcalls, leering)	"If you work hard enough in America, you can overcome anything." (i.e., failure to acknowledge or lack of unawareness of the systemic economic structures in the United States)[71]	A school counselor tells a Black student, "If you work hard, you can succeed like everyone else." (i.e., people of color are lazy and need to work harder)	Saying to an Asian American male, "As a woman, I know what you're going through."	"You don't look a day over ____."	"You just haven't found the right person of the opposite sex."[81]	"I am not anti-Semitic. I have a friend who is Jewish." (i.e., I believe I am not capable of bias)[57]	"But you look so normal." (i.e., deciding for others how extensive their disability is or isn't)

toward Black Americans; however, research since then has uncovered that microaggressions occur with similar negative consequences toward all marginalized societal groups.[60-62] *Micro* refers to the size of the transgression, not the magnitude of the harm.[60]

Microaggressions are not simply acts of political incorrectness, as is often suggested.[63] They are derogatory assaults directed at one's gender, ethnicity, or socioeconomic status.[63] People in marginalized societal groups may experience a significant cumulative effect of receiving multiple microaggressions over the course of a day from the media, strangers, colleagues, and even family members.

Discrimination reinforces the power and privilege discrepancies that perpetuate the cycle.[64,65] The psychological and physical consequences of microaggression are harsh and so pervasive that they are often taken for granted.[65] These include depression, anxiety, anger, somatic symptoms, blaming or distancing, migraines, heart disease, and autoimmune disorders. Microaggressions are a barrier to optimal interactions with patients.[60,62,66-69]

The three types of microaggression are **microinsults**, **microassaults**, and **microinvalidations** (table 4.9).[65,72,73]

- *Microinsults:* These are insensitive or rude remarks that convey contempt for the target. The transgressor may be unaware of the offensive nature of her comments and may believe she is paying the person a compliment.[72-76]
- *Microassaults:* These behaviors are most closely aligned with isms like sexism or racism. Assaults can be verbal, nonverbal, implicit, or explicit (i.e., intentional) discriminatory behavior. Avoidance behavior is also a microassault.[77,78]

TABLE 4.9   **Examples of Microinsults, Microassaults, and Microinvalidations**

	Microinsult	Microassault	Microinvalidation
Gender	"I didn't do well in Therapeutic Modalities, but, oh well, girls aren't supposed to be good at physics anyway, ha-ha."	Student informs AT faculty that he is a transgender male and in the process of changing his campus email and preferred name. Faculty person replies, "That's great. You will bring some diversity to our program because of your gender issues."	"I don't believe Dr. Doe was being sexist or racist with his comments. You're blowing this out of proportion."
SES	Student describing a patient refers to her as "white trash" as an indicator of SES.	To a fellow student who has just shared that he cannot afford to go on an outing with the class to see the Body World exhibit: "Aw, are you sure?"	"The book is expensive, but it shouldn't be an issue. Just have your parents pay for it."
Language	"Is there any way you could dial back the accent a bit? It really makes you sound unprofessional." [Assumption: *You cannot have an accent and be an AT.*]	"Go back to your country."	Teacher continues to mispronounce the name of a student even after the student has repeatedly corrected the teacher.
Race	"You're the first Black person I have had in my bio classes. It must be hard being an athlete and a biology major."	Student refers to Asian classmate as "Oriental"	"Race isn't an issue in our department—students just need to take better advantage of the resources on campus."
Age	Disparaging language like "old man," "gramps," "geezer," and "old bag" Describing minor forgetfulness as a "senior moment"	Preceptor directs an AT student to remove the hydrocollator from the "young lady" on the back table. (The patient is a 71-year-old woman.)	An AT working with a 71-year-old tennis player remarks in a slow high-pitched voice, "Sweetie, you look good for [your age]. You prove that age is just a number!"
Sexual or gender identity	"It's so gay that we can't get this heel lock to work correctly." (sexual identity)	"Do you know when you are planning top surgery?" (gender identity)	"You don't sound gay." "You don't look like a lesbian; you are so attractive." (sexual identity)
Religion and spirituality	A Native American student explains the significance of the sweat lodge ceremony, to which a classmate exclaims, "That's crazy."	"So, if you don't believe in God, what *do* you believe in?"	"As a minority, I understand how bad the Holocaust was for Jews."
Family structure	"Do you know your real parents?"	"It's as cold as a stepmother's kiss."	When letters sent home are addressed to "the parents of"
Ability	"I am totally spastic today."	Someone pushes the chair of a person using a wheelchair without asking permission.	"Everyone has some sort of disability."
Ethnicity	A student from Georgia (United States) explains to her Gen Med class that all the women she knew (including her family) ate white dirt called kaolin when they were pregnant, to which a classmate exclaims, "That's gross."	An athlete having his ankle taped is questioned by the AT: "Who put that crap between your toes?" The athlete replies, "My parents use it for athlete's foot." "Where are your parents from?" "Jamaica." The AT says, "Make sure you wash that crap off after practice. We use _____ in the United States."	Visiting athletic trainer assumes the Latino AT who is checking the filter behind the ice machine is a janitor even though he is wearing khaki pants and a golf shirt in the home team's colors.

- *Microinvalidations:* These comments are dismissive of the feelings or experiences of the person being addressed or denying one's own (possibly unconscious) biases toward a social group.[62,64,77,78]

We all have unconscious biases and we all are responsible for the effect our actions have on others, especially when it comes to interactions with our patients.[63] Athletic trainers may unknowingly commit microaggressions and negatively affect the patient–clinician relationship.[65] Social responsibility and respect are core values explicitly delineated for most health care professionals licensed in the United States. Ideally, those who embrace their professional values change behaviors that are harmful to patients through educative correction, or embracing ideals, information, and socialization as part of the professional education process.

Adverse Childhood Experiences

Adverse childhood experiences (ACEs) have a profound influence on a patient's health. A dose–response relationship exists in that the more ACEs a patient has experienced, the more significant the negative health consequences she experiences. Prolonged activation of the stress response results in toxic stress. Exposure to toxic stress in children (up to age 19) can cause delayed cognitive development and psychological (including anxiety, depression, suicide) and somatic symptoms. Higher incidence of asthma, infection, and obesity is associated with ACEs. In adolescents, internalized stress may cause or increase substance abuse and lead to increased prevalence of early pregnancy. In adults,

diabetes, cancer, and heart disease have been linked to ACEs. Adverse experiences early in life cause genetic changes at the molecular level called epigenetic change. Epigenetic change is transmitted to future generations as an inability to regulate the stress response.[79-81]

A physiological stress response is initiated when someone perceives or experiences a trauma that causes fear. Repeated stressors lead to chronically high levels of epinephrine, cortisol, and glucose, which damage blood vessels, increase blood pressure, and release glucose and increase appetite, leading to fat storage. In children and adolescents who experience chronic stress, neurodevelopment is negatively affected by surges of neurochemicals.[81,82]

Original ACE categories were childhood exposure to abuse (physical, emotional, sexual); neglect (physical, emotional); and household dysfunction (mental illness, substance abuse, incarcerated relative, divorce, domestic violence).[79,83] Racism, bullying, homelessness, witnessing violence, and living in foster homes were later added.[80] The original 1990 study participants were mostly White and college educated; 12% reported 4 or more ACEs, which puts one at double-digit risk for attempting suicide and drug injection.[83,84,90] ACE screening questionnaires ranging from simple (10 questions) to detailed are readily available on the Internet.

As a component of the psychosocial course in your professional education coursework, you will discuss ACEs and toxic stress, how to recognize them, and the referral guidelines for psychological conditions outside your scope of practice. However, you should also be cognizant of ACEs in routine interactions with patients, especially in secondary school and collegiate settings, because a majority of public school students

Sampling of ACE Questions Asked by Providers

- Did a parent hit you so hard that it left marks for more than a few minutes?
- Did a parent say hurtful things that made you feel bad, embarrassed, or humiliated more than a few times a year?
- Did other children say things behind your back, post derogatory messages about you, or spread rumors about you?
- Have you ever felt that your mother (or other important maternal figure) was emotionally unavailable to you? This could be for a variety of reasons, like military service, taking care of a sick relative, in school, or a business necessity.
- Was your parent (or other important parental figure) very difficult to please?
- Have there been times you didn't have enough to eat?
- Were you ever left unsupervised at an age or in situations when you should have been supervised?
- Have you ever felt that your family was under severe financial pressure?
- Have you spent time living in two or more households?
- Have you ever felt that you had to shoulder adult responsibilities?

have lower socioeconomic status, and poverty increases ACE accumulation.[84] Athletic trainers can be a part of a student-athlete's social support system by developing nurturing relationships over time. The data suggest that nurturing adults can remediate and proactively protect students from the effects of ACEs by helping them to foster resilience. Resilience is the psychological elasticity that enables people to recover quickly from significant adversity. Active listening, a core skill for all health care professionals, is helpful for patients who have had adverse experiences and contributes to a safe environment for patients. Holistic patient care improves patient outcomes.[79,84]

Social Determinants of Health

The CAATE supports the growing evidence that attending to social determinants of health enhances patient care and promotes exceptional patient outcomes. Social determinants of health are factors that contribute to health outcomes outside the athletic trainer's work setting, such as poverty; discrimination; access to transportation, recreation, health care, clean drinking water and air, healthy food, and housing; exposure to crime; food and housing insecurity; environmental toxins; and physical barriers for people with disabilities.[56,70,85,86] Research data reveal connections between social determinants of health and health equity.[70]

Let's consider poverty as an example. Poverty limits access to many resources, including those that help people buffer stressful events. This disadvantage causes stress, which promotes unhealthy coping mechanisms. These, in turn, contribute to the inequities in health care and musculoskeletal recovery that influence outcomes.[56,70]

Athletic training students must be mindful of social determinants of health in addition to the medical aspects of the care provided. Social determinants affect 80% of well-being. Medical care accounts for just 20% of patient health. Socioeconomic factors (40%), individual health behavior (30%), and environmental factors (10%) are responsible for the remainder. Psychosocial coursework in the athletic training educational program will help you engage patients skillfully when assessing social determinants of health and facilitate access to community services in a culturally sensitive manner.[70]

Health Disparities

In the United States, differences exist in how people experience health care delivery. Admittedly, there are personal and cultural differences in the way people view health, what they do about it, whom they seek out for help, and under what conditions they seek assistance. The size and type of the organizational structure and provider variability also contribute to differences that are particularly salient for members of marginalized groups.[87] The differences across social groups between prevalence of disease or injury, access to health care, and patient outcomes are called **health disparities**. Table 4.10 provides examples of health disparities.

Health Inequities

A health inequity arises from the social injustices that increase the vulnerability of marginalized groups. These are systematic barriers to optimal health and patient outcomes for members of these groups.[95] Inequity implies an ethical judgment or conflict.[97] Here's an example. It is a given that the proven treatment for ACL instability is ACL reconstruction, which increases function and quality of life and helps prevent the development of early osteoarthritis. Suppose that women were less likely to hear about ACL reconstruction as a treatment option than men were. This would make it less likely that they would have a friend or family member who chose ACL reconstruction surgery as a treatment option. If, in this hypothetical example, low participation in ACL reconstruction by women was also partially caused by low levels of provider education on this issue, this situation would be a preventable injustice. This then would be a health inequity.[96] Table 4.11 provides examples of health inequities.

Clinicians who embrace equity strive to remediate the systematic barriers under their control. An obstacle in this effort is that a sizeable number of Americans do not believe systemic inequities exist, especially with regard to race. Even when variables like access to care, socioeconomic status, and disease severity are controlled for racism and all the isms, the result is a lower quality of health care, including for routine services.[87,95]

Cultural Competence

Cultural competence means that a clinician renders care effectively in cross-cultural situations as a result of understanding social, cultural, and ethnic group differences and health inequities.[107-109] Lack of culturally competent care results in less than optimal patient outcomes.[5] There are five components to cultural competence (table 4.12).[105]

Traditional cultural competence education has focused heavily on cultural knowledge, including lists of communication skills, health beliefs, and generalized cultural facts and behaviors. For example, chapters with a focus on cultural knowledge often distinguish between skills and facts for caring for Filipino, Hispanic, or Native American patients. The implicit message is that cultural competence is acquired by memorizing lists of group profiles. Although it would behoove you to become familiar with traditional cultural facts and behaviors of the

TABLE 4.10   **Examples of Evidence-Based Health Disparities**

Health disparity	Evidence
Women report longer durations of pain and more severe pain and are more likely to develop complex regional pain syndrome.	Hoffman DE, Tarzian AJ. The girl who cried pain: A bias against women in the treatment of pain. *The Journal of Law, Medicine & Ethics.* 2001;29(1):13-27.[24]
Black children may experience increased frustration and decreased pain tolerance. Latino children may be reluctant to acknowledge pain.	Fortier MA, Anderson CT, Kain ZN. Ethnicity matters in the assessment and treatment of children's pain. *Pediatrics.* 2009;124(1):378-380.[88]
Women report higher postoperative pain after arthroscopic ACL reconstruction with less postoperative function.	Taenzer AH, Clark C, Curry CS. Gender affects report of pain and function after arthroscopic anterior cruciate ligament reconstruction. *Anesthesiology.* 2000;93(3):670-675.[89]
Religion plays a central role (meaning of pain, reason for pain, coping mechanism) in the pain experience of racial and ethnic minorities.	Shavers VL, Bakos A, Sheppard VB. Race, ethnicity and pain among the US population. *Journal of Health Care for the Poor and Underserved.* 2010;21(1):177-220.[90] Booker S. African Americans' perceptions of pain and pain management. *Journal of Transcultural Nursing.* 2016;27(1):73-80.[32]
Males demonstrate greater pain tolerance and less sensitivity to pain. Men and women respond differently to pain treatments.	Jarrett C. Ouch! The different ways people experience pain. *Psychologist.* 2011;24(6):416-420.[91] Hoffman DE, Tarzian AJ. The girl who cried pain: A bias against women in the treatment of pain. *The Journal of Law, Medicine & Ethics.* 2001;29(1):13-27.[24]
African-American, Hispanic, and Asian patients feel less respected than White patients by their physicians and have decreased trust in them.	Blendon R et al. Disparities in physician care: experiences and perceptions of a multi-ethic America. *Health Affairs.* 2008;27:507-517.[92]
African Americans and Asian Americans demonstrate greater pain sensitivity.	Booker S. African Americans' perceptions of pain and pain management. *Journal of Transcultural Nursing.* 2016; 27(1):73-80.[32] Kim HJ, Greenspan JD, Ohrbach R, et al. Racial/ethnic differences in experimental pain sensitivity and associated factors—cardiovascular responsiveness and psychological status. *PLoS One.* 2019;14(4):1-22.[30]
Native Americans have decreased pain responses and prevalence of several painful chronic conditions.	Palit S, Kerr KL, Kuhn BL, Terry EL, DelVentura JL, Bartley EJ, Shadlow JO, Rhudy JL. Exploring pain processing differences in Native Americans. *Health Psychology.* 2013;32(11):1127-1136.[93]
Pharmacodynamic and pharmacokinetic ethnic differences are documented in the literature.	Campbell CM, Edwards RR. Ethnic differences in pain and pain management. *Pain Management.* 2012;2(3):219-230.[28]

patients in your geographical area of employment and to expand your repertoire over time, there are several reasons why this approach lends itself to a rather myopic view of cultural values. As diversity increases in the United States, the number of cultural profiles you would need to memorize to be competent by this standard would be expansive. Considerable intraethnic group variability and differences due to the degree of individual acculturation

add to the complexity of this approach. Acculturation is the degree to which a family or group has assimilated into U.S. culture. Finally, culture is not limited to race and ethnicity.[5,53,109-110]

Most athletic training students and clinicians agree or strongly agree that they possess high awareness and skill proficiency in providing culturally competent care, despite the finding in medical education research that

TABLE 4.11 **Evidence-Based Health Inequities**

Health inequity	Evidence
Women experience longer ED waits than men.	Waters J. Just why do women face a fight for equal health? *Community Practitioner.* 2019;92(9):36-41.[26] Hoffman DE, Tarzian AJ. The girl who cried pain: A bias against women in the treatment of pain. *The Journal of Law, Medicine & Ethics.* 2001;29(1):13-27.[24]
In ED, White patients reporting pain were more likely to receive an opioid than Black, Hispanic, Asian, or other patients.	Lord B, Khalsa S. Influence of patient race on administration of analgesia by student paramedics. *BMC Emergency Medicine.* 2019;19(1):32.[99]
African Americans and, to a lesser degree, Hispanics are less likely to receive pain medication by student paramedics administering prehospital care.	Briggs E. Cultural perspectives on pain management. *Journal of Perioperative Practice.* Nov2008;18(11):468-471.[29]
African Americans receive a lower standard of care than White people when being treated for breast cancer, orthopedic problems, cardiovascular disease, pain, and end-of-life care.	Nelson S. Race, racism, and health disparities: What can I do about it? *Creative Nursing.* 2016;22(3):161-165.[49]
Nonwhite female members of sexual identity minorities are more likely to experience lower quality of health care. Gay nonwhite men and bisexual and lesbian nonwhite women are disadvantaged in many aspects of access to health care, including delayed care. Gay, lesbian, and bisexual White men and women also experience delayed care, but to a lesser degree; their overall health care experience appears more similar to that of their heterosexual counterparts.	Hsieh N, Ruther M. Sexual minority health and health risk factors: Intersection effects of gender, race, and sexual identity. *American Journal of Preventive Medicine.* 2016;50(6):746-755.[98]
Minority patients are less likely to be referred to an asthma specialist. Increased asthma morbidity, lower quality of care, and suboptimal asthma management regimens in adults and children are found in nonwhite (especially Hispanic) adult and pediatric patients.	Kharat AA, Borrego ME, Raisch DW, Roberts MH, Blanchette CM, Petersen H. Assessing disparities in the receipt of inhaled corticosteroid prescriptions for asthma by Hispanic and non-Hispanic white patients. *Annals of the American Thoracic Society.* 2015 Feb;12(2):174-183.[100]
Members of racial and ethnic minorities experience longer ED wait times.	Okunseri C, Okunseri E, Chilmaza CA, Harunani S, Xiang Q, Szabo A. Racial and ethnic variations in waiting times for emergency department visits related to nontraumatic dental conditions in the United States. *Journal of the American Dental Association.* 2013;144(7):828-836.[101]
Racial, ethnic, and socioeconomic factors (including environmental) in underserved neighborhoods negatively affects prevalence and management of pediatric asthma.	Woodley LK. Reducing health disparities in pediatric asthma. *Pediatric Nursing.* Jul/Aug2019;45(4):191-198.[102]
Multiple geographical health issues exist in rural America, primarily among people of color and American Indians. Opioid overdose deaths and suicides are also noted for rural, White male Americans.	Kozhimannil KB, Henning-Smith C. Racism and health in rural America. *Johns Hopkins University Press.* 2018;29(1):35-43.[103]
People with disabilities report that clinicians lack disability awareness and are uncomfortable working with them. Also, accessibility to health care facilities and services (examination tables, scales) are not adapted for people with disabilities.	Krahn GL, Klein Walker D, Correa-De-Araujo R. Persons with disabilities as a unique health disparity population. *American Journal of Public Health.* Apr 2015;105(S2):S198-206.[104]

TABLE 4.12 **Five Components of Cultural Competence**[105]

Component	Explanation	Sample behaviors
Cultural desire	Reflects the desire to learn from others and make a personal and professional commitment to embrace this construct rather than go through the motions. It is a mindset shift that sparks one's cultural development.	Have you read enough and exposed yourself to enough cultures outside of your own to be passionate about improving patient interactions and outcomes?
Cultural awareness	Examine and explore your own cultural and professional values to avoid judging others and imposing your values on patients	Recognize that culture is more than skin color.
Examine your cultural background and identities and identity intersections.
Learn about stereotypes and identify stereotypes you have held.
How do you communicate? (Explore personal space, facial expressiveness, gestures, and eye contact.)
Learn about how history and social constructs affect marginalized social and cultural groups, intersections, and isms in health care.
Take the IAT. Make a plan to be conscious of your biases and remediate patient interactions.
Be aware of cognitive overload and other stressors that affect provider interactions.
Cultural knowledge	Develop a solid foundational knowledge of health-related values and beliefs, the prevalence and incidence of disease, and efficacy of treatment to understand how patients make sense of illness or injury and how their beliefs and values guide their thinking and behaviors.	Read scholarly research and make an effort to seek out culturally based media and books.
Engage in conversation with friends and colleagues.
Invest in culturally based continuing education.
Cultural skill	Perform culturally based assessments, determine patient needs, and construct appropriate individualized therapeutic interventions.	Practice
Be vigilant
Use professional resources to perfect your skill
Are you using a cultural assessment tool?
Cultural encounters	Participate in cross-cultural interactions and form relationships with culturally diverse people.	More encounters decrease the likelihood of stereotyping.
Seek out opportunities for new experiences like cultural celebrations or religious services.
Cultural communication is a part of cultural encounters. Have you incorporated CLAS standards into your clinical practice?

confidence level does not have predictive value with regard to skills and abilities. This discrepancy is called unconscious ignorance. The actual abilities of both groups are likely inflated. Students' cultural awareness does not translate into cultural skill application. The demographic mismatch for athletic training students, clinicians, and

patients in the traditional clinical setting further contributes to the chasm that exists between having cultural awareness and possessing the ability, skill, and knowledge to effectively put it into practice. Specific education is required to understand the multifaceted aspects of the psychosocial, cultural, and even historical factors and the

FOUNDATIONAL SKILLS

Tools for Cultural Competence

The LEARN model is a framework for cross-cultural communication that helps build mutual understanding and enhance patient care.[111]

L: Listen

E: Explain

A: Acknowledge

R: Recommend

N: Negotiate

The RESPECT model[114,115] (Respect, Explanatory, Sociocultural context, Power, Empathy, Concerns, Trust and therapeutic concern) is a checklist for clinicians and a model for preceptor interactions with student clinicians. The model also reminds clinicians to assess their verbal and nonverbal interactions with patients.

Respect Demonstrate respect and validate the concerns of the patient.	"Hello, Ms. Smith. My name is Siobhan; my pronouns are she, her, hers. I am one of the athletic training students assigned to Mr. Smythe this semester from the university and I will be working with you today." "How would you like me to address you?" "Thanks for coming in today, how can I help?"
Explanatory model Ask how the patient understands the illness or injury.	"Please tell me how this started." "What do you think caused this?" "What makes it worse or better?" "What you have done for it?" "How has this situation affected athletics and daily life?"
Sociocultural context Ask how any sociocultural factors (including complementary/alternative medicine) affect the patient, including stressors, support, and resources.	"How has this situation affected athletics and daily life?" "Have you sought help for this from another healer besides me?" "Has anyone recommended a treatment that you have tried or considered?" "Who do you live with?" "Do they have the same last name as you do? What do they like to be called?" "Do they know about this injury?" "What is their view of it?" "Will they be able to take my call at work?" "Is there anything I need to be respectful of in caring for you?" "The school physician has hours this Wednesday evening. Will you have transportation to get here and back home?" "Will you be able to get in for treatments and rehabilitation for the next 2 weeks?" "Thanks for sharing that with me. We'll do our best to come up with an alternative to the custom orthotics that will improve your lower leg biomechanics, no worries."
Power Acknowledge power differences and perceptions. Act to empower the patient. Remove barriers. Share information with the patient. Negotiate the treatment options and plan.	"Hang on; let me grab the anatomical model to explain what is going on to you." "I understand that you are concerned about being at full strength for the upcoming games. I am sure we can work out something you'll be happy with to keep your skills sharp and your conditioning up while we get that pain moving out of here."

Empathy Verbally and nonverbally acknowledge the emotions and concerns of the patient and parent or guardian.	"Anyone would be bummed to miss this week and on top of that to be so sore, but we will get things moving as quickly as we can."
Concerns Ask open-ended questions about the patient's concerns and fears. Acknowledge concerns verbally and nonverbally.	"Moving forward, what concerns or fears do you have?" "Well, if anything comes up, please let me know." "How do you feel about what we have discussed?"
Trust and therapeutic concern Ensure construction of the therapeutic alliance that supports compliance, trust, and engagement.	"What questions can I answer?" "Sure, a number of athletes through the years have overcome this injury." "Feel free to shoot me an email or a text or just grab me if you have any questions moving forward." "I will be sure to get your parent/guardian in the loop as well." "It's my job to look busy, [chuckle]. But listen, you are not an interruption of my work; you are the reason for my work. Deal?" "Can you give me a minute to run this treatment plan by my preceptor? Then we'll get after it, OK?"

needs of cultural groups and learn how to best address them in clinical practice.[2]

Cultural assessment tools with acronyms have been developed to incorporate cultural sensitivity in patient assessment. Patient-centered assessment is conducted from a perspective that respects the values of the patient rather than the traditional values of the medical culture. The encounter is more open. The practitioner uses open-ended questions to develop trust, which hopefully encourages the patient to share to what extent his beliefs and values affect the reason he sought care.[2,19,38] The sidebar provides two tools to help you remember the order of the questions. Some adjustments may need to be made for athletic trainers working in traditional settings.

Cultural Humility

Several terms exist that express the idea of the evolution from competence to humility. This chapter uses the term "cultural humility" to describe the paradigm shift. Cultural humility, described first in 1998, is different from cultural competence.[109] The clinician striving for cultural humility must be committed to the historical realities of discrimination and the disparities that negatively influence care and perceptions of societal groups, both from society at large and within U.S. health care systems. Cultural humility also encompasses a commitment to lifelong cultural learning rather than simply memorizing profiles of cultural groups. Another tenet of cultural

humility is patient-centered care. Enabling patients to be the center of their care and true partners in the therapeutic relationship eliminates the need to be proficient in all the details of the health beliefs of every distinct cultural group.[109] The evidence of this commitment will be the clinician's active engagement in social justice for patients to remediate the inequality that is correlated to negative patient outcomes.[114] Poor cultural humility results in poor patient outcomes.[109]

Apology

Cross-cultural interactions may result in an interpersonal transgression that requires an apology. A timely, appropriate apology delivered in person in a contrite tone is viewed more positively than a delayed apology, and such an apology is a therapeutic essential for healing.[115-117]

In a sincere apology, the clinician must take responsibility and reference the specific offense (tables 4.13 and 4.14).[115-117] This demonstrates that he has experienced a level of contrition that will allow him to restore trust with the patient. An apology where the speaker does not assume responsibility is reported to be even more harmful because it lacks empathy. Finally, offering reparation (i.e., making amends) when appropriate, committing to refrain from repeating the hurtful behavior (i.e., remorse), and requesting forgiveness are important components of a sincere and effective apology. An apology without remorse is an excuse.[115]

TABLE 4.13   **Apology Dos and Don'ts**

Don't say this	Reason	Do say this
I am sorry that happened to you. I regret that [fill in the blank] happened. I am sorry.	This response lacks remorse and does not accept responsibility.	I am so sorry that I gave you a tape blister yesterday. I was rushing; there is certainly no excuse for Clinic 2 to make those kinds of errors, and now you have a painful, gaping hole on your heel. I will be more careful with my tape tension moving forward *and* I won't forget the heel and lace pad. I hope you can forgive me and give me a chance to make it right. Starting with dressing that wound. May I? Thanks, I appreciate you giving the rookie another chance.
A mistake was made.	This shifts the blame to an unknown entity rather than assuming responsibility.	I apologize for not speaking up earlier when the fencer made that rude remark. I was not monitoring the room as closely as I should have been. Quite frankly, I was stunned and when I realized what was said, she was gone. We have a no tolerance policy; I want everyone to feel safe. Rest assured that I will deal with this by day's end. I will be more vigilant moving forward. Can you forgive me?
I am sorry you feel that way. I am sorry you felt hurt. I am sorry you think I did something wrong. I am sorry if I offended you. I regret you felt upset.	This is not an apology; it shifts the blame onto the victim as if it is their fault for reacting and invalidates their experience.	I heard you had quite a time getting to the appointment I made for you. I apologize that I did not check with you about transportation. I am sorry you were upset and frazzled; I understand the frustration. I will be more mindful in the future in making sure you are taken care of. Is there anything I need to do to smooth this over with your instructor? Do you need a note or shall I send him an email on your behalf? I apologize again. Family takes care of family, right? I dropped the ball. It won't happen again.
I am sorry, *but* . . . . I am sorry, but in my defense	The word "but" negates everything that has just been said. This is a nonapology. "In my defense" shifts the blame onto the victim.	I am sorry I offended you when I used inappropriate pronouns. I regret that you felt invalidated by my oversight. I never want to make anyone feel that way. I should not have made an assumption; I should have asked. My patients' feelings are important to me. I want everyone to feel that the AT facility is a safe place. I am asking for your forgiveness; I will be much more vigilant moving forward.
I guess I should say I am sorry.	"I guess" is dancing around the apology.	I am sorry for not asking you directly.

TABLE 4.14   **Parts of an Apology**

Apology without conditions	Care for the victim's feelings	Remorse	Reparation or amends	Request forgiveness
I am so sorry that I gave you a tape blister yesterday.	I was rushing; there is certainly no excuse for Clinic 2 to make those kinds of errors and now you have a painful gaping hole on your heel.	I will be more careful with my tape tension moving forward *and* I won't forget the heel and lace pad.	Give me a chance to make it right. Starting with dressing that wound.	I hope you can forgive me. May I? Thanks, I appreciate you giving the rookie another chance.
I apologize for not speaking up earlier when the fencer made that rude remark.	I was not monitoring the room as closely as I should have been. Quite frankly, I was stunned and when I realized what was said, she was gone.	We have a no tolerance policy; I want everyone to feel safe. I will be more vigilant moving forward.	Rest assured that I will deal with this by day's end.	Can you forgive me?

Apology without conditions	Care for the victim's feelings	Remorse	Reparation or amends	Request forgiveness
I heard you had quite a time getting to the appointment I made for you. I apologize that I did not check with you about transportation.	I am sorry you were upset and frazzled; I understand the frustration.	I will be more mindful in the future in making sure you are taken care of.	Is there anything I need to do to smooth this over with your instructor? Do you need a note or shall I send him an email on your behalf?	I apologize again. Family takes care of family, right? I dropped the ball. It won't happen again.
I am sorry I offended you when I used inappropriate pronouns.	I regret that you felt invalidated by my oversight.	I never want to make anyone feel that way. I should not have made an assumption; I should have asked.	My patients' feelings are important to me. I want everyone to feel that the AT facility is a safe place.	I am asking for your forgiveness. Are we good?

CLINICAL BOTTOM LINE

- Cultural competence is a critical component of patient-centered care (PCC). An understanding of the historical contexts connected with the patient's experience, word choice, and empathy all directly affect patient outcomes.

- Cultural competency requires the practitioner to participate in self-reflection. This includes, but is not limited to, attitudes, beliefs, values, and social status. Cultural competency includes cultural humility, desire, awareness, knowledge, skills, and encounters.

- Athletic trainers should understand the context of historical realities of discrimination and the disparities that negatively influence care and perceptions of societal groups in order to mitigate potential inequities in patient–practitioner interactions.

- Privilege and microaggressions can affect patient–provider interactions and thus patient outcomes. Recognizing privilege and the construct of a microaggression can positively affect communication with patients.

- Applying cultural literacy considerations can advance communication with and understanding of patients and enhance patient-centered care.

 Go to HK*Propel* to complete the activities and case studies for this chapter.

Go to HK*Propel* to view videos of a culturally incompetent and culturally competent patient interaction.

CHAPTER 5

Health Care Administration and Health Care Informatics

Leamor Kahanov, EdD, ATC, LAT

CAATE STANDARDS

The following CAATE 2020 standards are covered in this chapter:

> Standard 62
>
> Standard 63
>
> Standard 65

CHAPTER OBJECTIVES

After reading this chapter, you will be able to do the following:

- Understand foundational concepts of health care administration

- Comprehend how national policies and regulations stipulate requirements of health care practices

- Understand the concepts of quality assurance and improvement

- Identify medical documentation guidelines and uses

- Understand insurance and billing concepts in athletic training

Health care administration is a relationship between colleagues, clinicians, patients, regulators, legislatures, and various stakeholders. The interplay between these constituents dictates the organizational environment, including culture, policy, and, most importantly, patient care and safety. The environmental change in health care is continuous, and thus our role in creating and sustaining organizations through health care administration is a pivotal platform for patient-centered care. Athletic trainers are often in a unique role that requires them to combine health care administration with clinical practice. As such, you must remain current with administrative happenings.

This chapter provides an overview of health care administration with foundational information on organizational structures, administrative objectives and duties, and the regulations, policies, and practices required to ensure patient care and safety. Health care administration and management encompass a wide net of responsibilities that vary for the athletic trainer depending on health care setting or employment environment. For more information on health care administration and management, you can further investigate the sources cited in each section.

Health Care Administration and Management

Health care administration in athletic training ranges from work in large health care conglomerates to smaller

63

settings such as privately owned physician's offices, rehabilitation clinics, and secondary school athletic training clinics. Regardless of the setting, optimal patient care and safety are the desired outcomes. Key components of health care administration are based on the following:

- Size and type of the organization
- Functional organizational structure
- External and internal factors
- Administrator roles and responsibilities

Each athletic training setting and employer environment is unique and requires different specific daily skills and tasks for facilitating patient care and client services.

Health Care Administration

Health care administration is the planning, direction, and coordination of medical and health services. Health care administrators may coordinate an entire facility, a specific clinical area or department, or a medical practice.[1-4] Health care administration varies in size and scope depending on the employment setting, but regardless of the workplace, administrators have the same role in coordinating or supervising the following (see also figure 5.1):[1,4,5]

- Budgets
- Services
- Administrative operations
- Facilities
- Personnel

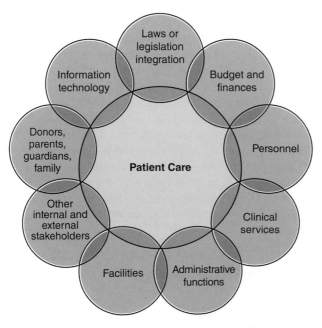

FIGURE 5.1   Health care administration roles.

Health care administration requires that athletic trainers monitor the quality of patient care and the fiscal health of the medical entity by managing stakeholder interests.[5] Routinely monitoring external and internal factors through planned assessments best addresses the quality of patient care and stakeholder interests (see the sidebar).

Health Care Management

Health care managers provide organization, leadership, and direction to help health care practitioners, staff, service personnel, and the organization provide medical services to patients.[1,2,4,6,7] The role of the manager is to ensure high performance from employees, fiscal solvency, and patient safety.[1,2,4,6] Critical to health care management is the integration of health care laws, regulations, and technology with human resources.[2,4,6,7-14]

Management positions are not relegated to top-level administration (i.e., senior management). Non-senior-management administration positions may include, but are not limited to, the following:

- Director of information management
- Floor manager (rehabilitation facility or hospital)
- Medical service coordinator
- Service coordinator
- Staff coordinator

Management positions depend on the size and complexity of the organization. Here are some of the most common organizational structures:[1,2,4,6]

- *Functional organizational structure.* This is a pyramid hierarchy with a strict chain of command and linear reporting (figure 5.2).
- *Team-based model (matrix model).* Groups of functional staff (e.g., nursing, rehabilitation, medical imaging) are assigned to a population, such as a college athletic training site, geriatrics, or marketing team (figure 5.3). Advantages include improved lateral communication.
- *Service line model.* People are appointed to oversee services (i.e., rehabilitation, mental health, cardiology; figure 5.4). This model allows managers to cross departments and provide more continuity between patients.

Regardless of the organizational structure, sound professional judgment is the key component of successfully completing managerial functions. Effective managers have three key qualities:[1-4,9,10,15]

1. Managing self: time-management, attention to personal space, appropriate responsiveness to

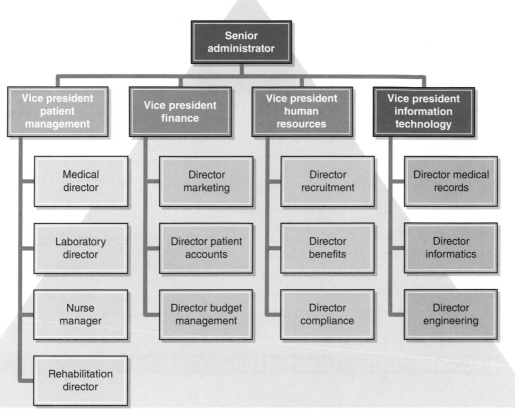

FIGURE 5.2   Functional organizational structure. The number and scope of positions depends on the size of the organization.

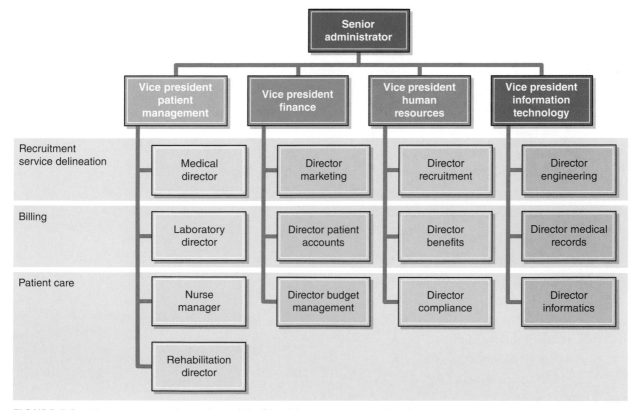

FIGURE 5.3   Matrix or team-based model of health care organizational structure.

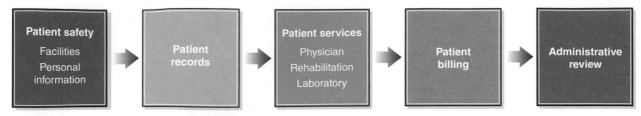

FIGURE 5.4   Health care service line model.

others, follow-through, positive attitude, and motivation

2. Management of the team, regardless of the hierarchical level:

   • Understanding managerial strategies and techniques

   • Delegating work tasks and modifications of assignments

   • Ensuring delivery of services

   • Managing talent and recruiting and retaining employees

3. Organizational level: Work with other managers and administrators to ensure organization performance; share information and collaborate with peers and supervisors

Health Policy and Laws

Athletic trainers, like any health professional or health care organization, must abide by laws, regulations, and professional policies, otherwise termed *health care policies*. The intent of health care policies is to provide direction for societal care, financial oversight, patient

External and Internal Factors of Health Care Administration

External Factors

• Demographic climate or population

• Accreditation

• Laws and regulations

• Stakeholders (e.g., parents, families, donors)

• Competitors

• Insurance carriers

• Technology

Internal Factors

• Budget

• Quality assurance

• Referral relations (physician, hospital, rehabilitation)

• Technology (e.g., electronic medical records [EMR], access)

• Stakeholders (board, patients or clients)

• Personnel talent

Internal Positions of Power

• Supervisor or department director

• Clinical staff

• Administrative staff (e.g., medical billing, financial staff, staffing managers)

• Maintenance staff

• Fiscal manager

• CEO or president

• Marketing

Major Federal Health Care Legislation

The Privacy Act of 1974[25]

- This act prohibits the disclosure of personally identifiable information maintained by the entity or institution without the consent of the individual.

- Employees have the right to access records maintained on themselves.

- Employees have the right to request amendments to their records, assuming that they can show that the records are not accurate, relevant, timely, or complete.

- This act establishes a code of fair information practices that requires agencies to comply with statutory norms for collection, maintenance, and dissemination of records.

Health Insurance Portability and Accountability Act (HIPAA) of 1996[26,40]

- Rules were enacted to allow for continuance of health insurance coverage in situations involving job changes or loss.

- Regulations were created to monitor electronic health care and set limits on disclosure of protected health information.

- Patients received the rights to their own health information, including the right to examine and obtain a copy of their health records and request corrections.

Health Information Technology for Economic and Clinical Health (HITECH) Act of 2009[29]

- This act enhanced enforcement of HIPAA with penalties for noncompliance.

- Patients are required to be notified if a breach of their protected information occurs.

- Patients must be allowed access to medical records in an electronic form.

Affordable Care Act (ACA) of 2010[38]

- Health care costs were lowered and coverage made accessible to people who were previously uninsured.

- Health insurance quality increased.

- All applicants for insurance coverage must be accepted regardless of preexisting conditions, sex, and ethnicity.

---

safety, and patient care. Health care policies may be federal, state, or institutional (e.g., employment setting, insurance, company). The following section identifies the federal policies relevant to athletic trainers. You should investigate state and institutional policies for your place of employment.

The United States health policies are unique in that government programs are prescribed only for certain vulnerable groups; however, the health policies monitor and legislate private and employer-based health care provisions.[16-44] Current health care policy in the United States is based on a historical focus on the following:

- Efficiency among types of health insurance
- Health care for vulnerable groups (e.g., elderly, people with lower socioeconomic status, veterans)

- Fiscal management of health care (national, state, local, individual)
- Patient safety

In addition to federal regulations and legislation, professional and organizational standards are used to create best practices in health care administration in the areas of patient care, safety, and information. Here are examples of some health care organizations and standards:

- *Commission on Systemic Interoperability:* organization charged with creating strategy so that patients and health care providers have access to health care records at all times

- *Health Level Seven International:* organization that creates accredited standards for the exchange, integration, and sharing of electronic health information

Comparison of International Health Care Policies

Here is a list of policies from other countries or regions that are comparable to HIPAA in the United States.[45]

- European Union: Data Protection Directive
- Canada: Personal Information Protection and Electronic Documents Act (PIPEDA)
- Mexico: Federal Law on the Protection of Personal Data
- Argentina:
  - Regulation 60 (DNPDP Disposition 60)
  - Data Protection Law 2000
- Brazil: Data Protection Bill of 2016
- Netherlands: Dutch Notification of Data Breach Law
- France: Digital Republic Act
- Germany: Federal Data Protection Act & Works Constitution Act
- Spain: Royal Decree 1720 of 2007
- Italy: Personal Data Protection Code
- Singapore: Personal Data Protection Act of 2012
- India: Privacy Rules 2011
- Philippines: Data Privacy Act of 2012
- Australia: Federal Privacy Act 1988
- New Zealand: Privacy Act 1993 (amended 2008)
- Taiwan: Computer-Processed Personal Data Protection Law
- China: Tort Liability Law
- South Africa: Protection of Personal Information (POPI) Act
- Russia: Personal Data Act 2006 (amended 2009)

- *International Telecommunication Union (ITU) e-Health Standards and Interoperability:* United Nations specialized agency for information and communication technology
- *JCAHO (Joint Commission: Accreditation of Healthcare Organizations):* commission that accredits nearly 21,000 health care organizations and programs in the United States to ensure patient safety
- *National Quality Forum:* nonprofit foundation that focuses on improvements with measures and standards to increase patient safety and improve health care outcomes
- *Public Health Data Standards Consortium:* consortium of federal, state, and local agencies to improve individual and community health through technology standards (nonprofit organization)
- *Workgroup for Electronic Data Interchange (WEDI):* formed by the Secretary of Health and Human Services to improve health care information exchange to enhance quality of care

Quality Assurance

The ultimate goal of health care organizations (departments, health care systems, clinics, centers) is to ensure beneficial patient outcomes and optimal functioning of the health care system. Patient outcomes must be routinely assessed from multiple vantage points to ensure patient safety and optimal service. This routine evaluation is called **quality assurance** or quality improvement. Several components called **key indicators** contribute to the overall outcome of a quality assurance program. These include factors such as patient and employee safety, optimal services provided, and desired patient or client outcomes (figure 5.5).[14,41,42]

Quality assurance assesses all of the key indicators in a systematic, continuous evaluation of measurable health care service.[7,14,21,42] **Continuous quality improvement** (CQI) is the term used for the ongoing loop of activi-

World Health Organization's Standardization of Terminology and Diseases

Health policy laws and insurance providers use standardized terminology to communicate. Standard terminology for injury, illness, insurance and legal policies are available at the following:

- WHO e-Health standardized terminology
- **International Classification of Diseases** (ICD-10 current edition)

ties intended to evaluate the key indicators; remediate or change noneffective elements of an organization, department, health care system, or rehabilitation center; and then reassess the changes to ensure that quality has improved (figure 5.6). CQI cycles vary by health care organization and may range in length from a week to a year based on the needs, size, and scope of the health care institution.

In CQI, members of the health care team work in concert to routinely and continually assess how the organization (e.g., department, institution, clinic) is doing and what can be done better. CQI is typically based on several key indicators:[20,35,42]

- Patient outcomes: Is the care benefiting patients?
- Efficacy: Is the care effective and financially feasible?
- Timing: Can we provide care in a timelier manner?

CQI requires that the culture of the health care institution embrace continued evaluation in order to improve care with a structured plan to evaluate the following:[20,42]

- Current organizational and structural practices
- Tools commonly used to determine if desired outcomes are being achieved
- Health care delivery and services.

Intervention into current clinical and organization practices occurs through the ongoing assessment loop. The assessment may be **qualitative** or **quantitative** in nature, but should establish the following in order to effectively evaluate health care services and the organization or system:[14, 20,42]

- Baseline for future evaluations
- Effective solutions
- Monitoring of changes to ensure improvements occur and are sustained
- Comparison of performances across institutions or departments

A quality assurance process identifies the organization's philosophy and assesses outcomes based on specified values that relate to the mission. Specific

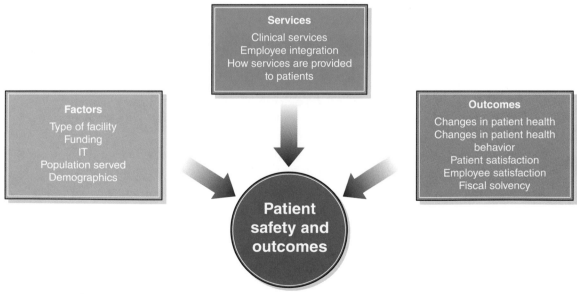

FIGURE 5.5   Quality assurance key indicators.

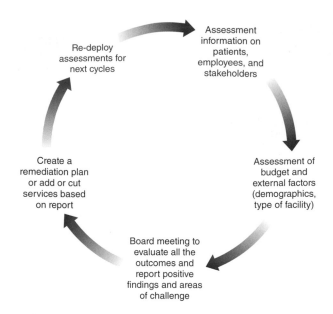

FIGURE 5.6   Continuous quality improvement model.

models (table 5.1) and assessment tools (table 5.2) are then developed based on the health care organization's mission, size, and scope.

Quality improvement models and assessment tools are used by people in specific roles to deliver and analyze the data. Key roles for quality improvement include the following:[7,20,21,35,42]

- Clinician to input medical records
- Operations manager for assessment: This person manages the day-to-day leader who organizes and drives the measurement; may be the department or institutional president or manager or a designee for measurement operations.

- Data entry clerk: This job may be done by a designated person or conducted by each employee.
- Data specialist: This person collects, analyzes, creates, and uses the QI tools; role may be performed by a designated employee or a separate hire.

Documentation and Medical Records

Documentation is only one component of information management and quality improvement, yet the skill is important for athletic trainers in all employment settings. Well-maintained medical records assist with clinical decision making and quality assurance. Documentation can be segmented into two purposes, medical records and administration, and serves the following purposes:

- *Professional standard.* Medical documentation is a professional standard practice as indicated by athletic training domain 6, Health Care Administration and Professional Responsibility.
- *Memory.* Documentation helps athletic trainers and medical professionals recall past care provided or administrative activities, particularly if these are seldom reviewed.
- *Legal protection for both the patient and practitioner.* The medical record provides written verification of medical care and administrative functions.
- *Communication.* Documentation provides an avenue for communication with other providers, patients, insurance, billing, and assessment regulators.

FOUNDATIONAL SKILL

Steps in Developing a Quality Assurance Plan

1. Identify the health care entity's desired outcomes. These can include reduced time lost from sport, work, or activities of daily living; patient satisfaction with services; fiscal solvency; and employee satisfaction.
2. Create or purchase assessment tools based on the desired outcomes.
3. Establish a time line for deployment of the assessment tools.
4. Train employees on the assessment tools, which may also include electronic medical records.
5. Establish a time line for the evaluation of the assessment outcomes.
6. Hold a board or administration meeting to evaluate the outcomes and identify strengths, opportunities, and challenges. The board makes an implementation plan for any changes in services or health care delivery.
7. Revise and reimplement assessments for the next cycle.

TABLE 5.1   **Quality Improvement and Assurance Models**

Models	Summary
Care model	Promotes high-quality disease prevention and management through the support of the provider or service and patient interactions. Patients are supported to take an active part in their care.
Lean model	Identifies the patients' wants and individually maps the customer values with process competency, time-efficiency, and cost-effectiveness
Model for improvement	Focuses on three questions to set the aim or organizational goal, establish measures, and select changes. It incorporates Plan-Do-Study-Act (PDSA) cycles to test changes on a small scale.
FADE	Focus on problem Analyze data Develop action plan for improvement Execute plan
Six sigma	A method of process improvement and problem reduction that uses one of two models for quality improvement: 1. Existing processes use DMAIC: define, measure, analyze, improve, control 2. New processes in development use DMADV: define, measure, analyze, design, verify

Data from Peer and Rakich (2000); Institute of Medicine of the National Academies (2006).

TABLE 5.2   **Quality Improvement Assessment Tools**

Assessment area	Tool examples	Distribution best practice
Patient safety	Patient satisfaction Safety and injury data Mistakes Patient confidentiality	Dependent on the setting Patient satisfaction surveys may be distributed directly after practitioner interaction or at the end of treatment. Biannual to annual collection of injury data, mistakes, and patient confidentiality analysis
Management	Financial status Facility usage Patient satisfaction	Conducted biannually or annually
Personnel	Employee satisfaction surveys Attendance information Safety and injury data Number and quality of professional development	Conducted biannually or annually
Patient satisfaction	Patient surveys Billing turnaround Waiting time Caregiver- or staff-to-patient ratios	Dependent on the setting Patient satisfaction surveys may be distributed directly after practitioner interaction or at the end of treatment. Biannual to annual evaluation of billing turnaround, waiting time, and caregiver- or staff-to-patient ratio
Clinical quality	Preventive measures (blood pressure, labs, imaging, health behaviors screening) Number of revisits Time and quality of return to activity or discharge Patient follow-up	Collected after each patient interaction Analyzed biannually or annually

Based on Hughes (2008); Peer and Rakich (2000); NQC Quality Academy (2017); National Health Expenditures (2014); Institute of Medicine of the National Academies (2006).

- *Critical decision making for treatment and rehabilitation.* Evaluation of medical documentation provides a basis of assessing diagnosis, prevention, and disease or injury outcomes in order to make initial or ongoing changes to clinical decisions.

- *Discharge decisions.* Medical documentation assists providers in assessing patient outcomes in order to appropriately discharge from the hospital, treatment, or rehabilitation.

- *Quality improvement or outcomes assessment.* The assessment of outcomes is critical to determining both administrative or department effectiveness and patient care efficacy.

- *Injury surveillance.* Documentation provides the data to review aggregate injury and illness information related to different populations (e.g., age, gender, sport) to assess trends of injury incidence and intervention.

- *Patient satisfaction.* Medical records should include patient satisfaction information to better inform providers or health care systems regarding care.

- *Referral services and continuity.* Documentation provides an avenue for communication with other providers regarding referral services in order to maintain patient service continuity.

- *Financial and insurance reimbursement.* Medical records provide the information to appropriately third-party bill for reimbursement or direct patient billing.

Forms of Medical Documentation

Medical documentation must follow federal, state, and organizational requirements. Specific athletic training documentation may vary between organizations or employment settings, but many of the documents are standard practice. This section identifies standard documentation for both medical and administrative purposes, as well as corresponding policies.

Standard Medical Documentation

The items included in standard medical documentation in athletic training depend on the employment setting. The following items may be included:

- Patient consent forms
- Physical examination forms
- Insurance information
- Emergency information
- Release of medical information:

  - FERPA (Family Educational Rights and Privacy Act)
  - HIPAA
- Permission to treat
- Injury or illness evaluation forms
  - SOAP note: charting by patient information
    - *Subjective:* description of provider's impressions of patient based on the patient's descriptions, motivation, mood, and communication.
    - *Objective:* measurable information, including tests, percentages, goals or objectives, and other data
    - *Assessment:* interpretation of the objective data
    - *Plan:* outline of course of treatment
  - Focus charting
    - Charting by exception
    - Narrative charting
    - Special reports: blood analysis, diagnostic imaging, surgical reports, cardiac assessments, strength testing, urinalysis, and communication from other professionals and practitioners.

Administration Records

Standard administrative documentation in athletic training may include items from the following list. Documentation is dependent on the employment setting. All of the administrative records may be used for quality assurance and improvement processes.

- Budget reports
- Nonmedical correspondence
- Equipment and inventory
- Government reports: required reports that may include patient and staff safety, patient or health entity outcomes, or other information depending on individual states
- Department performance reports: non-personnel key performance indicators for a department or health care system
- Personnel information
  - Performance evaluations
  - Salary
  - Employment application
  - Employment contract
  - Professional development

Medical Records and Information Technology Governance

Several U.S. laws were enacted to ensure a patient's right to privacy with respect to protected health information (PHI). Privacy laws cover the sharing of information with health care providers, who are bound to use it in the patient's best interest, and the maintenance of stored and transmitted information. Table 5.3 details specific purposes of PHI and administrative practice.

Newer technology trends, including social media and cloud storage, have changed the mode in which health care providers and entities share information. Vigilance to maintain PHI appropriately is thus a responsibility of both health care administrators and practitioners. PHI includes the following:

- Past, present, and future information
- Information generated or received by a health care provider or entity, an employer, a school, or a life insurance company

Documentation Systems

A clinical documentation system that details medical treatments can be analog or digital. Documentation systems in health care and the integration of information are crucial for coordinating medical practices and researching best practices and quality assurance (figure 5.7). Docu-

mentation must be standardized, accurate, timely, and patient specific. The primary types of documentation are as follows:

- Paper documentation
- EMR

Electronic Medical Records and Big Data

Electronic medical records (EMRs)—the digital equivalent of paper records or charts at a clinician's office—are currently best practices in health care settings because they provide the ability to do the following:[5,46]

- Coordinate medical services between providers with greater efficiency
- Mine data for coordinated care and health or service indicators
- Research
- Directly integrate billing systems
- Assimilate nonmedical administrative patient and organization assessment key indicators

EMRs typically contain general information such as treatment and medical history about a patient as it is collected by the individual medical practice.

The American Recovery and Reinvestment Act required that all public and private health care providers

TABLE 5.3 Medical Records and Patient Information Governance and Standards

Federal law or act	Purpose	Implementation
HIPAA	Ensure that patient health and medical information and records are private and protected	Secure medical records: providers must have a plan. Patients must be informed of their rights regarding medical records. When transferring patient information to other health care providers, clinicians must follow key practices.
American Recovery and Reinvestment Act	Requires that all public and private health care entities that receive Medicare or Medicaid reimbursement have electronic health care records (EHR/EMR).	Electronic health records may not be required in all AT settings that do not seek reimbursement, but EHR are a best practice and are required for reimbursement.
FERPA	Protects the privacy of student education records Applies to all schools that receive funds under an applicable program of the U.S. Department of Education	Parents or eligible students have the right to inspect and review the student's education record. Rights transfer to students at 18 years of age.
Health Level Seven (HL7)	An accredited protocol for the handling and exchange of information of medical and health care administrative records	A written protocol must be created and maintained that indicates the handling and exchange of information in the medical entity.

Meaningful Use of Electronic Health Records

The following are some objectives of meaningful use of electronic medical or health records (EMR/EHR):[57]

- Improve quality, safety, and efficiency
- Reduce health disparities
- Engage patients and family
- Improve care coordination and population and public health

To ensure that your patients' health and medical information and records are private and protected, the Health Insurance Portability and Accountability Act of 1996 (HIPAA) has rules about who can look at, receive, and use patients' health information and outlines measures for protecting the confidentiality, integrity, and security of the information.

Patient consent is one component of maintaining patient confidentiality while adhering to HIPAA guidelines. Informed consent is generally captured through a written signature that creates an agreement to provide medical intervention. Written consent is often obtained at varying points of medical and athletic training services, depending on the setting. In athletic environments and prior to office visits, informed consent is most often obtained from a new patient as a component of history and insurance paperwork. Additional informed consent is also provided when specialized intervention, treatment, special tests, or surgery is recommended. Written patient consent is required through signature for patients 18 years and older. Surrogates are allowed to sign on a patient's behalf for a minor (under 18). A legal designee can also be identified when a patient lacks decision-making abilities. In athletic training or emergency situations where the patient is unable to communicate, consent is implied, meaning that emergency life-saving procedures may be performed. In an athletic environment, the patient consent form often includes a clause indicating consent to treat should an emergency life-threatening situation occur. Medical records should include information regarding interventions. They are also a component of the obligation implied through a written patient consent. Patient information about interventions should include the following:

1. The diagnosis (when known) or potential diagnoses
2. Details regarding the intervention and reasons for intervention
3. Potential benefits of the intervention
4. Potential burdens or risks of both the intervention and forgoing the recommendation

The HIPAA Privacy Rule sets national standards to protect the privacy of individually identifiable health information and ensure the security of electronic personal health information (PHI). Under HIPAA, athletic trainers and health care facilities must do the following:

- Put safeguards in place to protect patients' health information
- Reasonably limit uses and sharing to the minimum necessary to accomplish the intended purpose
- Have agreements in place with any service providers who perform functions or activities on their behalf to ensure that the services providers (referred to as "business associates") use and disclose patients' health information properly and safeguard it appropriately
- Have procedures in place to limit who can access their patients' health records
- Maintain a training program for employees about how to protect the patients' health information
- Notify patients when a breach of medical information occurs and notify the public when more than 500 people are affected

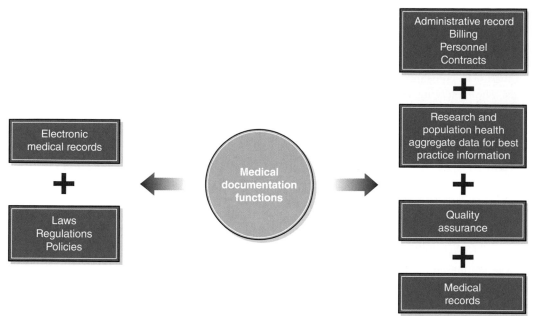

FIGURE 5.7 Documentation systems in health care.

and other eligible professionals adopt and demonstrate meaningful use of electronic medical records (EMR) by January 1, 2014, in order to maintain their existing Medicaid and Medicare reimbursement levels. Since that date, the use of electronic medical and health records has spread worldwide and shown its many benefits to health

Paper Documentation Dos and Don'ts

Paper documentation is no longer best practice since it precludes facilities from seeking reimbursement. However, facilities that continue to maintain paper documentation must follow the same best practices as EMR, paying particular attention to keeping records inaccessible to the public and employees who should not have access.

Do

- Maintain records in a locked area inaccessible to patients and employees who do not need access
- Use timed entries (The medical record should be dated, timed using a 24-hour clock, and legible.)
- Ensure that each record is signed by the person making the entry and done as soon as possible after patient engagements
- If there is a delay, record the time of the event, the delay, and the reasons for the delay
- Make sure entries are objective (history, assessment, clinical findings, decisions, actions)
- Document any noncompliance

Don't

- Place records in a place accessible to the public (includes sign-in sheets with or without privacy screen)
- Use abbreviations
- Use ambiguous terms
- Delete or alter the contents of clinical notes
- Make subjective comments that require interpretation (i.e., terms such as *heavy*, *occasionally*, or *mildly*)

organizations everywhere. Athletic trainers working in a setting that participates in Medicaid or Medicare reimbursement are required to have EMR.

EMR has improved the ability to monitor larger systems of information to assess medical and organizational best practices. The increasing use of population health management (PHM) to assess large amounts of patient information for best patient diagnosis, disease and injury prevention, and treatment or therapy is supported through an EMR that collects patient data. PHM is the collection of patient data across multiple health information technology resources. Combining the patient records or data into a single record allows providers to make optimal health care decisions based on patient data and best practices. EMR may also help improve both clinical and financial outcomes through **big data,**[47-51] a term used to describe a large volume of electronic information. The data can be analyzed and used for quality assurance and improvement, health care and population management predictions, and market analysis.[5,52,53] For the following reasons, EMR is considered a component of quality assurance:

- Maintains privacy and security of patient health information
- Manages the need of the identified population to decide which medical team is accountable to those patients
- Lowers patient and organizational costs by identifying trends

Big data is defined by three characteristics:[48-51]

1. *Volume:* the amount (quantity) of data collected and the number of sources
2. *Velocity:* the speed at which data is produced, which should be calculated so the system is not overwhelmed
3. *Variety:* the type of data collected from medical records, billing, text information, and assessment data to social media

All three characteristics are crucial to implementing the use of big data in a health care setting. The infrastructure must be present with the capacity to support the volume and velocity. The variety of data is based on the health care entity's quality assurance plan. Big data can be used to answer questions and identify issues to help develop evidence-based prevention, treatment, and training plans (see chapter 2).

Insurance, Third-Party Reimbursement, and Billing

Insurance reimbursement can be a complex issue in athletic training. A team effort is required to accomplish meaningful reimbursement. Insurance reimbursement is heavily regulated by federal and state guidelines. The National Athletic Trainers' Association (NATA) is a rich resource for regulatory information regarding insurance matters for athletic trainers.[54]

Insurance

Insurance is a contract between a client and an insurance company. This contract is represented by a policy in which a client or entity receives financial protection or reimbursement against losses from an insurance company. A client contracts with an insurance company through agreed-upon premiums (payments) for the client and service payments from the insurance company. Typically, an insurance company will pool the client's payments to make insurance payments more affordable and at the same time create a pool of funds to provide payouts to clients for their losses.

Billing and Reimbursement

Filing insurance claims immediately and correctly after medical service is necessary in order to receive reimbursement. Filing insurance claims requires several considerations:

FOUNDATIONAL SKILL

Are You Eligible to Bill as an Athletic Trainer?

In order to bill as an athletic trainer, you must meet the following requirements:[54]

- Be licensed, certified, or registered as an AT in the state where you are practicing or want to practice
- Have a National Provider Identifier (NPI)
- Use the taxonomy code for an athletic trainer (2255A2300X: SPECIALIST/TECHNOLOGIST - ATHLETIC TRAINER)
- Have an employer who bills for medical services (Some secondary school and university athletic training clinics do not bill for services.)

- State regulations regarding insurance billing
- State athletic trainer practice acts (what services an athletic trainer may bill for)
- Staffing and personnel dedicated to filing claims (typically a full-time position)
- Contracted agreements and rates with insurance companies for services
- Filing time lines

The services may be paid directly by the patient (fee for service) or through a third party. Third-party reimbursement is the process whereby providers or health care entities receive reimbursement from a policyholder's (patient's) insurance company for treatment or services provided. Several types of third-party payers exist (see figure 5.8).[6,55,56]

Insurance for athletes in secondary schools and colleges varies based on the institutional policies. The organization's governance should indicate which institutional insurance policies to use (see the following list). The governance process may include some or all of the participants in risk management, the principal or dean, president, and board. The athletic trainer needs to identify the process for approving insurance policies prior to instituting them and communicating with parents and students.

Three global types of insurance policies exist in athletic departments:

1. *Self-insurance.* Institution decides not to purchase insurance but instead pays for all health care costs out of pocket or from a saved account.
2. *Primary coverage.* The athlete, athletic department, or institution holds an insurance policy that is delineated as the health insurance plan that pays on claims first.
3. *Secondary coverage.* The injured athlete must first make a claim under his primary insurance policy. Any remaining direct medical costs are paid by the athletic department or institution. This may be combined with self-insured policies based on institutional policy.

The following insurance codes are commonly used by athletic trainers:[7,54]

Evaluation

- 97169 Athletic training evaluation, low complexity

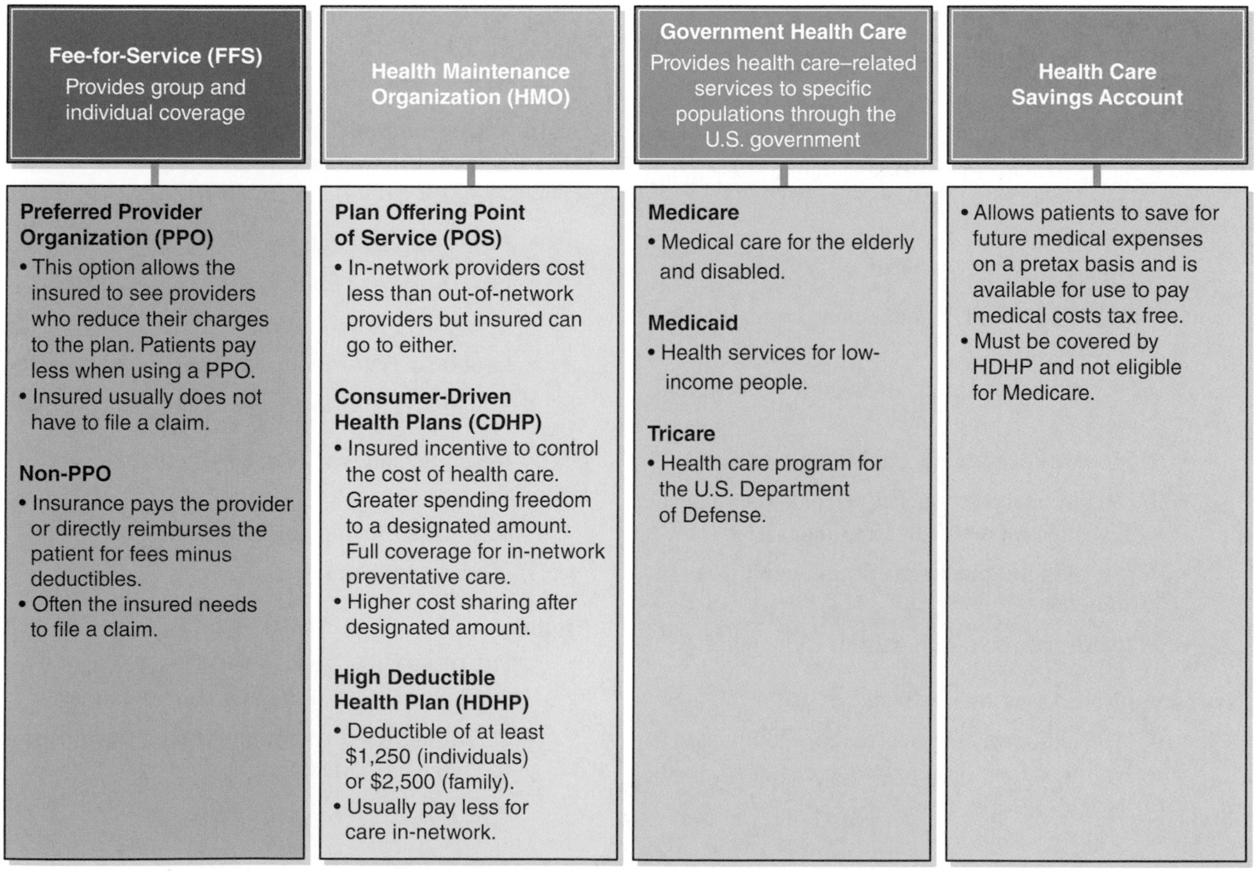

Fee-for-Service (FFS) Provides group and individual coverage	Health Maintenance Organization (HMO)	Government Health Care Provides health care–related services to specific populations through the U.S. government	Health Care Savings Account
Preferred Provider Organization (PPO) • This option allows the insured to see providers who reduce their charges to the plan. Patients pay less when using a PPO. • Insured usually does not have to file a claim. **Non-PPO** • Insurance pays the provider or directly reimburses the patient for fees minus deductibles. • Often the insured needs to file a claim.	**Plan Offering Point of Service (POS)** • In-network providers cost less than out-of-network providers but insured can go to either. **Consumer-Driven Health Plans (CDHP)** • Insured incentive to control the cost of health care. Greater spending freedom to a designated amount. Full coverage for in-network preventative care. • Higher cost sharing after designated amount. **High Deductible Health Plan (HDHP)** • Deductible of at least $1,250 (individuals) or $2,500 (family). • Usually pay less for care in-network.	**Medicare** • Medical care for the elderly and disabled. **Medicaid** • Health services for low-income people. **Tricare** • Health care program for the U.S. Department of Defense.	• Allows patients to save for future medical expenses on a pretax basis and is available for use to pay medical costs tax free. • Must be covered by HDHP and not eligible for Medicare.

FIGURE 5.8 Third-party insurance payers.

- 97170 Athletic training evaluation, moderate complexity
- 97171 Athletic training evaluation, high complexity
- 97172 Athletic training re-evaluation

Physical Medicine

- 97018 Paraffin bath therapy
- 97022 Whirlpool therapy
- 97024 Diathermy (e.g., microwave)
- 97028 Ultraviolet therapy
- 97032 Electrical stimulation, manual, each 15 minutes
- 97034 Contrast bath therapy, each 15 minutes
- 97035 Ultrasound therapy, each 15 minutes
- 97036 Hydrotherapy, each 15 minutes

Rehabilitation Codes

- 97110 Therapeutic exercises, each 15 minutes
- 97112 Neuromuscular reeducation, each 15 minutes
- 97116 Gait training therapy, each 15 minutes
- 97140 Manual therapy 1/> regions, each 15 minutes
- 97530 Therapeutic activities, each 15 minutes
- 97532 Cognitive skills development, each 15 minutes
- 97535 Self-care management training, each 15 minutes
- 97537 Community or work reintegration, each 15 minutes
- 97542 Wheelchair management training, each 15 minutes
- 97545 Work hardening or conditioning; initial 2 hours
- 97546 Work hardening; each additional hour
- 97750 Physical performance test or measurement, with written report, each 15 minutes
- 97760 Orthotic management and training, each 15 minutes
- 97761 Prosthetic training, each 15 minutes

Neurocognitive Assessments/Tests

- 96119 Neuropsychological testing: administered by technician, per hour of technician time, face-to-face

- 96120 Neuropsychological testing: administered by a computer, with qualified health care professional interpretation and report

Evaluation and Management Code

- 99211 Office/outpatient visit, established office visits

Application of Casts and Strapping

- 29240 Strapping; shoulder
- 29260 Strapping; elbow or wrist
- 29280 Strapping; hand or finger
- 29520 Strapping; hip
- 29530 Strapping; knee
- 29540 Strapping; ankle or foot
- 29550 Strapping; toes
- 29580 Unna boot
- 29581 Application of multi-layer compression system; leg (below knee), including ankle and foot
- 29582 Compression system; thigh and leg, including ankle and foot, when performed
- 29583 Compression system; upper arm and forearm
- 29584 Compression system; upper arm, forearm, hand and fingers

Health Care Common Procedure Coding System (HCPCS) Level II Codes

- A6441-A6457 Bandages or dressings
- E0110-E0118 Crutches
- E0720-E0770 TENS
- E1800-E1841 Orthopedic devices
- L1500-L2999 Orthotic devices (lower extremity)
- L3650-L4130 Orthotic devices (upper extremity)

UB 04 Revenue Codes Used by Athletic Trainers in Hospitals

- 0940 Other therapeutic services
- 0951 Athletic training

Modifier

- GP Billing for services provided as part of an outpatient physical therapy plan of care
- 25 Billing for a re-evaluation and treatment on the same day (Medicare)

• KX Medicare patient who has exhausted their benefits for rehabilitation services (The clinician is "certifying that the services rendered are medically necessary.")

Refer to the Centers for Medicare and Medicaid Services webpage for additional modifiers and their explanations. Prior to billing, athletic trainers should consult the International Statistical Classification of Diseases and Related Health Problems.[1-4,35]

CLINICAL BOTTOM LINE

• Health care administration requires the oversight and coordination of budget, facilities, services, operations, and personnel to ensure healthy patient outcomes and safety. Health care administrators should focus on three qualities of an effective manager: self-management, team management, and organizational level management. Organizational structures include functional, team-based, and service line models that are chosen based on best organizational fit.

• The Privacy Act of 1974 coupled with the Health Insurance Portability and Accountability Act (HIPAA) of 1996 ensure the protection of personal medical information and the dissemination of those records through traditional and electronic means. Patients have the right to access their medical records and request amendments when documentation exists.

• Quality assurance and improvement are used to evaluate all components of health care services to determine patient safety and treatment and service outcomes. Performance indicator ratings will determine if changes in any care component require attention, change, or future re-evaluation. Quality assurance requires continuous assessment in a loop to evaluate the following:
  • Current organizational and structural practice processes
  • Tools commonly used to assess desired outcomes
  • Health care delivery and services

• HIPAA and FERPA guidelines indicate that medical records must have safeguards such as a locked filing cabinet in a place inaccessible to patients or electronic records with password protection located where patients cannot see the screen or access the information. Procedures should be in place to limit who can access patients' health information.

• Insurance for athletes may be one of three types (dictates the ability or type of billing available to athletic trainers):
  • Self-insurance
  • Primary coverage
  • Secondary coverage

 Go to HK*Propel* to complete the activities and case studies for this chapter.

Go to HK*Propel* to download a foundational skill check sheet for writing SOAP notes.

CHAPTER 6

Management, Planning, and Professional Development

Leamor Kahanov, EdD, ATC, LAT

CAATE STANDARDS

The following CAATE 2020 standards are covered in this chapter:

Standard 65

Standard 67

Standard 68

Standard 88

Standard 91

CHAPTER OBJECTIVES

After reading this chapter, you will be able to do the following:

- Understand the foundations of management and leadership

- Recognize the components of planning

- Apply finance and budgeting principles

- Identify implications of risk management

- Define advocacy as a component of professional practice

Athletic trainers gain the technical skills and knowledge they need to provide health care to a diverse patient or client population within the context of an organization. The organization may be a for-profit (e.g., medical equipment producer or for-profit health care clinic), public (e.g., secondary school athletic department), or health care entity (e.g., outpatient physical therapy clinic). Regardless of the business type, organizations must communicate their identity (**mission** and **vision**) and a plan for achieving their goals (**strategic plan** and **operational plan**). Athletic trainers are often in the position of assisting with the planning of an organization, whether as the owner of a clinic, the head athletic trainer, or a department leader. Understanding and enacting planning is crucial to creating an employee culture and achieving the desired organizational outcomes.

This chapter provides an overview of organizational planning, leadership, management, and the relationship between advocacy and resources. The foundation of any organization is its mission, vision, and strategic and organizational plans. The implementation of those plans is subject to fiscal and facility resources and leadership style. This chapter provides contextual and foundational information regarding management, leadership, and financial budgeting in health care. Because planning, leadership, and finance are complex, seek additional information if your job involves organizational management in athletic training.

Management and Leadership

Management and leadership are two different functions within an athletic training environment. **Management** involves creating and managing policies and organizing, planning, and controlling resources to ensure the solvency of the organization. These functions are often interconnected, requiring adept skill from the manager.[14] **Leadership** is the ability to influence others through vision and direction. Leaders are often not involved in operational functions.

Management

Management is an operational function for an institution, such as a high school, hospital, rehabilitation clinic, sales company, or other public or private entity. The difference between the manager of an organization and a clinician with a patient load is the breadth of responsibility. Practitioners are responsible for the patient and patient outcomes, and managers are responsible to many stakeholders, including the patients, organization, state regulatory authority, board of directors, and other internal and external groups. Managers must consider the needs of a group rather than individual clients; thus, they must understand different components of management to best govern and ensure reduced risks to the institution or company, both legally and fiscally.

Components of Management

Various theories exist in the study of management[1-6] (this chapter covers power and authority); however, extended investigation of management is beyond the scope of this chapter. Foundationally, management is separated into three distinct roles:

1. *Interpersonal.* Management of relationships requires a host of skills that include understanding nonverbal behaviors, varying communication styles for different people and personalities, resolving conflict, using creative problem solving to address relationship issues, and garnering legitimacy with constituents through technical expertise.[7,8]

2. *Knowledge or informational.* Management of information requires astute communication skills to use and disseminate information to various internal and external stakeholders in order to facilitate organizational business. Knowledge or informational management has several components, including the acquisition, dissemination, and disposal of information. Digital platforms have increased the difficulty of controlling information.[9-13] Managing digital information for the benefit of the patient or clients and people in the organization has become increasingly complex and requires a careful communication plan with and among all constituents to ensure ease of access.[2]

3. *Decisional.* Managers are often in the position of making decisions; however, they must employ a comprehensive strategy that covers rules, regulations, and plans for making decisions. Managers should communicate this strategy to the people in the organization so that critical decisions are well thought out and constructed to minimize negative effects on the entity. In addition, a rule of order for making decisions is critical to ensure that employees buy in and patients or clients act on any plans.[14,15]

Operational components of management in athletic training often include human relations, data management, strategic planning, operational planning, policy creation, resource management, information management, and risk management. The operational components routinely intersect with management roles, and an adept manager understands the intersectionality (figure 6.1).

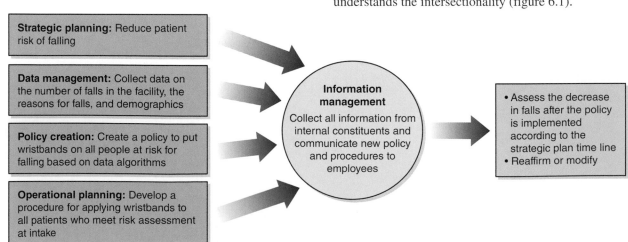

Strategic planning: Reduce patient risk of falling

Data management: Collect data on the number of falls in the facility, the reasons for falls, and demographics

Policy creation: Create a policy to put wristbands on all people at risk for falling based on data algorithms

Operational planning: Develop a procedure for applying wristbands to all patients who meet risk assessment at intake

Information management

Collect all information from internal constituents and communicate new policy and procedures to employees

• Assess the decrease in falls after the policy is implemented according to the strategic plan time line
• Reaffirm or modify

FIGURE 6.1 Example of intersection between roles and functions of management.

Power

Leadership, power, and authority are separate components of management that function independently of each other. A leader may be an influential employee who speaks for the group or the visionary president of a company who has the support of the employees. Power also varies based on the person. It may be based on a person's title, or position of power, which enables him to have authority over another employee.[16] People with positional power often affect the pay, vacations, and upward mobility of other employees and thus have an expressed legitimacy in the role based on potential negative or positive effects on personnel. However, power and authority sometimes reside with an employee who does not have a title or position of power. The power and authority roles are defined differently in each organization based on the people employed in that business, company, or institution.[16] Power is therefore transient and is defined by both the person who is in a position of power and the employees, based on the organizational dynamic. Power is exchangeable and routinely re-evaluated by employees to determine the best people to engage for communicating and advancing ideas or change. To understand organizational culture and facilitate operations, you must learn about the positions of power. Table 6.1 identifies the different positions of power. Organizational structure is complex, and a detailed discussion is beyond the scope of this chapter.

Leadership

Leadership is a profoundly studied phenomenon with more than 200 definitions and yet is the least understood aspect of management.[17,18] Although the needed skills can be acquired, a large component of leadership is innate communication, interpersonal skills, and a self-understanding that enhances interactions with others.[17,18] As in other fields, leadership in athletic training requires **emotional intelligence**, which is the awareness of and capacity to control one's own emotions and manage the emotions of others through interprofessional relationships. Good leaders need emotional intelligence coupled with a distinct motivational and employee or organizational plan to achieve desired outcomes for their clients and institution.[3] A plan for managing personnel may be individual, departmental, or institutional, depending on the needs of the organizational culture. Details of specific techniques are beyond the scope of this chapter; you should pursue further study to become an effective leader in athletic training.

Leadership is the influence over others or the art of motivating others to achieve a common goal.[19-20] Leaders can often be identified as such by their peers and are not necessarily in named positions of power (e.g., head athletic trainer, supervisor, or vice-president). Leaders in health care must employ multiple behaviors given the unique and varied responsibilities of patient and client care and peer and supervisor relations.[20-22]

TABLE 6.1 Positions of Power

Power	Definition	Examples
Legitimate power	Identified position that gives employee the ability to make decisions for the organization	Head athletic trainer Clinical director Vice-president of sales
Expert power	Perception by others that someone possesses superior knowledge or skills	Premier researcher in concussions A rehabilitation technique named after the inventor Person wrote a book on a subject 40 years in athletic training education
Informational power	A person who possesses desired information. This is short-term power because the person typically does not have influence or positional power.	The staff athletic trainer who has been asked to put together an inventory system and has budget and IT information; this is a short-term project.
Reward power	Motivation is garnered by offering financial incentives.	Clinic owner who uses transactional leadership to provide raises annually
Connection power	Someone who obtains favors by having friends or people of influence in his professional network	Often used to obtain employment through references by a person in a position of influence in the industry
Referent power	Charisma; the ability to provide personal approval or acceptance to another person. This is the most valuable type of power and transcends leadership types.	Someone who obtains a fellow colleague's accolades when her work is well done, regardless of financial or employment status

Leadership and management are distinctly different functions. Leadership qualities typically transcend the organizational setting, whereas managers are identified only in an employment context.[20]

Leaders

- Are visionary and are often identified as fast movers or evoking too much change
- Are not limited by current organizational culture to solve problems or advance policy
- Are strategic thinkers
- Demonstrate contextual intelligence
- Take initiative for change or problem solving

Managers

- Uphold the status quo
- Use organizational policy to make decisions
- Are limited to the culture and precedent of the organization
- Have little influence over the mission and vision of the organization or policy creation

Leadership styles are complex, and leaders use different styles based on each unique situation (table 6.2). An adept leader in athletic training is able to address employees, patients or clients, and other internal and external constituents by understanding the different leadership styles and knowing which style comes naturally to her and which are best in different situations, regardless of preference.

Planning

Planning is a key component of managing and leading an organization, department, or team. Identifying the common direction, goals, and desired outcomes helps leaders provide services and rally the employees in a common direction that is understood and valued. The way in which the vision and mission for an organization, department, or team are created, reviewed, and ratified is based on the leadership type; this process may be dictatorial with a transactional leader or team based with a collaborative leader. Regardless of leadership type, a vision and mission are required to create a strategic plan to guide employees and assist in supporting the organizational culture.

Planning is sequential in nature and depends on developing a mission, vision, strategic plan, and operational plan (figure 6.2). These plans are typically reviewed on a routine basis that is specific to the institution or company. Planning cycles vary and may be as short as a month or as long as 5 years depending on the needs of the institution or company.

1. The mission and vision are long-standing foundational planning structures that are reviewed

TABLE 6.2 Types of Leadership

	Definition	Leadership focus
Collaborative or team leadership	Coordination and collaboration of an identified team that has the independence to make decisions. Teams make decisions for the organization with a designated team leader.	The team is the focus of power.
Consensus	Teams are part of a larger network that integrates information to develop decisions. All team members are provided with equal authority.	Network focused
Servant leadership	The leader participates in subordinate work responsibilities. Listening and problem solving are emphasized to develop trust.	Others' needs are addressed first.
Situational leadership	The leader determines the type of leadership necessary for differing situations. For example, the leader may be a participant, observer, motivator, or delegator depending on the situation.	Focus depends on the needs specific to each situation.
Transactional	Hierarchical structure where leaders influence behaviors of subordinates through rewards and penalties. Focus is on avoiding mistakes.	Organizational needs are the primary focus.
Transformational	Leader motivates others through optimism and encouragement. Values include creativity and promoting understanding for the organization's needs.	Environment of the organization is the primary focus.

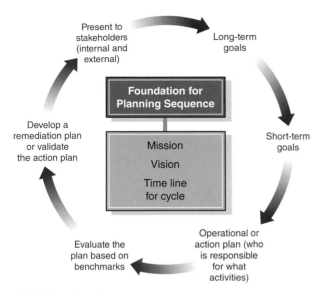

FIGURE 6.2 Planning sequence.

every 5 to 10 years to ensure that the organization is current.

2. The strategic plan is often created for a multiyear period to achieve designated outcomes and meet organizational goals.

3. After an organization determines its mission and vision, long-term goals are created with embedded short-term goals to achieve desired outcomes.

4. An action plan is developed to determine who will lead long-term and short-term initiatives.

5. Benchmarks are created to determine the success of the long- and short-term goals, and then an evaluation is made of the outcomes to determine continuance of the strategic plan.

6. Typically, the evaluation includes either a remediation plan to better affect outcomes or a validation of plans reported to stakeholders of the organization.

7. The cycle begins again.

The sidebar Interplay Between Mission Statement, Vision Statement, Strategic Plan, and Operational Plan (see page 86) provides examples of wording used in different settings.

Mission Statements

A mission statement drives the actions of the organization.[23,24] It is an expression of the organization's purpose, both today and in the foreseeable future. Specific objectives are derived from the mission statement. Three components constitute a mission statement:

1. What we do
2. Whom we serve
3. How we serve them

Vision Statements

The next step in planning requires a vision statement that focuses on the future of the organization and its aspirations.[25] The purpose of the vision statement is to provide a directional framework for the organization and employees based on the identifying aspirational change. Vision statements have four components:

1. Identification of the organization
2. Identification of the service provided
3. Identification of the service population
4. Identification of the aspirational identity

Strategic Planning

Strategic planning is often created by senior management teams, but depending on the leadership style, it may include a network of people in the organization (called consensus leadership). Athletic trainers who are responsible for a department or area may also need to create or implement strategic planning. Strategic plans are created using the mission statement to identify organizational goals, internal and external outcomes, benchmarks for achieving those outcomes, and a timeline for completion. The strategic plan is then used to create operational plans for the organization, department, or area.

Operational Planning

An operational plan, also known as a work plan or action plan, is an outline of the short- and long-term goals of the organization. It can vary depending on the mission, vision, and time line for the strategic planning cycle. The operational plan identifies the people responsible for completing the short- and long-term goals. Components that should be included in an operational plan for an athletic training room at a high school, for example, include the following:[5,6]

- Scope of services
  - Type of individual services
  - Hours of operation
  - Type of coverage for an athletic program (e.g., in season, out of season, travel vs. no travel)
- Facility and personnel coverage [16,26-46]
  - Use of data to determine coverage (high use vs. low use of facility or clinic)
- Policies
  - Emergency plan and policies
  - Inventory and supply routine evaluation and purchasing system
  - Equipment review, capital purchase plan
  - Hygiene of facilities
  - Personnel and human resource policies

Interplay Between Mission Statement, Vision Statement, Strategic Plan, and Operational Plan

The following examples illustrate how mission statements, vision statements, strategic plans, and operational plans work in different athletic training settings.

High School Athletic Training Room

Mission: to provide student-athletes with services in four areas:

1. Injury prevention
2. Recognition, evaluation, and treatment of injuries and illnesses
3. Rehabilitation and reconditioning of injuries
4. Health and wellness education

Vision: to provide student-athletes with the highest-quality health care by staying on the leading edge of health care practice in sports medicine.

Strategic Plan
1. Provide quality patient care
   a. Safe return to participation
   b. Return to participation within 90% range of average in literature
   c. Maintain connection as primary responsibility with local health care system
   d. Work with coaches to educate new coaches, parents, and athletes on safe return to participation and the importance of treatment or rehabilitation adherence
2. Partner with the local university to support student clinical education

Operational Plan
1. Hold meetings with parents and coaches twice a semester to educate them on safe practice and adherence
2. Provide daily updates on injured athletes to coaches and parents
3. Obtain clinical contract for physicians, emergency services, radiography, and so on with local health care system

Medical Company

Mission: to provide the finest overall value in mobility equipment for people with disabilities and mobility impairments
Vision: to be the world leader in the design, development, and manufacture of the best quality, highest performing, and most adaptable and affordable prosthetic products with the strongest warranties

Strategic Plan
1. Increase market recognition of company by 50% for excellence in quality affordable prosthetic products
   a. Develop a marking plan aligned with product quality information
2. Enhance current product durability to a 10-year wear pattern

Operational Plan
1. Change marketing management team and add to the international team
2. Alter image and graphic elements by 2022
3. Deliver new warranty on all products by 2022
4. Produce 5 new robotic prosthetics by 2027

Health Care Rehabilitation System

Mission: to serve the community as a regional leader in rehabilitation services through 4 major areas:

1. Quality patient care
2. Rehabilitation research
3. Education and training of sports medicine professionals
4. Assistive technology

Vision: to be a trusted leader in caring for people and advancing health

Strategic Plan

1. Provide quality patient care
    a. Capture 20% of the market share in 4 years
    b. Receive patient satisfaction ratings of 4/5
2. Produce research in rehabilitation
    a. Produce 20 publications a year
    b. Receive 1 million a year in grant funding
    c. Give 45 presentations a year
3. Partner with all educational programs in a 90-mile radius to support clinical student education in 4 years
4. Provide assistive technology advocacy

Operational Plan

1. Create staffing policy to ensure low-risk management, high patient satisfaction, and low burnout rate
2. Research policy for funding, grant revenue, and support for publications and presentations
3. Obtain clinical contracts with local secondary schools
4. Identify relationship with assistive technology company to obtain free or reduced equipment for low-income patients

Benchmarking

Benchmarking in health care is setting goals or targets to assess and create best practices or evaluate the operational plan.[47,48] The short- and long-term goals typically have a defined outcome for which the goal is successful or unsuccessful. Benchmarking may be both internal and external.

Internal benchmarking: sets targets for the organization

- Example 1: 80% of athletes will be back to participation within the standard time frame for healing.
- Example 2: The number of patients in the rehabilitation clinic will increase 10% from last year.

External benchmarking: sets targets against other organizations

- Example 1: The rehabilitation clinic will be voted best clinic by the regional association for rehabilitation clinics.

- Example 2: The athletic training clinic will have the greatest coverage of sports compared to the local competitors.

Benchmarking is the link between operational and strategic planning. Setting a defined outcome for short- and long-term goals in the operational plan assists with determining direction and success of the strategic plan. Adherence to benchmarks can influence policy that may, in some cases, guide initiatives for strategic or operational plans. For example, if the practice of greeting every patient with a bottle of water when he walks in the door is proven to help the organization exceed the benchmark of retaining 80% of patients until discharge, a policy may be created that every patient must receive a bottle of water on intake.

Conversely, the external or mandated policy—often governmental laws or accreditations—may influence benchmarking and strategic plans. For example, bloodborne pathogen regulations require the creation of a policy and plan with a benchmarking of an operational goal where less than 1% of patients and employees will encounter blood-borne pathogens. This policy and concomitant benchmark may never have been created without external requirements.

Operational planning, benchmarking, analysis, and policy are components of strategic planning necessary to an organization's success, and the connection between

them helps regulate and direct employee actions. Assessing the connection between benchmarks, strategic plans, organizational operations, and policies needed to conduct business is critical for ensuring employees understand their roles in the context of the working environment. Table 6.3 provides examples linking operational planning, benchmarking, analysis, and policy planning.

TABLE 6.3   Intersection Between Operational Planning, Benchmarking, Analysis, and Policy Planning

Operational plan	Benchmark	Analysis	Policy plan
Optimize return to work for police force by incorporating preventive care and fitness that includes optimizing ergonomics with equipment	80% of active duty police will be back to work within the standard time frame for healing.	Results indicated that 90% of the active duty police returned to work within the standard time frame for healing.	Continue to require preventive care and fitness for all active duty police.
Increase revenue for rehabilitation clinic through social media marketing on Facebook over next 6 months	The number of patients in the rehabilitation clinic will increase 10% from last year.	The number of patients declined 2% over 6 months.	Change strategy and update social media marketing to include current platforms like Snapchat, Reddit, and Instagram.

FOUNDATIONAL SKILL

SWOT Analysis

SWOT analysis examines the organization's strengths, weaknesses, opportunities, and threats (or challenges). A SWOT analysis typically occurs prior to strategic and operational planning to assess the environment and help guide the mission and vision of the organization. An example of a SWOT analysis is provided here:

	Rehabilitation clinic	Collegiate athletic training clinic
Strength	Revenue up 25% with 25% more of the regional market	Respectful environment; positive coordination with coaches and administration
Weakness	Low personnel morale and high employee turnover	Electronic record keeping that articulates with health care systems, university, and PPE portal. Not all employees use EMR due to lack of coordination.
Opportunities	Strong patient satisfaction and brand recognition	Capitalize on respect and recognition of knowledge with administration to change EMR system
Threats	Turnover may decrease patient satisfaction and overall clinic rating	Poor communication with coaches and administration and possible lapse in medical care is due to poor EMR. Inability to communicate with health care entities increased time to return in 20% of injuries.
Potential goals	Increase employee morale with flexible scheduling and educational opportunities.	Overhaul EMR.
Potential operational plan	Institute morale survey to assess the effect of flexible scheduling and educational opportunities.	Provide a detailed plan, including budget of EMR overhaul, with benefits and detriments.
Potential benchmarks	25% decrease in employee departure over 1- and 3-year time frames.	Decrease time to return lag by 10% over 1- and 3-year time frames.

Policies

A policy is the articulation of a rule or set of rules that are to be followed for an organization. Policies may be regulatory and have punitive consequences if not followed or may be used to identify best practices for the organization. Typically, a policy is used to direct employees or patients or clients to manage and decrease both physical and financial risk. In comparison, a procedure is a series of steps to follow as a required approach to circumstances that commonly arise in an organization. For example, a physician's office may have a policy that all employees must wash their hands prior to engaging with a new patient. The connected procedure would state that employees should enter the patient room, greet the patient, and wash their hands for 30 seconds in front of the patient.

The creation of policy in a health care entity may be due to internal operational needs or regional, state, or national legal requirements. Policies are enacted to ensure desired outcomes and minimize risk to employees, patients, or the legal and financial status of the organization. Examples include blood-borne pathogen policies to help prevent infections or HIPAA regulations that help to secure personal patient information.[49] Other internal policies may include an emergency action plan or procedures to close the facility after a workday. The intent of all policies is to ensure the safety, security, and legal protection of the health care entity.[49]

Facility Planning

Facility planning is the process of managing, designing, and facilitating the function and use of a space. In athletic training, facility planning is specific to the type of health care organization and includes multiple areas of thoughtful usage planning. Typical facility planning in athletic training includes the following:

- Patient accessibility to all facilities in adherence with the Americans with Disabilities Act (ADA) requirements
- Emergency management and access to emergency personnel and automated external defibrillators; access to the outside for facilities with sport field or courts[1]
- Storage of large and small equipment, medical supplies, and transportation vehicles
- Displaying of licenses, certifications, or professional standards (may be organization or state requirements)
- Medication storage and distribution (see chapter 23 for legal specifications on pharmaceuticals)

- Electrical safety
- Office space adequate for staffing and private conversations
- Record keeping space for security and confidentiality

On occasion, athletic trainers have the opportunity to participate in the development of new facilities or the renovation of facilities. More often, they will need to identify ways to use the current space to best accommodate annual policy changes and patient or staffing service delivery. These issues should be considered in the context not only of space planning but also of budget planning.[46,52]

Facility planning is also a component of strategic planning and operational planning. Annual assessment of facility needs includes internal and external policy updates, regulation updates, personnel changes, and addition of equipment, services, and patients or clients. An annual review of adherence to ADA standards and patient and employee safety (e.g., alarms, fire extinguishers, items in need of repair that may be hazardous) must also be considered as part of the annual facility planning. Changes or modification to facilities as part of the annual facility planning may affect budget; therefore, the two planning components necessitate coordination as part of the strategic planning process. Facility planning should be completed annually to reflect routine changes in policy and staff and patient populations and ensure that renovations and updates are planned and identified for long-term budgeting.

Policy changes may also affect facility usage and budgetary needs. Changes to policies may occur externally (e.g., from government or association regulators) and internally (e.g., policy changes).[16,50-52] Table 6.4 is a nonexhaustive list of policies that should be reviewed annually to determine if facility changes are needed.

Budgeting

Budgeting means planning to manage the financial resources of the health care setting. It is highly tied to the type of organization, whether public, private, nonprofit, or profit generating.[1] The process for each setting differs depending on what is included in the operating budget.[52,53] The following may be included:

- Salaries
- Insurance
- Equipment maintenance
- Purchasing of equipment and expendable items
- Supporting professional development and memberships

TABLE 6.4 Policies and Planning That May Affect Facilities

Policy	Example	Planning
Blood-borne pathogens (BBP)	New BBP policy internally indicates that a disposal container for sharps and biohazardous material must be present next to any patient area, table, or rehabilitation equipment.	Budgeting should be done to increase the number of biohazard and sharps containers in the facility. Long-term budgeting is needed to hang containers on the walls in inconspicuous areas.
HIPAA, FERPA, or other privacy policies	Changes to the HIPAA guidelines require more privacy on entry into the health care facility.	Budget should allow for the annual cost of upgrading a digital system so that patients may sign in independently and do not have to identify themselves verbally where others may hear their names and birth dates.
Employee safety	A high employee injury rate occurred last year. Investigation into the reason indicated that the new tile at the entry was slippery and the cause of 50% of the slips and falls.	Budgeting should be done to replace the tile long term. Short-term (annual) budgeting should be done for mats that create a walkway onto carpeted areas.
Handwashing	An audit of the health care facility identified that only one handwashing station exists for the entire 3,000 square feet rehabilitation area.	Long-term budgeting should be done for new multiple sink areas. Short-term budgeting should be done to place hand-sanitizing stations around the perimeter of the rehabilitation area.
Patient supervision	The current height of the staff desks disallows for patient supervision while making medical notes.	Short-term budgeting solution is to purchase standing desks. Long-term solution is to place floor-to-ceiling windows in the office.
Emergency action planning (EAP)	The internal assessment of the EAP indicated that the location of the high school athletic training room, which lacks outside access, increases time to an injured athlete by 10 min.	Long-term budget includes adding an outside door. Short-term solution with budgetary implications is adding a satellite facility closer to the outside locations.

- Travel
- Office support (e.g., supplies, printing)

Budgeting is a component of resource planning that covers everything from purchase of expendable items to salaries. Resource pressures drive the organization's ability to provide care and effectively manage a facility, including personnel,[55] and the economics of the health care industry directly affect its management of services. For example, athletic trainers in health care settings that bill for services have a financial process that mirrors a for-profit industry, where revenue drives services. Other athletic trainers may be employed in a governmental education system that identifies the cost of services with a static financial amount of funding, for which operations are then aligned.

There are different ways to create budgets (table 6.5). Given that athletic training occurs in many settings, selecting the right type of budgeting for your environment is key to resource allocation. Organizations often have a required budgeting type, but in others, you may be able to discuss the best fit with stakeholders. You can have significant input about the best budgeting system to maximize effectiveness for resource allocation.

Budgets can be further segmented into different components, such as institutional requirements for funding based on state or federal regulations. Athletic trainers should speak with the organization's finance department to determine requirements of that organization or state prior to developing a budgeting plan. Typical budget components include the following:

- Operating budget
- Capital budget
- Personnel budget

TABLE 6.5 **Types of Budgeting**

Budget type	Definition	Benefits	Challenges
Zero-based budgeting	A budget where all expenses are detailed and justified prior to approval of an annual budget	Useful in service entities such as government and public education	Time consuming to develop the model and inflexible when unexpected expenses occur
Static budgeting	A budget with predetermined income and expenses that does not anticipate changes	Good model for budgets with one expected outcome (may be good for high school or college/university with a static budget)	Very rigid and doesn't account for changes that occur in income or expenses
Flexible budgeting	A budget that allows for multiple income models and adjusts expenses accordingly	Useful when income is hard to predict or variable; may be good for small health care clinics	More difficult to prepare with multiple models
Lump-sum budgeting	Nonspecific approach to budgeting with general categories for spending; lacks detail	Very flexible approach to budgeting, leaving high degree of discretion to budget manager	Lacks detailed analysis of expenditures and may support a status quo budgeting that lacks efficiency and becomes out of date
Line-item budgeting	Budget that emphasizes a list of itemized expenditures (e.g., supplies, salaries, equipment)	Offers simplicity and saves time in preparation of the budget	

Operating Budget

An operating budget is a detailed account of all revenue and expenses that are used to facilitate services for a designated period, typically 1 year. Operating budgets have two components: expenses and revenue.

- An **expense** is the amount paid for an item or service. Expenses may include equipment, salaries, insurance, electricity, Internet, or consulting work.

- **Revenue** is the organization's income or earnings. Revenue can include payments for services from clients or insurance companies or an allotment provided by a government entity.

Health care settings that bill for services, such as physician offices, hospitals, rehabilitation clinics, and some athletic training clinics, will have expenses and revenues. Health care settings that do not bill for services, such as a nonprofit health centers, high schools, and some college athletic training rooms, may only have expenses applied against a budgeted allowance for an academic year. The following are examples of items included in an operating budget:

- Travel for continuing education

- Operating supplies (e.g., tape, wraps, ultrasound gel)
- Drug screening equipment
- Ambulance services for athletic events
- Insurance
- Contracts with physicians or other medical services

Capital Budget

A capital budget is a component of a larger budget that identifies fund allocations for large, permanent items that meet a cost threshold. Cost thresholds to determine whether an item is a capital expense are defined by the organization and may be $5,000 or more. Capital budgets include all expenses for major purchases for a fiscal year. In athletic training, these may include record management systems, therapeutic modalities or exercise equipment (e.g., ultrasound machines, treadmills), or furniture or facility improvements (purchasing high-low tables or new computers). To ensure appropriate fiscal management, the athletic trainer in charge of managing budgets must confer with the institution to obtain the criteria, which may include a monetary amount and type of purchase.

Personnel Budget

The salary, wages, and benefits related to labor are forecasted for 1 year in a personnel budget. Labor costs may include salary, insurance, taxes, benefits, overtime, discharge and recruitment, and hiring costs. Each organization manages personnel budgets differently. Occasionally, personnel budgets are managed by the organization at a central finance location. Likewise, personnel budgets may be the purview of the division (e.g., athletic training, rehabilitation, athletics) where the director is responsible for maintaining the personnel budget and making decisions on salary.

Purchasing

Purchasing is the process of paying for goods or services. In an organization, purchasing of items is based on the budget allotment for the division or organization, and the person responsible for purchasing must meet the mission, goals, and desired outcomes of the workplace. For example, purchasing expendable medical equipment or continuing education for an employee would fit within the strategic plan and goals for a health care system that provides patient care. In contrast, purchasing a vehicle for an ambulatory clinic would not meet requirements to fulfill the plan or goals and may be denied.

Purchasing is a highly integrated process. The person responsible must manage the budget with needs, goals,

and outcomes to ensure she is adhering to the organizational mission. Operationally, the purchasing agent for the organization must ensure she is purchasing responsibly, which requires an accounting of current equipment and supplies called inventory.

Many digital inventory systems are available that make it easy to account for expendable and capital items. Athletic trainers should investigate the best digital system to purchase for their employment setting with all relevant stakeholders (e.g., division head, purchasing agent, employees in the division). A routine assessment of inventory use and equipment quality is necessary to determine the ongoing need for **expendable** and **capital equipment**. Inventory assessment is needed when planning for the following fiscal year's budget.

A needs assessment, which is separate from inventory, is required for making the strategic plan. Conducting a needs assessment involves identifying gaps between the current state of the facility or institution and its desired or aspirational state. For example, the athletic training facility or clinic may need new carpeting and furniture to upgrade the environment and promote positive morale among employees, potentially driving more patients into the facilities. The needs assessment then drives the budget request to incorporate capital items such as carpet and furniture into the budget decision process, where critical decisions are made on what is affordable to the institution or company (figure 6.3).

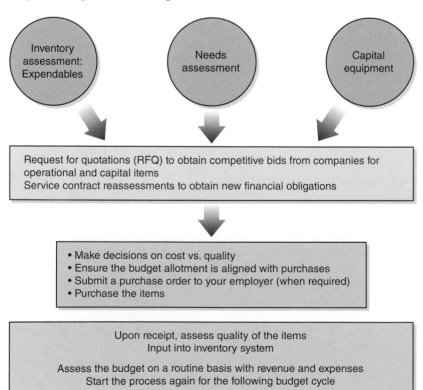

FIGURE 6.3 Decision tree for purchasing.

Key Component to Managing Inventory

- Choose a central storage location where inventory can be controlled.
- Automate the inventory process (many products available).
- Maintain authorized access for people trained in coding when removing inventory.
- Create a reminder-benchmark system for repurchasing when inventory hits a predetermined low quantity.

Risk Management

Risk management is the identification, evaluation, and prioritization of risks to an organization or institution that is then mediated by policy, budget, or other application of resources to mitigate potential harm to the organization, employees, or patients or clients. Assessing risk to an organization is part of a strategic plan. In athletic training, risk management is often considered in the context of identifying risk factors for athletic participation or return to activities, such as heart health, concussions, falls, and reinjury. In the context of an organization, risk factors encompass a host of additional components:

- Legally adhering to governmental regulations (e.g., blood-borne pathogens regulations)
- Legally adhering to contracts with partners or patients or clients (e.g., providing qualified athletic trainers for high school events, notifying patients of special test results)
- Notifying patients or clients and employees of their rights and adhering to those rights (e.g., HIPAA, FERPA)
- Ensuring facilities are safe
- Ensuring care providers are appropriately licensed and provide appropriate care
- Ensuring the organization is fiscally sound or has adequate revenue to provide services and pay employees

Legal assistance or organizational counsel is often involved with interpreting regulations, contracts, and partnerships to assist with policy making to mitigate risk to the organizations. Athletic trainers are an important part of risk management in providing appropriate care to patients, maintaining medical and communication records, facilitating acknowledgment of patient rights, managing employees, identifying unsafe facilities, and managing budgets. Athletic trainers, depending on their role and employment environment, must have adequate communication with organizational stakeholders to articulate potential risks to the organization and fold those risks into the ongoing strategic planning process. Mitigating risk often requires policy making and evaluation of data and policy. Appropriate medical care and adherence to governmental and organizational regulations are the responsibility of all practitioners.

Advocacy

Advocacy in any health care profession commonly has two aspects: patient advocacy and professional advocacy.

Patient advocacy is when a health care provider assists a patient with communicating and obtaining information regarding his health, enabling him to make informed decisions. The role of the health care provider in assisting the patient to obtain this information is controversial because it may be seen as interfering in the patient's ability to make an informed decision. Another area of patient advocacy involves research; athletic trainers can play a role in safeguarding and protecting participants when they are involved in research.[56] The athletic trainer often must make ethical and subjective decisions as to whether to advocate for a patient. For example, advocating for a particular treatment with an insurance company may be best for the patient but affect future insurance coverage and affordability.

Professional advocacy is an individual or group interest to facilitate the goals of the profession or safety of people served by that profession.[57-60] Professional advocacy may be a component of creating public policy; it can take the form of lobbying state or national governmental entities for regulation, licensure, or certification or may entail informing employers, boards, or communities of the abilities and duties of a professional.[58-60] Changes in laws, specifically the Affordable Care Act, insurance reimbursement, or state regulations, may necessitate that athletic trainers inform and educate the community on their role in various settings. Professional advocacy is often employed to raise awareness of professional practice.[58-60]

FOUNDATIONAL SKILL

National Athletic Trainers' Association Advocacy Position

The National Athletic Trainers' Association (NATA) considers professional advocacy to be a responsibility of athletic trainers to advance professional practice. The NATA provides the following framework of responsibilities for athletic trainers when advocating for the profession:

1. Inform the public and legislatures as to the importance of the profession as a component of a health care team[16,57]

2. Serve as an educator or advocate with other health care professionals as part of a health care team

3. Inform other health care providers of the knowledge, skills, and abilities of athletic trainers

CLINICAL BOTTOM LINE

- Leaders and managers maintain different roles in an organization. Leaders are typically visionary and managers are operational and detail oriented. Many leadership and management styles exist and are based on personal style, organizational needs, and external influences. Ultimately, the success of an organization is maintained by a symbiotic relationship between leaders and managers in developing the organizational culture and supervising employees.

- Strategic planning is the foundation for the mission and values of an organization or institution. A well-defined strategic plan is often based on a SWOT analysis to determine operational goals and benchmarks. In addition, budget expenditures are predicated on the strategic plan to ensure continuity with the mission of the organization or institution.

- Finance and budgeting principles in athletic training are dependent on the facility and organization. Depending on the budget type, expenditures may include salary, insurance, operating costs, equipment, travel, and continuing education. The budget for each entity will vary based on the needs of the organization.

- Risk management in athletic training requires the identification of risk factors in the context of medical practice, the organizational effect, and patient outcomes and safety. Athletic trainers participate in risk management through providing appropriate care to patients, maintaining medical and communication records, facilitating acknowledgment of patient rights, managing employees, identifying unsafe facilities, and managing budgets. Communication with organizational stakeholders to articulate potential risks to the organization and fold those risks into the ongoing strategic planning process is a component of an athletic trainer's duties.

- Advocacy can be defined two ways: (1) patient advocacy, where the provider empowers patients to make personal health decisions while guiding and supporting their rights through the medical and insurance system, and (2) professional advocacy, where providers help inform the general public and governmental agencies on the roles and benefits of the health care profession.

 Go to HK*Propel* to complete the activities and case studies for this chapter.

PART II

Injury and Illness Prevention and Wellness Promotion

The athletic trainer's role in injury and illness prevention is the focus of part II. The information provided in these chapters highlights important concepts for students starting in their first clinical rotations in athletic training educational programs. Although each chapter provides information on distinct areas of prevention strategies, students should consider the interconnectedness of prevention concepts in order to provide holistic, patient-centered care. Part II provides introductory information on blood-borne pathogens, preparticipation examinations (PPE), weather monitoring, hydration, taping and bracing, nutrition, fitness and wellness, and protective equipment fitting. Chapter 7 on blood-borne pathogens provides the foundational understanding for infectious diseases, and chapter 8 focuses on strategies and procedures for best practice in preventing injury and illness. Chapters 9 and 10 focus on the components of fitness, wellness, and nutrition that contribute to the prevention of injuries and illness. Chapters 11 and 12 discuss protective equipment and its use and taping and bracing procedures for best protecting patients and athletes in their activities and recovery. All the concepts provided in part II should be used together to provide optimal preventive care.

CHAPTER 7

Blood-Borne Pathogens

David C. Berry, PhD, MHA, AT, ATC
Ellen K. Payne, PhD, LAT, ATC, EMT

CHAPTER OBJECTIVES

After reading this chapter, you will be able to do the following:

- Define and identify the purpose of the Occupational Safety and Health Act and the Occupational Safety and Health Administration (OSHA)
- Define blood-borne pathogens and infectious disease and delineate what constitutes other potentially infectious materials
- Identify, examine, and appraise the epidemiology, transmission, signs and symptoms, vaccination, and occupational risk of infection due to common blood-borne pathogens and other potentially infectious materials
- Define and identify the occupational risk of infection due to common blood-borne pathogens and other potentially infectious materials
- Explain how to minimize this occupational risk of infection where applicable, including precautions, engineering controls, personal protective equipment, and housekeeping policies
- Recognize the need for an exposure control plan and design one to be used in different athletic training settings
- Describe, develop, and implement training guidelines and elements specific to blood-borne pathogens under the OSHA standards
- Describe, develop, and implement procedures for reporting exposure to blood-borne pathogens

CAATE STANDARDS

The following CAATE 2020 standards are covered in this chapter:

Standard 66

Standard 91

Blood-borne pathogens are pathogenic **microorganisms** that are present in human blood and can cause disease in humans. These pathogens include, but are not limited to, hepatitis B virus (HBV) and human immunodeficiency virus (HIV). **Other potentially infectious materials (OPIMs)** fall under three categories:

1. Human body fluids: semen, vaginal secretions, cerebrospinal fluid, synovial fluid, pleural fluid, pericardial fluid, peritoneal fluid, amniotic fluid, saliva, blood, and all body fluids in situations where it is difficult or impossible to differentiate between body fluids

2. Any unfixed tissue or organ (other than intact skin) from a human (living or dead)

3. Human cell or tissue cultures that contain HIV, organ cultures, and HIV- or HBV-containing culture medium or other solutions; blood, organs, or other tissues from experimental animals infected with HIV or HBV

Protecting health care providers against the health risks associated with exposure to blood and OPIMs is the responsibility of the U.S. Department of Labor, specifically the Occupational Safety and Health Administration (OSHA). In 1992, OSHA authorized workplace regulations to protect all at-risk employees, not just health care providers, from potential exposure to blood-borne pathogens. Revised in 2001 to address the Needlestick Safety and Prevention Act,[1] these regulations outlined in the standards apply to all organizations who have employees with reasonably anticipated occupational exposure to blood or OPIMs.

Occupational exposure is "reasonably anticipated skin, eye, mucous membrane, or parenteral contact with blood or OPIM that may result from the performance of the employee's duties."[2] OSHA standards identify how organizations can minimize or eliminate occupational exposure through the use of personal hygiene, **personal protective equipment (PPE)**, engineering and work practice controls, injury surveillance and continuous quality improvement, and continuous training.[2]

This chapter describes in detail requirements of OSHA's Bloodborne Pathogens Standard (found in Title 29 of the Code of Federal Regulations). It also offers insight on what employers must do to protect workers who are occupationally exposed to blood or OPIMs and what athletic trainers can do to protect themselves when they come into contact with blood or OPIMs on the job.

Means of Pathogen Entry

For an occupational exposure to a blood-borne pathogen, the pathogenic agent must enter the host via one of four means (table 7.1):

1. **Direct contact**
2. **Indirect contact**
3. **Airborne contact**
4. **Vector-borne contact**

In the health care setting, direct and indirect contact are the two most common means of exposure. These exposure routes include exposures through the inadequate or inappropriate use of PPE (e.g., gloves) and inappropriate workplace behaviors. In rare cases, exposures occur through needlesticks or cuts from other sharp instruments contaminated with an infected patient's blood or through contact of the eye, nose, mouth, or skin with a patient's blood. Important factors that influence the overall risk for occupational exposures to blood-borne pathogens include the number of infected people in the patient population and the type and number of blood contacts. Most exposures do not result in infection. After a particular exposure, the risk of infection may vary with factors such as the following.[3]

- The pathogen involved (e.g., HBV, HCV, HIV)

Occupational Safety and Health Administration

With the Occupational Safety and Health Act of 1970, Congress created the Occupational Safety and Health Administration (OSHA) to ensure safe and healthful working conditions by setting and enforcing standards and providing training, outreach, education, and assistance. OSHA is part of the U.S. Department of Labor. Under the Occupational Safety and Health Act, organizations have the responsibility to provide a safe workplace.

Employer Responsibility
- Follow all relevant OSHA safety and health standards.
- Find and correct safety and health hazards.
- Inform employees about chemical hazards through training, labels, alarms, color-coded systems, chemical information sheets, and other methods.
- Notify OSHA within 8 hours of a workplace fatality or within 24 hours of any work-related inpatient hospitalization, amputation, or loss of an eye.
- Provide required personal protective equipment at no cost to workers.
- Keep accurate records of work-related injuries and illnesses.
- Post OSHA citations, injury and illness summary data, and job safety and health posters.
- Guarantee they will not retaliate against any workers who use their rights under the law.

Employee Rights
- Work in conditions that do not pose a risk of serious harm.
- Receive information about chemical and other hazards, methods to prevent harm, and OSHA standards that apply to their workplace.
- Review records of work-related injuries and illnesses.
- Receive copies of test results done to find and measure hazards in the workplace.
- File a complaint asking OSHA to inspect their workplace if they believe there is a serious hazard or that their organization is not following OSHA rules. This complaint must be filed within 30 days of the alleged retaliation.

TABLE 7.1 **Means of Pathogen Entry**

Means	Description	Example
Direct contact	Occurs if infected blood from one coworker splashes into the eye of another coworker or by directly touching the body fluids of an infected person	Percutaneous or mucosal contact
Indirect contact	Occurs when a person touches an object that contains the blood or OPIMs of an infected person, and that fluid then enters his own body at a correct entry site	Sharing items such as razors and toothbrushes
Airborne contact	Occurs when person inhales infected droplets that have become airborne	Exposure to bacteria or virus through coughing and sneezing
Vector-borne contact	Transmitted by an animal	Exposure to infected animals such as dogs, raccoons, insects, and bats

- The type of exposure (i.e., direct, indirect, or airborne in health care)
- The amount of blood (or OPIMs) involved in the exposure (i.e., an adequate amount must be present)
- The amount of virus in the patient's blood at the time of exposure
- Susceptibility of a person to the pathogen (e.g., lack of vaccinations)

Common Pathogens

Pathogens are infectious microorganisms that enter the human body and cause infection. Blood-borne pathogens are found in human blood and transmitted through blood. Common pathogens that must be addressed here include various forms of hepatitis and human immunodeficiency virus (HIV).

Hepatitis

Hepatitis means inflammation of the liver. Toxins, certain drugs, certain diseases, heavy alcohol use, and bacterial and viral infections can all cause hepatitis. Hepatitis is also the name of a family of viral infections that affect the liver; the most common types are hepatitis A (HAV), hepatitis B (HBV), and hepatitis C (HCV).[4] For a summary of types of hepatitis, see table 7.2.

TABLE 7.2 **Summary of Hepatitis Types**

	HAV	HBV	HCV
Transmission	Direct contact via feces Commonly occurs with poor sanitary conditions and when good personal hygiene is not practiced. People can get hepatitis A by drinking contaminated water or eating contaminated food.	Direct contact Indirect contact	Same as for HBV
Signs and symptoms	Fever Fatigue Loss of appetite Nausea **Emesis** Abdominal pain Dark urine Clay-colored stool Joint pain Jaundice	Fever Fatigue Dark urine Clay-colored stool Abdominal pain Loss of appetite Nausea Emesis Joint pain Jaundice	70%-80% of people with acute hepatitis C do not have any symptoms Fatigue Abdominal pain Poor appetite Jaundice Mild to severe liver damage, including **cirrhosis** and liver cancer
Vaccination	Yes	Yes	No vaccination Research underway for development of a vaccine

Human Immunodeficiency Virus

Human immunodeficiency virus (HIV) is the virus that leads to acquired immunodeficiency syndrome (AIDS) if not treated. Unlike with some other viruses, the human body cannot get rid of HIV completely, even with treatment. Once HIV is contracted, a person has it for life. According to the Centers for Disease Control and Prevention (CDC), the risk of occupational exposure to HIV infections appears to be minimal:[3]

- The average risk of HIV infection after a needle-stick or laceration exposure to HIV-infected blood is 0.3% (about 1 in 300).
- The average risk after exposure of the eye, nose, or mouth to HIV-infected blood is estimated to be 0.1% (1 in 1,000).
- The risk after exposure of nonintact skin to HIV-infected blood is estimated to be less than 0.1%. A small amount of blood on intact skin probably poses no risk at all. There have been no documented cases of HIV transmission due to an exposure involving a small amount of blood on intact skin.

Table 7.3 provides a summary of HIV.

Exposure Control Plan

Organizations where personnel are deemed to have an occupational risk to blood or OPIMs must have a system for reporting exposures in order to quickly evaluate the risk of infection, inform personnel about available treatments to help prevent infection, monitor personnel for side effects of treatments, and determine if an infection occurred and what the possible long-term consequences are. An **exposure control plan (ECP)** is intended to reduce occupational exposure to blood-borne pathogens and OPIMs and provide a safer work environment by outlining the detailed policies, procedures, and processes to eliminate or minimize chances of an occupational exposure. An ECP must contain the following:

TABLE 7.3   **Summary of HIV**

Transmission	Having anal or vaginal sex with someone who has HIV without using a condom or taking medicines to prevent or treat HIV. Sharing needles or syringes, rinse water, or other equipment (works) used to prepare drugs for injection with someone who has HIV. HIV can live in a used needle up to 42 days, depending on temperature and other factors. Less common modes of HIV transmission:[5] • From mother to child during pregnancy, birth, or breastfeeding • Being stuck with an HIV-contaminated needle or other sharp object (mainly a risk for health care workers)
Signs and symptoms	Early HIV • Fever • Chills • Rash • Night sweats • Muscle aches • Sore throat • Fatigue • Swollen lymph nodes • Mouth ulcers Late HIV • Rapid weight loss • Recurring fever or profuse night sweats • Extreme and unexplained tiredness • Prolonged swelling of the lymph glands in the armpits, groin, or neck • Diarrhea that lasts for more than a week • Sores of the mouth, anus, or genitals • Pneumonia • Red, brown, pink, or purplish blotches on or under the skin or inside the mouth, nose, or eyelids • Memory loss, depression, and other neurologic disorders
Vaccination	None

- **Exposure determination**: who is at risk based on job classification where exposure to blood or OPIMs may occur without regard to the use of PPE
- Schedule and methods of implementation of various methods of exposure control including, but not limited to, the following:

- **Universal precautions** to prevent contact with blood or other potentially infectious materials
- Engineering and work practice controls to eliminate or minimize employee exposure
- Personal protective equipment when risk of occupational exposure remains after institution of engineering and work practice controls

EVIDENCE-BASED ATHLETIC TRAINING

Recommendations for Application of Standard Precautions for the Care of All Patients in All Health Care Settings

Application	Recommendations
Hand hygiene	After touching blood, body fluids, secretions, excretions, or contaminated items Immediately after removing gloves Between patient contacts
Personal protective equipment (PPE): gloves	For touching blood, body fluids, secretions, excretions, and contaminated items For touching mucous membranes and nonintact skin
Personal protective equipment (PPE): gown	During procedures and patient-care activities when contact of clothing or exposed skin with blood or body fluids, secretions, and excretions is anticipated
Personal protective equipment (PPE): mask, eye protection (goggles), face shield	During procedures and patient-care activities likely to generate splashes or sprays of blood, body fluids, and secretions, especially suctioning and endotracheal intubation During aerosol-generating procedures on patients with suspected or proven infections transmitted by respiratory aerosols, wear a fit-tested N95 or higher respirator in addition to gloves, gowns, and face and eye protection.
Soiled patient-care equipment	Handle in a manner that prevents the transfer of microorganisms to others and the environment. Wear gloves if equipment is visibly contaminated. Perform hand hygiene.
Environmental control	Develop procedures for routine care, cleaning, and disinfection of environmental surfaces, especially frequently touched surfaces in patient-care areas.
Textiles and laundry	Handle in a manner that prevents transfer of microorganisms to others and the environment.
Needles and other sharps	Do *not* recap, bend, break, or hand manipulate used needles. If recapping is required, use a one-handed scoop technique only. Use safety features when available. Place used sharps in puncture-resistant container.
Patient resuscitation	Use a barrier device, bag valve mask (BVM), or other ventilation devices to prevent contact with mouth and oral secretions.
Respiratory hygiene and cough etiquette	Instruct symptomatic people to cover mouth and nose when sneezing or coughing. Use tissues and dispose of them in a no-touch receptacle. Observe hand hygiene after soiling of hands with respiratory secretions. Wear a surgical mask if tolerated or maintain spatial separation of >3 ft (1 m) if possible.

Adapted from Siegel et al. (2007).

- Handwashing facilities should be available. If not feasible, an appropriate antiseptic hand cleanser should be used in conjunction with clean cloth or paper towels or antiseptic towelettes. When antiseptic hand cleansers or towelettes are used, hands shall be washed with soap and running water as soon as possible.
- Hepatitis B vaccination
- Postexposure evaluation and follow-up
- Communication of hazard to employees and training
- Record keeping of the standards

The organization is responsible for ensuring that a copy of the ECP is accessible to personnel at all times. The ECP should be reviewed and updated at least annually and whenever necessary to reflect new or modified tasks and procedures that affect occupational exposure and new or revised employee positions with occupational exposure.[2]

OSHA identifies standards of compliance that address several specific items that must be incorporated into an ECP to eliminate or minimize any chance of accidental occupational exposure:

- Precautions (e.g., standard, universal, body substance isolation)
- Engineering and work practice controls
- Personal protective equipment
- Housekeeping

Precautions

Precaution guidelines have been established to prevent the transmission of infectious agents in health care settings. **Standard precautions (SPs)** integrate and expand on universal precautions and **body substance isolation (BSI)** to include organisms spread by the following:[6]

- Blood
- All body fluids, secretions, and excretions except sweat, regardless of whether they contain blood
- Nonintact skin
- Mucous membranes

Today, SPs include a group of infection prevention practices that apply to all patients, regardless of suspected or confirmed infection status, in any setting where health care is delivered. These include hand hygiene; use of gloves, gown, mask, eye protection, or face shield (depending on anticipated exposure); and safe injection practices. Equipment or items in the patient's environment that are likely to have been contaminated with infectious body fluids must also be handled in a manner that prevents transmission of infectious agents.

Engineering and Work Practice Controls

Engineering and work practice controls are procedures and techniques that eliminate or minimize employee and work site exposure to blood and OPIMs.

- **Engineering controls** isolate or remove the blood-borne pathogens hazard from the workplace; examples are sharps disposal containers, self-sheathing needles, and safer medical devices, such as sharps with engineered injury protections and needleless systems.
- **Work practice controls** reduce the likelihood of exposure by altering the manner in which a task is performed; an example is prohibiting recapping of needles by a two-handed technique.

According to OSHA, engineering controls must be examined and maintained or replaced on a regular schedule (yearly) to ensure their effectiveness. Organizations must plan to create constant improvements in minimizing occupational risk,[8] often through the use of new technologies.[7] An example of occupational risk is injuries due to needles and other sharps, which have been associated with transmission (limited) of HBV, HCV, and HIV to health care personnel.

Required engineering and work practice controls in an athletic training environment or health care setting may include the following general working conditions:[9]

- Handwashing facilities should be readily accessible to employees. When provisions of handwashing facilities are not feasible, the organization should provide either an appropriate antiseptic hand cleanser in conjunction with clean cloth or paper towels or antiseptic towelettes. When antiseptic hand cleansers or towelettes are used, hands should be washed with soap and running water as soon as feasible.
- Employees should wash hands immediately or as soon as feasible after removal of gloves or other PPE.
- Following contact with blood or OPIMs, employees should immediately wash hands and any other contaminated skin with soap and water or flush mucous membranes with water.
- Contaminated needles and other contaminated sharps should not be bent, recapped or removed unless the organization can demonstrate that *no* alternative is feasible or that such action is

required by a specific medical or dental procedure. Such bending, recapping, or needle removal must be accomplished through the use of a mechanical device (figure 7.1) or a one-handed technique. Shearing or breaking of contaminated needles is prohibited.

- Immediately or as soon as possible after use, contaminated sharps should be placed in appropriate containers until properly reprocessed (figure 7.2). These containers must be:
  - Puncture resistant
  - Labeled or color-coded by this standard
  - Leakproof on the sides and bottom
- Eating, drinking, smoking, applying cosmetics or lip balm, and handling contact lenses are prohibited in work areas where there is a reasonable likelihood of occupational exposure.

- Food and drink shall not be kept in refrigerators, freezers, shelves, or cabinets or on countertops or bench tops where blood or OPIMs exist.
- All procedures involving blood or other potentially infectious materials shall be performed in such a manner as to minimize splashing, spraying, spattering, and generation of droplets of these substances. For example, mouth pipetting and suctioning of blood or other potentially infectious materials is prohibited.
- Specimens of blood or other potentially infectious materials shall be placed in a container that prevents leakage during collection, handling, processing, storage, transport, or shipping. The container for storage, transport, or shipping shall be labeled or color-coded according to OSHA guidelines and closed before being stored, transported, or shipped.
- Equipment that may become contaminated with blood or OPIMs shall be examined before servicing or shipping and must be decontaminated as necessary, unless the organization can demonstrate that decontamination of such equipment or portions of such equipment is not feasible.

Personal Protective Equipment

Personal protective equipment (PPE) is specialized clothing or equipment worn by athletic trainers and other health care providers for protection against a hazard (figure 7.3). General work clothes (e.g., uniforms, pants,

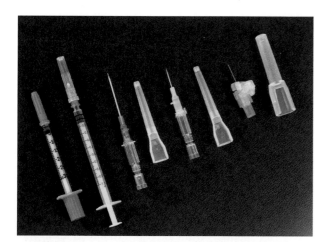

FIGURE 7.1   Safety-engineered needles.

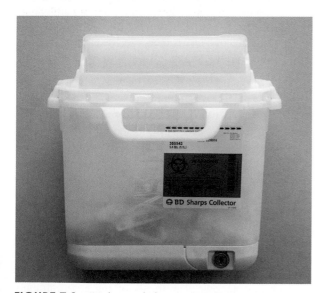

FIGURE 7.2   Biohazard sharps container.

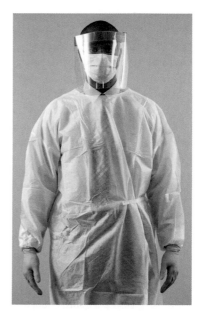

FIGURE 7.3   Proper PPE, such as eye protection, masks, gloves, and gowns, can help prevent the spread of potentially infectious organisms.

FOUNDATIONAL SKILL

Using PPE

Remember these four elements when using PPE:

1. Don PPE before any direct contact with patients. When donning PPE, the recommended sequence is (1) gown, (2) mask or respirator, (3) protective eyewear, and (4) gloves.
2. Be mindful that the combination of PPE used, and therefore the sequence for donning, is determined by the situation.
3. Once PPE is donned, be mindful not to spread contamination.
4. Once the tasks are completed, remove the PPE carefully and discard in an appropriate receptacle, then immediately perform hand hygiene before moving on to the next patient.

shirts or blouses) not intended to function as protection against a hazard are not considered to be personal protective equipment.

PPE is considered appropriate according to the standard if it does not

permit blood or other potentially infectious materials to pass through to or reach the employee's work clothes, street clothes, undergarments, skin, eyes, mouth, or other mucous membranes under normal conditions of use and for the duration of time which the protective equipment will be used.[2]

Therefore, items such as everyday glasses and contact lenses are not considered PPE because protective eyewear has solid side shields. In athletic training, the most commonly used PPE are gloves and breathing devices (i.e., resuscitation or bag valve mask); however, this is anecdotal, not scientific.

When available and reasonable, employees should be able to choose between several comparable and effective safety devices or PPE (e.g., gloves, protective eyewear, mask, gowns) to suit individual work practices, body sizes, and comfort. Under OSHA regulations, organizations should clean, launder, and dispose of required PPE at no cost to the employee. Additionally, organizations should repair or replace PPE as needed to maintain its effectiveness at no cost to the employee.[2]

Gowns, Aprons, and Other Protective Body Clothing

Gowns, aprons, and other protective body clothing are used to protect the health care provider's arms and exposed body areas and prevent contamination of clothing. Use of these items is mandated by the OSHA Bloodborne Pathogens standard. Clinical and laboratory coats or jackets worn over personal clothing for comfort to identify a professional role are not considered PPE.[7]

Isolation gowns are worn in combination with gloves and other PPE when indicated. Gowns are usually the first piece of PPE donned. Full coverage of the arms and body front, from the neck to the mid-thigh or below, ensures that clothing and exposed upper body areas are protected. Gowns should be removed before leaving the patient care area to prevent possible contamination of the environment outside the care area. They should be removed in a manner that prevents contamination of clothing or skin.

Masks

Masks are used for three primary purposes in health care organizations:

1. Placed on health care personnel to protect them from contact with infectious material from patients
2. Placed on health care personnel when engaged in procedures requiring a sterile technique to protect patients from exposure to infectious agents carried in a health care worker's mouth or nose
3. Placed on coughing patients to limit potential dissemination of infectious respiratory secretions from the patient to others (i.e., respiratory hygiene and cough etiquette)

Masks may be used in combination with protective eyewear to protect the mouth, nose, and eyes. Alternatively, a face shield may be used to provide a complete protection for the face. Masks come in various shapes (e.g., molded and nonmolded), sizes, filtration efficiency, and method of attachment (e.g., ties, elastic, ear loops). Health care organizations may find that different types of masks are needed to meet individual health care personnel needs.[7]

Protective Eyewear

Infectious pathogens can be transmitted through various mechanisms; among these are infections introduced through the mucous membranes of the eye (conjunc-

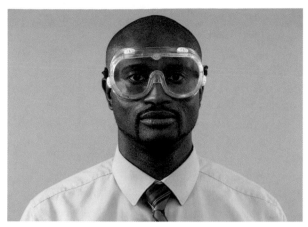

FIGURE 7.4 Safety goggles should protect the tops, sides, and bottoms of the employee's orbit.

tiva). Therefore, OSHA mandates that masks be worn in combination with eye protection devices, such as goggles, glasses with solid side shields, or chin-length face shields, whenever splashes, spray, spatter, or droplets of blood or OPIMs may be generated or when eye, nose, or mouth contamination can be reasonably anticipated.[2] The type of protective eyewear chosen (e.g., goggles or face shield) depends on the circumstances of exposure, other PPE used, and personal vision needs.[7]

Personal prescription eyewear does not provide optimal eye protection, and should not be used as a substitute for protective eyewear.[10] Professionals who use prescription eyewear should wear either prescription safety glasses or goggles that fit snugly over personal prescription lenses (figure 7.4). Depending on the organization and occupational risk, athletic trainers may have access to disposable eyewear and nondisposable eye protection.

Gloves

Gloves can protect both patients and health care personnel from exposure to infectious pathogens in the following situations:

- Anticipating direct contact with blood or body fluids, mucous membranes, nonintact skin, and other potentially infectious material
- Having direct contact with patients who are colonized or infected with pathogens transmitted by the contact route
- Handling or touching visibly or potentially contaminated patient care equipment and environmental surfaces

Nonsterile, single-use disposable gloves are made of a variety of materials (e.g., latex, vinyl, nitrile). The selection of glove type for nonsurgical use is based on different factors, including tasks to be performed, anticipated contact with chemicals and chemotherapeutic

agents, latex sensitivity, sizing, and facility policies for creating a latex-free environment.[7] Over the years, many health care workers have developed a latex sensitivity; therefore, latex gloves are no longer recommended (NIOSH Latex Allergy Prevention Guide).[11] Nitrile gloves are preferable for clinical procedures requiring manual dexterity that involve more than brief patient contact. Before donning nonsterile, single-use disposable gloves, consider covering open wounds or sores and remove any jewelry that might pierce the gloves. After donning the gloves, inspect them for tears. If gloves become torn or punctured while you are working with a patient, remove and replace them as soon as possible.

It may be necessary to change gloves during the care of a single patient to prevent cross contamination. It also may be necessary to change gloves if the patient interaction also involves touching equipment that may lead to indirect contact. Discarding gloves between patients is necessary to prevent transmission of infectious material. Remember to discard gloves in the nearest appropriate receptacle based on the ECP. Gloves must not be washed or decontaminated for reuse because microorganisms cannot be removed reliably from glove surfaces and continued glove integrity cannot be ensured.

Barrier Devices

Barriers such as resuscitation masks, face shields, and bag valve masks (or bag valve devices) limit exposure to blood, body fluids, secretions, and vomitus by provider mouth-to-mask, mouth-to-barrier ventilation. Barrier devices are safe, simple, and efficient in the hands of a basic-trained rescuer. The use of a mouth-to-mask ventilation device is recommended for out-of-hospital ventilation by a single rescuer, and the device should be part of the rescuer's standard equipment. When used by basic-trained rescuers, mouth-to-mask ventilation devices fulfill the requirements of safe, simple, and efficient care.[12] Bag-valve mask ventilation is efficient if performed by well-trained rescuers, but it leads to a low ventilation quality in the hands of a less experienced rescuer. It should be emphasized that regular training every 6 to 12 months is necessary to perform proper ventilation.[12] The bag valve mask with a HEPA filter is the device of choice when treating a patient with a potential respiratory condition as it further limits the risk of exposure for the rescuer. Athletic trainers are urged to have bag valve masks as part of their standard emergency care equipment. These devices are intended for one-time use on a specific patient and should be properly disposed of once they have been used.

Personal Hygiene

As previously stated, health care organizations should provide handwashing facilities that are readily accessible

FOUNDATIONAL SKILL

Removing Protective Gloves

1. With both hands gloved, (figure 7.5a) grasp one glove near the cuff and (figure 7.5b) pull the glove from the wrist toward your fingertips until it folds over. Be careful not to touch bare skin when reaching inside of the glove.

2. Carefully grasp the fold of the glove and pull the glove away from your body until it is pulled off of your fingertips, turning the glove inside out (figure 7.5c). Be careful not to flip any particles from the glove as it is removed.

3. Place and hold the removed glove in the palm of your gloved hand (figure 7.5d). Keep it wadded up as much as possible so as to more easily complete steps 4 and 5.

4. Using the ungloved hand, carefully insert two fingers into the cuff of the gloved hand (figure 7.5e). Slide your fingers under the glove and toward your fingertips until the glove folds over, then turn the glove inside out while also encasing the other contaminated glove (figure 7.5f). Avoid touching the outside of the glove.

5. Grasp the fold of the glove and fully remove it from your hand (figure 7.5g). Be careful not to flip any particles that may contaminate the area. Many germs are spread when personal protective equipment is removed.

6. Properly dispose of the gloves. Do not contaminate trash areas, especially when handling harmful substances or chemicals.

7. Thoroughly wash your hands with soap and water to ensure that any contamination from the glove removal is eliminated.

Note: Extra disposable gloves should be available, and gloves should always be changed between patients.

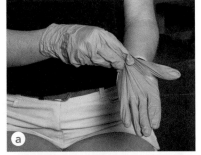

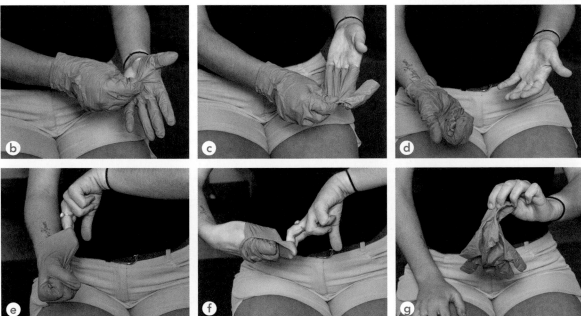

FIGURE 7.5   Glove removal steps.

Reprinted by permission from M. Cleary and K. Walsh Flanagan, *Acute and Emergency Care in Athletic Training* (Champaign, IL: Human Kinetics, 2020), 37.

to employees. A **handwashing facility** provides an adequate supply of running potable water, soap, and single-use towels or air-drying machines.[2] Keeping hands clean through improved hand hygiene is one of the most important steps taken to avoid getting sick and spreading germs to others.[13] Personal hygiene (i.e., handwashing) is believed to help in reducing the transmission of infectious pathogens[14] and health care–associated infections.[13,15]

Handwashing, which is defined as washing hands with soap and water, is indicated before making contact with patients and donning gloves and after contact with any intact skin, body fluids or excretions, nonintact skin, or wound dressings, as well as after removal of disposable gloves.[13] Handwashing is recommended in the following situations:

FOUNDATIONAL SKILL

Handwashing

Here are the steps for properly washing your hands (figure 7.6):

1. Remove all jewelry.
2. Wet hands with clean, running water (warm or cold), turn off the tap, and apply soap.
3. Lather hands by rubbing them together with the soap. Be sure to lather the backs of the hands, the fingers, and under the nails.
4. Scrub hands for at least 20 seconds. Need a timer? Hum the "Happy Birthday" song from beginning to end twice.
5. Rinse hands well under clean, running water.
6. Dry hands using a clean towel or air-dry them.

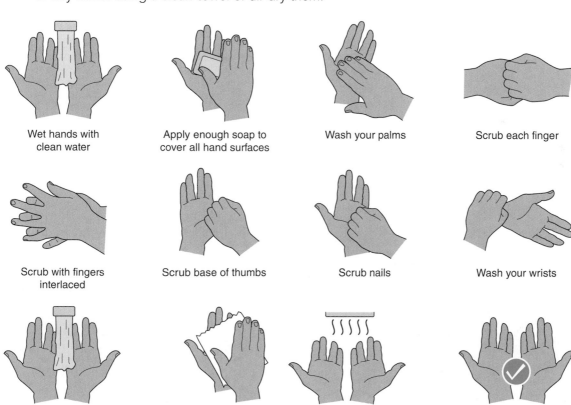

Wet hands with clean water

Apply enough soap to cover all hand surfaces

Wash your palms

Scrub each finger

Scrub with fingers interlaced

Scrub base of thumbs

Scrub nails

Wash your wrists

Rinse off soap with clean water

Dry hands with towel, tissue, or dryer

Hands are clean

FIGURE 7.6 Handwashing steps.

Adapted from Centers for Disease Control and Prevention (2002).

- Before, during, and after preparing food
- Before eating food
- Before and after caring for someone who is sick
- Before and after treating a cut or wound
- After using the toilet, changing diapers, or cleaning up a child who has used the toilet
- After blowing your nose, coughing, or sneezing
- After touching an animal, animal feed, or animal waste
- After handling pet food or pet treats
- After touching garbage or taking out the trash

Washing hands with soap and water is the best way to reduce the number of germs on them in most situations.

If soap and water are not available, use an alcohol-based hand sanitizer containing at least 60% alcohol.

Allow the hand sanitizer to air-dry on your hands and avoid removing excess hand sanitizer with a towel. Alcohol-based hand sanitizers can quickly reduce the number of germs on the hands in some situations, but sanitizers do not eliminate all types of germs and might not remove harmful chemicals.

Housekeeping

According to OSHA, organizations should ensure that the worksite is maintained in a clean and sanitary condition. The organization should determine and implement a plan with an appropriate written schedule for cleaning and the method of decontamination based on the location within the facility, type of surface to be cleaned, type of soil present, and tasks or procedures being performed in the area.[2]

EVIDENCE-BASED ATHLETIC TRAINING

Hand Sanitizers

Studies have found that sanitizers with an alcohol concentration between 60% and 95% are more effective at killing germs than those with a lower alcohol concentration or non-alcohol-based hand sanitizers.[16,17] Non-alcohol-based hand sanitizers may not work equally well for all classes of germs, cause germs to develop resistance to the sanitizing agent, merely reduce the growth of germs rather than destroy them outright, or be more likely to irritate skin than alcohol-based hand sanitizers.[16,17]

Although alcohol-based hand sanitizers can inactivate many types of microbes very effectively when used correctly,[18] people may not use a large enough volume of the sanitizer or may wipe it off before it has dried.[16] Furthermore, soap and water are more effective than hand sanitizers at removing or inactivating certain kinds of germs.

Note that many studies show that hand sanitizers work well in clinical settings like hospitals, where hands come into contact with germs but are not heavily soiled or greasy. However, hands may become very greasy or soiled in community settings, such as after people handle food, play sports, work in the garden, or go camping or fishing. When hands are heavily soiled or greasy, hand sanitizers may not work well; handwashing with soap and water is recommended in such circumstances.[13]

EVIDENCE-BASED ATHLETIC TRAINING

NATA Position Statements

Two NATA position statements are important to consider when reviewing and updating an organization's policies and procedures related to blood-borne pathogens and infection control. The first is the NATA position statement on skin diseases, which addresses many important aspects of infection control for the athletic trainer.[19] This includes housekeeping and hygiene practices that should be included in the policy and procedure manual to prevent the spread of disease. The statement also addresses education of stakeholders, including administrators, coaches, athletes, and custodial staff, on these important policies. The second NATA position statement, Management of Acute Skin Trauma, lists supplies needed to protect the athletic trainer and patient when dealing with open wounds.[18] Treating acute skin trauma is just one of the many scenarios where athletic trainers need to wear PPE and practice standard precautions.

Warning Labels and Signs

Warning labels must be affixed to containers of regulated waste, refrigerators, and freezers containing blood or OPIMs (figure 7.7) and to other containers used to store, transport, or ship blood or OPIMs. Also, they must meet certain requirements. The organization should post signs at the entrance to work areas recognized by the standard.

Decontamination

Specific procedures and protocols defined by the organization's ECP must be followed on a daily basis by facility employees in accordance with OSHA standards.

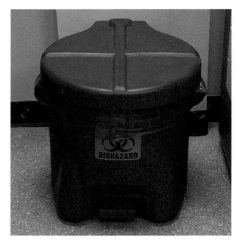

FIGURE 7.7 Proper location of a biohazard warning label.

- All equipment and environmental and working surfaces must be cleaned and decontaminated after contact with blood or other potentially infectious materials.

- Contaminated work surfaces must be decontaminated with an appropriate disinfectant after completion of procedures, immediately or as soon as feasible when surfaces are overtly contaminated or after any spill of blood or OPIMs, and at the end of the work shift if the surface may have become contaminated since the last cleaning.

- Protective coverings, such as plastic wrap, aluminum foil, or imperviously backed absorbent paper used to cover equipment and environmental surfaces, should be removed and replaced as soon as feasible when they become overtly contaminated or at the end of the work shift if they may have become contaminated during the shift.

- All bins, pails, cans, and similar receptacles intended for reuse that have a reasonable likelihood of becoming contaminated with blood or OPIMs must be inspected and decontaminated on a regularly scheduled basis and cleaned and decontaminated immediately or as soon as feasible on visible contamination.

- Broken glassware that may be contaminated must not be picked up directly with the hands. It should be cleaned up using mechanical means, such as a brush and dust pan, tongs, or forceps.

Sharps Containers and Usage Standards

Sharps Containment System
- Easily accessible
- Closable
- Puncture resistant
- Leakproof on sides and bottom
- Labeled or color-coded

Requirements for Use
- Located as close as is feasible to the immediate area where sharps are used or can be reasonably anticipated to be found
- Maintained upright throughout use
- Replaced routinely and not be allowed to overfill
- Closed immediately before removal or replacement to prevent spillage or protrusion of contents during handling, storage, transport, or shipping (when moving containers of contaminated sharps from the area of use)
- Not opened, emptied, or cleaned manually or in any other manner that would expose employees to the risk of percutaneous injury

- Reusable sharps that are contaminated with blood or OPIMs should not be stored or processed in a manner that requires employees to reach by hand into the containers where these sharps have been placed.
- All soiled or contaminated items should be handled using PPE and precautions; decontamination using commercial cleaning solutions should follow the manufacturer's recommendations.

Spill Cleanup

Cleaning and decontamination of spills of blood or OPIMs should be prompt and with observance of standard precautions guidelines by trained people with the appropriate equipment. When a spill occurs, the first, and probably most significant, step is spill containment. Continue cleaning the spill by following the steps in the sidebar Cleaning and Decontamination of Spills of Blood or OPIMs.

Contaminated Laundry

According to OSHA standards, contaminated laundry should be handled as little as possible with a minimum of agitation. The standard goes on to state that handling of contaminated laundry should be done as follows:[21]

- Bag laundry or place it in a container at the location where it was used. Do not sort or rinse laundry in the location of use.
- Place and transport laundry in bags or containers labeled or color-coded in accordance with OSHA standards. When a facility uses universal precautions in the handling of all soiled laundry, alternative labeling or color-coding is sufficient if it permits all employees to recognize the containers as requiring compliance with universal precautions.
- If laundry is wet and presents a reasonable likelihood of soaking through of leaking from the bag or container, place it in bags or containers that prevent soak-through or leakage of fluids to the exterior.
- Use protective gloves and other appropriate PPE whenever handling contaminated laundry.

Exposure Incident

An exposure incident occurs when a provider experiences a "specific eye, mouth, other mucous membrane, non-intact skin, or parenteral contact with blood or other potentially infectious materials that result from the performance of an employee's duties,"[2] often as a result of a needlestick, sharps injury, or improper or faulty PPE usage. When an exposure occurs, follow these postexposure recommendations and, more importantly, the organization's ECP.[2]

- Remain calm. Wash the needlestick, sharps wound, and any remnants of blood or OPIMs with soap and water.
- Flush splashes of blood or OPIMs reaching the nose, mouth, or skin with tap water.
- Flush splashes of blood or OPIMs to the eyes with clean water, saline, or sterile irrigation solution from the inside out.

FOUNDATIONAL SKILL

Cleaning and Decontamination of Spills of Blood or OPIMs

1. Don gloves, at a minimum. If there is potential for splashing, consider donning a gown, mask, protective eyewear, and gloves (in this order).
2. Soak up blood or OPIMs using any absorbent material (paper towels, cloth towels) or commercially designed hazardous material containment kits. Large, sharp objects (i.e., glass) should be removed using tongs or other devices that limit risk.
3. Place the contaminated sharps waste in a sharps container.
4. Wet the surface using a ratio of 1-1/2 cups (350 mL) liquid chlorine bleach to 1 gal (4 L) of freshwater solution (1 part bleach per 9 parts water, or about a 10% solution) or a disinfectant approved by the Environmental Protection Agency for 10 minutes.
5. Soak up the solution using an absorbent material or commercially designed hazardous material containment kits.
6. Place the contaminated waste in a properly labeled or color-coded container.
7. Let the area air-dry. Dispose of any PPE in a properly labeled or color-coded container.
8. Wash hands.

- Immediately report the incident to the department supervisor responsible for managing exposure incidents. Prompt reporting is essential, since postexposure treatment may be necessary and should be started as soon as possible.

- Immediately seek confidential medical evaluation and treatment from a licensed health care provider, following the recommended guidelines established by your facility's ECP. This medical care should be provided free of charge. Medical treatment may include postexposure prophylactic medication and counseling, which includes recommendations for avoiding transmission and prevention of HIV. All medical treatments prescribed should follow appropriate current U.S. Public Health Service recommendations.

- Within 15 days, you will receive a copy of the physician's written opinion of your medical evaluation. The report will identify whether an HBV vaccination was recommended and whether or not you received the HBV vaccination or were informed of any medical conditions resulting from exposure to blood that require further evaluation or treatment.

All work-related needlestick injuries and cuts from sharp objects that are contaminated with another person's blood or OPIMs must be recorded. The case information must be recorded on the OSHA 300 Log as an injury. All incident reports must include at least the following:

- Date of the injury
- Type and brand of the device involved (syringe, suture needle)
- Department or work area where the incident occurred
- Explanation of how the incident occurred

Prompt reporting of an exposure incident or needlestick is also important for several other reasons.[22] It helps prevent the spread of blood-borne infection between other providers and family and friends. Reporting an exposure allows for testing of the blood of the source person to determine HBV and HIV infectivity if his status is unknown and he grants permission for testing. As the exposed employee, you have the right to be informed of any tests results regarding the source person.

Training

OSHA's mission is to prevent workplace deaths, injuries, and illnesses. Organizations seeking to fulfill OSHA's mission often also strive to create a culture of safety. An organizational culture of safety is created through the following:[7]

- The actions management takes to improve patient and personnel safety
- Personnel participation in safety planning
- The availability of appropriate protective equipment
- Influence of group norms regarding acceptable safety practices
- The organization's socialization process for new personnel

Organizational education or training is a key standard addressed under OSHA. OSHA states that organizations must train each employee about occupational exposure during working hours at no cost to the employee. The person conducting the training session must be knowledgeable about the covered subject matter as it relates to the workplace and provide opportunity for interactive questions and answers with the providers.

CLINICAL BOTTOM LINE

- OSHA standards are not an option; they are required for all health care professionals in all settings. Athletic trainers should work with their supervising physician, administration, and custodial staff to make sure all requirements are met.

- The OSHA standards require employers and employees to consider the ECP, SPs, engineering and work practice controls, PPE, housekeeping, vaccinations, postexposure follow-up, training, and record keeping when preparing and implementing their policies and procedures.

- Athletic trainers should be knowledgeable about potential blood-borne pathogens, their routes of transmission, and how to prevent exposure in the workplace.

 Go to HK*Propel* to complete the activities and case studies for this chapter.

Go to HK*Propel* to (1) view a video of proper exam glove removal and (2) download foundational skill check sheets for removing protective gloves and properly washing your hands.

CHAPTER 8

Prevention Strategies and Procedures

Ellen K. Payne, PhD, LAT, ATC, EMT

CAATE STANDARDS

The following CAATE 2020 standards are covered in this chapter:

Standard 70

Standard 81

Standard 83

Standard 85

CHAPTER OBJECTIVES

After reading this chapter, you will be able to do the following:

- Summarize the goals and objectives of the preparticipation examination (PPE)

- Explain the types of PPEs and the required and recommended components

- Identify important resources to use when planning and implementing PPEs

- Describe the referral process and decision making with potentially disqualifying conditions

- Summarize thermoregulatory mechanisms within the body

- Discuss methods for preventing heat-related illnesses

- Discuss methods for preventing cold-related conditions

- Discuss ways to prevent lightning-related deaths or injuries during outdoor activities

- Summarize the principles of ergonomics and its importance in injury prevention

Prevention of injuries and sports-related illnesses and conditions is an essential component of an athletic trainer's job duties and responsibilities. Prevention is a skill that differentiates athletic trainers from other health care providers who work with patients only after illness or injury has occurred. It is such an important aspect of an athletic trainer's daily responsibilities that it encompasses all of Domain I of the Board of Certification's Practice Analysis.[1] Several chapters in this textbook cover different aspects of injury and illness prevention:

- Chapter 7: Blood-Borne Pathogens
  - Provides information on preventing disease transmission
- Chapter 10: General Nutrition Concepts and Sports Nutrition
  - Discusses the role of diet in injury and illness prevention and provides information on disordered eating
- Chapter 11: Protective Equipment
  - Addresses the role of various protective equipment in injury prevention
- Chapter 12: Taping and Bracing
  - Addresses the role of taping, wrapping, and bracing in injury prevention

- Chapter 13: Emergency Planning in Health Care
  - Discusses the role of emergency planning in preventing injuries and provides details about how to create an emergency action plan (EAP)

This chapter focuses on prevention through the use of preparticipation examinations, environmental illness prevention programs, and ergonomics. Although not all injuries and illnesses can be prevented, the items addressed in this chapter can greatly help mitigate the risk of many injuries and illnesses common in athletic training.

Preparticipation Physical Examination

The **preparticipation physical examination** (PPE) is one of the most commonly used mechanisms in the recognition and prevention of potential injuries and illnesses in the athletic population. In general, PPEs serve two main functions:

1. Protecting the athlete
2. Protecting the organization

A thorough and complete PPE allows the athletic trainer and other members of the health care team to identify people with preexisting injuries or conditions and those at risk for a vast array of potential injuries or conditions through sports participation. This identification allows potential red flags to be addressed prior to participation and other, less severe items to be addressed before they turn into something serious. PPEs also assess the athlete's readiness for activity through fitness testing and a general health screening. Again, potential issues such as lack of aerobic fitness can be addressed early, before an injury occurs. Lastly, PPEs help protect the organization, limiting liability for the athletic trainer, team physician, and the organization's administration. PPEs can serve as a time for athletes to receive information on a variety of health-related topics and sign waivers or assumption of risk forms if necessary. The purpose of the PPE is to "facilitate and encourage safe participation, not exclude athletes from participation."[2]

Typically, the PPE is conducted in one of two ways:

1. *Individual office visit.* Office visit PPEs are done one athlete at a time, usually directly scheduled with the physician by the patient or his parent or guardian. The PPE can be conducted by the team physician or the family's personal physician (or health care home). The individual office visit at the athlete's health care home is the recommended location and method for conducting PPEs.[2]

2. *Group-based assessments.* Group-based assessments can be used when the medical team has full access to the athlete's complete medical records[2]—for example, in college athletics. This method can also be used on a limited basis for secondary school athletes who do not have access to a primary care physician or a health care home. Group-based assessments are conducted with a team approach, which allows physicians, athletic trainers, nurses, and other health care providers to assist in the process. A recommendation for group-based physicals is that providers complete the entire physical examination on the athletes they see as opposed to working a station and examining athletes in the assembly-line fashion seen in many old-school PPEs.[2,3] The one-provider approach allows for the possibility of building a rapport with the athlete, which can help athletes be honest when answering the provider's questions. It also allows for continuity during the evaluation, which can help the provider identify and link any abnormal findings that present across components.

Table 8.1 outlines the advantages and disadvantages of each approach.

Both types of PPEs have advantages and disadvantages. Station-based examinations, or mass physicals, conducted in the school's gymnasium or locker rooms are not recommended because of privacy issues and lack of access to athletes' complete medical records. Individual office visit physicals conducted at an urgent care or retail medical facility are also not recommended because the physician and other health care providers do not have access to the athlete's complete health histories and other pertinent information for making decisions.

Whenever possible, the institution's required PPE forms should be made available to parents and guardians

Goals of the PPE

- Assess and determine general physical and psychological health
- Identify any potentially life-threatening or disabling conditions
- Identify other conditions that could alter performance
- Obtain baseline data, including vital signs and fitness testing
- Provide an opportunity to educate athletes on health-related topics
- Satisfy liability and insurance requirements

TABLE 8.1   **Advantages and Disadvantages of Individual Office Visits and Group-Based PPEs**

	Individual office visits	Group-based assessments
Advantages	• Private visit • Previous relationship with primary care physician • Continuity of care	• Lower cost • Physicians are familiar with sport requirements • May have some specialist on site for immediate referral
Disadvantages	• More expensive • Typically not fully covered by insurance • Physician may not be familiar with sport requirements • Not all athletes have a primary care physician or health care home	• Lack of privacy • Athletes can be uncomfortable discussing personal topics in this setting • Lack of continuity of care

Based on Bernhardt and Roberts (2019); Walsh Flanagan and Cuppett (2017); Conley et al. (2014); Lehman and Carl (2017).

prior to the PPE appointment. This allows them time to thoroughly complete the medical history component with the athletes in advance.[6] It also gives parents and guardians an opportunity to complete any insurance information. Ideally, these are electronic forms.

The PPE should be completed by a physician (MD or DO) or advanced practice provider (nurse practitioner or physician assistant) in conjunction with other health care providers as needed.[2] Some states or organizations require that the form be signed by a physician, while others allow other health care providers to complete the PPE.[7] Regardless of who conducts the PPE and signs the form, clearance decisions are ultimately made by the organization's team physician.

Components of a PPE

The PPE format includes a focused systems-based history and physical examination with specific history questions and other components for identifying issues that are known to affect sports performance and participation. No matter where or by whom the PPE is conducted, it should contain the following components:

Medical History
- Personal history
- Family history
- Wellness questions

Physical Examinations
- Medical examination
- Cardiovascular screening
- Orthopedic screening
- Wellness screening

When conducted as a group-based PPE, these components can be further divided into the following items:

- Registration
- Vitals station
  - Height and weight
  - Vital signs
  - Vision screening
- General medical examination
  - History review
  - Physical examination
- Specialty examination
  - Orthopedic assessment
  - Other system-based examination
- Optional additional components (see following list)

Organizations often add components to meet their needs:

- **Baseline concussion testing**
- Body composition assessment
- Fitness testing
  - Flexibility and range of motion
  - Aerobic capacity
  - Anaerobic capacity
  - Strength testing
- Drug testing (performance enhancing or recreational)
- Blood analysis
- Electrocardiograms (ECG)

History

The history component of the PPE form and examination is one of the most important aspects.[2,11] The form must be thoroughly completed by the patient and her parent or

EVIDENCE-BASED ATHLETIC TRAINING

Important Resources for Planning and Implementing PPEs

Many resources are available for athletic trainers who are planning and implementing PPEs for their organizations.

PPE Monograph

The *PPE: Preparticipation Physical Evaluation,* also known as the PPE monograph,[2] is a comprehensive document that includes detailed referenced information on the following:

- Organization and administration of the PPE
- System-based physical examination
- Special population considerations
- Determining clearance
- Working with athletes with special needs
- Examples of forms (now in both English and Spanish)

The goal of this document is to help standardize the PPE process among providers and organizations. The PPE monograph was authored in collaboration with the American Academy of Family Physicians, American Academy of Pediatrics, American College of Sports Medicine, American Medical Society for Sports Medicine, American Orthopaedic Society for Sports Medicine, and American Osteopathic Academy of Sports Medicine. The PPE monograph is the primary resource for all physicians, athletic trainers, and other health care providers involved with PPEs.

NATA Position Statement

Another important resource to refer to when planning PPEs is the NATA position statement Preparticipation Physical Examinations and Disqualifying Conditions.[5] This document outlines PPEs from an athletic trainer's perspective and provides recommendations for conducting PPEs, along with the research justifying the recommendations. It includes research and recommendations to consider when planning and conducting PPEs.

IOC Consensus Statement

Although most athletic trainers are not working day-to-day with Olympic level athletes, the International Olympic Committee (IOC) consensus statement on periodic health evaluation of elite athletes provides information on PPE or periodic health evaluation (PHE) at that level of athletics.[8] An interesting difference is the committee's recommendation for **electrocardiograms (ECG)**. This could be partly due to the difference in the international population and the risk factors for sudden cardiac death, which are currently not present in the U.S. population.[3,8-10] The committee did not endorse the use of routine echocardiograms or other testing as part of the routine physical examination. Another difference is the recommendation for routine **urinalysis** and iron testing (for female athletes) during the examination. When examining the difference between the IOC recommendations and those of other organizations, you should consider the difference in the population screened, resources available during the examination, and the number of athletes screened.

guardian and reviewed by the sports medicine team. This component of the form should include personal medical history, family medical history, and routine wellness questions. As stated previously, access to the athlete's complete medical records is important. This allows for improved accuracy of available medical history. Additionally, a parent or guardian should assist in the thorough completion of the medical history component of the PPE form to ensure the information is as complete and accurate as possible. Although the PPE does not replace an annual physical examination with the athlete's personal physician, the routine wellness questions are important because this may be the only time she sees a health care provider all year.[2,5]

The PPE history component should address the following:

- Questions about general health, mental health, a complete review of systems, and previous musculoskeletal injuries and surgeries
- History questions that address both family and personal history related to cardiovascular health
- A detailed review of concussion history to allow the practitioner to identify athletes at high risk for concussion and to allow for some informational concussion education at this time[11]
- Review of medication and supplementation use (The PPE gives the provider an opportunity to question the athlete about recreational drug or steroid use and discuss banned substances.)
- Nutrition and eating habits[12]
- Mental health status and any appropriate referrals

Physical Examination

The physical examination should include vital signs; vision screening; and cardiovascular, respiratory, neurological, musculoskeletal, dermatological, and general medical screenings. The goal of this examination is to determine if an athlete can safely participate in his chosen sport without undue risk.[3] Depending on how the PPE is conducted, different providers may perform different components of the examination. For example, you may take the athlete's vital signs and the school nurse may be responsible for conducting the vision screening. As discussed earlier, ideally, the same physician should conduct the cardiovascular, neurological, musculoskeletal, and general medical examinations.[2,3] Additional examinations

may be warranted based on the athlete's history such as obtaining a baseline peak flow measurement for an athlete with asthma or other respiratory condition.

The details of the complete physical examination are beyond the scope of this textbook. For details of the system-by-system examination, please refer to recommendations from Miller and colleagues,[3] Lehman and Carl,[6] and Mirabelli and others;[13] for the most comprehensive guideline on the PPE, please refer to the PPE monograph,[2] which contains consensus recommendations endorsed by multiple medical societies.

Additional Components

Beyond the standard recommended physical examination, many organizations add other components to their PPE. Table 8.2 presents a summary of some of the additional components frequently completed during the PPE.

Athlete Education

Athletic trainers or other health care professionals may also use the PPE as a time to provide basic patient education and counseling on a wide variety of health-related topics.[2,3,16] This may be formal or informal education. As an example of formal education, schools may complete state-required concussion education programs in conjunction with PPEs. The school nurse may use this time to informally talk to students about high-risk behaviors and where to seek additional information and help.

Paperwork

The last component of the PPE process is usually a review of paperwork. Athletes and their parents or guardians should complete the following:

Health-Related Topics for Patient Education During the PPE

Here are some health-related topics to discuss during the PPE:[2,3,16]

- Concussions
- Proper nutrition and weight management
- Dietary supplements
- Banned substances
- High-risk behaviors
  - Tobacco use (including vaping)
  - Alcohol use
  - Driving while impaired or distracted
  - Recreational drug use and abuse
  - Unprotected sex
- Mental health
- Sexual health
- Resources available in the community

TABLE 8.2 **Additional PPE Components**

Component	Evidence
Electrocardiograms (ECG) and other noninvasive cardiac screening tests	• ECGs are frequently proposed as a component of PPEs at the secondary and collegiate levels to help detect cardiac abnormalities that could lead to sudden cardiac death. • Due to financial cost and the rate of false positive, ECGs and other tests are not recommended as part of the routine PPE unless there are red flags in the athlete's personal or family history or abnormal findings during the physical examination.[2,3,5,9-11] • This recommendation is different for elite-level athletes. At this level, resources are more abundant and fewer athletes are screened.[8]
Routine blood work and urinalysis	• These are not recommended for all athletes,[2] but have been recommended for elite-level participants.[8] • The NCAA requires all student-athletes to show the results of sickle cell trait test or sign a waiver declining the screening.[14] The NATA position statement also recommends confirming sickle cell trait status in all athletes.[5] Sickle cell trait status is now screened at birth in all 50 states.
Baseline concussion testing	• Baseline testing allows for individualized comparison before and after the head injury score and helps aid in return-to-play decisions. • Both the Standardized Assessment of Concussion (SAC) and the Sport Concussion Assessment Tool version 5 (SCAT5) can be used in baseline testing. Many other options are available as well. • Computerized neurocognitive testing is another option for baseline concussion testing, with ImPACT being the most commonly used.[15] • At the current time, concussion experts do not consider baseline testing mandatory for all athletes.[16] • Whether or not baseline testing occurs during the PPE, obtaining the athlete's medical history related to concussion should be a standard part of the PPE process.
Fitness assessment	• This may involve testing flexibility, range of motion, aerobic capacity, anaerobic capacity, and strength. • This assessment is different from the general musculoskeletal examination performed by the physician during the standard PPE physical examination to determine possible injury or conditions that require follow-up prior to the start of the season. • These are additional components, often assessed by the athletic trainer, strength and conditioning coach, team coach, or another member of the sports medicine team. • One popular component is the Functional Movement Screen (FMS). FMS results are proposed to help predict future injury; therefore, baseline testing during the PPE would allow athletic trainers and strength and conditioning coaches to identify susceptible athletes and work with them before an injury occurs. At this time, the evidence to support the use of FMS to predict injury is mixed.[17,18] No medical organization, including the NATA, recommends FMS screening during the PPE. Letafatkar and colleagues may have summarized it best when they said that "more research is still necessary before implementing the FMS into a pre-participation physical examination (PPE) for athletics, but due to the low cost and its simplicity to implement, it should be considered by clinicians and researchers in the future."[19]

• Emergency contact information
• Insurance information
• Informed consent
• Assumption of risk

• HIPAA or confidentiality release
• Any required waivers

The forms used for the PPE may be mandated by the state secondary school athletic federation or the individual districts if no state mandate exists. For example, Pennsylvania requires that a state form called the Comprehensive Initial Pre-Participation Physical Evaluation (CIPPE) be completed for each athlete. The NCAA does not require a standardized form across member institutions. The decision is left to the discretion of the team physician and the athletic training staff. Many institutions of all levels refer to the PPE monograph for template PPE forms.

PPE-Recommended Guidelines

Beyond the required and recommended components of the PPE, you should take other important recommendations into consideration when planning and implementing PPEs. Each sponsoring organization (e.g., NCAA, state secondary school athletic federation, youth sports league) has different requirements and recommendations for PPEs. No national standards or mandates exist for PPEs, just recommendations from various professional organizations.[2,7] For example, Pennsylvania dictates the timing of and form (CIPPE) used for secondary school physicals. The NCAA also has its own timing recommendations, but it leaves many other aspects of the PPE to the discretion of the team physician and the athletic training staff. Youth sports have no national requirement that PPEs be conducted, but individual teams and leagues may have their own recommendations and requirements.

Timing

Ideally, PPEs should be conducted 4 to 8 weeks prior to the start of the preseason to allow plenty of time for additional testing, follow-up appointments, or treatments if needed.[2,3,5,6] Returning athletes who compete in fall sports could complete the PPE in the late spring before leaving for summer vacation. Then in the summer, PPEs could be offered for new students, including freshman and transfers. Additional PPE dates would be set, following similar guidelines, for winter and spring sport athletes. Realistically, this system is not always feasible. Sometimes PPEs are conducted 1 or 2 days before the start of the preseason. If this is the case, athletes should not be

allowed to participate until the PPE is completed and they have received clearance from the team physician. This may mean a delayed start to the season for that athlete if follow-up appointments are needed.

Frequency

The frequency of the PPE is dictated by state requirements, the level of participation, and league or conference rules. Currently no evidence is available to dictate exactly how frequently PPEs should be conducted.[2] In general, it is recommended that an athlete complete a new PPE at each level of participation. This means when an athlete goes from high school to college, a complete PPE is warranted. Many organizations require an annual PPE, or at least an annual review of the athlete's medical history, vital signs, and any problem areas.

Requirements for PPEs for secondary school sports vary by state. Some states require comprehensive PPEs to be conducted annually, while others allow for just an annual review of the athlete's medical history and vital signs. The NCAA requires new student-athletes to complete a physical when entering the intercollegiate athletic program.[14] After that initial PPE, the NCAA recommends taking an annual updated history and measuring height, weight, and blood pressure. A complete PPE is recommended only for student-athletes with a change in their history or health status. Regardless of the level of participation, insurance information should be updated at least annually and with any changes in coverage.

Interpreting PPE Results and Proper Referral

Red flags raised during the PPE, including affirmative answers to any cardiac screening questions, need additional follow-up. This may be as simple as the team physician reviewing the responses again with the athlete and her parent or guardian, if needed, to clarify a response before the end of the PPE screening. If various specialists attend a group-based physical event, the concern may be addressed during the PPE. For example, an orthopedic surgeon could assess the stability of an athlete's shoulder

PPE Clearance Categories

Clearance is divided into 1 of 5 categories:[2]

1. Cleared with no restrictions
2. Cleared with a recommendation for further evaluation or treatment (e.g., rehabilitation exercise for a previous ankle sprain)
3. Not cleared until additional testing, evaluation, or treatment is complete
4. Not cleared for certain activities or sports
5. Not cleared to participate in any sport or physical activity

and determine if she needs a follow-up appointment or just needs to do strengthening exercises with the athletic trainer. Some PPE findings may also involve referral to the appropriate specialist at a later date. Athletes demonstrating signs of a mental health condition or suspicions of disordered eating should be referred to the appropriate specialist.[12] Athletes with known conditions, such as a heart murmur or diabetes, should also be cleared by the specialists who care for them before they receive clearance to participate. Regardless of whether a red flag is raised, every PPE form should be reviewed by the organization's athletic trainer and team physician prior to determining medical clearance.

The athletic trainer and team physician can assist with referrals to proper specialists for follow-up consultation and ensure there is good communication between all stakeholders. Timing the PPEs well before the start of the sports season allows the athlete to complete a potential referral process without missing the preseason. The team physician, in consultation with the appropriate specialist, has the final say on medically clearing an athlete for participation or lifting any restriction placed on him. It should be noted that clearance is not a static determination; the athlete's clearance level may change based on the status of his condition and the presence of new information. When something arises from the PPE, good communication must be maintained between the team physician, athletic trainer, the athlete, and his parent or guardian, if necessary.[2]

The purpose of the PPE is to help identify potential issues and refer athletes for additional testing and treatment if available, not to disqualify them from participation. That said, some conditions may disqualify certain athletes from certain activities. Your goal is to find the right activity for the athlete based on the medical restrictions placed on him by the specialist and the team physician.[13] For example, certain conditions could limit an athlete's ability to safely play football, but he may be able to play another sport without risk. The team physician and organization have the legal right to restrict an athlete from participating in sports as long as the decision made is based on the best medical evidence available.

An example of a disqualifying condition is the loss of one of a paired organ, which may limit the athlete's involvement in contact and collision sports. Cardiovascular conditions may also limit participation. If diabetes is not controlled properly, it could limit the athlete's participation. The team physician, consulting specialists, and athletic trainer should work with the patient and his parents or guardians as a team to make the best decision for his long-term health. Ultimately, the decision is in the hands of the team physician for the acceptable level of risk that may be taken.

Thermoregulatory Mechanisms

This section was written by Angela Hillman, PhD; Assistant Professor of Exercise Physiology; Ohio University.

Thermoregulation is the body's ability to maintain a normal **core temperature**, which is rigorously maintained at approximately 37°C (99°F). The human body produces heat from physical activity, as well as digestion. Unfortunately, the human body is quite inefficient at producing energy, which results in large amounts of heat production (up to 75% of energy produced). When more heat is produced than is lost through thermoregulation, body temperature rises; hyperthermia results when core body temperature rises over 38°C (100°F).

Thermoregulation is controlled by the hypothalamus, the body's thermostat. When changes in temperature are sensed, the hypothalamus makes necessary changes to maintain core temperature. Messages are sent from the hypothalamus to effector organs, such as skin arterioles, sweat glands, skeletal muscles, and eccrine glands, which results in vasoconstriction or vasodilation, sweating, shivering, or changes in metabolism based on the direction of core temperature change.

Maintaining core body temperature is a delicate balance of heat exchange as the body tries to match losses with gains. Table 8.3 provides examples of each portion of the heat exchange paradigm. Evaporative cooling is the most important form of thermoregulation for humans.

TABLE 8.3 **Heat Exchange**

	Definition	Heat gain	Heat loss
Radiation	Heat loss or gain from a warmer to cooler body or environment	Standing outside in direct sunlight	Being in a room cooler than your body temperature
Conduction	Being in direct contact with a surface	Standing on a blacktop or a turf field	Wearing an ice vest or ice pack against the body
Convection	Movement of air molecules across the surface of your body	Sitting in front of a fire or space heater	Being in front of a fan or outside with a breeze
Evaporation	Heat loss through water vapor on the skin's surface	N/A: Heat is only lost through evaporation.	Sweating

Without it, body temperatures can rise to dangerous levels and be potentially fatal.

The effectiveness of these methods for heat loss depends on a number of factors, including the **thermal gradient**, or the difference in the temperature of the environment and the body. Marathons are typically run in the fall and spring in early morning because the thermal gradient is greater, allowing for better thermoregulation by the participants. Similarly, lower humidity levels allow for greater evaporative cooling; therefore, **relative humidity** is an important factor. Air movement and evaporation lead to better cooling and the degree of direct sunlight affects the amount of radiant heat gain. Finally, clothing is an often overlooked yet important factor for maintaining thermoregulation, especially during exercise. When exercising in the heat, it is important to wear comfortable, breathable clothing that allows for evaporative and convective heat loss, while also minimizing radiant and conductive heat gain.[20]

Hyperthermia

This section was written by Angela Hillman, PhD; Assistant Professor of Exercise Physiology; Ohio University.

Hyperthermia, or elevated core temperature, poses a serious challenge to the body's cardiovascular system. During exercise, particularly in warm environments, sweating results in the loss of fluid from the blood (dehydration). Sweating is the most important way for the human body to maintain thermoregulation. Sweating demands that blood flow be directed to the skin (vasodilation); however, exercise also demands that blood flow be directed to the muscles. During exercise in warm environments, dehydration leads to decreases in skin blood flow and sweating.[21,22] A subconscious decision is made to either maintain sweating or exercise capacity, and we know that exercise performance is compromised with dehydration, even when people are unaware of their hydration level.[23] However, at a certain point after prolonged exercise, the body will stop sweating in order to maintain cardiac output, which can lead to heat stroke.

Many factors affect the way the cardiovascular system responds to exercise in hyperthermic environments. Two of the most important factors are fitness level and acclimatization, which provide many of the same benefits. People with higher fitness levels have lower resting and preexercise core temperatures[24] and heart rates, as well as greater plasma volume.[25] In addition, people who are more fit begin sweating sooner, have higher sweat rates, and can maintain these sweat rates for longer.[26] Many of these fitness-related adaptations can also be conferred on an athlete through **acclimatization**. Additional factors affecting hyperthermia include body composition and hydration. Higher body fat percentage results in lower skin temperature[27] and thus may lead to greater heat stor-

age. Finally, hydration is a key component in maintaining plasma volume for sweating and should be considered on an individual basis.

Prevention of Hyperthermia

Prevention of hyperthermia, rather than treatment, should be the primary focus of athletes, athletic trainers, and coaches. A number of preventive strategies are useful for preparing athletes for exercising in hyperthermic environments:

- Ensuring baseline fitness
- Acclimatization
- Avoiding high-risk conditions
- Maintaining hydration

As noted previously, higher fitness levels afford people with better thermoregulatory mechanisms to deal with hyperthermia. This is one of the reasons athletes should condition prior to the start of official preseason practice in the summer. Following attainment of a baseline level of fitness, acclimatization should be used for athletes who intend to compete in the heat. Acclimatization should be a gradual progression of exposure to and exercise in the heat for 7 to 14 days[28,29] under the direction of trained personnel who monitor the athlete's core temperature and sweat rates (see figure 8.1).

In addition to the benefits provided by fitness level, heat acclimatization also matches fluid needs with thirst.[26] Avoidance of high-risk situations, including providing cooling stations when wet-bulb globe temperatures (WBGTs) are above 30°C (86°F) and limiting exposure when WBGTs are above 33.4°C (92.1°F), are all important components of preventing heat illness.[31] WBGT guidelines should be region specific and based on the following criteria:

- Environmental conditions
- Intensity of activity
- Heat-acclimatization status
- Equipment and clothing
- Fitness of the athlete
- Age of participant

See table 8.4 for an example of WBGT guidelines.

Heat-related conditions can be prevented with careful planning, weather monitoring, and stakeholder education. Chapter 14 addresses the emergency care steps for athletes suffering from heat illness.

Hydration

Maintaining **hydration** is key for conserving evaporative heat loss; however, many factors can influence hydration, including caloric and carbohydrate content, temperature,

Area of practice modification	Practices 1-5		Practices 6-14
	Days 1-2	Days 3-5	
# of practices permitted per day	1		2, only every other day
Equipment	Helmets only	Helmets and shoulder pads	Full equipment
Maximum duration of single practice session	3 hours		3 hours (a total maximum of 5 hours on double session days)
Permitted walk-through time	1 hour (but must be separated from practice by 3 continuous hours)		
Contact	No contact	Contact only with blocking sleds or dummies	Full, 100% live contact drills

FIGURE 8.1 Preseason heat-acclimatization guidelines. Note: Warm-up, stretching, cool-down, walk-through, conditioning, and weight room activities are included as part of practice time.

Reprinted by permission from Korey Stringer Institute, "Heat acclimatization." https://ksi.uconn.edu/prevention/heat-acclimatization.

TABLE 8.4 Example of Wet-Bulb Globe Temperature Guidelines and Activity Guidelines*

WBGT reading	Rest or break guidelines
Under 82.08°F (27.88°C)	Normal activities: Provide three separate rest breaks per hour of at least 3 min each during workout.
82.0°F to 86.98°F (27.88°C to 30.58°C)	Use discretion for intense or prolonged exercise. Watch at-risk players carefully. Provide three separate rest breaks per hour of at least 4 min each.
87.08°F to 89.98°F (30.58°C to 32.28°C)	Maximum practice time should be under 2 hr. For football: Players are restricted to helmet, shoulder pads, and shorts during practice. All protective equipment must be removed for conditioning activities. For all sports: Provide four separate rest breaks per hour of at least 4 min each.
90.0°F to 92.08°F (32.28°C to 33.38°C)	Maximum practice time should be under 1 hr. No protective equipment may be worn during practice. No conditioning activities should be done. Provide at least 20 min of rest breaks during the hour of practice.
Over 92.18°F (33.48°C)	Cancel exercise and outdoor workouts. Delay practices until a cooler WBGT reading occurs.

*This example originates from Georgia High School Athletics Association wet-bulb globe temperature guidelines. It is applicable only for those who practice, condition, train, or compete under similar environmental conditions.

Based on Casa et al. (2015): Korey Stringer Institute; Georgia High School Association.

and **gastric emptying** rate. Sweat rates can range from 1 to 2 L/hr.[37] Unfortunately, human gastric emptying rate is only approximately 1 to 1.2 L/hr at maximum; therefore, at the highest sweat and gastric emptying rates, it becomes impossible for the person sweating to replace fluid losses without developing **dehydration**. Various studies have shown that athletes are already dehydrated at the start of their activity.[25,38-40] Even when fueled optimally, if athletes

ignore their water consumption, their performance can be jeopardized, and the risk of heat-related injury increases. To prevent heat-related illnesses, athletes must drink plenty of fluid before, during, and after physical activity; avoid over exercising in hot weather; and stop exercising at any sign of heat exhaustion.[35]

Fluid replacement is a modifiable factor that can reduce the risk of developing heat illness. Ideally, athletes should strive to maintain **euhydration**, with body mass losses of less than 2% during exercise.[35] The easiest method for assessing hydration is to measure body mass before and after exercise.[41] Using a sweat rate calculator based on these body mass changes provides athletes with the volume of fluid that should be replaced during activity. Changes in body mass should be measured on a regular basis, since values from three consecutive days are needed to establish a baseline.[42] In addition to weight changes, urine color charts are frequently used by athletes to assess hydration. These charts were developed and validated as a field assessment of hydration,[43] and appear to be valid during hyperthermic exercise.[44] Although assessment of urine color has some flaws, this method is very easy for athletes to use (see figure 8.2). The best advice is any shade darker than that of a yellow crayon may indicate that the athlete will start to experience fatigue, impaired performance, muscle cramping, and increased risk for heat injury. To prevent hyponatremia, a clear shade of urine is not required. However, to increase accuracy, athletes should also measure urine specific gravity (USG) and monitor the number of voids in a day.[45]

Urine Color Chart

Hydrated

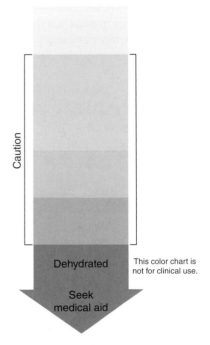

FIGURE 8.2   Urine color chart.

Pre- and postactivity weight checks are one of the best ways to monitor hydration status for both levels of dehydration and overhydration. The weight lost or gained during activity can be directly associated to fluid lost or gained (respectively) from their body. For every 1 lb (.5 kg) lost, athletes will require 16 to 24 fl oz (475-710 mL) of fluid to replace their weight. Again, weight loss up to 2% body water is appropriate. As mentioned previously, athletes should never gain weight during sport. Athletes who gain weight between weight checks are drinking too much and need to be educated on the dangers of hyponatremia.

To avoid developing hyponatremia, athletes must maintain hydration by consuming fluids more frequently rather than trying to replace large amounts of fluid loss all at once. **Hyponatremia**, or low blood sodium levels (<135 mEq/L), is a potentially fatal condition that can occur in athletes such as long-distance runners and cyclists, rowers, American football players, and members of the military,[46] particularly when **hyperhydration** occurs prior to or during exercise. Many of the symptoms of hyponatremia can be similar to those of dehydration. Athletes may confuse headaches and muscle cramping for signs of dehydration and make the serious error of drinking even more water. There have been episodes of athletes drinking 2 gal (8 L) of water and 2 gal of Gatorade after a single practice, which ended in hyponatremia and death.[47] A timely diagnosis and quick treatment are the two main components to successful treatment of hyponatremia. These patients should be referred for a higher level of care immediately.

Athletic trainers must be able to tell the difference between dehydration and overhydration, since patients' lives hang in the balance.[35] Although this chapter provides general hydration guidelines, athletic trainers should individualize hydration strategies for each client and each practice or game environment. Two great practical places to start in educating clients on managing their hydration status are pre- and postactivity body weight checks and urine color.

Hypothermia and Cold-Related Conditions

Cold-related injuries and conditions seem to get less attention in the medical literature and media than heat-related conditions, but they can be a serious threat to the health and safety of athletes. Depending on the location, some athletic trainers may see more practice and competition days with the possibility of a cold-related complication than a heat-related problem. For example, in the northeastern United States, spring sports such as lacrosse start practicing outside in January or February when the weather is still wintry.

EVIDENCE-BASED ATHLETIC TRAINING

Prevention of Heat Illnesses

Here is a summary of ways to help prevent heat-related conditions in athletes:[28,31,34-36]

- Identify at-risk people during PPEs:
  - People with larger muscle mass
  - People with a previous history of heat related illnesses
  - People taking certain medications or supplements
  - People who are not physically fit
  - Overweight people
  - People with sickle cell trait
- Withhold an athlete who has a fever, viral infection, serious rash, or other illness or condition that could make her more prone to heat illness until the condition has fully resolved.
- Ensure proper hydration and nutrition.
- Ensure adequate rest and sleep.
- Make sure proper acclimatization steps are taken.
- Monitor the weather and adjust practice and competitions as needed.
  - Assess the WBGT at the specific practice or competition site using a digital heat stress monitor (figure 8.3) or calculating it (see Foundation Skill).
- Ensure athletes are wearing the proper attire for the weather and adjusting their attire and equipment based on the weather.
  - Athletes should wear loose-fitting, lightweight, and light-colored clothing.
  - Limit practice in helmet and shoulder pads when the weather is hot and humid.
- Monitor all athletes, but especially those at higher risk, for the signs and symptoms of heat illness.
- Ensure medical staff are onsite during conditioning, practices, and games.
- Onsite medical staff should have the authority to alter schedules or practices, including increasing rest breaks, changing practice time, reducing equipment worn during practice, and withholding certain people from practice based on medical conditions or environmental conditions.
- Create guidelines for outdoor practices and competitions during heat and humidity.
- Ensure the organization's EAP is up to date and that all involved personnel are aware of their role in implementing it.
- Educate coaches, administrators, parents, and athletes on heat-related conditions (early identification) and the organization's policies related to heat and activity.

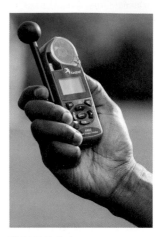

FIGURE 8.3   Heat stress monitor.

FOUNDATIONAL SKILL

Calculating WBGT

The formula for calculating WBGT is as follows:

$$WBGT = 0.7\,TW + 0.2\,TG + 0.1\,TD$$

TW = wet bulb temperature, which indicates humidity

TG = globe temperature, which indicates radiant heat

TD = ambient air (dry) temperature

The body is good at producing heat, and most activity allows for adequate heat production and dissipation. Problems arise when heat loss exceeds the heat production generated by metabolism. The body responds to a decrease in core temperature by constricting the peripheral blood vessels to reduce heat loss through the skin and by diverting blood away from colder areas. This is done to ensure that the brain, heart, and other vital organs receive warm blood. This protective mechanism also puts the athlete at greater risk for cold injuries such as frostnip and frostbite by diverting warm blood away from the extremities.[48] As this mechanism progresses, the temperature of the skin decreases, sweating stops, and shivering begins. **Shivering** is an involuntary response to decreased core temperature in an effort to generate heat through muscle contractions.

Heat loss can occur from radiation, evaporation, convection, and conduction. Cold temperatures, in conjunction with wind or dampness, can increase the chances of hypothermia and other cold-related conditions. **Hypothermia** is defined as a core temperature below 35°C (95°F). Cold-related conditions are divided into three categories:[49]

1. Decreased core temperature (hypothermia)
2. Freezing injuries of the extremities
3. Nonfreezing injuries of the extremities

Athletic trainers can help prevent hypothermia and cold-related conditions by doing the following:[14,49-51]

- Ensure athletes wear the proper apparel for the weather. Athletes should do the following:
  - Include both waterproof and windproof fabrics as appropriate
  - Layer clothing and adjust articles of clothing to maintain body temperature
  - Cover areas at risk for cold-related conditions (e.g., wearing a hat and gloves)
  - Wear fabrics made of materials that maintain their warmth when wet (e.g., wool, synthetic fabrics like polypropylene)
- Ensure athletes avoid overexertion and sweating during activity.
- Maintain athletes' hydration levels.
- Ensure adequate nutrition.
- Counsel athletes to avoid alcohol, nicotine, and caffeine.
- Ensure athletes receive adequate rest and sleep.
- Identify at-risk athletes during the PPE and increase monitoring of them during activity. At-risk people include the following:
  - Athletes with a history of previous cold injury

FOUNDATIONAL SKILL

Sweat Rate Calculator

To calculate an athlete's sweat rate, take the following measurements:

1. Weigh the athlete before exercise after she voids the bladder (A).
2. Have the athlete exercise for an hour (for exercise time of 30 minutes, multiply the end sweat rate by 2). If the athlete drinks during exercise, be sure to measure the volume of liquid consumed to incorporate into the following math (D).
3. Weigh the athlete postexercise (B) in the exact clothing worn preexercise to calculate sweat rate (G) and the amount of fluid needed to be consumed during and postexercise to maintain hydration (G).

Plug the numbers from the preceding measurements (A-G) into the following formula:

- A. Body weight preexercise: _____ [lb/2.2 = kg]
- B. Body weight postexercise: _____ [lb/2.2 = kg]
- C. Change in body weight (A − B): _____ g [kg × 1,000 = g]
- D. Volume of fluid consumed: _____ mL [oz × 30 = mL]
- E. Sweat loss (C + D): _____ mL [oz × 30 = mL]
- F. Exercise time: _____ [min or hr]
- G. Sweat rate (E / F): _____ [mL/min or mL/hr]

To convert sweat rate (G) back into ounces, do the following:
    G / 30 = oz

- Women (although most people who die from hypothermia are men)[52]
- Black people
- Lean people
- Lower fitness levels
- Older people (>65 years)
- Children
- Those with a comorbidity, such as Raynaud's syndrome, poor circulation, diabetes, or anorexia
- Those on certain medications
- Monitor the weather conditions.
- Limit time outdoors during cold, wet, and windy conditions (see figure 8.4).
- Perform frequent outdoor temperature checks.
- Create guidelines for outdoor practices and competitions during cold weather.
- Educate coaches, administrators, parents, and athletes on cold-related conditions (early identification) and the organization's policies related to cold weather and activity.

Be aware of both athletes and spectators when practices and competitions take place outside, especially when wind and dampness can exacerbate cold-related conditions. Athletic trainers also need to be cognizant that swimmers can develop hypothermia from being in the water too long, even when the temperature outside is warm.[48,51,53] Additionally, hypothermia can develop in a patient who is in hypovolemic shock from severe bleeding or in conjunction with other types of shock. This is why athletic trainers are taught to keep patients warm as part of the general treatment for shock.

Just like with heat-related conditions, cold-related conditions can be prevented with careful planning, weather monitoring, and stakeholder education. In the traditional athletic training setting, good prevention should mitigate these conditions from developing in athletes. Chapter 14 addresses the emergency care steps for athletes who develop cold-related conditions.

Lightning

Lightning is a serious environmental threat to participants in outdoor activities. It is attributed to an average of 47 deaths per year[54] and 300 documented injuries.[48] It can occur any time of the year, but is most frequent in the period from early spring to fall when thunderstorms are more common. Lightning deaths are most common in June, July, and August,[55] which are also the peak months for outdoor summer activities. Lightning can occur in the winter as well.[50,56] Lightning deaths have been reported during soccer, golf, running, baseball, and football,[55] but lightning activity can happen during any outdoor event. Athletic trainers working with the military athletes should also be especially diligent when monitoring for lightning activity because of their frequency of outdoor training.[57] In the United States, lightning strikes are most common in Florida, Texas, the Gulf States, southern states, Colorado, and the southwest, but they can occur anywhere.

Temperature (°F)

Calm	40	35	30	25	20	15	10	5	0	−5	−10	−15	−20	−25	−30	−35	−40	−45
5	36	31	25	19	13	7	1	−5	−11	−16	−22	−28	−34	−40	−46	−52	−57	−63
10	34	27	21	15	9	3	−4	−10	−16	−22	−28	−35	−41	−47	−53	−59	−66	−72
15	32	25	19	13	6	0	−7	−13	−19	−26	−32	−39	−45	−51	−58	−64	−71	−77
20	30	24	17	11	4	−2	−9	−15	−22	−29	−35	−42	−48	−55	−61	−68	−74	−81
25	29	23	16	9	3	−4	−11	−17	−24	−31	−37	−44	−51	−58	−64	−71	−78	−84
30	28	22	15	8	1	−5	−12	−19	−26	−33	−39	−46	−53	−60	−67	−73	−80	−87
35	28	21	14	7	0	−7	−14	−21	−27	−34	−41	−48	−55	−62	−69	−76	−82	−89
40	27	20	13	6	−1	−8	−15	−22	−29	−36	−43	−50	−57	−64	−71	−78	−84	−91
45	26	19	12	5	−2	−9	−16	−23	−30	−37	−44	−51	−58	−65	−72	−79	−86	−93
50	26	19	12	4	−3	−10	−17	−24	−31	−38	−45	−52	−60	−67	−74	−81	−88	−95
55	25	18	11	4	−3	−11	−18	−25	−32	−39	−46	−54	−61	−68	−75	−82	−89	−97
60	25	17	10	3	−4	−11	−19	−26	−33	−40	−48	−55	−62	−69	−76	−84	−91	−98

Wind (mph)

Frostbite occurs in: 30 min   10 min   5 min

Windchill (°F) = 35.74 + 0.6215T − 35.75($V^{0.16}$) + 0.4275T($V^{0.16}$)

T = air temperature (°F)   V = wind speed (mph)

FIGURE 8.4 Wind chill chart.

The risk of lightning injury or death can be mitigated with proper planning for weather-related emergencies. As chapter 13 discusses, a policy for lightning should be included in the organization's EAP. To prevent lightning injuries, do the following:[28,58,59]

- Have all athletes and spectators remain indoors during lightning activity.
- Evacuate outdoor venues to a safe location during lightning activity.
  - Identify safe locations in advance, including permanent structures with four walls, a roof, plumbing, and electrical wiring.
  - Buses or cars with metal roofs and the windows rolled up can serve as a safe alternative if no other safe structure can be identified.
  - Sheds, three-sided shelters, tents, picnic pavilions, and other similar structures are not deemed safe locations. People should move to predetermined safe shelters when lightning activity is present.
- If no appropriate shelter or vehicle is available, such as the possible case in trail running or military settings, seek shelter:[50]
  - Away from open areas where you are the tallest object
  - Away from exposed ridges or solitary trees
  - Away from water
  - In a forested area among trees, bushes, or rocks
- Designate one person to be the weather watcher to monitor changing conditions and determine when the event should be postponed or resumed.
  - This person should have the unchallengeable authority to make weather-related safety decisions.
- Monitor the weather with a local, reliable source.
  - The National Weather Service (NWS), along with other commercial, real-time lightning detection services, can be used to monitor the weather.
  - Handheld lighting detectors can also be part of the weather monitoring process.[60] These devices should not replace the designated weather watcher and NWS monitoring.
- Require everyone to remain inside until 30 minutes after the last lightning strike or sound of thunder.
  - Timing must restart with each subsequent lightning strike or sound of thunder.
- Notify athletes and spectators when severe weather is imminent and clear the venue in advance to allow everyone to enter the designated safe areas before the storm begins.
- Educate coaches, administrators, parents, and athletes on lightning safety, the organization's policies, locations of safe structures, and timing during a lightning storm.
- Remember the slogan "When thunder roars, go indoors."

Little new information has been published related to lightning safety for athletic trainers since the NATA position statement from 2013.[58] The Korey Stringer Institute provides succinct, up-to-date information on lightning safety, specifically during athletic events.[61] Another great resource is the NWS website, which provides comprehensive information on lightning safety, including emergency planning tool kits for youth and community sports organizations.[54]

Ergonomics

Ergonomics is an important part of injury prevention for athletic trainers, especially those working in nontraditional settings. Ergonomics for the athletic trainer can be defined as "designing the job, equipment, and work area to fit the employee for optimal safety and production."[62] The Occupational Safety and Health Administration (OSHA) recommends ergonomics as a way to prevent many musculoskeletal disorders.[63] The causes of these disorders or injuries include repetitive tasks, bending and lifting, reaching overhead, and working in awkward body positions. By fitting the job to the person, athletic trainers can accomplish the following:[63]

- Decrease the amount of stress on the worker's body
- Decrease the amount of muscle fatigue the worker experiences
- Reduce the number and severity of injuries suffered at the workplace
- Increase worker productivity
- Decrease time lost from work

Many industry-specific resources can be found on the OSHA website.

These twelve principles by Dan MacLeod summarize ergonomics:[64]

1. Work in neutral postures.
2. Reduce excessive force.
3. Keep everything in easy reach.
4. Work at proper heights.
5. Reduce excessive motion.
6. Minimize fatigue and static load.

7. Minimize pressure points.

8. Provide clearance.

9. Move, exercise, and stretch.

10. Maintain a comfortable environment.

11. Make displays and controls understandable.

12. Improve work organization.

Ergonomic assessment has become increasingly important as athletic trainers work in more diverse settings.[62] Often it is not enough to simply assess the client; the athletic trainer must also look at her work environment and how it could influence injury. Athletic trainers should be familiar with basic ergonomic assessments based on employment setting. Figure 8.5 provides an example of an ergonomic check sheet for an office worker. Athletic trainers tasked with doing ergonomic assessments can refer to the OSHA website and their employer for more information.

FIGURE 8.5   Basic ergonomic check sheet.

Item	Specifics	Yes	No	Action taken
Chair	Base • Five-point base with castor wheels • Swivel			
	Seat • Padded • Waterfall front • 2 or 3 finger-breadth between knees and edge of seat • Thighs parallel to the floor when seated • Knees at 90 degrees • Feet flat on the floor			
	Backrest • Padded • Supports the upper back perpendicular to the floor • Apex of lumbar support positioned at or slightly below the beltline			
	Armrests • Shoulders relaxed and level • Elbow at 90 degrees • Fits under workstation or allows for positioning close to the work surface • Adjustable			
Workstation	There is clearance for thighs and sufficient legroom (2 to 3 in., or 5-8 cm).			
	Foot area is clear of obstacles.			
	Height is equal to seated elbow height.			
	No sharp edges			
	Frequently used items are within easy reach.			
	Minimal reaching above the shoulder			
	Minimal reaching below the shoulder			
	Surface space is adequate.			
Keyboard	Neutral wrist position			
	Located close to the body			
	Relaxed arm position during keyboarding			
Mouse	Fits user's hand			
	Neutral wrist position			
	Located close to keyboard and at same level			
	User maintains a loose grip.			

Item	Specifics	Yes	No	Action taken
Monitor	Positioned directly in front of user			
	Top of screen is at or below eye level.			
	Screen is tilted perpendicular to the floor.			
	Viewing distance is a comfortable 18-24 in. (46-60 cm).			
	Glare is minimized.			
Accessories	Document holder • Positioned in front of user • Stable			
	Position cables and cords to prevent tripping.			
Work habits	Take breaks (3-5 min every 20-40 min).			
	Monitor keyboarding behavior (high impact, deviated or extended wrist).			
	Minimize static or awkward postures.			
	Limit highly repetitive tasks.			

Adapted by permission from Eric Shaver, *Performing Office Ergonomics Self-Evaluations* February 27, 2015. ©Eric F. Shaver, Ph.D.

CLINICAL BOTTOM LINE

- PPEs serve multiple functions, including identifying potentially life-threatening or disabling conditions, identifying other conditions that could alter performance, obtaining baseline data, providing an opportunity to educate athletes on health-related topics, and satisfying liability and insurance requirements.

- Athletic trainers need to be familiar with the PPE requirements and recommendations for the setting they are working in. Aspects of PPEs vary by state, level of competition, and league or conference.

- Injuries and illnesses due to environmental conditions, including heat, cold, and lightning, can be prevented through careful planning and preparation, weather monitoring, and stakeholder education.

- Athletic trainers working in many settings, especially the nontraditional setting, can use the principles of ergonomics to prevent injuries.

 Go to HK*Propel* to complete the activities and case studies for this chapter.

Go to HK*Propel* to download a foundational skill check sheet for completing an ergonomic assessment.

CHAPTER 9

Fitness and Wellness

Angela Hillman, PhD

CAATE STANDARDS

The following CAATE 2020 standards are covered in this chapter:

Standard 56

Standard 58

Standard 61

Standard 79

Standard 80

Standard 82

Standard 87

CHAPTER OBJECTIVES

After reading this chapter, you will be able to do the following:

- Identify the role of a physically active lifestyle and exercise on health
- Select, administer, and interpret tests to assess fitness
- Design individualized exercise programs
- Understand how to establish client or patient relationships and direct clients through exercise programs
- Assess safety issues related to exercise and understand the precautions to take

The World Health Organization (WHO) defines health as "a state of complete physical, mental and social well-being and not merely the absence of disease or infirmity."[1] Therefore, living a healthy life entails consuming a nutritious diet (see chapter 10), regular exercise (described in this chapter), social interaction, mental stimulation, and mental well-being. Regular exercise, as this chapter shows, is important for overall health; however, each of the other components of health is equally important, but perhaps overlooked. For instance, mental well-being is important for overall health because it teaches people to be productive, cope with the stresses of life, make meaningful connections, and contribute to work and society. Physical activity and exercise can do these things as well and work in concert with the other components to ensure a healthy life.

Role of Exercise in Maintaining a Healthy Lifestyle

Traditionally, if asked the relationship between exercise and health, most people would respond that it is beneficial to the heart and muscles. Although this is true, there are many other important health benefits of exercise and leading an active lifestyle, including disease prevention and improved cognition and mental health.

Health Benefits

Exercise has many important health benefits. The most significant of these is that high fitness levels are linked with decreased all-cause **mortality**.[2] In particular, those who change from being physically inactive to active have decreased mortality. On the other hand, people who were previously active but decrease their activity levels have a greater risk of cardiovascular disease.[3] It also appears there is no bad time to start exercising, since the benefits occur even in those who don't become physically active until their fourth to sixth decade of life.[4] The benefit of exercise for health is attainment and maintenance of a high level of cardiorespiratory fitness (CRF). As we'll see throughout this chapter, high CRF is the most important factor in maintaining health and longevity. A **dose–response relationship** exists between physical activity and mortality (figure 9.1),[5,6] with no observable upper limit of benefit for higher levels of activity and fitness;[2] therefore, physical activity and exercise are vital in everyday life.

Disease Prevention

Cardiorespiratory fitness (CRF) is most closely linked with long-term health[2] because of decreased risk for development of conditions such as coronary artery disease,[7] diabetes,[8] stroke,[9] and cancer.[10] Exercise strengthens the **autonomic nervous system**,[11] which controls resting heart rate and blood pressure. This, along with improved function and control of blood vessels,[12] helps decrease the risk for **hypertension** and stroke. In addition, exercise promotes the attainment and maintenance of

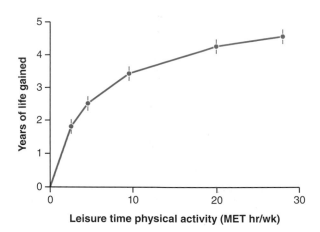

FIGURE 9.1 Dose–response relationship between physical activity and mortality.

Reprinted from S.C. Moore, "Leisure Time Physical Activity of Moderate to Vigorous Intensity and Mortality: A Large Pooled Cohort Analysis," *PLoS Medicine* 9, no. 11 (20191): e1001335. This article is under Creative Commons License (CC BY).

optimal blood lipid levels,[13-16] decreasing the risk of cardiovascular disease. Another important component in the protection against disease is the immune system, which regulates the body's inflammatory state. Chronic, low-grade inflammation is common in many diseases, such as obesity, diabetes, cardiovascular disease, and cancer.[17] Although exercise is known to temporarily increase inflammation in the body, regular exercise and increased CRF are associated with decreased systemic inflammation,[18] which is protective against these diseases.[19]

Perhaps the most important mechanism of higher CRF and disease prevention is that of weight management and blood glucose regulation. Overweight and obesity are independent risk factors for many diseases,[20] including

EVIDENCE-BASED ATHLETIC TRAINING

The Effect of Leisure-Time Physical Activity on Mortality

Leisure-time physical activity (LTPA) includes daily living activities such as walking, dancing, biking, and hiking. It may also include planned exercise but is typically not considered to include activity done during work (i.e., physical or manual labor jobs) or transportation (i.e., walking or riding a bicycle to and from work). In a recent study, Saint-Maurice and colleagues explored the relationship between LTPA and mortality. The authors surveyed 315,059 participants and categorized them into three groups: maintainers (those who participated in consistently stable LTPA over time), increasers (those who increased LTPA from adolescence or later in adulthood), and decreasers (participants who had higher LTPA in early adulthood but reduced activity later). They analyzed all-cause mortality, cardiovascular disease (CVD), and cancer mortality risk of the participants and found that consistent exercise contributed to lower all-cause mortality and CVD mortality risk. Importantly, the decreasers group had increased risk for all-cause and CVD mortality. The authors also found that at least 2 hours per week of LTPA resulted in 14% lower risk of cancer mortality. Increasing LTPA later in life led to a 16% decrease in cancer mortality risk. These results demonstrate that it's never too late to begin and reap the benefits of exercise.[4]

type 2 diabetes. In combination with physical inactivity, the conditions increase disease risk.[19] Exercise alone can lead to a 2% to 3% reduction in body weight;[21] however, in overweight or obese people, the recommended amount of weight loss is 10%. Weight loss should occur at a rate of 1 to 2 lb (0.5-1 kg) per week, which is safe and likely to be maintained for at least a year.[21] Successful weight loss likely requires dietary changes, such as reduced caloric intake, which should be facilitated by a registered dietician. (See chapter 10 for a full discussion of nutrition.)

Approximately 30.3 million U.S. adults (12.2% of the population) had diabetes in 2015; of these, 90% to 95% were type 2 diabetes.[22] Type 2 diabetes is considered a **lifestyle disease** because it typically manifests as a result of increased body mass, low physical activity levels, **insulin resistance**, and even smoking. More than half of all new diagnosed cases of diabetes occur in people aged 45 to 64, an age that correlates with decreased physical activity and increased disease risk. Indeed, nearly 41% of those diagnosed with diabetes were physically inactive.[22] The role of exercise in type 2 diabetes is very clear: It is a first-line treatment and a primary component of prevention strategies, along with dietary modifications.[23] Regular exercise helps maintain weight and can even prevent the development of type 2 diabetes in at-risk patients,[24,25] primarily by training muscles to take up and use glucose, thus decreasing insulin resistance.[26] Most importantly, a combination of resistance and aerobic exercise is necessary to see a significant change in **hemoglobin A1c**.[27]

Cognition and Mental Health

CRF and exercise also affect other markers of health, such as cognitive function, sleep, and depression. Higher levels of CRF aid memory and reduce declines in cognitive function.[28] It appears that physical activity early in life helps maintain memory and cognition;[29] however, starting exercise later in life is also beneficial.[30] Exercise positively affects sleep, particularly in middle- and older-aged people, although a consensus has not been reached for younger people.[31] Although little data exist, research indicates that as CRF levels decline, such as occurs with aging, incidences of sleep problems increase,[32] making maintenance of CRF vital. With regard to mental health, greater CRF is associated with lower symptoms of depression, more so in men than in women.[33] Additionally, maintaining higher CRF later in life can help prevent the onset of depressive symptoms.[34] Please see chapter 19 for more information related to mental health.

Definition of Exercise

Exercise is defined as any sustained activity for the purpose of increasing or maintaining fitness. This contrasts with physical activity, which is movement of daily living that is not structured specifically for fitness. The health benefits of exercise have been recognized since ancient times[35] and continue to be studied today. Exercise can be taken in many forms, from aerobic (endurance or cardio) to resistance (weight lifting) and high-intensity interval training, and even flexibility and neuromotor training.

Aerobic Exercise

Aerobic exercise is often referred to as endurance or cardio exercise. "Aerobic" means a process that requires oxygen and refers to the necessity of oxygen to meet energy demands of the working muscles. Therefore, not all aerobic exercise is created equal; some is more physically demanding, requiring larger oxygen consumption than others. For example, walking and jogging are both considered aerobic exercise, but they demand different levels of oxygen by the muscles. Aerobic exercise is the primary form used when trying to increase or maintain high CRF levels.

Resistance Training

Resistance training (i.e., strength training or weight lifting) is a form of exercise where the muscles contract against an external force in order to increase strength, tone, and endurance. This external force could simply be body weight, such as in doing push-ups, or it may be machines, free weights, or resistance bands. Resistance training is important for maintaining muscular fitness and preventing and treating diseases.

Flexibility and Neuromotor Training

Flexibility and **neuromotor** training are often neglected when thinking of exercise and its importance to health. Flexibility is the ability of a joint to move through its full range of motion. Although previously thought to aid in injury prevention, flexibility is not believed to play as strong a role as general fitness. Nevertheless, flexibility is important in certain sports (e.g., gymnastics, dance) and performing activities of daily living; therefore, you should assess and prescribe exercises that focus on improving or maintaining flexibility. Neuromotor training is exercise that incorporates balance, coordination, and **proprioception**. Just like with flexibility, it leads to improved quality of life, especially in later decades.

Standardized Testing in Fitness and Wellness

Health-related physical fitness testing is frequently used to determine current health status while providing baseline fitness data for exercise prescription and future testing. A wide variety of physical fitness components can be tested, each with its own set of laboratory and field-based tests. A comprehensive health and fitness assessment includes measures of the following:

- Height
- Weight
- Heart rate
- Blood pressure
- Body composition
- Cardiorespiratory fitness
- Muscular fitness
- Flexibility and neuromotor ability

To obtain the most accurate results from your testing, provide your clients with pretest instructions such as the following at least one day before testing:

- Wear appropriate and comfortable clothing for the exercises to be conducted, including athletic shoes.

- Drink plenty of fluid in the 24 hours prior to testing, stopping 2 hours before.
- Avoid alcohol and caffeine for at least 8 hours before testing.
- Avoid consumption of large meals 2 hours before testing.
- Avoid strenuous exercise in the 12 hours before testing.
- Get adequate sleep (6-8 hours) prior to testing.

Prior to beginning any exercise testing or programming, participants should be cleared to begin exercise either by completing health history forms and physical readiness questionnaires (such as the PAR-Q[36]) or receiving clearance from their physician. During this time, assessment of resting vitals (such as height, weight, heart rate, and blood pressure) should be obtained. Any body composition analysis (see the section Body Composition) should also be done before conducting exercise testing.

FOUNDATIONAL SKILL

Measuring Height

1. Using a stadiometer, have the client stand with the back flush against the ruler.
2. Ask the client to take in a full breath and hold it.
3. Adjust the stadiometer to the top of the client's head (figure 9.2) and read the result.

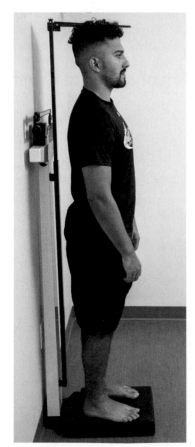

FIGURE 9.2 Measuring height using a stadiometer.

FOUNDATIONAL SKILL

Measuring Resting Heart Rate

1. Ask the client to sit quietly in a comfortable position with the arm resting in a supported position.

2. Locate the radial pulse by placing your index and middle finger at the base of the thumb, next to the tendon (figure 9.3).

3. Using a stopwatch, count the number of heart beats felt in 15 seconds. Multiply this number by 4 to get the heart rate for 1 minute.

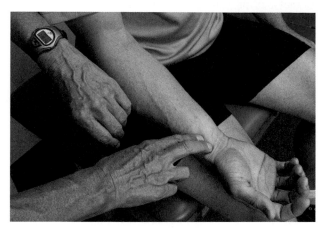

FIGURE 9.3   Locating the radial pulse to measure heart rate.

Cardiorespiratory Fitness

Cardiorespiratory fitness (CRF) is the measure of the ability of the heart and lungs to take in oxygen and distribute it through the body to the working muscles during prolonged exercise. The **gold standard** measure of CRF is maximal oxygen consumption, or **$\dot{V}O_2$max**. This is a measure of the maximal volume of oxygen the lungs can take in and the working muscles can distribute and use. $\dot{V}O_2$max can be assessed either directly in a well-equipped laboratory or indirectly with field-based methods. Laboratory-based methods require expensive equipment that can analyze inspired and expired air during an exercise test to exhaustion (**indirect calorimetry**). In addition, these tests require trained personnel to conduct the tests and analyze and interpret the results; therefore, they are not always ideal or feasible. It may often be easier to use a field-based method, which can estimate $\dot{V}O_2$max, either by measuring the response of heart rate to exercise, such as the Rockport walking test, or from performance during a timed run or distance, such as the 1.5-mi (2.5-km) run, 12-minute run, or the beep test (table 9.1). These field-based tests are ideal because they are inexpensive, requiring only heart rate monitors and stopwatches, and can be easily conducted and interpreted. They also allow larger groups of people to be tested at the same time, such as team sport athletes or military personnel. For example, the 1.5-mi run is part of the physical fitness testing for the Navy, Air Force, and Coast Guard. Similarly, the physical fitness test for the Marines includes a 3-mi (5-km) timed run, while the Army requires a 2-mi (3-km) timed run.

Muscular Fitness

Muscular fitness is an important component of overall health and physical fitness that affects other body systems and functions, such as bone health,[41,42] glucose regulation,[43] metabolism and weight management,[44] and the ability to carry out activities of daily living. Like CRF, muscular fitness can also predict all-cause mortality from disease[45] as well as the development of depression.[46]

Muscular fitness includes the following aspects:

- *Strength:* the ability of the muscle to exert maximal force
- *Endurance:* the ability of the muscle to contract a submaximal load for an extended period of time
- *Power:* the ability to produce a high rate of force over a short period of time

Tests of muscular strength typically include fewer repetitions with higher loads, endurance tests include lower load and higher repetitions, and measures of power include explosive movements and sprints. See table 9.2 for examples of muscular fitness tests for both upper and lower body across the life span. Like the tests of aerobic fitness, many are used for testing in the military, as well as in the NHL and NFL.

Keep safety in mind when conducting tests of muscular fitness. Excessive force production or repetitions are more likely to result in injury or muscle damage; therefore, you should make modifications for untrained and older populations, ensuring that tests are appropriate for

TABLE 9.1   **Examples of Cardiorespiratory Fitness Tests**

	Rockport walking test	Cooper 1.5-mi run	12-min run	Beep test
Test principle	Participants walk 1 mi (1.6 km) as fast as possible. Heart rate is recorded for 10 sec after completion and $\dot{V}O_2$max is calculated.	Participants run 1.5 mi (2.5 km) as fast as possible. $\dot{V}O_2$max is estimated from the time it takes to run 1.5 mi. The faster the time, the higher the $\dot{V}O_2$max.	Participants run for 12 min. $\dot{V}O_2$max is estimated from the total distance covered in 12 min. The farther the distance run, the higher the $\dot{V}O_2$max.	Participants complete repeated sprint intervals with decreasing rest time between intervals. $\dot{V}O_2$max is estimated from distance covered.
Test objective	Walk 1 mi as fast as possible	Complete the 1.5-mi distance as quickly as possible	Run as far as possible in 12 min	Complete as many intervals as possible
Population or application	Untrained or unfit populations; not ideal for well-trained people	Experienced exercisers or team sports; not ideal for untrained populations	Experienced exercisers or team sports; not ideal for untrained populations	Team sport athletes (e.g., soccer, field hockey)
$\dot{V}O_2$max calculation	**Females** $\dot{V}O_2$max = 139.168 − (0.388 × age) − (0.077 × weight in lb) − (3.265 × walk time in min) − (0.156 × heart rate)[37,38] **Males** $\dot{V}O_2$max = 139.168 − (0.388 × age) − (0.077 × weight in lb) − (3.265 × walk time in min) − (0.156 × heart rate) + 6.318	$\dot{V}O_2$max = (483 / time) + 3.5[39]	$\dot{V}O_2$max = (35.97 × mi) − 11.29[39]	$\dot{V}O_2$max = (maximal sprint speed × 6.65 − 35.8) × 0.95 + 0.182[40]

TABLE 9.2   **Examples of Muscular Fitness Tests**

	Muscular strength	Muscular endurance	Muscular power
General population			
Upper body	Handgrip dynamometer[47] One-repetition maximum[48]	Push-ups YMCA bench press[49]	Seated medicine ball throw
Lower body	One-repetition maximum[48]	Wall squat	Vertical jump Broad jump
Athletes			
Upper body	One-repetition maximum bench press or shoulder press	YMCA bench press[49]	Seated medicine ball throw[50] Bench press power[50]
Lower body	One-repetition maximum leg press or leg extension	SPARQ hurdle jump tests Wall squats	Vertical jump Broad jump Margaria-Kalamen power test[51]
Older adults			
Upper body	Handgrip dynamometer[47]	Arm curl test[52]	Seated medicine ball throw[53]
Lower body	Chair stand test[52]	30-sec chair stand[52]	8-ft up and go test[52]

EVIDENCE-BASED ATHLETIC TRAINING

Athletic Training Position Statement: Safe Weight Loss and Maintenance Practices in Sport and Exercise

The National Athletic Trainers' Association issued a position statement on safe weight loss and maintenance practices in sport and exercise. This statement was created by a panel of experts who reviewed the related literature and made recommendations based on the available evidence. Because athletic trainers are often a primary source of information on nutrition and weight loss for athletes, patients, and clients, they must have knowledge of appropriate nutrition, body composition assessment methods, and weight management practices. The position statement concludes that body composition assessment should occur in the most scientifically valid way possible, in a hydrated state, and should be used to determine safe body weight and body composition goals for each athlete or client. In addition, total calorie intake recommendations should be made based on measurement of **basal metabolic rate**, physical activity levels, and desired body composition and weight goals. Finally, athletic trainers should recommend a balanced diet that provides sufficient calories and nutrients, including daily quantities of carbohydrate, fat, and protein, for athletes and clients.[57]

FOUNDATIONAL SKILL

Measuring Waist and Hip Circumferences

Use a spring-loaded (i.e., Gulick) tape measure for circumference measurements, which standardizes tape tension on the skin and improves consistency of measurements.

For waist circumference, do the following:

1. Ask the client to stand in a relaxed position, with the arms at the sides and feet together.
2. Take a horizontal circumference measure at the narrowest part of the body, between the umbilicus and xyphoid process (figure 9.4a).

For hip circumference, do the following:

1. Ask the client to stand in a relaxed position, with legs slightly apart, about 4 in. (10 cm).
2. Take a horizontal circumference measure at the widest part of the body, including the buttocks (figure 9.4b). This may be just below the gluteal fold.

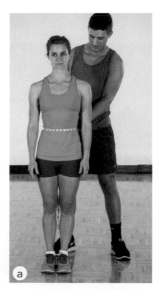 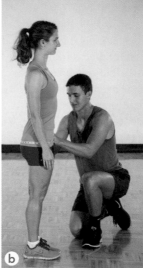

FIGURE 9.4   *(a)* Waist and *(b)* hip circumference measurements.

your client's age and ability. You should become familiar with the testing environment, including the equipment and instruction, before conducting the tests to ensure valid results.

Body Composition

Excessive body fat, particularly when located around the abdomen, is associated with many chronic conditions, such as type 2 diabetes, cardiovascular disease, and metabolic syndrome.[54] According to the National Health and Nutrition Examination Survey, an estimated 32.7% of U.S. adults are overweight, 37.9% are obese, and 7.7% are extremely obese.[55] Body composition changes can occur by decreasing fat mass, increasing fat-free mass (i.e., muscle), or, most likely, doing a combination of both. The American College of Sports Medicine (ACSM) recommends a minimum of 150 minutes per week of moderate-intensity exercise for a modest amount of weight loss to improve health and 200 to 300 minutes of exercise per week for long-term weight loss.[56]

Body composition can be assessed in a variety of ways with varying levels of accuracy. Simple methods for gauging disease risk include measuring circumferences, such as hip-to-waist ratio. This method assesses the amount of fat a person carries around the midsection; it is not a direct measure of body fatness, but rather of fat distribution. Fat stored in this area is a strong indicator of disease risk and mortality.[58]

Lab-based methods for assessing body composition include the measurement of fat below the surface of the skin (subcutaneous), body volume either by air or water displacement or tissue density (densitometry), or bioelectrical impedance.

Skinfold

Skinfolding is a technique that estimates body fat percentage from several thickness folds of skin and subcutaneous fat across the body (figure 9.5). This technique is based on the principle that these individual thickness folds are a good representation of the fat distribution across the body.[59] The accuracy of the skinfolding technique requires a high level of expertise by the practitioner, proper landmark location and measurement, and appropriate use of estimation equations based on sex, race, and physical fitness level. If all factors have been maximized, the typical error rate for skinfolding is ±3.5%.[60]

Densitometry

The densitometry technique involves measuring body volume and calculating whole-body density and thus body composition (fat). Three techniques are typically used: water displacement, air displacement, and bone densitometry.

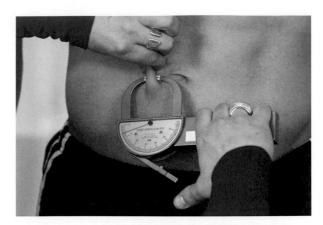

FIGURE 9.5 Skinfolding technique.

- **Hydrodensitometry,** also called underwater weighing, is based on Archimedes' principle, which states that the amount of water displaced by an immersed body is equal to the weight of the body. Body density is calculated from this measurement. Because bone and muscle are denser than fat, the higher the body density, the lower the body fat percentage. In this technique, the client is submerged underwater while exhaling as much air out of the lungs as possible (figure 9.6). This method can be uncomfortable for the client and it requires specialized equipment and the measurement of residual lung volume in order to be the most accurate.

- **Plethysmography,** or air displacement, uses the same principles as underwater weighing. The client sits in a closed chamber (i.e., the Bod Pod; figure 9.7), and body volume is measured. Clients typically tolerate this method better than underwater weighing, and it has similar levels of accuracy.[61]

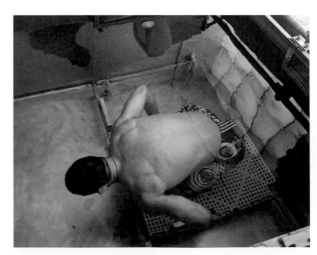

FIGURE 9.6 Hydrodensitometry using load cells and platform.

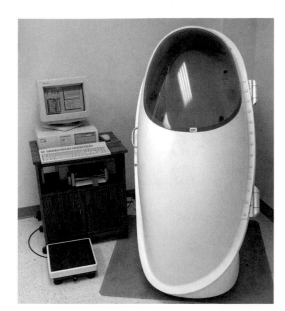

FIGURE 9.7 Bod Pod equipment for plethysmography.

- **Dual-energy X-ray absorptiometry (DEXA)** uses low-radiation X-rays to measure tissue density. This technique is used to measure bone mineral content but can also provide the density of fat tissue in the body (figure 9.8). Although DEXA is the gold standard for bone mineral density and provides fairly accurate body fatness measures,[62] it is not typically used solely for body composition because it is expensive and exposes people to radiation, albeit in small amounts.[63]

Bioelectrical Impedance

Bioelectrical impedance is a noninvasive and low-cost technique that estimates body fat percentage by sending a low-level electrical current through the body and measuring the resistance to the flow of the current (**impedance**). This gives a measure of total body water from which body fat percentage can be calculated. Higher levels of water and thus of muscle lead to lower impedance values and lower body fat percentages. Therefore, hydration is a key component of this test. If a client is dehydrated, he will appear to have higher body fat percentage. Conversely, overhydrated people will appear to have lower body fat percentage. Additionally, there are many types of bioelectrical impedance machines, the most popular being handheld devices and scales (figure 9.9). Although the handheld devices measure only the impedance between two hands holding the device, a simple scale measures the impedance between two legs. Scales that have both upper and lower body contact points measure whole-body impedance and are therefore more accurate. To increase the accuracy of body fat estimates from bioelectrical impedance, the test should ideally be conducted in the morning. Clients should do the following:

- Maintain a standing position for 5 minutes prior to the test to avoid body fluid shifts.
- Adequately hydrate in the day prior, stopping fluid and food intake at least 2 hours before the test.
- Urinate before the test.
- Avoid exercise for 8 hours prior to the test.

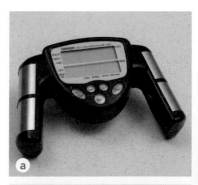
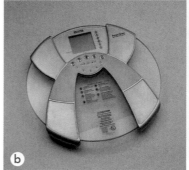
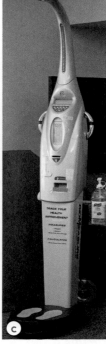

FIGURE 9.9 (a) Handheld, (b) scale, and (c) whole-body versions of bioelectrical impedance machines.

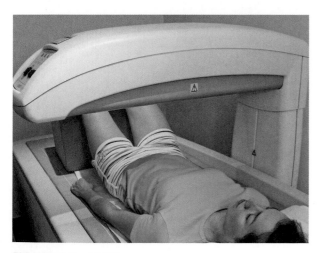

FIGURE 9.8 DEXA scan.

BSIP/Getty Images

Flexibility

No one test can be used to assess the flexibility of all the joints in the body, since joints are task specific and have different ranges of motion (ROM). However, when thinking of flexibility tests, most people automatically think of the sit-and-reach test because of its widespread use. The sit-and-reach test assesses the flexibility of both the hamstrings and the lower back, although it is a better indicator of hamstring than lower back flexibility.[64] The modified version of the sit-and-reach test takes arm length into account. The chair version[52] is more appropriate for older populations or those who have a previous hip, knee, or back injury.[65] The skin distraction test (figure 9.10) is a better measure of lower back flexibility that is useful and easy to conduct. The back scratch test (figure

9.11), also used in older populations, measures shoulder flexibility[52] and is one of the only tests of upper body flexibility outside of goniometry (see the Foundational Skill sidebar General Procedures for Taking Goniometric Measurements in chapter 16). Goniometry directly measures the passive ROM of a joint using a handheld device, such as universal goniometers, digital inclinometers, or even smartphone applications (see table 16.2 for ROM for each joint). Goniometry is especially important for measuring ROM before and after injury or postoperative outcomes,[66] particularly for elbow and knee joints. Accurate assessment by goniometry requires skill and can be enhanced with practice.[67] The advantage of smartphone applications is that they appear to be reliable[68] and can be used by both skilled and novice practitioners.[69]

FOUNDATIONAL SKILL

Measuring Lower Back Flexibility With the Skin Distraction Test

1. With the client standing, locate the right and left posterior superior iliac spines. At the intersection of the line between these two landmarks and the spine, place a small mark.
2. Measure 15 cm (5.9 in.) superior to this point and place a second mark (figure 9.10a).
3. Ask the client to bend as far forward as he comfortably can and measure the distance between the two marks (figure 9.10b).

Although normative values do not exist for all age groups, average skin distraction for 15- to 18-year-old males is 6.7 ± 1.0 cm and 5.8 ± 0.9 cm for 15- to 18-year-old females.[70]

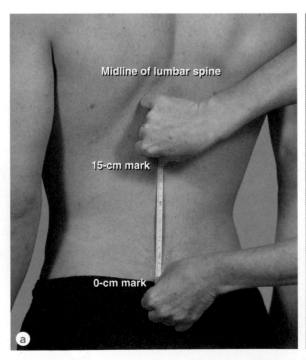
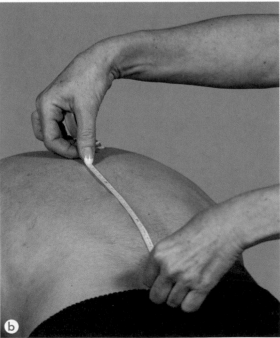

FIGURE 9.10 Skin distraction test to assess lower back flexibility.

Measuring Shoulder Flexibility With the Back Scratch Test

1. Ask the client to place one hand behind her head with the palm touching her back and the fingers pointed downward.

2. Next, ask her to place the other arm behind her back, with the palm facing outward and the fingers upward.

3. Ask her to reach as far as possible down the middle of her back with the top hand and as far up the back with the bottom hand as possible, attempting to touch or overlap the middle fingers of both hands.

4. Measure the distance between the tips of the middle fingers (figure 9.11). If the fingertips touch, then the score is zero. If they do not touch, measure the distance between the fingertips (a negative score); if they overlap, measure by how much (a positive score).

5. Allow two practice attempts and then test two times. Stop the test if the client experiences pain. Published normative data are available only for adults 60 or older,[52] although some data exist for other age groups.[71]

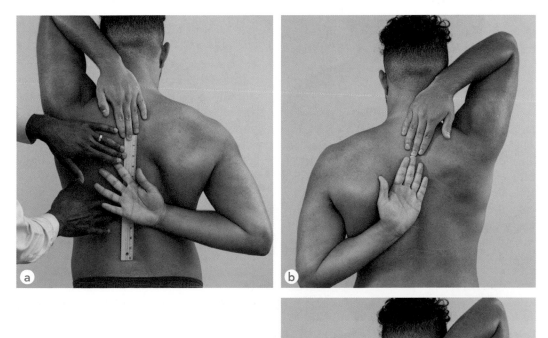

FIGURE 9.11 The back scratch test where client score is (a) negative, (b) zero, (c) positive.

Neuromotor Ability

Neuromotor ability is a measure of balance, coordination, gait, agility, and proprioception.[72] Although it was not previously a focus of comprehensive fitness plans, neuromotor ability was incorporated into the most recent ACSM position stand on designing exercise programs[73] and the Physical Activity Guidelines for Americans.[74] Testing for neuromotor ability is important for establishing a baseline for assessing improvements or changes.

Unipedal Stance Test

The unipedal stance test, often referred to as the single-leg standing balance test, is a measure of static balance ability that requires very little equipment to complete and can be conducted in a variety of settings. The test is completed twice, once with both eyes open and again with both eyes closed; each result provides information on fall risk, especially in older populations, and health-related fitness in all adults.[75] The test may also be useful in predicting risk of noncontact lower-extremity injury in athletes.[76] Normative data for a wide age range also exist, making the test applicable to many people.[77]

Functional Reach Test

The functional reach test is a test of dynamic balance, determining maximum distance reached past arm's length without losing balance. A yardstick or measuring stick is placed at shoulder height at the end of the participant's reach. With feet firmly planted, the participant reaches as far as possible along the measuring stick for three trials, with the scores averaged (figure 9.12). The scores can be used to classify older people into fall risk categories.[78] It can also be used in older athletes, who still experience changes in balance with aging even though they are physically active.[79]

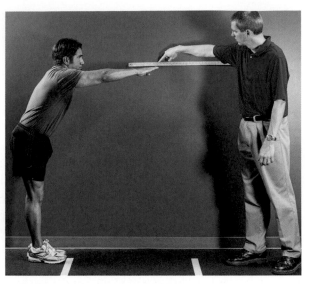

FIGURE 9.12 Functional reach test.

Star Excursion Balance Test

The star excursion balance test is a measure of dynamic balance that requires people to balance on one leg while reaching in each of eight directions with the other leg (figure 9.13). The objective of the test is to reach as far as possible along the scale with the moving leg.[80] The test is widely used for physically active people or athletes, but it is not intended for those at risk for falls. It may also be used in rehabilitation settings, particularly for working with ankle injuries[81] or determining injury risk and assessing recovery during rehabilitation.[82] Because completing all directions on both legs can be quite time consuming, a modified version with only three directions exists. The modified version has been proven valid and realiable[83] and allows for comparison with the Y-balance

---

FOUNDATIONAL SKILL

Test Procedures for Unipedal Stance Test

1. Determine dominant leg by having the client kick a ball.
2. Ask the client to cross his arms across the chest. For the eyes open test, ask him to focus on a point on the wall at eye level.
3. While standing barefoot on the dominant leg, ask the client to raise his other foot off the floor. Start a stopwatch immediately when the foot leaves the floor.
4. Terminate the test when the client does any of the following:
   a. Uncrosses or uses his arms for balance
   b. Moves the raised foot away from the midline or touches the floor
   c. Moves the weight-bearing foot for balance
   d. Exceeds 45 seconds
   e. Opens the eyes during a closed eye test
5. Administer three trials each with eyes open and closed, using the best time from each for the client's score.

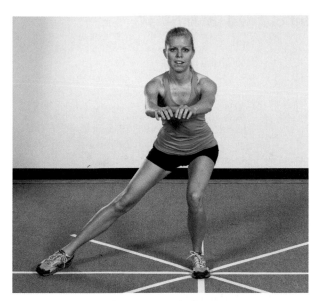

FIGURE 9.13 Star excursion balance test.

test,[84] which also measures dynamic balance in three directions, but appears less useful for injury prediction.[85]

Designing a Fitness Program

Exercise prescription is both a science and an art, because it requires knowledge and proper application of this knowledge. Although a plethora of science and data exist to aid athletic trainers in prescribing exercise, not all people respond the same way to that prescription, nor are all capable of the same movements or activities. Athletic trainers should adjust exercises and programming to their individual clients and strive for excellent communication skills when directing exercises, which is more of an art.

Amount of Exercise Needed

Regardless of the type of exercise done, the current Physical Activity Guidelines for Americans recommend 150 minutes per week of moderate-intensity exercise or

75 minutes per week of vigorous-intensity exercise.[74] Exercise intensity is often defined in terms of **metabolic equivalents** (METs), where 1 MET is the energy expenditure of sitting. See table 9.3 for examples of common MET values for different exercise intensities. A compendium of MET values also exists that contains more than 800 types of exercise, household, and work-related activities.[86]

FITT Principle

When designing exercise programs, exercise physiologists typically use the FITT principle, which stands for frequency, intensity, time (duration), and type (mode). Each component of physical fitness has a FITT prescription based on recommendations from the American College of Sports Medicine[73] and the Physical Activity Guidelines for Americans.[74] See table 9.4 for a summary of the FITT principle for each of the physical fitness components discussed in this chapter.

Overload, Progression, Specificity

In addition to typical prescription guidelines, for an exercise program to be successful at increasing or maintaining fitness levels, a few conditions must be met. First, the programming must include **progression**, or changes in the prescription over time. To see benefits and improvements, an exercise program needs variety and change that the body can adapt to; otherwise, stagnation will occur and improvements will likely not be seen. Progression of exercise typically has three phases:

1. *Initial conditioning phase.* This phase may be necessary for those who are not physically fit or currently active. It may last 1 to 6 weeks, where exercise intensity is low and small progression occurs. If a client has a baseline level of fitness, is currently active, and is accustomed to the modes of exercise in her prescription, this phase can be skipped.

TABLE 9.3 **Examples of Exercise Intensities and MET Values for Common Activities**

Exercise intensity	Low	Moderate	Vigorous
MET value	<3.0	3.0-5.9	>6.0
Examples	Light walking (up to 2.5 mph) Light stretching or Hatha yoga Light household chores	Brisk walking (2.5-4 mph) Bicycling to work or for pleasure (<10 mph or 30-50 Watts) Doubles tennis Dancing Golf Resistance training	Jogging or running Group fitness class Rowing Sports activities and competitions (football, soccer, racquetball, hockey) Shoveling snow

TABLE 9.4 **FITT Principle for Each Component of Physical Fitness**

	Frequency	Intensity*	Time	Type*
Cardiopulmonary	>3-5 days/week	Moderate to vigorous	20-60 min/day	Continuous, purposeful exercise using large muscle groups
Muscular fitness	2-3 days/week	60%-70% 1RM (moderate to vigorous) for novice to intermediate exercisers >80% 1RM (vigorous to very vigorous) for well-trained and experienced exercisers <50% 1RM for muscular endurance	No specific duration required; however, allowing for 1-3 min rest between sets is advised. 48-hr rest between sessions for any single muscle group is recommended. 8-12 repetitions are recommended for improving strength. 15-25 repetitions are recommended for improving endurance. 2-4 sets of each exercise are recommended.	All major muscle groups Multijoint exercises are recommended to be completed before single-joint exercises (i.e., upright rows before biceps curls).
Flexibility	2-3 days/week, daily preferred	Hold each stretch to the point of feeling slight discomfort.	Static stretches should be held for 10-30 sec each. Each exercise should be performed 2-4 times.	Stretching all major muscle groups is recommended. Static, dynamic, or PNF stretching
Neuromotor	2-3 days/week, daily preferred	Effective intensity has not been determined.	20-30 min per day or 60 min per week	Yoga Tai chi Balance boards

*See table 9.3 for further explanation of intensity and exercise types.[73,74,87]

2. *Improvement phase.* This phase typically lasts 4 to 8 months. The rate of progression is faster than for the initial conditioning phase. Progressive overload is applied during this phase.

3. *Maintenance phase.* This phase is used to preserve fitness once a client has reached her desired fitness level at the end of the improvement phase. Theoretically, this phase would be endless. It requires variety in programming to counteract boredom and stagnation.

People might move between the improvement and maintenance phases if they are changing activity levels. For example, if someone is physically fit, then decides to train for a marathon, this will likely result in him moving from maintenance back to improvement. This is because the nature of the training (volume) is different from what he currently does to maintain fitness. Should he wish to continue competing in marathon races, he would likely maintain that volume; however, if not, he may move to a new type of activity and hence improvement stage, or simply decrease his training volume to his previous maintenance level.

The next and perhaps most important part of exercise prescription is **overload**, or a progressive and systematic increase in the load, duration, or frequency of exercise. "Progressive" is the key word in terms of overload, since the increase should be made in either duration or intensity (not both simultaneously) and should not be too large. Typically, increasing exercise duration by 5 to 10 minutes or intensity by 10% per week is recommended for cardiorespiratory and resistance training.[87] Unfortunately, because the long-term effect of flexibility or neuromotor exercise on health has not been fully studied, no guidelines for progressive overload are available for them.

The final important principle for exercise prescription is that of **specificity**, meaning that the benefits of exercise occur to the systems of the body carrying out the exercise. For aerobic endurance exercise, this might be the lungs and exercising muscles. For resistance training, this would be the group of muscles used or focused on. Specificity is especially important for sports training. For example, a sprinter would complete training that included many sprints and short bursts of activity but would not complete endurance-type exercises in preparation. Similarly, swimmers often participate in land-based training once a week to help with muscular endurance.

Instructing a Patient Through Fitness Exercise

Just as exercise prescription is a combination of an art and science, so too is instructing clients through their exercise routines. Clear communication and instruction and safety are the most important parts of working with clients. First, you must ensure you've selected the most appropriate exercises for the client and that she feels comfortable completing them. Although the textbook description of a squat says to stand with feet hip-width apart, that position might not be comfortable for your client, and you should make adjustments. Ensuring the client is comfortable is an important first step to maintaining safety and ensuring she stays injury free.

Clear Communication

A clear line of communication between yourself and the client is imperative. You should ensure not only that your instructions are clear, but also that your client is willing to communicate any concerns or issues with you. Suggestions for establishing a good client relationship include the following:

- Start a session by asking the client how he felt after his previous session.
- Ask about his preference for exercises. What did he like or dislike from the previous experience?
- Explain test results in lay terms, avoiding scientific jargon the client is not likely to understand.
- Try to frame poor results in a positive way to motivate initiation and adherence to exercise programs.

Additionally, in order to stick with an exercise program, the client really needs to understand the benefits.

This is often called the "buy in." The client needs to understand why these exercises are important and why he should do them. Rather than explaining the science, explain the benefits. For example, the science of squatting is that it uses the thighs and glutes, which are large muscle groups that burn plenty of calories when exercised. Although many people might care about calories burned, learning the personal long-term benefit of doing squats, such as having looser fitting pants, might be a more appropriate motivator for other clients.

Show-Tell-Do

Next, employ the show-tell-do method for instructing exercises, especially resistance training techniques. As the first step implies, you'll show your client the exercise she will complete, preferably with 4 to 6 repetitions or attempts. Do your best not to tell her what to do or not do at this time. Simply demonstrate the action. Next, allow the client to practice the exercise while you explain the steps for successful completion. While explaining the steps, focus on what she should be doing rather than what not to do, which may confuse her. Have a dialogue with the client about what muscles she feels are being used. This will help her make the connection between the actions, expectations, and muscles. Allow the client 2 or 3 sets of training or 4 to 6 attempts to get used to the activity.

Feedback

Providing helpful feedback during training sessions is essential. Positive comments on how well a client is doing during an activity is key to providing a constructive experience. You may also want to make recommendations on activities to be changed, such as ensuring the client is breathing through all activities instead of holding his breath. Make sure to give your recommendations in a positive manner. When the client demonstrates the change, provide encouragement and positive reinforcement.

It is also a good idea to reflect with the client after each activity to gauge its effects or his feelings toward the activity. You can ask questions about how the exercise benefited him or what he needs to pay greater attention to during the exercises. These questions will help keep the client focused on you and the exercise, rather than on the gym or surrounding environment. You also need to know if your client feels comfortable completing the exercise without your assistance, which he will likely do at some point. If the client does not feel comfortable, go back to the show-tell-do for that exercise or consider changing the activity to a more appropriate one.

Safety Precautions and Hazards

Exercise is generally regarded as safe for most people; however, it can provoke cardiovascular events in susceptible populations, including athletes. This is especially true if someone has a positive medical history for cardiovascular disease, has previously smoked, or has had an episode of fatigue or flulike symptoms.[88] Additionally, there are **contraindications** to exercise testing, especially for those with a medical history. When conducting exercise tests, athletic trainers should be familiar with contraindications to avoid emergent situations during testing. Importantly, there are a number of ways to ensure exercise is safe for all people and to help clients avoid injury, including properly warming up and cooling down following exercise and avoiding environmental extremes.

Contraindications

There may be situations and reasons why exercise testing is not recommended for a client. These can be absolute or relative.

- An *absolute contraindication* means no physical exercise or testing should occur, since it could put the person being tested in a life-threatening situation. Typically, these are disease-related conditions, such as an acute myocardial infarction or unstable angina.

- A *relative contraindication* means that caution should be exercised when testing people displaying these signs. People exhibiting relative contraindications can exercise; however, the exercise physiologist or athletic trainer should use her best judgment when proceeding. Generally, if the benefit outweighs the risk with these people, exercise is indicated. For example, someone with extreme systolic blood pressure will likely benefit from exercise, since it lowers blood pressure through vasodilation. Similarly, someone with high blood glucose will likely benefit from exercise; however, it should be supervised to ensure her safety during and after.

See the following sidebar for a list of absolute and relative contraindications to exercise testing.

Contraindications to Exercise Testing

There are several absolute and relative contraindications to exercise testing:[89-91]

Absolute
- Acute myocardial infarction (within 2 days)
- Unstable angina not previously stabilized by medical therapy
- Uncontrolled cardiac arrhythmias causing symptoms or hemodynamic compromise
- Symptomatic severe aortic stenosis
- Uncontrolled symptomatic heart failure
- Acute pulmonary embolism or pulmonary infarction
- Acute myocarditis or pericarditis
- Acute aortic dissection
- Acute systemic infection, accompanied by fever, body aches, or swollen lymph nodes

Relative
- Left main coronary artery stenosis
- Moderate stenotic valvular heart disease
- Electrolyte abnormalities
- Severe arterial hypertension
- Tachyarrhythmias or bradyarrhythmias
- Hypertrophic cardiomyopathy and other forms of outflow tract obstruction
- Mental or physical impairment leading to inability to exercise adequately
- High-degree atrioventricular block
- Ventricular aneurysm
- Chronic infectious disease (mononucleosis, AIDS, hepatitis)
- Uncontrolled metabolic disease (diabetes, thyroid)

Warm-Up and Cool-Down Procedures

Warm-up and cool-down procedures should be used in all exercise sessions. A warm-up before exercise achieves the following:

- Ensures a gradual increase in heart rate
- Increases muscle and body temperature to prepare the body for exercise
- Helps prevent delayed-onset muscle soreness[92,93]

An active cool-down achieves the following:

- Allows for a gradual lowering of heart rate
- Provides the means for lactate clearance from the muscles, aiding in recovery[94,95]

In addition to helping clients through warm-up and cool-down, use a gradual progression of exercise volume.

UV Exposure

Exercising in outdoor environments poses potential health risks in a number of ways, including UV exposure, air temperature, and air quality. UV exposure is beneficial in that it stimulates the body's production of vitamin D.[96] However, exposures of even 15 minutes can cause the skin to become more sensitive to light and damage,[97] resulting in skin damage and increased risk for cancer.[98] Avoiding exercise during peak time (10 a.m. to 4 p.m.) is advised to prevent overexposure.[99] Additionally, the use of sunscreen to block UV radiation is imperative. Although 96% of athletes believe sunscreen use prevents cancer, 50% never use it and only 75% use it three times per week or less.[100] Additionally, many people wear fewer pieces of clothing to ensure comfort during exercise, resulting in greater exposure of the skin to UV rays,[98] making sunscreen use even more important.

Ambient Temperature

Ambient temperature, both extreme heat and cold, can result in illness, injury, or even death. Hot environments are typically a greater safety issue to humans than cold. This is because the muscles produce large amounts of metabolic heat, which can raise internal body temperature. If more metabolic heat is produced than can be lost through **thermoregulation**, body temperatures will elevate further. Additionally, if sweat rates are high, people can become dehydrated, which will further elevate body temperature and increase heat illness risk (see chapter 8 for a more in-depth review).

Although more deaths occur during cold weather than in other conditions,[101] in most cases, exercising in cold environments does not pose any health or performance issues. The greatest risk is development of upper respiratory tract infections, hypothermia, and frostbite. Hypothermia can develop when heat loss is greater than heat production, decreasing the body's internal temperature. Similarly, frostbite can occur when skin is exposed to cold weather, in part because blood flow is diverted to the muscles during exercise. It is imperative to use clothing as a mitigation strategy. In cold environments, people should dress in layers to reduce heat loss and provide insulation. For hot environments, people should wear clothing that allows for optimal thermoregulation through air flow and sweating, yet covers skin to avoid excessive UV exposure.

Air Quality

Air quality during exercise may pose health hazards that surpass the benefits of the exercise itself.[102] This is in part due to increased breathing rates during exercise and the tendency to breathe through the mouth during higher-intensity exercise. Mouth breathing bypasses the nasal passages, which normally reduce pollutants from the air we

EVIDENCE-BASED ATHLETIC TRAINING

The Effect of Air Quality on Physical Activity Behavior of Adults

Air quality is known to affect health (see Air Quality), especially particulate matter, which can be inhaled during exercise. However, little is known about the effect air quality has on physical activity behaviors. Because most adults don't get the recommended levels of physical activity or exercise, reluctance to exercise due to poor air quality could exacerbate this issue. A meta-analysis of air quality studies showed that for every one unit increase in particulate matter concentration in the air, there was an increase in the odds of physical inactivity by 1.1% among U.S. adults.[104] The authors also found that people mitigated the poor air quality by decreasing time spent in outdoor physical activity and increasing leisure-time inactivity. It is unknown if the participants made up for decreased outdoor time by exercising indoors, but the authors concluded that for this to happen, more time and money must be spent in developing cost-friendly and accessible workout facilities for the population. This is particularly imperative in developing countries with large pollution and air-quality issues, such as China and India.[104]

breathe. Exposure to poor air quality during exercise may lead to headaches, increased risk of developing asthma or exacerbating asthma symptoms, as well as increased risk of death from lung cancer and cardiovascular disease.[103] Generally, the long-term benefits of exercise outweigh the dangers of pollution; however, people should avoid exercising in areas and times of high pollution, such as cities and during rush hour. Monitoring air quality before exercise is also advised. This can be done by consulting the Internet or one of many weather applications.

CLINICAL BOTTOM LINE

- Exercise and physical activity are important for maintaining lifelong health and decreasing all-cause mortality risk. Importantly, for sedentary people, increasing physical activity levels leads to similar benefits in reduced disease and mortality risk as maintaining high levels of fitness throughout the life span.

- Athletic trainers should use appropriate exercise tests to evaluate the fitness of clients and athletes. They should follow testing with evidence-based exercise prescription to meet the client or athlete's fitness and body composition goals.

- Exercise prescription is both science and an art. Athletic trainers should establish and maintain strong relationships with athletes and clients, focusing on open communication. This will enable the athletic trainer to guide clients through their exercise routines, make adjustments based on their feedback, and ensure they are reaching their goals.

- Maintaining a safe environment during exercise is imperative for the health and well-being of clients and athletes. This involves avoiding extreme environmental temperatures, UV exposures, and poor air quality, as well as wearing the appropriate clothing.

 Go to HK*Propel* to complete the activities and case studies for this chapter.

Go to HK*Propel* to (1) view videos of several fitness and wellness tests and (2) download foundational skill check sheets for measuring height, resting heart rate, and shoulder flexibility.

CHAPTER 10

General Nutrition Concepts and Sports Nutrition

Ellen K. Payne, PhD, LAT, ATC, EMT

Jennifer Doane, MS, RDN, CSSD, LDN, ATC

CAATE STANDARDS

The following CAATE 2020 standards are covered in this chapter:

Standard 55

Standard 83

CHAPTER OBJECTIVES

After reading this chapter, you will be able to do the following:

- Define the six essential nutrients and their roles in the body
- Describe the different energy-producing nutrients, including carbohydrate, protein, and fat, and their role in energy production
- State daily requirements for carbohydrate, protein, and fat for active people
- Define select micronutrients and describe their role in nutrition
- Explain the concept of fueling athletes and other physically active people for their specific activity
- Describe the importance of hydration and compare when to use sports drinks versus water to meet hydration needs
- Discuss the importance of nutrition in the healing process
- Define low energy availability, including the female athlete triad and relative energy deficiency in sport (RED-S)
- Explain the role of dietary supplements and their various key types, including amino acids, energy drinks, protein powders and bars, and omega-3s
- Identify resources to help clients select dietary supplements

In addressing the nutrition concerns of physically active people, athletic trainers need to do more than simply recommend that their clients eat a balanced diet. Fueling athletes and other physically active people for optimal performance is a difficult and complex task. The topic of nutrition can often be unclear and confusing due to the barrage of available information, both evidence based from sound practitioners and unsubstantiated claims from questionable sources. Athletic trainers need to filter through complex nutrition information and educate active clients on healthy, evidence-based ways to optimally fuel to support performance and healing.

Nutrition is the act or process of nourishing or being nourished; specifically, it is the processes by which a person takes in and uses food substances that are necessary for human function. For athletes and physically active people, being optimally nourished determines not only their health status but also their performance. Focus on proper fueling for athletes has recently increased, and many coaches, teams, and individual athletes see nutrition as a barrier to cross in order to achieve success in sport.[1,2] The National Collegiate Athletic Association (NCAA) deregulated meals and snacks in 2014, leaving room for programs to make greater strides toward providing proper fuel for all athletes.[2-5]

Regardless of whether you are designing a nutrition program for an elite athlete, recreational athlete, factory worker, dancer, or any other active person, the six essential nutrients remain the same:

1. Carbohydrate
2. Protein
3. Fat
4. Vitamins
5. Minerals
6. Water

When assisting a person with fueling strategies or medical nutrition therapy concerns, you should work with a **registered dietitian (RD)** who is also a **certified specialist in sports dietetics (CSSD)**.[6] Work to form an interprofessional team with a RD/CSSD, the team physician, and possibly mental health experts to provide comprehensive care for active people at all levels. This chapter provides an overview of nutrition consideration for athletes and other physically active people.

Energy and Nutrition Needs

To assist people with adequate fueling, it is important to understand the body's energy systems. The energy system a person uses directly affects his optimal fueling needs. The predominant nutrients that determine successful fueling are carbohydrate and fat. The entirety of all the chemical processes that convert the essential nutrients we consume in our food into energy in our bodies is called **metabolism**. Many genetic factors affect metabolism, but the best way a person can maximize the potential of his metabolism is to eat consistently throughout the day and consume adequate portions.

Although fat provides more energy toward **aerobic** activity when a person is working within a low- to moderate-intensity aerobic capacity for any duration of time, it takes on a larger role in fueling when activity starts to surpass 2 hours in duration, such as with ultraendurance athletes.[13,14] For both **anaerobic** exercise and high-intensity aerobic training, **glucose** is the main source of energy.

Only one energy or fuel really counts in the body: **adenosine triphosphate (ATP)**. The body primarily produces ATP by breaking down carbohydrate and fat. Through both anaerobic and aerobic pathways, the body can generate ATP for energy. The anaerobic pathways range in energy production from seconds up to 2 minutes;

EVIDENCE-BASED ATHLETIC TRAINING

Nutrition Position Statements

The National Athletic Trainers' Association (NATA) has published four position statements related to nutrition and dietary concerns of athletes and other physically active people. These official position statements provide best-practice recommendations related to

- fluid replacement,
- guidelines for safe weight loss and management,
- the evaluation of dietary supplements, and
- disordered eating in athletes.[7-10]

They were written by a panel of experts in the specific areas who conducted a systematic review of the literature related to each topic and made recommendations based on the evidence available. You should review these statements, evaluate the recommendations in terms of their applicability to your institution's unique situation, and incorporate them into your facility's policies and procedures manual if feasible. As changes in the recommendations are released, you must stay abreast of them to ensure your organization provides best possible patient care. These position statements are found on the NATA website and are referenced throughout this chapter.

Additionally, be aware of the joint position statement released by the American College of Sports Medicine, Academy of Nutrition and Dietetics, and Dietitians of Canada, *Nutrition and Athletic Performance*.[11] This paper outlines the organizations' current evidence-based recommendations and guidelines in the field of sports nutrition. It is a great resource for athletic trainers who wish to learn more about sports nutrition, as well as a reference for many nutrition-related questions.

For nutrition questions for the general population, use the *Dietary Guidelines for Americans 2015-2020*.[12] This evidence-based document is updated every 5 years by the U.S. Department of Health and Human Services and U.S. Department of Agriculture. The focus areas of this document are basic nutrition, healthy eating patterns, and the association between diet and health.

the aerobic energy production of ATP can be infinite if exogenous energy sources are supplied adequately. Table 10.1 provides a summary of the energy systems.

Remember that neither the aerobic nor the anaerobic metabolic pathways function completely alone at any given time. To that end, the body simultaneously uses energy from carbohydrate or fatty acids throughout any activity. A person's muscles, and, to some extent, liver, supply the carbohydrate from glycogen stores. The **fatty acids** come mostly from **triglycerides** stored inside the muscles, but also partly from triglycerides released from the body's fat stores in adipose tissue. Both glucose and fatty acids are delivered to the muscles through the blood.

Macronutrients

A combination of **macronutrients** (carbohydrate, protein, and fat) in a person's diet creates optimal fueling for physical activity and sport performance. Due to varying components of activity duration, activity intensity, and a person's level of physical conditioning, a one-diet-fits-all approach is not enough to keep a person healthy or at the top of her performance. You should understand the three macronutrients and how the body uses them to provide fuel for activity. Table 10.2 provides the macronutrient recommendations.

Carbohydrate

The main carbohydrate found in the body is glucose. There are two types of carbohydrate:

- **Complex carbohydrates** are polysaccharides or long chains of carbohydrates containing more than 10 monosaccharide units. Whole grains, starchy vegetables, and legumes are examples of complex carbohydrates.

- **Simple carbohydrates** are formed from 10 or fewer monosaccharides and are found as oligosaccharides, disaccharides, and monosaccharides in our food. Dairy products, fruit, and sucrose are examples of simple carbohydrates.

Regardless of the carbohydrate consumed through food, only three monosaccharides (glucose, fructose, and galactose) are absorbed through the small intestines and travel through the body. Their end result in the human body is glucose. Glucose in the human body either becomes a component in the blood (blood glucose) or is

TABLE 10.1 **Summary of the Energy Systems**

Energy system	Oxygen needs	Duration	Type of fuel	Example of exercise
ATP-PC	No	Approx. 10 sec	Phosphocreatine (PC)	Coming out of the blocks for a sprint
Glycolysis	No	Less than 2 min	Carbohydrate	200-m race
Oxidative (aerobic) from carbohydrate	Yes	Approx. 90 min	Glucose and glycogen	Half-marathon
Oxidative (aerobic) from fat	Yes	Days	Fatty acids and triglycerides	Ultradistance events

TABLE 10.2 **Macronutrient Recommendations**

	General population	Athletes	Recovery	Other
Carbohydrate	45%-65% of total daily calories (or at least 130 g/day)	5-10 g/kg/day (g per kg body weight per day)	1.0-1.5 g/kg within 2 hr and the subsequent 2-hr time frame	Carbohydrate loading: 10-15 g/kg/day
Protein	0.8 g/kg/day	1.2-2.0 g/kg/day	1.0-1.5 g/kg (immediately following and 2 hr after exercise)	Per meal/snack: 0.25-0.30 g/kg (approx. 15-25 g protein)
Fat	At least 20% of total calories consumed (not less than 10% to prevent fatty acid deficiency)	1 g/kg/day	N/A	N/A

stored in the liver (liver glycogen) or muscles (muscle glycogen). **Glycogen**, a long chain of glucose molecules linked together, is the main source of energy for working muscles. When glycogen levels are low due to an underconsumption of the carbohydrate sources that provide glucose, performance suffers. To increase access to all forms of glucose or glycogen, a person must consistently consume carbohydrate-rich foods throughout the day: whole-grain breads, quinoa, brown rice, peas and beans, whole fruits, vegetables, milk, yogurt, and sport food options, such as sports drinks and high-carbohydrate bars.

During activities done at a higher intensity that surpass the ability of the heart and lungs to supply oxygen to working muscles, the body relies chiefly on glucose for fuel. Thus, activities such as sprinting will eventually deplete glycogen stores. Yet, when engaging in lower-intensity activities, the body can meet the muscles' oxygen demands and thus use glycogen more conservatively. Nonetheless, all activities at all intensity levels require some level of glucose (glycogen) for fuel, and these stores ultimately become depleted. Any pace of activity cannot be sustained without replenishing glycogen stores. A person will slow his pace when his carbohydrate supplies are depleted. During this last-ditch effort to keep moving, the liver releases some of its glycogen, which serves as a short-term backup, but this level of activity cannot be sustained. In the end, the athlete will "hit the wall" and be forced to stop his activity due to a lack of carbohydrate for fuel, not of a depletion of fatty acids for aerobic energy.

Carbohydrate loading is a practice that competitive and elite athletes use to supersaturate their muscles with optimal glycogen levels. It is not intended for people who exercise less than 90 minutes per workout at a low intensity; however, competitive or elite athletes who exercise at a high intensity for more than 90 minutes at a time may benefit from carbohydrate loading.[15,16] Older versions of the practice advised that athletes gradually increase carbohydrate intake over a full week while simultaneously tapering physical activity. However, it has been found to be just as beneficial to increase carbohydrate intake within recommended levels during the 36 hours prior to activity.[17] This practice is less disruptive to training schedules and more adaptive to individualized activity and fueling programs.

Protein

A protein is a chain of **amino acids**, which are the individual building blocks for protein structure. The type of protein made and its function are determined by the sequence and types of amino acids present in its structure. There are two types of amino acids:

1. Essential amino acids, which must be consumed through our diet

2. Nonessential amino acids, which are synthesized by the body

From a food standpoint, based on amino acid structure, there are complete and incomplete proteins. Complete proteins contain all the essential amino acids, whereas incomplete proteins are missing one or more essential amino acids. The type of protein consumed is especially important for those choosing a vegetarian lifestyle. Many plant-based proteins are incomplete in nature; thus, vegetarians must be more diligent about their food choices to maintain optimal health. Another aspect of animal- versus plant-based proteins is their **biological value**. Animal sources of protein typically have a high biological value as compared to plant-based sources. In studies, only soy has been shown to have a biological value similar to animal-based protein sources.[18]

How much protein a person's body uses during exercise (endurance exercise and heavy weightlifting) depends on the intensity and duration of the exercise being performed, the person's fitness level, and the glycogen stores in the muscles at the time of activity. However, it is a myth that protein fuels a person's muscles. Protein is an inefficient source of fuel compared to carbohydrate (glycogen/glucose) and fatty acids (muscle triglycerides). When glycogen stores are at optimal levels, protein contributes no more than 5% of fuel needs. The vast majority of protein serves structurally for those functions previously mentioned.

Muscle building is a supply and demand process. Thus, the way to make muscle cells grow is to put a demand on them. They will respond by taking up nutrients, including amino acids, so that they can grow or **hypertrophy**. People need a primary fuel source of carbohydrate (glucose/glycogen) to fuel their working muscles. Without proper carbohydrate and fat for fueling, a person may be on the road to breaking down the very muscle they are trying to build. Although muscle-protein breakdown dominates during heavy exercise, muscle growth escalates after exercise. The muscles use the available amino acids to repair and build, and the net effect of these changes is muscle protein synthesis (MPS). Optimal nutrient timing before or during and after resistance training can minimize muscle-protein breakdown and muscle damage during exercise. It can also optimize muscle growth and repair until the next training session.

In short, protein is not an efficient fuel source, and is used by the body throughout every 24-hour cycle.[11] Athletes should consume protein from a source with high biological value every 3 or 4 hours.[11,18] Increased protein consumption can be helpful during the onset of activity, for weight management, at the start of higher-intensity training, and during rehab or recovery postinjury.

Fat

The third macronutrient is fat. This essential nutrient is absorbed from our food and has many important functions in the body. It is not true that any dietary fat turns into body fat once consumed. The functions of fatty acids in the body involve the following:

- Cell structure (lipoproteins)
- Transport of fat-soluble vitamins
- Energy source
- Energy storage
- Protect or pad the body from injury
- Temperature regulation and insulation
- Synthesis for steroid hormones

Although the supply of fat is almost unlimited from the food people consume, the ability of the muscles to use fat for energy is not. Recall that for a working muscle to burn fat, oxygen and glucose must be present. That is, a person must have adequate muscle glycogen stores to keep up with the energy demands of her sport. When working at a rate that allows the heart to supply ample oxygen to working muscles, the muscles must rely heavily on body fat stores to meet aerobic energy needs. When increased exercise intensity limits the oxygen being supplied to cells, body fat (muscle triglycerides) continue to contribute energy, but the muscles need glucose in order for the anaerobic pathway to continue.

There are two essential fatty acids: omega-6 and omega-3 fatty acids. Examples of common sources are nuts (omega-6) and fish (omega-3). The two specific fatty acids are important because of their anti-inflammatory, cardioprotective, and **antithrombotic** properties. A balanced intake is essential for optimal health. In overall health and wellness, omega-3 fatty acids have been shown to help prevent coronary heart disease, hypertension, diabetes, obesity, and cancer. Omega-3 fatty acids hold extra value for athletes and other physically active people because they have been shown to counteract the inflammatory state brought on by exercise.

Active people and recreational athletes should include fish oils in their fat intake. They should look for sources with an **eicosapentaenoic acid (EPA)** and **docosahexaenoic acid (DHA)** content of about 1 to 2 g per day at a ratio of 2:1, respectively. A more individualized approach should be undertaken for competitive and elite athletes. All athletes should consume a balance of fatty acids; this can be achieved by substituting olive oil or canola oil for other sources of omega-6. Omega-3 fatty acids are essential for the overall health of athletes and should be a focus when including dietary fat in a daily eating plan.

Micronutrients

Micronutrients are the vitamins and minerals that must be obtained from our food in order to maintain optimal health. Many vitamins and minerals are of importance to athletes and physically active people for various reasons. Although all micronutrients are unique and important in the diet, the areas of energy metabolism, healing, and bone health are of the utmost importance for athletes and physically active people.

Vitamins

There are two classifications of **vitamins**: water-soluble and fat-soluble.

- Water-soluble vitamins can be absorbed and transported through an aqueous environment. If consumed or supplemented in excess, these vitamins are typically eliminated by the kidneys in urine. Water-soluble vitamins include the B-complex vitamins and vitamin C.

EVIDENCE-BASED ATHLETIC TRAINING

Postactivity Fueling

The recovery phase after activity is the most important aspect of an athlete's fueling regimen. If the energy used in activity is not replaced, the athlete will begin his next bout of activity in a deficit. Especially within the 2 hours postactivity, the athlete's muscles soak up carbohydrate to replace those used throughout his activity. Missing this recovery of muscle energy can set any athlete up for performance decline and fatigue. Athletes should consume 1.2 g of carbohydrate per kg of body weight immediately after activity as well as again 2 hours postactivity.[11,19] This means consuming 55 g of carbohydrate for every 100 lb (45 kg).

Protein is also an essential nutrient for postactivity fueling because of its role in the structural repair of muscles. Athletes should consume protein immediately after activity up until the 4 hours prior to resuming activity. Athletes should limit protein intakes to no more than 0.40 g of protein per kg of body weight at any one meal or snack.[20] The most ideal ratio of carbohydrate to protein in a snack or meal is 4:1.[20]

Phytonutrients

Phytonutrients are beneficial chemicals that come from plant-based foods. These substances have health-promotion properties (such as improving heart health or promoting immune function) but cannot be defined as either vitamin or mineral. Although this chapter does not cover phytonutrients in depth, you should know that these substances exist and that they are very beneficial to overall health. Eating a variety of plant-based foods can ensure the intake of a wide variety of phytonutrients. Some great examples of plant-based foods with phytonutrients are green tea, berries, leafy greens, and citrus fruits.

• Fat-soluble vitamins require the presence of fat in the body (see the previous section Fat) to be absorbed and transported. The fat-soluble vitamins A, D, E, and K are best consumed with dietary fat to achieve optimal levels in the body.

Table 10.3 summaries specific vitamins.

Vitamin D

Vitamin D is called the sunshine vitamin because ultraviolet rays can be converted to vitamin D in our skin. Low levels of vitamin D in the winter (and less sunny) months can be a contributing factor to seasonal affective disorder or low mood levels. Maintaining adequate calcium and

TABLE 10.3 Vitamin Sources for Promoting Healing and Immune Function

Vitamin	Recommended dietary allowance	Excellent sources (≥20% daily value, or DV) based on standard serving size	Good sources (≥10% DV) based on standard serving size
Vitamin A	9-13 years: 600 mcg 14+ years: 900 mcg (male); 700 mcg (female)	Beef liver, sweet potato, pumpkin, cantaloupe, sweet red bell peppers, mangoes, broccoli, apricots	Herring, tomato juice, ricotta cheese
Folic acid or folate	9-13 years: 300 mcg 14+ years: 400 mcg	Beef liver, spinach, black-eyed peas, cooked rice, asparagus, enriched spaghetti	Cooked broccoli, raw spinach, avocado, white bread, kidney beans, green peas, boiled mustard greens
Vitamin B$_{12}$	9-13 years: 1.8 mcg 14+ years: 2.4 mcg	Clams, trout, sockeye salmon, beef liver, haddock, some fortified breakfast cereals, sirloin	Milk, Swiss cheese, beef, ham, egg
Vitamin C	9-13 years: 45 mg 14-18 years: 75 mg (male); 65 mg (female) 19+ years: 90 mg (male); 75 mg (female)	Red or green bell peppers, orange juice, orange, grapefruit juice, kiwi, broccoli, Brussels sprouts, grapefruit, tomato juice, cantaloupe, cabbage, cauliflower, potato, tomato	Spinach, green peas, pumpkin, prune juice, peaches, potatoes, summer squash, yellow corn, edamame, okra, butternut squash
Vitamin D	Children: 600 IU (15 mcg) 14-70 years: 600 IU (15 mcg) 70+ years: 800 IU (20 mcg)	Cod liver oil, swordfish, sockeye salmon, tuna fish, orange juice fortified with vitamin D (check label), yogurt fortified with 20% DV vitamin D, milk	Egg (in the yolk), sardines
Vitamin E	9-13 years: 11 mg 14+ years: 15 mg	Wheat germ oil, sunflower seeds, almonds, sunflower oil, safflower oil, hazelnuts	Peanuts, corn oil, spinach

vitamin D intake is a primary way to promote optimal bone health. Peak bone mass is the stage at which the bones have reached their highest level of bone density. Peak bone mass generally occurs between the ages of 18 and 25 years for most people.[21] This important milestone determines bone health throughout the life span. One thing to consider is that the majority of teenagers and young adults do not have the most optimal nutrient intakes, especially nutrient-dense foods that contain calcium and vitamin D. See table 10.3 for vitamin D intake recommendations.

Vitamin D supplements should not be taken without counsel from a professional. Physician testing for vitamin D levels for at-risk people is relatively easy.[11] Note that anyone living in northern latitudes will have a very difficult time maintaining vitamin D levels because of the lack of sun, especially during the winter season. Other at-risk populations include people with dark skin, the elderly, and people who frequently wear sunscreen. For optimal absorption, vitamin D supplements should be taken with the largest meal of the day that includes added fat, such as salad dressing, olive oil, nuts and seeds, avocado, or trans-fat-free margarine spreads.[22,23]

Maintaining adequate levels of circulating vitamin D is crucial to both optimal health and performance. An RD can be your best source when deciding on an optimal dose. If adequate, serum levels will range from 30 to 100 nmol/L in healthy people.[24-26] Note that although 30 to 50 nmol/L are considered optimal by most medical providers, this amount differs from the Institute of Medicine's recommendations for bone and overall health in healthy people.[25]

B Vitamins

B vitamins are essential micronutrients that regulate the formation of the body's energy pathways and the muscle-building process. Without them, the body would not be able to convert the energy in our food to energy within the body. B vitamins should be a key focus area for athletes and other physically active people due to their increased demand for cellular energy when performing their activity.

The marketing of vitamin B inaccurately promotes the idea that B vitamins work in our body to metabolize macronutrients (especially carbohydrate and fat), making it seem that these vitamins have calories and give you more energy. In truth, the B vitamins do not have any caloric or energy component to their structure and operate only as cofactors to the body's aerobic and anaerobic metabolic pathways. Although B vitamins are required for energy production, they are not the most essential nutrient for directly providing energy to the cells.

Active people do need more B vitamins than sedentary ones. This does not mean that a well-balanced diet cannot support this additional requirement for athletes and physically active people. The largest food source both for muscle energy and of B vitamins is complex carbohydrates. Active people following a low-carbohydrate diet may not be obtaining adequate B vitamins. See table 10.3 for intake recommendations for B vitamins.

Minerals

Minerals are one of the six essential nutrients. They are divided into two categories—major and trace—based on

---

Antioxidants

Antioxidants have been widely studied. You should understand where they come from in food, their role in health and wellness, and their importance in the healing process. A person may supplement with antioxidants to reduce muscle soreness after exercise; however, research indicates low to moderate evidence of antioxidants assisting with this.[27] The main benefit of antioxidants is that they are the molecules that interact with free radicals.

Free radicals are atoms or groups of atoms with an odd (unpaired) number of electrons that are formed when oxygen interacts with certain molecules. Their presence results in cellular damage and even cell death. In short, oxygen is bad for cells in the human body. Think of bruises on a piece of fruit. You drop your apple, the cells get damaged, oxygen gets into your apple, and the cells turn brown and die, leaving a brown spot on your apple. The same thing happens in our bodies when the cell walls are damaged and oxygen enters the cell. Antioxidants effectively end the chain reaction of cellular damage caused by free radicals.

Antioxidants are found in fruits, vegetables, and whole-grains. Foods and substances particularly rich in antioxidants are citrus fruits, berries, and green tea. Meeting the recommendation of eating five or more fruits and vegetables per day will help people meet recommended intakes for a variety of antioxidant nutrients.[11]

the amount required in the diet (table 10.4). Calcium and iron are two of the most important minerals for physically active people. In general, minerals are an important part of the diet due to their role in many physiological functions.

Calcium

Calcium, a major mineral, is important for both bone health and muscle contractions. To achieve adequate calcium intake, focus on consuming low-fat dairy products, such as milk and yogurt, as well as other fortified foods, such as breakfast cereal. Certain vegetables also contain some calcium, such as collard greens, kale, spinach, and broccoli.

Iron

Iron is an important mineral that serves to move oxygen throughout the body by the use of hemoglobin and myoglobin. This is important because a depleted reserve of oxygen hinders any muscle's ability to perform at optimal levels.[28,29] Running low on iron, or being deficient, has not been reported as much of an issue for sedentary people, recreational athletes, or active people who are exercising at moderate levels.[11] It is typically female athletes, endurance athletes, elite athletes, and athletes consuming a vegetarian diet who are at the highest risks for depleted iron stores. For elite athletes, intense physical activity may cause both increased iron losses in sweat, feces, and urine and physical trauma, which leads to the destruction of red blood cells.[11,29,30]

Iron deficiency, called **anemia**, is diagnosed primarily by low levels of serum ferritin. Measuring the serum ferritin provides a specific look at a person's level of iron stored in the body. If iron-deficiency anemia is diagnosed through blood work, the best course of treatment is increasing values by taking a dietary supplement of ferrous sulphate.[31] It is very hard to correct a deficiency through increased dietary intakes alone. However, with that said, people should not supplement iron randomly. If a person is suspected of being anemic, she should schedule an appointment with her personal physician or the team physician.

Fluids

Water, one of our six essential nutrients, is just as important for optimal performance as a person's fueling strategies with carbohydrate, protein, and fat. It is the structural base for all cells and body fluids. Water serves many important roles in the body:

TABLE 10.4 Daily Values (DV) for Minerals and Sources for Select Minerals

Mineral	DV	Excellent sources (≥20% DV) based on standard serving size	Good sources (≥10% DV) based on standard serving size
Calcium	1,000 mg	Yogurt, cheese, milk, calcium-fortified orange juice, calcium-fortified soy milk, some brands of tofu made with calcium sulfate	Canned salmon with bones, cottage cheese, turnip greens, raw kale, soybeans
Iron	18 mg	Oysters, white beans, dark chocolate	Sardines, kidney beans, beef, tofu, spinach, lentils, chickpeas
Magnesium	400 mg	Pumpkin seeds, almonds, spinach, soybeans, black-eyed peas, Brazil nuts, cashews	Kidney beans, peanuts, brown rice, wild rice, walnuts
Phosphorus	1,250 mg	Turkey, pumpkin seeds, sunflower seeds, cheese (Swiss, cheddar, provolone), Brazil nuts, sesame seeds, milk, beans (white, yellow, pink, navy, pinto, lima), quinoa, almonds, wild rice	Beef, ricotta cheese, edamame
Potassium	3,500 mg	Radishes, beans (white, black, lima, pink, kidney, pinto, soybeans, French), turkey, orange juice, peaches, potatoes, bananas, yam, tomatoes	Apricots, cod, halibut, Brussels sprouts, milk, artichokes, vegetable juice, brown rice, winter squash, beef
Zinc	15 mg	Oysters, red meat	Poultry, fish, beans, cashews; diets high in protein provide substantial amounts of zinc.

Putting Evidence-Based Nutrition Guidelines Into Practice

- Complex carbohydrates should be the base of every diet. Choosing plant-based sources of grains, fruits, and vegetables can help active people follow a low-fat diet and obtain an optimal balance of macronutrients to support their energy needs.
- Choose foods for their **nutrient density**, not just calories. Each food a client chooses to eat should include a multitude of micronutrients and other phytochemicals to provide for both optimal performance and long-term health.
- Be consistent! This applies to many things in life, but especially to metabolism. For optimal metabolism, it is best to eat six to eight times evenly and consistently throughout the day. Clients should consume their first meal within 1 hour of waking. That will start their engine (metabolism) very quickly!
- Clients should drink early and often, following their thirst throughout the day. If an athlete can, he should weigh in before and after practice for optimal postpractice rehydration. Urine color can also be a great parameter to watch throughout the day (see figure 8.2).

- Transports nutrients
- Aids digestion
- Normalizes blood pressure
- Regulates body temperature
- Optimizes muscle function
- Lubricates joints

The water in a person's blood is especially important because it serves to keep her at top performance. For additional information on hydration and how it is related to heat illness and athletic performance, please review the content in chapter 8.

Recommended water intake is as follows:

- Men: 2.4 to 3.7 L per day
- Women: 2.1 to 2.7 L per day

Sports Drinks

For most people, sports drinks provide no benefit. Sugar drinks can be one of the leading causes of obesity and chronic disease in any population. However, for athletes, sports drinks may serve a purpose. Sports drinks are a water-based fluid that also contribute carbohydrate and electrolyte sources to respectively fuel and assist in hydration of working muscles. Most active people participating in less than 60 minutes of continuous activity will not require sports drinks.[7] When a person goes beyond 60 minutes of continuous activity or if the environment warrants, then sports drinks may become necessary.

The single most important factor to a functional sports drink is that it leaves the gastrointestinal tract quickly and without upset and enters the person's circulation, where it both replenishes glycogen stores and spares the use of energy stores, which will allow for continued fueling of sport. An optimal sports drink should contain at least 4% but no more than 8% carbohydrate. A sports drink with more than 8% carbohydrate (such as 100% fruit juice, regular sodas, and fruit punch drinks) will have a much slower absorption time than those with 4% to 8% carbohydrate. Neglecting this seemingly small detail can cause gastrointestinal cramping, nausea, bloating, and diarrhea.

Other than its water base, the other essential component to a performance-enhancing sports drink is electrolytes. **Electrolytes** are micronutrients that separate into ions in solution, thus acquiring the capacity to conduct electricity. The main electrolytes that are mandatory for optimal cellular hydration and functions are sodium, potassium, chloride, calcium, magnesium, and phosphate. Sodium plays the largest role in hydration because of its specific work to aid muscle contractions and cellular hydration status. This is an area of sports nutrition where defining who classifies as an athlete is very important in determining which guidelines to follow. Sports drinks are necessary only for activity of moderate- to high-intensity for greater than 60 minutes or for exercise in a very hot and humid environment. For everything else, water is the best choice for optimal hydration.

Nutrition for Optimal Healing

When an injury occurs, there are different stages to the healing process. Each of these stages requires an intake of essential nutrients above and beyond the daily requirements in order for optimal healing to occur.[11] For injuries that are significant in their nature, especially postoperatively, the additional energy required can be 15% to 30% more than the patient's resting energy expenditure.[36] Even something like ambulating on crutches can increase a patient's energy needs significantly throughout a day.

FOUNDATIONAL SKILL

Schedule of Hydration Before, During, and After Exercise

Before Exercise
- 2-4 hours before exercise
- 5-10 mL/kg
- Elicits pale yellow or lighter urine color

During Exercise
- 0.4-0.8 L/hr
- Hydration must be individualized to each athlete.
- Some weight loss is to be expected, but weight loss greater than 2% of body weight can impair performance.
- Athletes should not gain water weight during exercise; this can increase the risk of hyponatremia.

After Exercise
- Replace up to 150% of weight lost
- Roughly 16 to 24 fl oz (475-710 mL) per lb body weight

EVIDENCE-BASED ATHLETIC TRAINING

Chocolate Milk

Chocolate milk is a popular postactivity drink. It's not the chocolate that is the key, but rather the simple carbohydrates found in the natural milk sugar galactose (lactose/glucose) and the added sugars of sucrose (glucose/fructose) that provide the two most optimal sources for replenishing the glycogen stores of depleted muscles.[32,33]

Research has continually identified chocolate milk as an optimal recovery fuel beverage.[11,18,27,32-35] The optimal times for consuming chocolate milk are immediately after exercise and again 2 hours postactivity.[11,18,27,32-35]

There are four components to chocolate milk that make it one of the best choices as a recovery fuel after a workout or sport activity:

1. *Fluids.* During recovery, hydration is important. Athletes should be replacing approximately 150% of the weight lost during their sport or activity with fluids.[8] Having athletes consume 12 to 24 fl oz (355-710 mL) of chocolate milk to meet their recovery fuel needs will also replace some hydration lost during activity or sport. Consuming approximately 16 to 24 fl oz (475-710 mL) will replace 1 lb (0.5 kg) of weight lost. Consuming more chocolate milk than is required for meeting recovery fuel guidelines isn't necessarily better, so if an athlete has lost more than 1.5 lb (0.7 kg) of weight throughout his session, he should use water or sports drink to recover the remainder of his fluid balance.

2. *Type of carbohydrate.* The galactose (lactose and glucose) and sucrose (glucose/fructose) sources of carbohydrate (CHO) in milk are the fastest CHO types to be absorbed and so quickly go to work replenishing CHO stores of those working muscles.[32,33]

3. *Type of protein (PRO).* For optimal MPS, the branched chain amino acids are important.

4. *CHO-to-PRO ratio.* The CHO-to-PRO ratio shown to best refuel the glycogen stores of working muscles is roughly 4:1. Since chocolate milk has 32 g CHO to 8 g PRO, it is a perfect recovery beverage.[11,27,34,35]

To individualize a chocolate milk dose for an athlete, follow the recovery fuel guidelines of 1.0 to 1.5 g CHO per kg body weight and 0.25 to 0.30 g PRO per kg body weight.[11,34,35]

Bottom line: Make sure patients do not cut their calorie intake too short or else they may decrease their body's ability to heal optimally.

Protein is important in the healing process because the body needs more protein for repairing existing cells and potentially building new cells at the site of an injury. Especially if needing to be immobilized, there can be a tendency to lose lean mass, which would have negative effects on a patient's power and speed in the long run. A patient's postinjury protein intake should be between 1.6 and 2.0 g of protein per kilogram of body weight per day. All dietary needs should be addressed individually with each patient. Because many people already consume upper limits of protein daily, it is likely that the patient may already be consuming adequate amounts of this essential nutrient for healing. Patients who may potentially need to increase protein intake after an injury are endurance athletes, women, and vegetarians.

Carbohydrate cannot be overlooked in the healing process, and during the healing process, most calories should come from complex carbohydrates. The level of carbohydrate consumed should be very individualized to sport or activity, degree of injury or trauma, and the expected time frame of recovery so as to prevent unwanted weight gain.

Many essential nutrients can help in the inflammation process:[11]

- Omega-3s and antioxidants assist directly with decreasing inflammation and promoting healing.
- Vitamin C is vital for wound healing and cellular repairs.
- Vitamin A greatly aids cellular growth when the body is required to make new cells at the site of an injury.
- Vitamin D works with calcium to promote bone health and is an important nutrient for the body's immune system.[37]
- Zinc is important for wound healing and immune function.[38,39]

Patients should eat fruits and vegetables in a rainbow of colors in order to obtain the optimal blend of vitamins and minerals to promote healing. Foods with suboptimal nutritional content can hinder the healing process. Alcohol consumption, smoking, and poor sleep are also factors that decrease the body's ability to heal optimally.[40]

Low Energy Availability

Athletic trainers may be the first health care providers to recognize and intervene with many nutrition- and dietary-related conditions. Treatment of conditions related to lower energy availability may be beyond your scope of practice, but you should know how to recognize signs and symptoms, make proper referrals, and assist with treatment plans prescribed by the team physician, RD, and other members of the sports medicine team. As with all aspects of sports medicine, the team approach is generally the best.

The conditions discussed in the following sections all relate to inadequate energy balance. Energy balance seems simple on the surface: energy in, energy out. However, maintaining optimal energy balance is a more complex situation because bodies have many adaptations to **low energy availability**. Although disordered eating patterns definitely influence a person's dietary intakes, they are not the sole reason she may suffer the consequences of low energy availability. For details on differentiating aspects of disordered eating and evaluating a client for a clinical eating disorder, please see chapter 19. It is worth mentioning here that the NATA position statement *Preventing, Detecting, and Managing Disordered Eating in Athletes* is an evidence-based resource for practicing athletic trainers.[10]

Inadequate consumption of essential nutrients is a contributing factor to many medical and health-related concerns. Any person who is performing very strenuous exercise or not consuming adequate calories will be at potential risk for developing low energy availability or a relative energy deficit. The term "relative" can be used in some cases because it is possible for an athlete to be physically unable to consume adequate calories for his sport, such as in the case of an athlete training for an ultramarathon. It might seem obvious, but it must be stressed that an energy deficit will have many negative consequences on health and, for athletes, performance.

Female Athlete Triad

The **female athlete triad** was the first defined condition that could be related to low energy availability. It was first defined as a progression of an energy deficit that leads to menstrual cycle disruption and ultimately may be causative to bone mineral losses, stress fractures, or the occurrence of osteoporosis. This triad was made more three dimensional and expanded so that the sequelae of symptoms is now more of a spectrum related to the variations and degrees of physiological changes occurring. The current recommendations for the triad define variations of low energy intakes versus clinical eating disorders, oligomenorrhea to amenorrhea, and ranges of bone mineral loss across a spectrum (figure 10.1).[10,11,41,42]

Since a defining characteristic of the female athlete triad is the presence or absence of menstrual cycles, it is relatable only to physically active women. In this population, the development of amenorrhea due to low energy availability causes a greater risk of stress fractures occurring. Although stress fractures or low bone mineral

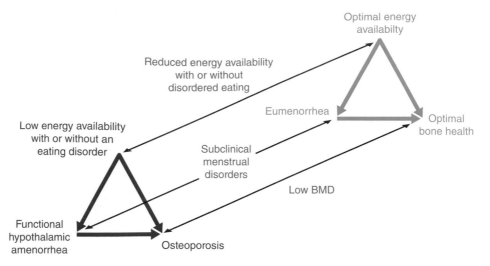

FIGURE 10.1   Female athlete triad.

density can affect any active person's sport participation, you should focus on the lifelong effects of the potential development of osteopenia or osteoporosis when discussing the triad with your clients. Your ultimate goal is to promote long-term health and wellness.

Suspicions of the female athlete triad should be part of a differential diagnosis when a menstrual cycle is absent for more than 3 months. Any woman who has experienced disruptions to her menstrual cycles for this magnitude or longer should be evaluated by a health care provider specializing in sports medicine and the female athlete triad.

The goal with any treatment is the resumption of normal menses and thus improved bone mineral density. The two main factors in treatment are increased caloric intakes and decreased caloric expenditure through reduced exercise. However, overall treatment goals may also include maintaining adequate body fat stores as well as ensuring a desirable level of daily calcium (between 1,000 and 1,500 mg per day). Due to the multiple conditions present, as well as the potential for a clinical eating disorder, take a team approach to care and work with the team physician, an RD, and a mental health professional.

These screening questions are recommended as part of the sport preparticipation examination (which is covered in detail in chapter 8):[41]

- Have you ever had a menstrual period?
- How old were you when you had your first menstrual period?
- When was your most recent menstrual period?
- How many periods have you had in the past 12 months?
- Are you presently taking any hormone replacement (estrogen, progesterone, oral birth control pills)?
- Do you worry about your weight?

- Are you trying to lose or gain weight?
- Has anyone recommended that you gain or lose weight?
- Are you on a special diet?
- Do you avoid certain types of foods or food groups?
- Have you ever had an eating disorder?
- Have you ever had a stress fracture?
- Have you ever been told you have low bone density (osteopenia or osteoporosis)?

Return to play after treatment for the female athlete triad is determined by the treating physician and based on a complex and comprehensive combination of health status, cumulative risk assessment, participation risk, sport, and decision modifiers.[41,43] Work with the treating physician and follow any reported guidelines to help a client return to play.

Relative Energy Deficiency in Sport (RED-S)

Although the female athlete triad first identified the topic of low energy availability, there has been a recent focus by the International Olympic Committee (IOC) on the effect of low energy availability on a full range of body physiology.[42] In its consensus statement, the IOC applied the physiological changes related to an energy deficit to all athletes, both male and female.[42] The IOC has taken special efforts to notice the female athlete triad as one spoke of the wheel of **relative energy deficiency in sport (RED-S)**. However, RED-S has expanded to include the physiological effects of low energy availability across all body systems (see figure 10.2).

For evaluating medical risk of RED-S, the IOC provides a three-level, color-coded system.

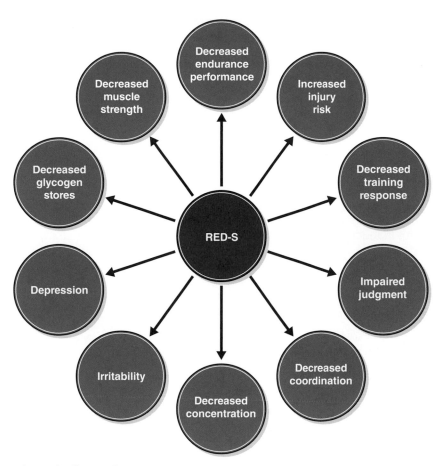

FIGURE 10.2 Physiological effects of RED-S.

1. *Green light.* The green light factors constitute the lowest risk. When physiological systems are evaluated, this level is determined when a provider's physical assessment finds healthy eating practices, normal metabolic functions, ideal bone mineral density, and a fully functioning musculoskeletal system.

2. *Yellow light.* When health risks are determined in an assessment, then an athlete may be considered in the zone of yellow light and her sport participation may be reduced or discontinued until she can achieve markers of optimal health. Some considerations for this level are significant decrease in body fat percentage, primary amenorrhea, reduced bone mineral density, abnormal lab values for hormone profiles, and physiological effects on the cardiovascular system, such as bradycardia.

3. *Red light.* The red light level of assessment warrants holding any athlete from participating in sport until medical clearance is obtained. The presence of a clinical eating disorder, serious medical condition (e.g., abnormal ECG), and

hemodynamic instability warrant anyone to be limited from sports activity.

Lastly, regardless of status, one large factor to successful treatment is patient compliance. Any noncompliance or lack of progress in treatment should be further evaluated and discontinuation of sport participation considered.

Dietary Supplements

Athletes and other physically active people often use **dietary supplements** as an ergogenic aid to enhance their sport performance. An **ergogenic aid** is any "training technique, mechanical device, nutritional ingredient or practice, pharmacological method, or psychological technique that can improve exercise performance capacity or enhance training adaptations."[44] Some supplements taken for promotion of health can be as basic as a multivitamin/mineral and others can be thought to be sport-enhancing, such as caffeine.

Supplement Regulation

Anyone considering a nutritional supplement must be educated on the lack of regulations of the industry. The

Resources on Dietary Supplements and Nutrition

Visit the websites of these organizations for good information on dietary supplements and nutrition:

World Anti-Doping Agency

NSF International's Certified for Sport

USP Dietary Supplement Verification Program

National Institute of Health

Drug Free Sport

U.S. Anti-Doping Association

Food and Nutrition Information Center (FNIC)

President's Council on Fitness, Sports, and Nutrition

American College of Sports Medicine

American Council on Exercise

Centers for Disease Control and Prevention

Sports, Cardiovascular and Wellness Nutrition (SCAN)

Collegiate and Professional Sports Dietitians Association

National Collegiate Athletic Association

Gatorade Sports Science Institute

bottom line with nutritional supplements of any kind is that they are produced in a buyer beware market. In 1994, the Dietary Supplement Health and Education Act (DSHEA) eliminated regulations prior to the release of dietary supplements, which allowed nutritional supplements to become a billion-dollar industry almost overnight. The largest negative effect of reduced regulation is that a manufacturer can put a nutritional supplement on the market with very little or even zero testing of its safety, quality, and efficacy.[45] In the early 2000s, the Food and Drug Administration (FDA) did add some regulations that disallowed disease claims on a dietary supplement label. The most recent changes came about in December 2006 with the Dietary Supplement and Nonprescription Drug Consumer Protection Act. This bill requires manufacturers of dietary supplements and nonprescription drugs to notify the FDA about serious adverse events related to their products.

One thing all people should look for with their nutritional supplements is the United States Pharmacopeia (USP) seal of quality assurance or one of many other assurances of third-party testing. To date, third-party testing programs are voluntary but are the only way to ensure the content and quality of a dietary supplement. For athletes, an unregulated dietary supplement may cause them to fail a drug test and disqualify them from competition. The negatives of poor regulation may outweigh the potential benefits to health or performance gained by taking a nutritional supplement.

Many questions should be asked *prior* to using any dietary supplement:

- Is it proven?
- Is it safe?
- Is it recommended?
- For athletes, is it legal?
- For athletes, is it banned?

For most competitive athletes, including collegiate, regulations exist regarding the use of dietary supplements and performance-enhancing ergogenic aids; some are banned from use.[9] The NCAA has a list of banned substances for use by collegiate athletes.[46]

Almost all athletes use or have used a vitamin or mineral nutritional supplement to enhance their sport performance.[47] However, with evidence lacking to show positive effects of these supplements, the **placebo effect** is likely to be responsible.[48,49]

Amino Acids

Twenty amino acids can be consumed through diet, and nine are essential. Amino acids are promoted as enhancing sport performance in a variety of ways, such as increasing the production of anabolic hormones, modifying fuel use during sport, preventing adverse effects of overtraining, and preventing mental fatigue.[9,11] Each amino acid has a different job, and the way amino acids are strung together determines the functionality of a protein.

For athletes and physically active people, the most functional amino acids are the branched-chain amino acids isoleucine, leucine, and valine.[11] However, conclusive evidence does not exist to recommend their use. Lastly, protein-based nutritional supplements, including amino acids, are a large group of nutritional supplements that can be cross contaminated with banned substances. Are protein and amino acid supplements harmful? Not likely, if they are consumed in moderation and evaluated for safety and legality of ingredients. However, they are definitely not a necessity.

Energy Drinks and Preworkout Energy Powders

Energy drinks have been mass-marketed to become one of the most popular drinks across the United States. Preworkout energy powders have also increased in popularity. These powders usually include a proprietary blend of ingredients that are based around high amounts of caffeine or stimulants, simple carbohydrates, and mixture of vitamins and minerals. The stimulant ingredients have caused many athletes and physically active people to use them for an energy boost to get through their day. When using this energy boost to assist their sport performance, however, they could run into many issues.

- Caffeine is a banned substance for NCAA competitive athletes at levels greater than 15 mcg/mL in urine.[46] This corresponds to ingesting about 500 mg, or the equivalent of 6 to 8 cups of brewed coffee; when consumed 2 to 3 hours before competition, it can produce a positive drug test.
- If they use energy drinks as a meal replacement, people may be missing vital nutrition from whole foods. The only real source of fuel for our energy systems is carbohydrate with a backup of fatty acids. If a person is feeling fatigued, the first place to look for energy should be from whole-food sources.

There have been some documented benefits of moderate caffeine use as an ergogenic aid. The goal for intakes is 2 to 6 mg of caffeine per kg body weight, or 1 to 3 cups of brewed coffee.[7,11,50] As a stimulant, the effects of caffeine will peak at approximately 1 hour post consumption. For people who have habitually consumed caffeine, the effects of caffeine will be blunted and possibly nonexistent. Individual tolerances can be very varied, leading to different responses to the use of caffeine or stimulants as a nutritional supplement for sport.

The potential benefits of caffeine are as follows:

- Decreased pain and perception of fatigue
- Decreased perceived exertion during submaximal resistance training
- Improved performance in endurance and sustained high-intensity training or competitions with consecutive high-intensity bouts lasting longer than 90 seconds
- Increased body coordination, ability to focus and concentrate, and sustained training intensity

The potential risks of caffeine are as follows:

- Caffeinated products may contain unlabeled or unclear amounts of banned stimulants like synephrine that when added to unknown amounts of caffeine can result in serious health consequences, including death.
- High levels of caffeine (i.e., 6 to 9 mg of caffeine per kg of body weight) can cause gastrointestinal issues, nausea, or shaking, as well as overstimulation that can negatively affect training, sleep, and performance.
- It's addictive! When consumed consistently, in levels as low as 100 mg a day (1 cup of brewed coffee), people can get addicted to caffeine. Subsequent removal of caffeine can cause withdrawal symptoms such as headache, fatigue, depression, irritability, insomnia, increased or irregular heart rate, and increased blood pressure.
- Without adequate fluids, caffeine can cause undesirable effects to thermal regulation, increasing the risk for heat illness.

Many nutritional products can also contain "other ingredients," or proprietary blends, which may contain banned substances for various sports organizations or very negative substances for overall health, such as stimulants. Clients should ask themselves the following questions prior to using an energy drink supplement to see if it will really benefit their health and performance:

- Does the drink contain herbal ingredients that will potentially result in a positive on a drug test or be harmful to my health?
- Will any of the ingredients in the products have adverse reactions or interactions with any prescription or over-the-counter medications?
- Does research show any evidence toward the claims being made for performance enhancement or health promotion?
- Does the product have a Nutrition Facts or Supplements Facts panel? Listed ingredients? If not, avoid this product!
- Does it contain "other ingredients" or a proprietary blend? If so, avoid this product!
- For athletes, are there any "other ingredients" that may be on a banned substance list for competitive sport?

- Have I done all I can with food-based nutrition interventions to achieve my desired goals?

Despite a popular belief that stimulants are helpful, research findings are conflicted, especially related to any benefits for sport performance and metabolism.[11,51] The largest touted positive effect is that caffeine consumption spares glycogen by causing a release of free fatty acids to be used as fuel. Thus, time to fatigue is extended and an athlete can perform for longer. However, there are just as many studies that do not show that caffeine has a significant impact on fuel use or fat oxidation.[51] The previously mentioned glycogen sparing effect has been seen only with elite-level and highly trained athletes.

In short, all people would do well to remember that caffeine is a drug. Overall, for energy drinks, caffeine, and stimulant preworkout drinks, the client, the athletic trainer, and the RD/CSSD should work together to determine if supplemental caffeine is appropriate, weighing all of the potential benefits and risks.

Protein Powders and Bars

The use of protein powders and bars has skyrocketed among all populations, but especially among athletes and physically active people. With many fad diets focused on higher levels of protein intake, the market is saturated with all types and formulations of protein found in powders and bars. The most popular is whey protein, which has been shown to play a large part in muscle protein synthesis. However, most animal-based proteins of a high biological value have also shown positive results for MPS. Soy is the only plant-based protein to show similar results to whey protein, although more research needs to be conducted, so it should not be counted out for enhancing MPS.[18]

Although protein powders and bars can be another group of nutrition supplement that have high levels of cross contamination and potentially contain banned substances, they can also be very functional. The dose and timing of the protein consumed play the largest roles in nutritional efficacy.[11,18] Powders can be a convenient and easy way to space out protein consumption throughout the day. Many people may not be accustomed to eating protein in the morning or may not give themselves enough time to prepare and eat a breakfast with protein. Mixing up a shake or putting some protein powder in their oatmeal can be a quick fix to full-day protein spacing. Protein bars offer portability and convenience for many sport and activity settings.

Omega-3s

One of the most important essential fatty acids is omega-3 polyunsaturated fatty acids (PUFAs). Research has demonstrated that these essential fatty acids perform many functions, such as decreasing the production of inflammatory eicosanoids, cytokines, and reactive oxygen species; supporting immunomodulatory effects; and attenuating inflammatory diseases.[52] Although a number of studies have assessed the efficacy of omega-3 PUFA supplementation on red blood cell deformability, muscle damage, inflammation, and metabolism during exercise, their full influence on exercise performance is still up for debate.[52-54] Some research has recommended the consumption of EPA and DHA of approximately 1 to 2 g per day, at a ratio of EPA to DHA of 2:1, to reduce exercise-induced inflammation and improve overall cell health.[55-57]

The recommendations for dietary intakes for most adults are approximately 8 oz (230 g) of seafood per week, more specifically fatty foods such as salmon, tuna, swordfish, or sardines. Consuming this amount of seafood each week will provide about 500 mg of EPA and DHA each day.[12] People who are not getting seafood in their diet may choose to take a nutritional supplement. As a general rule, the recommendations all advise a minimum intake in the range of 250 to 500 mg combined EPA and DHA each day for healthy adults.[12] However, higher amounts are often recommended for certain health conditions.

EVIDENCE-BASED ATHLETIC TRAINING

Do Omega-3s Help Patients Recover From Concussions?

Animal studies have demonstrated that there are potential anti-inflammatory benefits for recovery from a traumatic brain injury and that there can be a potential reduction in inflammation with high doses of omega-3s.[58-60] It is an understatement to say we need more research, especially in human populations. But, from what we know about omega-3s and their general functions, it would not be a negative practice to suggest supplementation either before injury as a preventive measure or after a concussion has occurred to promote optimal health and potentially a reduction in the inflammatory process.

CLINICAL BOTTOM LINE

- Athletic trainers should take a team-based approach to meeting their clients' nutrition needs, working with an RD who is ideally a CSSD as well. Other members of the sports medicine team frequently include the team physician and a sports psychologist or other member of the mental health profession.

- Meeting the nutrition needs of athletes and other physically active people involves more than just balancing the client's energy expenditures through the intake of carbohydrate, protein, and fat. Key micronutrients and fluids also play an important role in successful fueling for optimal sport performance. What is needed for each essential nutrient can vary based on many factors.

- Myths abound about nutrition, fad diets are promoted in the news, and supplements are available for purchase through the more than billion-dollar nutrition products industry. Since everyone seems to be selling something, athletic trainers should educate clients about proper nutrition based on information supported by the evidence. Many great resources are available to help with this task, including multiple position statements and reputable websites.

- Athletic trainers should be aware of low energy availability conditions to better assist patients in receiving the proper referral in a timely manner.

 Go to HK*Propel* to complete the activities and case studies for this chapter.

CHAPTER 11

Protective Equipment

Ellen K. Payne, PhD, LAT, ATC, EMT

CAATE STANDARDS

The following CAATE 2020 standard is covered in this chapter:

Standard 60

CHAPTER OBJECTIVES

After reading this chapter, you will be able to do the following:

- Describe legal considerations as they relate to protective equipment

- Identify agencies and organizations involved with the use of protective equipment

- Discuss issues related to selecting, issuing, and maintaining protective equipment

- Discuss various types of protective equipment commonly used in sport and activity

- Explain the proper fitting of select protective equipment and related foundational skills

- Understand equipment and techniques used in emergency equipment removal

- Explain the removal of select protective equipment and related foundational skills

One of the primary responsibilities of athletic trainers is the prevention of injuries. The use of protective equipment is one of the main ways to mitigate risk and help prevent injuries before they occur. Knowledge and skills related to **protective equipment** use is one of the areas that sets athletic trainers apart from other allied health care providers who work with physically active people. Athletic trainers must be able to do the following:

- Advise athletes, clients, patients, coaches, parents, and other stakeholders on the selection of protective equipment

- Correctly fit equipment per the manufacturer's guidelines

- Safely remove emergency equipment

Athletic trainers are experts in the area of injury prevention, and other members of the sports medicine team look to them for leadership and guidance when working with protective equipment, which is often complex.

Protective equipment is an evolving field; new developments in technology change how equipment is designed and manufactured and sports rules and regulations change to reflect the evidence and needs of each sport.[1-5] Protective equipment used in sports must be continuously adapted to meet these requirements. Take the football helmet, for example, which evolved from a moleskin hat with earflaps to today's state-of-the-art, high-tech designs.[6] No piece of sporting equipment has changed so much or received so much media attention over the last 100 years. Part of your job is to stay updated on changes in the field and make sure athletes have access to protective equipment that meets their individual needs and their sport's rules and regulations.

The use of protective equipment is frequently associated with collision sports, such as football, ice hockey, and lacrosse, and sports with the risk of injury from high-velocity impact, such as baseball and softball. In truth, most athletes use some type of protective equipment to prevent injuries, although they may not think of the item in that way, like shoes. This chapter focuses primarily on general protective equipment used in traditional sports, but you are responsible for learning about the unique equipment used by all your clients. This includes in nontraditional settings, such as motor sports, the military, and industrial settings, which may have different rules and regulations for the use of protective equipment.

Legal Issues

Athletic trainers should not replace equipment managers. Both have important roles when working with protective equipment to keep clients safe. To ensure best practices

Agencies and Organizations Involved With Standards, Regulation, and Certification of Protective Equipment

American National Standards Institute (ANSI)

The mission of ANSI is to enhance quality of life and the global competitiveness of U.S. businesses by promoting and facilitating voluntary consensus standards and conformity assessment systems and safeguarding their integrity.[8]

Athletic Equipment Managers Association (AEMA)

The purpose of the AEMA is to promote, advance, and improve the profession of equipment managers in all of its many phases.[9]

Hockey Equipment Certification Council (HECC)

HECC's mission is to seek out, evaluate, and select standards and testing procedures for hockey equipment for the purpose of product certification.[10]

Occupational Safety and Health Administration (OSHA)

The mission of OSHA is to assure safe and healthful working conditions for working men and women by setting and enforcing standards and providing training, outreach, education, and assistance.[11]

ASTM International

ASTM International, formerly known as the American Society for Testing Materials, sets the standards for protective equipment, including athletic shoes, baseball and softball equipment, body padding of equestrian events, eyewear, and helmets for a variety of sports.[12]

CSA Group

The CSA Group, formerly known as the Canadian Standards Association, is an independent, nonprofit member-based association dedicated to advancing safety, sustainability, and social good. The organization is internationally accredited for standards development, testing, and certification. It provides consumer product evaluation and education and training services.[13]

National Operating Committee on Standards for Athletic Equipment (NOCSAE)

The NOCSAE sets standards for the certification and recertification of equipment in the following sports: baseball, softball, football, hockey, lacrosse, polo, and soccer.[14]

Sports and Fitness Industry Association (SFIA)

The Sports and Fitness Industry Association (SFIA), formerly the SGMA, is the trade association of leading industry sports and fitness brands, suppliers, retailers, and partners. Its mission is to promote sports and fitness participation and industry vitality by focusing on core product areas in industry.[15]

in protective equipment use, your job description should differentiate between your role and that of the equipment manager. Although there can be some overlap in responsibilities, as an entry-level athletic trainer, you will not be adequately trained to be an equipment manager; if you would like to take on this role, you will need additional training and certification. Athletic trainers should perform or supervise the following duties:

- Ensure clients have access to the best available equipment
- Properly fit equipment for each athlete
- Instruct clients on the use of the equipment and warn them of potential risks of its use or misuse
- Maintain the equipment per the manufacturer's recommendation

You may not be directly responsible for every aspect of equipment selection and fitting, but you should recognize when something is amiss and work to rectify the situation. Failure to do so could result in a negligence lawsuit for breach of duty. The CAATE educational competencies related to protective equipment outline the knowledge an entry-level athletic trainer should possess.

The use of protective equipment in the sports setting is not regulated by the federal government.[7] Guidelines could be different for athletic trainers working in nontra-ditional settings, such as in industry, where OSHA regulations would apply to safety equipment. In traditional settings, protective equipment use is regulated through sports leagues and associations, with enforcement designated to coaches and league officials. Third-party organizations outside the sports' leagues and associations certify that various equipment meet the set technical standards. The following sidebar lists agencies and organizations involved with standards, regulation, and certification of protective equipment.

Documentation

Proper documentation is an important aspect of working with protective equipment. The equipment manager, coach, or athletic trainer should maintain a detailed inventory of all protective equipment. When issuing equipment at the beginning of the season, keep a detailed record to help prevent a first-come-first-serve approach to distributing items, which could cause athletes at the end of the line to receive improperly fitted items.[2] You should maintain a record of all annual inspections and yearly maintenance of protective equipment, along with a record of any repairs completed. Lastly, document all client education on the proper use of protective equipment. More information on documentation for athletic trainers can be found in chapter 5.

EVIDENCE-BASED ATHLETIC TRAINING

Athletic Training Position Statements

The National Athletic Trainers' Association (NATA) has published seven position and consensus statements related to patient care and use and removal of protective equipment. These official position statements are found on the NATA website and are referenced throughout this chapter. They provide best-practice recommendations related to

- dental and oral facial injuries,
- exertional heat illness,
- cervical spine injuries,
- cervical spine injuries in American tackle football,
- concussions,
- preventing sudden death in sport, and
- emergency planning in athletics.[16-18,21,90,91]

The statements are created by a panel of experts in the specific areas who systematically review the evidence-based literature related to each topic and make recommendations. You should review these statements and incorporate the recommendations into your facility's policies and procedures manual and emergency action plan, when feasible. The recommendations made in the position statements do not dictate care, but they should be independently evaluated for their applicability to each institution's unique situation. You must stay abreast of changes in recommendations as they are released to ensure your organization provides the best possible patient care. In today's litigious society, failure to stay up to date on best-practice recommendations could open you up to a lawsuit.

Product Liability

Protective equipment also falls under the legal area of **product liability**. Product liability holds manufacturers responsible for product defects in equipment. Any warranty will be void if the equipment is used incorrectly or is altered in any way, so you should educate clients on proper use of equipment. Athletic trainers, coaches, and athletes should not modify protective equipment. An injury that can be attributed to modified equipment can result in legal action against the person who modified the equipment.

Selecting and Issuing Protective Equipment

When selecting protective equipment or educating stakeholders on the selection of protective equipment, ensure that the equipment purchased meets the appropriate agency's certification, as well as safety standards and league requirements. These standards vary by sport and sponsoring organization, and you should consult league manuals or handbooks for official requirements. Even among certified products, the quality and price can vary. Select equipment appropriate for the client's age, size, and level of play. Just because something costs the most does not mean it is the best product available. Before purchasing protective equipment, you should research the available products because of the ever-changing nature of the market. Only purchase equipment from a known, reputable manufacturer.

As stated previously, protective equipment should not be issued on a first-come-first-serve basis.[2] The equipment should meet the needs of the individual client and fit him properly. Take care to not simply pass down older equipment to younger, less-experienced athletes.[22] Any equipment being passed down should be inspected and in good repair.

During the process of issuing equipment, instruct clients on the proper fit, function, and use of the equipment. Do not make assumptions about the client's prior use and knowledge of the equipment, no matter the level of play the client is participating in. In the ever-changing world of protective equipment, clients need to be educated about proper fit, correct use, and benefits of protective equipment, along with any new features.[3,5,18-20,23-27] During the issuing of equipment, clients should read all warning labels and sign any assumption of risk waivers. For example, football and lacrosse helmets must have a NOCSAE warning label attached to the outside of the helmet, which should be read by the player and parent or guardian prior to signing a statement that the warning has been read and the client understands the warning. Additionally, document all client education on the equipment. Before completing the issuing process, instruct clients whom to notify if equipment fit changes or damage occurs to the equipment during the course of the season.

Maintenance and Recertification

Protective equipment should be inspected at least annually and maintained and cleaned per the manufacturer's guidelines. All defective equipment should be discarded or repaired promptly. All maintenance and repairs should be completed by the equipment manager or another trained person. Recertification should be done based on the manufacturer's guidelines and the certifying agency's standards. Using reconditioned helmets is a safe way that teams can save money on equipment.[28] You should document all inspections, maintenance, and recertifications. See the NFHS website for a concise and up-to-date list of licensed reconditioners.[29]

Basic Application of Protective Equipment

Since technology, industry standards, and league rules are frequently changing, comprehensiveness in this section is difficult. This section highlights common protective equipment and its key features. In general, all protective equipment should be fitted and maintained per the manufacturer's guidelines. The type of protective equipment required or recommended depends on the sport, level, and league. Chapter 12 addresses commercially available protective braces and sleeves and custom-created devices.

Head and Face Protective Equipment

Head and facial injuries can be severe and traumatic. Sports such as football, rugby, ice and field hockey, and soccer, among others, are considered high risk for orofacial trauma.[30] The use of protective equipment, such as helmets, face masks, mouth guards, and eye protection, can help prevent serious orofacial trauma from occurring in sports. Although some protective equipment is standard and mandated for sports (e.g., helmets and face masks in football), other items are currently only recommended (e.g., mouth guards in basketball). You should educate various stakeholders in both required and recommended protective equipment due to the potential seriousness of orofacial injuries during activity and sport.

Helmets and Headgear

Properly fitted helmets help reduce the incident of head and orofacial injuries by redistributing impact forces throughout the helmet.[2,5,23,31,32] Helmets have the following components:

- Hard outer shell: typically made from polycarbonate or other plastic composites
- Foam liner: made from various foams for cushioning properties

In general, the thicker the liner, the greater its potential to dissipate the forces, but lining material and the stiffness of the shell also play a role in the performance of the helmet.[31] Although there has been some discussion of multiuse helmets, because of the unique needs and varying requirements of most sports, they are impractical at this time.[30]

Helmets can protect either the head alone or the head and the face. The helmet that protects both the head and the face is a full-face helmet (figure 11.1). Full-face helmets are frequently used in motor sports, mountain biking, and skiing. Regular helmets can incorporate different face masks or visors depending on the sport or even the position within the sport. All helmets and attached accessories need to meet the standards and regulations set for that sport. No matter the type of helmet, it should never be used to intentionally make contact with another player or as a weapon. Serious injury or even death can occur from improper use of a helmet. Client education plays an important role in making sure the helmet is used as intended.

Headgear does not have a hard outer shell like a helmet; it is made of soft padding material. This can be a thin foam headband. Headgear is typically used in rugby, soccer, and boxing. The evidence to support the effectiveness of headgear to prevent head and facial injuries in these sports is mixed, and additional research is needed in this area.[5,18,25,33,34]

Football Helmets No other piece of protective equipment has garnished as much attention as the football helmet. The football helmet has developed over time in response to player needs, rule changes, and advances in technology and design. With continued research and product development, we have not seen the end of the evolution of the football helmet. New manufacturers and helmet models continue to enter the market.[35]

At all levels of football (youth to professional), the NOCSAE-certified helmet is required for competition. Preliminary research has demonstrated that helmetless practices may reduce the number of head impacts an athlete sustains, so a helmet might not be required for all practices.[36] The objective of the football helmet is to dissipate forces to prevent skull fractures and other orofacial trauma. Helmets must be able to withstand multiple player-to-player collisions and multiple impacts with the ground and other surfaces. The ability of the helmet to prevent concussions in football has been hotly debated. At the current time and with the current design, there is inconclusive evidence to support the idea of helmets preventing concussions in all situations, and additional research is warranted.[5,18,20,34,37,38]

All football helmets issued should meet the technical and safety standards set by NOCSAE. Here are some helmet manufacturers with NOCSAE-approved helmets:[35]

- Riddell models: Speed, Revolution Speed, Speed Icon, Foundation
- Schutt Sports models: Air XP Pro VTD II, DNA Pro+, Vengeance DCT, Vengeance VTD
- Xenith models: Epic+, X2E+, Epic, X2E

Additionally, independent researchers at Virginia Tech have developed a rating system for football helmets to help consumers purchase helmets with confidence.[39] Whether new or reconditioned, helmets are required to have a warning sticker attached directly to the outside (figure 11.2).

A variety of football helmets are sold with different technologies and features to meet the needs of individual players. Some helmets incorporate inflatable bladders, high-tech padding, and impact data sensors in an effort to better protect athletes. No matter the design of the football helmet, the helmet and face mask must be secured with a four- or six-point chin strap. All helmets should be fitted and maintained based on manufacturer's recommendations. The general steps to fitting a football helmet are addressed in the Foundational Skills sidebar. After the initial fitting and issuing of the helmet, it should be routinely assessed for continued fit and any possible damages.[2,22,27]

Ice Hockey Helmets Helmets are mandated in all levels of hockey for male and female players, but face masks or visor requirements vary by level and league. Unlike football helmets, hockey helmets typically need to withstand a singular impact, and the type of impact

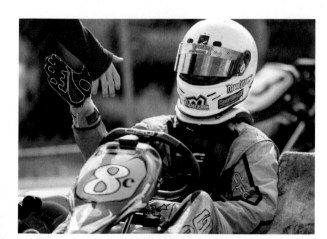

FIGURE 11.1 Example of a full-face helmet.

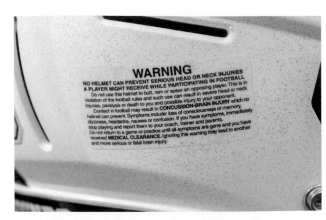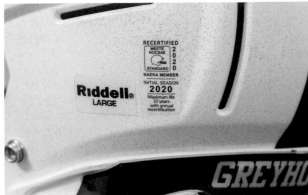

FIGURE 11.2   NOCSAE warning label.

is different. In ice hockey, a helmet must protect from a high-velocity impact from a puck or stick and low-velocity impact such as the player's head contacting the boards or ice. Hockey helmets must meet CSA or HECC technical and safety standards. Regardless of the manufacturer or model of the helmet, all helmets should be fitted and maintained based on manufacturer's recommendations and assessed for continued fit and any possible damages over the course of the season.

Lacrosse Helmets   In lacrosse, helmets are required for field players in men's lacrosse and the goalkeeper on both men's and women's teams. Field players in women's lacrosse are required to wear approved eye protection but not helmets. All lacrosse helmets must meet NOCSAE technical and safety standards and are designed to withstand repeated high-velocity impacts. Independent researchers at Virginia Tech have developed a rating system for lacrosse helmets to help consumers select one with confidence.[43] Lacrosse helmets have an attached face mask and a four-point buckling system to ensure the helmet stays in place. Clients should be educated about proper fit and avoid excessive tilt.[44] Regardless of the manufacturer or model of the lacrosse helmet, the helmet should be fitted and maintained based on manufacturer's recommendations and assessed for continued fit and any possible damages over the course of the season.

Head Protection in Other Sports   Helmets and headgear are standard protective equipment in many other sports and activities. The choice of equipment for individual clients varies depending on position or activity. For example, due to the high risk of head and facial injuries in softball and baseball, helmets and sometimes full-face masks are required for batters, players at bat, and base runners. These helmets are designed to withstand high-velocity impact from a thrown or batted ball and must meet NOCSAE technical and safety standards. Other sports with position-dependent helmet requirements include goalkeeper in field hockey and women's lacrosse and batsmen in cricket.

Helmets in cycling are designed to withstand one singular impact: the athlete contacting the ground or another object. USA Cycling requires all athletes to wear a properly fitted helmet for both competitions and training.[45] Many states require children and adolescents to wear helmets during recreational bike riding as well. In downhill skiing and snowboarding, where helmets are required in competition, there is strong evidence to support their use.[37] Helmets are also required in motor sports and equestrian events. In sports where helmets are not required, such as rodeo, they are frequently included as recommended protective equipment.[46] Athletic trainers working in the nonathletic setting such as industry and the military may see a variety of specialized helmets or hard hats. If you are working in one of these settings, familiarize yourself with technical requirements, fit, and maintenance.

Face Masks

Face masks, or face guards or shields, can be part of standard protective equipment or used postinjury to prevent additional injuries during healing. Postinjury face masks distribute forces from impact over a large area, therefore protecting the injured area from receiving the force. Currently little evidence is available on the use of postinjury face masks.[30]

Here is what is known about face masks as standard protective equipment:

- Face masks are used to protect the client's face and eyes from flying objects and collisions with other players. When used properly, face masks can reduce the risk of facial and dental injuries.[2,34,53-55]

- A variety of face masks are available, and the choice depends on the sport and even the position played within that sport.

- Face masks can be bar (e.g., football), cage (e.g., ice hockey), or mesh wire (e.g., fencing; see figure 11.4).

Fitting a Standard Football Helmet

Here are the steps to fit a standard football helmet:[2,40-42]

1. Measure the circumference of the client's head 1 in. (2.5 cm) above the eyebrows with a cloth measuring tape (figure 11.3*a*) and then select the appropriate size based on the manufacturer's sizing chart.
2. Place the helmet on the client, inflate any air bladders or liners if applicable, and secure the chinstrap (figure 11.3*b*). The helmet should be snug.
3. The forehead pad should be 1 in. above the client's eyebrows. Adjust the air as needed.
4. Jaw pads should sit snugly against the client's face. Adjust jaw pads as needed.
5. With a properly fitted helmet, the ear holes on the helmet should align with the client's ears and the base of the skull should be covered in the back (figure 11.3*c*).
6. The face mask should be 3 finger widths from the nose and not obscure the client's vision (figure 11.3*d*).
7. To ensure proper fit, rotate the helmet on the client's head. The client's hair, skin, and head should move with the helmet as a unit. This ensures the helmet is snug, but it should not be so tight it causes discomfort.
8. When you press down on the top of the helmet, the client should feel pressure on the crown of the head, not the brow.
9. The chinstrap should be centered and snug. Adjust if needed.

Additional tip: Wetting the client's hair prior to fitting will replicate a sweaty head from play and provide a better fit.

Remember to always consult the manufacturer's guidelines for fitting each helmet model.

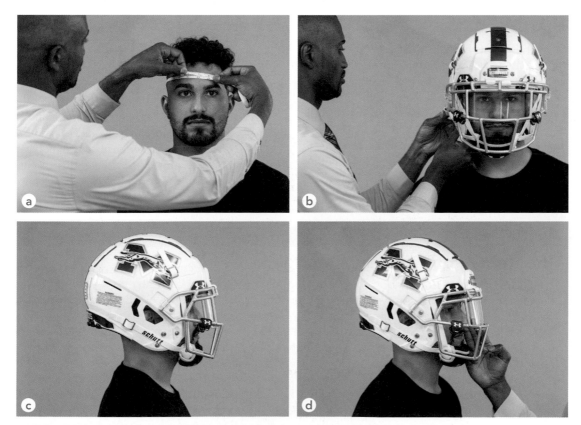

FIGURE 11.3   Fitting a football helmet.

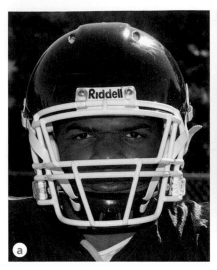 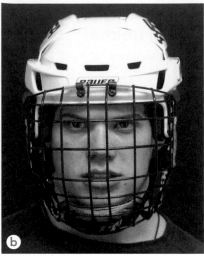 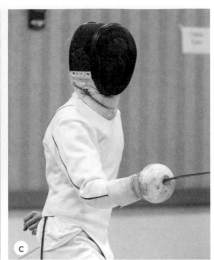

FIGURE 11.4 *(a)* Bar, *(b)* cage, and *(c)* mesh wire face masks.

- Face masks can be built into the helmet or added separately.
- Any face masks used should be approved for the specific sport and worn with the helmet, if applicable.
- When fitting a face mask, ensure that it does not obscure the client's vision or sit too close to the face and that it covers the entire face.

Eye Protection

Many eye injuries are preventable with the use of properly fitting protective eyewear. The American Academy of Pediatrics and the American Academy of Ophthalmology recommend the use of protective eyewear in all sports where there is a risk of eye injury.[56] The following sidebar provides a list of high-, moderate-, and low-risk sports for eye injuries. Even with recommendations, few sports mandate the use of eye protection. Although the benefits of protective eyewear are well documented,[3,30,47,57,58] when given a choice, many athletes refuse to wear them, often citing comfort or vision obstruction. Protective eyewear should be mandatory for clients who are functionally one-eyed.[56]

Eye protection should be made from polycarbonate plastic, which is both highly durable and impact resistant and is approved for the type of sport in question.[58] The recommended thickness is 3 mm.[30] Protective eye shields, or visors, can also attach directly to helmets in some sports (e.g., football and men's lacrosse). Visors must be clear to allow athletic trainers and other medical personnel to assess the client's eyes, unless the client has a medical condition warranting a tinted visor. Protective eyewear should be inspected frequently and replaced when cracked or yellowing. Contact lenses, prescription glasses, and street-wear sunglasses provide little to no eye protection and should not be worn as the sole eye protection. In some sports (e.g., women's lacrosse), cage-like eye protection can be worn instead of polycarbonate plastic goggles to protect the athlete's eyes from impact from a ball or stick (figure 11.5).

EVIDENCE-BASED ATHLETIC TRAINING

The Debate on Protective Headgear

Headgear is frequently used in rugby, boxing, and soccer, but currently no standards are in place for testing and certifying these types of headgear. Evidence supporting the use of padded headgear to prevent concussions is mixed, especially since the mechanism of injury can vary so greatly.[5,18,34,38,47-50] Debate exists as to whether wearing protective headgear will make athletes more aggressive in their style of play based on a false sense of security. Headgear may be beneficial in protecting against lacerations, abrasions, and other soft-tissue injuries in these sports.[25,48] What can be agreed on is the need for equipment standards and additional research on headgear.[18,50-52] When counseling athletes on the possible use of headgear during sports like soccer, make sure you address the potential benefits and risks.

Risk Categories for Sport-Related Eye Injury for the Unprotected Player

High Risk
- Baseball and softball
- Basketball
- Boxing
- Cricket
- Fencing

- Field hockey
- Ice hockey
- Lacrosse
- Martial arts, full contact

- Paintball
- Rifle or BB gun
- Squash and racquetball
- Street hockey

Moderate Risk
- Fishing
- Football

- Soccer
- Tennis and badminton

- Volleyball
- Water polo

Low Risk
- Cycling
- Martial arts, noncontact

- Skiing
- Swimming and diving

- Water skiing
- Wrestling

Eye Safe
- Gymnastics
- Track and field (Javelin and discus have a small but definite potential for eye injury that is preventable with good field supervision.)

Adapted by permission from P.F. Vinger, "A Practical Guide for Sports Eye Protection," *Physicians Sportsmedicine* 28, no. 6 (2000): 49-69.

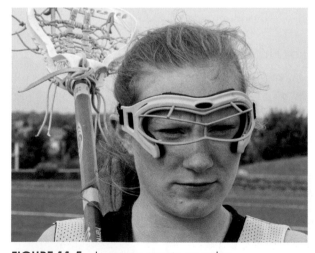

FIGURE 11.5 Lacrosse sports goggles.

Mouth Guards

Mouth guards are required protective equipment in many sports and recommended in more. The primary purpose of a mouth guard is to act as a shock absorber and dissipate force throughout the surrounding structures. The use of a properly fitted mouth guard has been well documented to reduce orofacial injuries, including teeth fractures and luxations, orofacial fractures, jaw dislocations, and soft-tissue injuries.[16,18,25,30,47,59-61] Despite what was once thought true, little evidence exists supporting the ability of mouth guards to reduce the rate or severity of concussions.[16,18,38] Mouth guards are required in collision and contact sports, such as football, ice and field hockey, lacrosse, and boxing. The American Dental Association (ADA) also recommends mouth guards in other sports, such as basketball, volleyball, skiing, and surfing.[62]

All mouth guards used in sports should meet ANSI/ADA standards.[63] They are typically made of ethylene vinyl acetate (EVA). The recommended thickness of mouth guards is 4 mm.[59] A mouth guard that is too thin does not adequately absorb or transmit force; one that is too thick can affect speech and respiration and is uncomfortable for the athlete.

Table 11.1 summarizes the advantages and disadvantages of each type of mouth guard. No matter the type of mouth guard, it should cover all upper teeth, including the posterior ones. Mouth guards should not be altered beyond the manufacturer's instructions. To aid in enforcement of proper use, mouth guards should be colored, not

TABLE 11.1   **Different Types of Mouth Guards**

Type of mouth guard	Description	Advantages	Disadvantages
Stock	Stock guards require no modifications and are ready for immediate wear.	Easily fits over braces Inexpensive Readily available	Poor fit and easily dislodged Can disrupt normal breathing and speech Least protective
Boil and bite	Boil and bite guards are softened in hot water and then placed in the client's mouth to allow for some customization (figure 11.6a).	Inexpensive Form-fitted	Deteriorates over time May not last entire season Places pressure on cheeks and gums if not fitted well
Custom	Custom-fabricated mouth guards require dental impressions made by a dental professional and then are either vacuum formed or heat-pressure formed (figure 11.6b). After dental impressions are made, vacuum formed mouth guards can be fabricated by an athletic trainer in the clinic.	Accurate fit Increased comfort Increased compliance	Most expensive Several trips to the dentist may be required.

clear or white. More information about preventing and managing oral and dental injuries can be found in the NATA position statement on the subject.[16]

Independent of the type selected for use, mouth guards must be cared for properly:[60]

- Mouth guards should be rinsed with soap and water or mouthwash before and after each use and allowed to air dry.
- When not in use, the mouth guard should be stored in a hard, well-ventilated container.
- Clients can use a toothbrush and toothpaste to clean mouth guards.

- Mouth guards should not be stored in outdoor spaces, like in a car glove box, because heat can distort its shape.
- Mouth guards should be inspected for tears or distortion and replaced if damaged.

Ear Protection

Ear protection serves one of three major functions in sports:

- Protecting the external ear from shearing forces in sports like wrestling, boxing, and water polo (figure 11.7a)

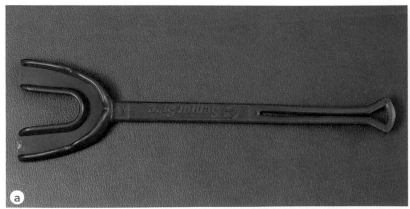
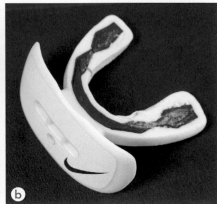

FIGURE 11.6   Two types of mouth guards: *(a)* boil and bite guard and *(b)* custom fabricated guard.

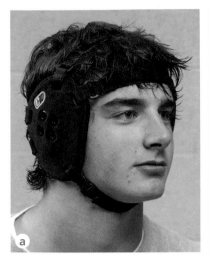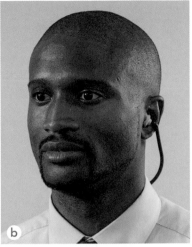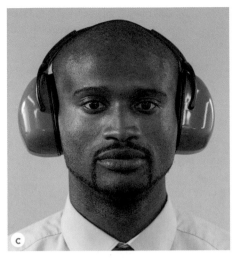

FIGURE 11.7 *(a)* External ear protection, *(b)* internal ear protection, and *(c)* hearing protection.

- Protecting the inner ear from damage in water sports such as swimming and surfing (figure 11.7*b*)
- Protecting hearing in nontraditional sports such as shooting and motor sports and in the industrial setting (figure 11.7*c*)

Protective Equipment for the Spine and Torso

The use of protective equipment for the spine and torso varies greatly by sport and position within a sport. Protective equipment is most frequently used in collision sports or sports where the player can be hit by a projectile. Protective equipment for the spine and torso is designed to dissipate forces, protect vital organs, and pad bony areas of the body. All protective equipment for the spine and torso should be fitted to the individual client per the manufacturer's guidelines.

Throat Protection

Although throat injuries are uncommon in traditional athletic events, they can be very serious, even fatal. Throat protectors are required for goalkeepers in lacrosse, ice hockey, and field hockey; baseball and softball catchers; and some field players in field hockey. Throat protection can be built into the helmet or can be attached to the helmet as a separate piece (figure 11.8). Throat protectors are designed for impact protection from a puck, ball, or sticks. Throat protection is especially important in ice hockey, considering the danger presented by skate blades.

Commercially available neck laceration protectors are also available for use, but they are not required in all levels and positions. Even with a neck protector in place, there is still the risk of a laceration in ice hockey.[64]

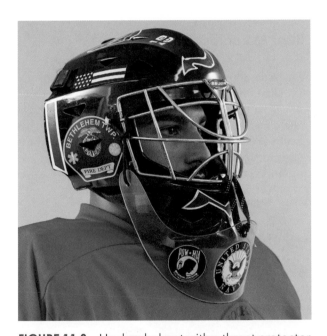

FIGURE 11.8 Hockey helmet with a throat protector.

Sports Bras

Sports bras began as modified jock straps. Although their production is a billion dollar industry, research has only recently focused on an effort to improve the design and effectiveness of sports bras.[65] The goal of the sports bra is to prevent movement of the breasts during physical activity and, therefore, prevent trauma to the breast tissue and discomfort during physical activity. Sports bras have been shown to be more supportive during activity than other alternatives.[66] A well-fitted sports bra should not impede sports performance and can improve function.[66,67]

In general, sports bras secure the breasts against the body. The bras accomplish this through various elastic fabrics, molded cups, supportive bands around the base of the bra, and, to a lesser extent, the straps. There are two types of sports bras on the market:

- Encapsulating sports bras use cups to support each breast separately.
- Compressive sports bras squeeze the breasts against the chest.

Although sports bras need to be supportive, they should not be so tight as to restrict the client's breathing. Sports bra selection should be based on chest circumference, cup size, and the activity it will be worn during (e.g., a less supportive bra is needed for walking than for running). Correct bra size is important to prevent skin irritation and allow the bra to be effective.[66,68] In contact and collision sports, padded sports bras can be worn for additional protection from impact. Some sports allow for additional protection of the breasts through plastic chest protectors (e.g., women's ice hockey).

Chest Protectors

Chest protectors are worn in collision sports and sports with the possibility for high-velocity hits from a ball or a puck. For example, chest protectors are required for baseball and softball catchers (figure 11.9) and goalkeepers in field hockey and lacrosse. NOCSAE standards have recently been developed and implemented for chest protectors for use in baseball and lacrosse to protect against **commotio cordis**.[69]

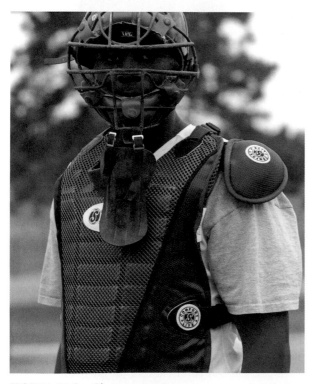

FIGURE 11.9   Chest protector.

Shoulder Pads

Shoulder pads are worn to protect the bony protuberances and joints of the shoulder complex in collision sports. Promising research supports the ability of shoulder pads to protect the head during shoulder-to-head contact in ice hockey.[70] Although shoulder pads are best known for their use in football, ice hockey, and lacrosse, they can also be used in nontraditional sports like skiing, boardercross, and BMX. Shoulder pads are specific to each sport and even the position within the sport. All shoulder pads should be fit based on the manufacturer's guidelines. Ideally, shoulder pads protect the athlete without compromising the athlete's range of motion.

Football Shoulder Pads   Currently, there are two types of shoulder pads for football players: cantilevered (figure 11.10) and noncantilevered. Selection varies by position played and the need for shoulder range of motion versus protection. Cantilevered pads are bulkier and worn by players in constant contact with others. Noncantilevered pads are worn by quarterbacks and receivers since they allow for more motion and less protection. New, high-tech shoulder pads are coming on the market as technology advances. The new shoulder pads are lighter and more streamlined. Neck protection (i.e., neck rolls) can be added to remind athletes not to hyperextend the neck (figure 11.11). Rib pads and other accessories can be added per the manufacturer's guidelines.

Shoulder Protection in Other Sports   Shoulder pads are required protective equipment for men's lacrosse (figure 11.12) and both men's and women's ice hockey (figure 11.13). These shoulder pads are fitted similarly to football shoulder pads, but you should always consult the manufacturer's recommendations. Many nontradi-

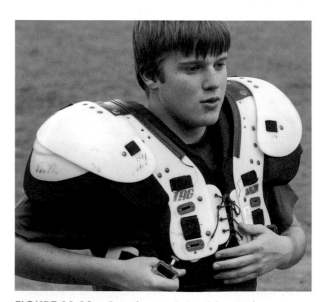

FIGURE 11.10   Cantilevered shoulder pads.

Fitting Football Shoulder Pads

1. Shoulder pad sizing is typically based on chest circumference, shoulder width, and weight. After obtaining measurements, select the proper size based on the manufacturer's guidelines.
2. The tips of the shoulder pads should cover the lateral aspect of the shoulder.
3. All shoulder pads should cover the deltoids, clavicles, chest, and scapula.
4. The neck opening should allow for adequate movement of the neck without excessive sliding. This can be assessed by having the client extend his arms overhead.
5. Straps should be snug but not binding.

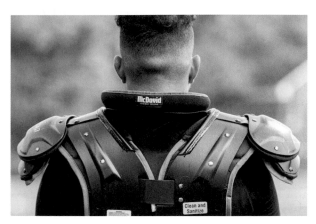

FIGURE 11.11 Football neck roll.

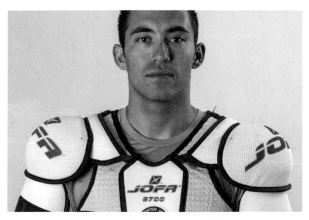

FIGURE 11.13 Ice hockey shoulder pads.

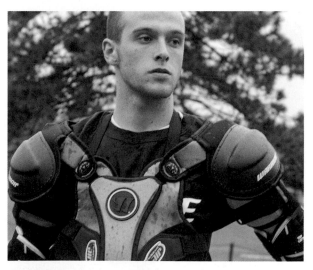

FIGURE 11.12 Lacrosse shoulder pads.

tional sports, such as motocross, skiing, boardercross, BMX, and other X Games–type sports recommend or require shoulder pads for protection. Other sports, such as rugby, allow for sport-specific padded shirts for added protection.[71]

Rib, Spine, and Back Protectors

Rib, spine, and back protectors are used in various sports. Rib protectors, or flak jackets, and back protectors are often attached to football shoulder pads to add protection to the area (figure 11.14). Spine and back protectors are also commonly worn in snow sports and motorcycle racing, among other sports. Padded shirts

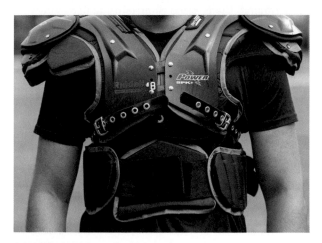

FIGURE 11.14 Football rib protector.

can also be worn under uniforms to add protection. Rib, spine, and back protectors can have a soft or hard outer surface, depending on the athlete's needs and the sport's requirements.

Hip and Buttock Pads

Hip and buttock pads are typically used in collision sports to provide extra padding to bony protuberances, such as the iliac crest, greater trochanter, and coccyx (figure 11.15). All padding must be the right size for the client and positioned in the proper place to be effective. In some sports, the pads are placed in special pockets within the uniform pants (e.g., football); in others, the protection can come from padded shorts (e.g., hockey, skiing, cycling). Many athletes also wear padded compression shorts under uniform shorts for additional comfort.

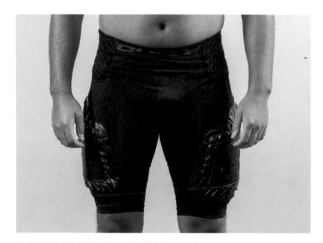

FIGURE 11.15   Football hip pads.

Groin and Genitalia Protection

The protective athletic cup and the appropriate athletic supporter (i.e., jock strap), athletic brief, or compression shorts are used to protect the external genitalia in male clients. Athletic cups are designed to protect from blunt force trauma. Bieniek and Sumfest state that "although data regarding the effectiveness of cups in reducing the incidence of genital trauma is lacking, the use of athletic cups remains logical" (p. 1488).[72] Various sizes and types of athletic cups are commercially available and vary based on the requirements of the sport. Athletic cups fit tightly against the body to provide maximum protection.

Protective Equipment for the Upper Extremities

Many types of pads are used to protect the upper extremity, and the need varies based on sport and position played and previous injury to the area. Pads, which are custom-constructed by the athletic trainer, are useful in these areas, but you must consult league rules for the type of materials that are allowed. The following section addresses some commonly used protective equipment for the elbow, forearm, wrist, and hand.

Arm Protectors and Pads

Wrist, forearm, and elbow pads and protectors are common in collision sports and sports with high-velocity projectiles (e.g., baseball and softball while the athlete is batting; figure 11.16). Be cognizant of the materials used when fabricating custom pads or selecting commercially available equipment. Many sports have specific requirements for the type of padding and protectors used. Arm protectors and pads can be used to prevent injuries or to protect an existing injury.

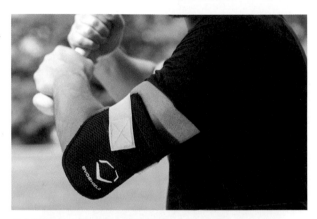

FIGURE 11.16   Baseball elbow guard.

Gloves

Gloves are used in many sports to protect participants' hands and fingers from injury. Commonly padded gloves are used in collision sports (e.g., football linemen, ice hockey [figure 11.17], and men's lacrosse)

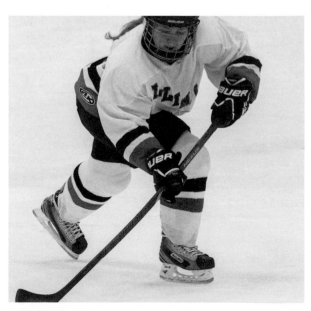

FIGURE 11.17   Ice hockey gloves.

or for additional protection for goalkeepers (e.g., field hockey and women's lacrosse goalkeepers). Gloves are also frequently used to increase grip in sports such as baseball and softball, but these thin gloves provide little protection for injury.

Protective Equipment for the Lower Extremities

Many different types of protective equipment for the lower extremities are available for use by sports participants. The need for such equipment varies based on sport or activity, position within the sport, and possibly previous injury to the area. The following sections summarize important information about thigh pads, kneepads, shin guards, and footwear.

Thigh Pads

Thigh pads are typically used in collision sports or to protect a previous injury during healing. They can be held in place in special pockets within uniform pants or with wraps or sleeves. Padded compression shorts can also be used to protect the thigh and upper leg in sports that do not require specialized padding.

Kneepads

Kneepads are worn in sports with potential for direct blows to the knee (e.g., volleyball; figure 11.18) and in collision sports (e.g., football). Depending on the sport, kneepads can have a soft or hard outer surface. They can be held in place with an elastic band, elastic straps, or special pockets in pants. Kneepads are also common in

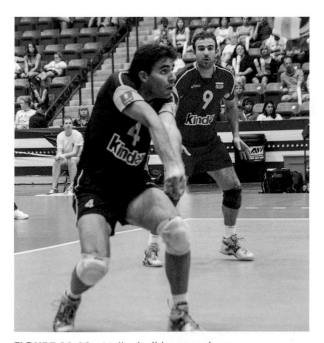

FIGURE 11.18   Volleyball kneepads.

nontraditional settings for clients whose job requires an extensive amount of kneeling.

Shin Guards

Shin guards are required protective equipment in a few sports (e.g., soccer and field hockey; figure 11.19) and position dependent in others (e.g., goalkeepers in field hockey and lacrosse). Shin guard use is recommended in many sports, but athletes do not usually comply unless use is mandated.[73] Shin guards are important because of the potential for **acute anterior compartment syndrome**, which can be very serious, even limb threatening. Some important facts about shin guards include the following:

- Shin guards protect athletes from direct impact from a ball or puck or a kick from another player.
- Soccer shin guards must meet NOCSAE standards.
- To be effective, shin guards must fit correctly. They should cover the lower leg from below the tibial tuberosity to just above the ankle mortise and should not impede ankle range of motion.
- Commonly, athletes wear shin guards that are too small and do not provide adequate protection.

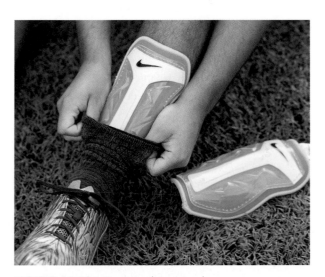

FIGURE 11.19   Soccer shin guards.

Shoes and Socks

Almost all athletes wear some protective equipment in competition or training when considering footwear. Socks and shoes are also important protective equipment for nontraditional clients (e.g., work boots for factory employees or military personnel). Work shoes are more than just comfort items, fashion statements, or part of the uniform; they are essential in injury prevention.[74] Shoes and socks should be selected for the specific sport or activity on hand.

Socks   Socks are important for preventing blisters, athlete's foot (i.e., tinea pedis), and cold-related conditions (e.g., frostbite). Socks should fit properly—those that are too tight can crowd the toes and those that are too loose can cause blisters. Socks should be made of synthetic materials, as opposed to cotton, to allow for the wicking of moisture away from the foot to prevent athlete's foot or other infections. Synthetic or wool socks can also help maintain warmth, even when the sock is wet.

Shoes   Shoes are an important component of protective equipment for physically active people in both traditional and nontraditional settings. The proper shoes for the activity can help prevent various injuries, including ankle sprains, turf toe, and crush injuries. Shoes also improve performance by increasing traction and efficiency. Customers have many choices when selecting shoes, and not all shoes are created equal. When counseling clients on shoe options, advise them to select a shoe created for their sport and their foot type.[75] You should also attempt to keep up to date on various trends for shoes and running like barefoot running and minimalist shoes.

Athletic shoes have many components (figure 11.20):[76]

- *Cleats:* molded rubber or screw-in type depending on sport and playing surface; designed to increase traction and performance
- *Collar:* inside back portion of the shoe that provides comfort around the ankle
- *Eyelets:* holes the shoelaces pass through
- *Last:* foot model over which a shoe is constructed; can be straight, curved, or semicurved
- *Heel counter:* an inflexible internal support in the rear of the shoe
- *Medial post:* component within the midsole that is firmer than the rest of the midsole

- *Midsole:* material that sits between the upper and outsole and provides cushioning and protection from impact forces
- *Outsole:* rubber part of the shoe that makes contact with the ground; provides traction and protection
- *Quarter panel:* material that makes up the sides of the shoe
- *Shank:* part of the shoe under the arch that makes the middle portion of the shoe more resistant to torsion and flexion; metal-shanked shoes often seen in the industrial setting
- *Sock liner:* inside of the shoe that makes contact with the foot
- *Toe box:* front area of the shoe where the toes sit; metal-toed shoes often seen in the industrial setting
- *Tongue:* flap of soft fabric that fits over the top of the foot to protect it from pressure caused by the laces
- *Upper:* leather, fabric, or mesh part of the shoe that encases the foot and protects it from dirt and rocks; contains the eyelets for laces

Customized, Off-the-Shelf, and Athletic Trainer-Made Protective Equipment

Customized protective equipment is designed and made to fit the individual client. Examples of common customized protective equipment in sports include mouth guards and some braces, such as ACL knee braces. Customized equipment generally has a higher cost and increased production time when compared with off-the-shelf options.

Tips for Buying and Wearing Shoes

- Clients should try on shoes later in the day, when their feet are at their largest.
- Clients should have their feet measured each time they buy shoes because foot size can change as people age.
- When trying on shoes, clients should wear the type of sock that they will wear when participating in sport and bring their orthotics with them, if used.
- There should be approximately a thumb's width of distance between the client's longest toe and the top end of the shoe.
- Shoes can be laced in different patterns to provide additional support or decrease pressure put on certain areas of the foot.
- To prevent blisters or other discomfort, clients should be instructed to break shoes in gradually.
- Running shoes should typically be replaced every 300 to 500 mi (485-800 km).

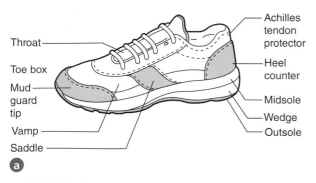
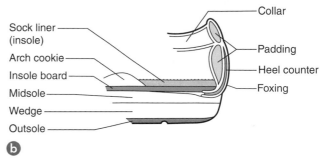
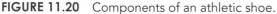

FIGURE 11.20   Components of an athletic shoe.

Custom protective wear also requires additional personnel to produce the equipment. However, customized protective equipment does allow for a better fit and possibly better user compliance because of that fit.

Off-the-shelf protective equipment is premade and requires no modification prior to use. Examples of typically used off-the-shelf protective equipment include most pads, braces, and sleeves. These items come in standard sizes but may not fit the client as well as a custom-made option.

Another option you have when choosing protective equipment is designing and constructing items yourself. Outside of fabricating mouth guards, little research is available on the construction of protective equipment. Athletic trainers typically construct protective pads postinjury when custom or off-the-shelf items do not meet the need. The construction of protective equipment is definitely something that cannot be taught in a textbook alone; there is an art to creating protective pads. In general, custom-constructed protective pads involve the following:

- Soft padding such as felts or foams
- Hard materials such as thermomoldable plastics
- Can be held in place with athletic tape, elastic wraps, or sleeves

When using hard materials, consult sport and league rules. Remember that custom-constructed protective equipment does not come with any manufacturer warranty or legal protection for the person creating the equipment. You should be cautious of the legal liability of constructing protective equipment, especially if injury occurs during use.

Emergency Removal of Protective Equipment

Although athletic trainers aim to protect clients from injury, sometimes that is not possible. When an injury occurs, you must be able to remove any protective equipment in a timely manner, whether on the field or in the clinic. Emergency medical services (EMS) personnel and the emergency department staff will look to your skills and expertise in equipment removal. Emergency equipment removal policies and steps should be outlined in the site-specific emergency action plan (EAP) for your institution or facility.[17,19-21,77,90,91] Athletic trainers and other stakeholders who will be involved with the process need to practice these skills at least annually. [17,19-21,78-80,90,91] You should be well versed on the intricacies of the protective equipment worn by your clients and the tools needed to remove it. As equipment changes, you must stay current with the developments and updates in the field.

Emergency equipment removal is warranted when a patient has a potential head or spine injury or requires CPR.[24,91,92] It also needs to be completed prior to or during emergency cooling of a patient with heat stroke, when possible.[22,80] All protective equipment (helmet and shoulder pads) should be removed prior to transport to the hospital at the earliest possible time if the resources available (e.g., personnel, equipment) allow it.[90,91] This is a change from the previous school of thought that recommended removing only the face mask prior to transport, unless other variables (e.g., the need to do CPR) warranted the removal of additional equipment. At minimum, the face mask should be removed prior to every emergency transport, regardless of respiratory status.[91] Emergency equipment removal prior to transport allows for improved patient care on the field and during transport. It also allows the practitioners most familiar with and trained in equipment removal to do the actual procedure.

Emergency Removal of Football Equipment

New helmet and shoulder pad designs are on the market to allow for easier emergency equipment removal. You should be aware of the workings of both traditional and new designs and well versed in the type of equipment your clients use. Have the following tools available for emergency equipment removal:

EVIDENCE-BASED ATHLETIC TRAINING

Protective Equipment and Heat Illnesses

Although protective equipment is designed to reduce the risk of certain injuries in sports, it can also put athletes at increased risk for exertional heat illnesses.[7,20,80-82] Protective equipment increases the weight the athlete has to move during activity and prevents sweat evaporation and efficient cooling. To reduce the risk of exertional illnesses, proper acclimatization procedures should occur during the preseason to gradually phase in the use of protective equipment. During practices and competitions in the heat, athletes should be allowed to remove protective equipment (e.g., helmets) during rest periods to help facilitate cooling. Recommendations for proper acclimatization and prevention of heat illnesses are provided in chapter 8. If an athlete is demonstrating signs and symptoms of heat illness, protective equipment should be removed as soon as possible. Research has demonstrated that core body temperature decreases faster in athletes wearing shorts, underwear, and socks than in athletes wearing standard football equipment during cold-water immersion.[81] However, if the protective equipment cannot be quickly removed for any reason, cooling should not be delayed. Make sure you are familiar with the protective equipment and practice emergency equipment removal in an effort to decrease the time needed to prepare the athlete for cold-water immersion.

- Cordless screwdriver (recommended tool for face mask removal[19,83-85])
- Manual screwdriver
- Manufacturers' quick release tools
- Various cutting tools (e.g., trauma shears, Trainer's Angel, FM Extractor, pruning shears)

Steps for helmet removal, traditional face mask removal, and removal of a quick-release mounting system are listed in the following sidebar. The first step in all of these skills is for one rescuer to maintain in-line stabilization. The face mask should be removed or tilted back for helmet removal. Remember, when removing the helmet,

FOUNDATIONAL SKILL

Steps for Face Mask and Helmet Removal

Steps for Traditional Face Mask Removal

1. Use the cordless screwdriver, if possible, to remove the 2 screws for the side loop straps while another rescuer stabilizes the patient's head (figure 11.21a).*
2. Remove the screws for the top loop straps.*
3. Lift the face mask off the helmet (figure 11.21b).

*When attempting to remove the screws, if one or more of the screws cannot be simply unscrewed, continue to the next screw until all the screws that can be successfully unscrewed are removed. Then use a backup cutting tool to cut any remaining loop straps. See the preceding list of cutting tools. You should be familiar with the proper use of the various cutting tools.

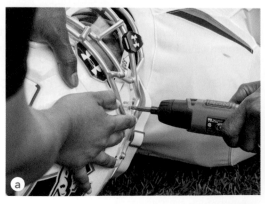 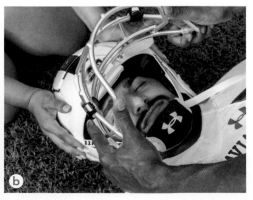

FIGURE 11.21 Traditional face mask removal.

Steps for Quick-Release Face Mask Removal[86]

1. Use the Quick Release tool or another pointed object to depress the pin in the side-mounted Quick Release clips (figure 11.22).
2. Pull the clips directly away from the helmet.
3. Remove the top mounted clips with a screwdriver or cutting tool.
4. Remove the face mask.

Steps for Football Helmet Removal[19]

1. Remove the face mask.
2. Cut the chin strap off (don't unsnap it as it could cause head movement) (figure 11.23a).
3. Remove the cheek pads, if necessary.*
4. If the helmet contains an air bladder, remove the air from the bladder with a deflation needle or blade to loosen the fit of the helmet.*

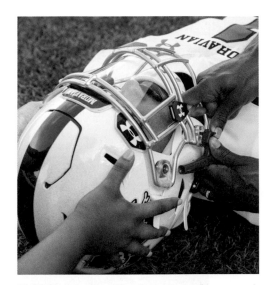

FIGURE 11.22   Quick-release face mask removal.

5. The athlete's jersey and shoulder pads should be cut now in preparation for removal.
6. Cervical spine stabilization should be transferred from the rescuer at the head to another rescuer, who assumes cervical spine control from the front (figure 11.23b).
7. The rescuer at the head then grasps the helmet from the sides and spreads the helmet out while rotating it up to facilitate removal (figure 11.23c).
8. Shoulder pads should be removed immediately after the helmet to maintain neutral alignment of the cervical spine.

*The need for these steps and process to complete them should be determined in advance based on the type of helmet worn. You should be familiar with the techniques for removal of different types of helmets worn by your athletes.

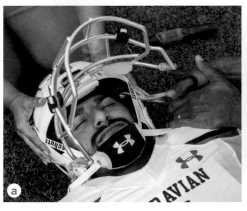 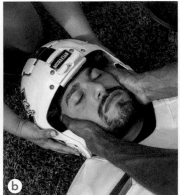 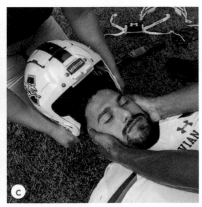

FIGURE 11.23   Football helmet removal.

the shoulder pads must be removed as well to maintain cervical spine alignment.[19,91]

Football shoulder pads can be removed in multiple ways, and three ways are highlighted here:

1. Flat torso removal technique: requires 2 to 4 rescuers
2. Elevated torso removal technique: requires 4 or more rescuers
3. Separating the shoulder pads when using Riddell RipKord shoulder pads: requires 2 or 3 rescuers. Research has demonstrated that the Riddell RipKord shoulder pads are easier and faster to remove than traditional shoulder pads.[78,88]

For removal of both traditional and Riddell RipKord shoulder pads, practice decreases removal time and spinal movement. The following sidebar lists steps for removal of traditional and Riddell RipKord shoulder pads.

Steps for Traditional Shoulder Pad Removal

1. After removal of the helmet (see above), cut the jersey (figure 11.24a), shoulder pad straps (figure 11.24b), and center (figure 11.24c) in preparation for removal. Be aware of additional equipment that may be secured to the shoulder pads, such as rib pads or collars.

2. The rescuer holding cervical spine stabilization from the front of the client will continue to do so (see helmet removal steps previously listed).

3. The rescuer at the head, and ideally two other rescuers, should remove the shoulder pads by carefully siding them out from under the athlete (figure 11.24d).[11]

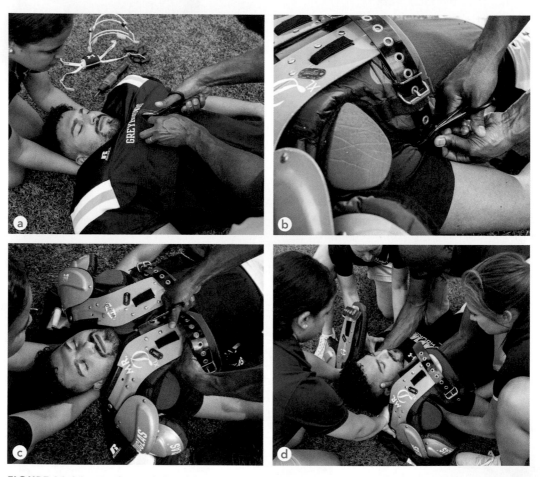

FIGURE 11.24   Traditional shoulder pad removal.

Steps for Riddell RipKord Shoulder Pad Removal

1. Cut and pull the RipKord (figure 11.25).
2. Cut center strap and all additional straps.
3. Pivot the shoulder pads out from beneath the client.[88]

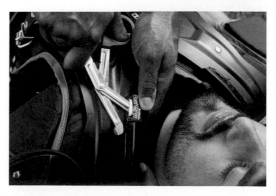

FIGURE 11.25   Riddell RipKord shoulder pad removal.

Emergency Removal of Equipment in Other Sports

Athletic trainers responsible for the care of any athlete wearing protective equipment should be familiar with the proper removal of the equipment in case of an emergency. You should stay abreast of changes in equipment design. Practice of emergency equipment removal is not limited to football and should include all sports with protective equipment.

Currently, quick-release protective equipment is unavailable for lacrosse or ice hockey. As with football, if removing the athlete's helmet, you should remove the shoulder pads as well to maintain spinal alignment.[19,90] Note that lacrosse face masks are not as easily removed as those in football or hockey.[19] Athletic trainers working with lacrosse players should have both a cordless screwdriver and cutting tools available for face mask and helmet removal. The steps for the removal of various lacrosse helmets, face masks, and shoulder pads are similar to those used to remove football equipment, but you will need to familiarize yourself with the equipment the athletes under your care will be using.

CLINICAL BOTTOM LINE

- Athletic trainers must ensure that equipment fits properly and is used correctly.
- Athletic trainers should refer to the manufacturer's guidelines for equipment fitting, maintenance, and recertification.
- Clients must have access to the appropriate equipment for their sport or activity based on sports' league or association requirements.
- Athletic trainers must provide education on the proper use of protective equipment.
- Athletic trainers should have a working knowledge of the equipment needs for all athletes in sports under their care.
- Protective equipment can be custom made for an individual client, purchased off the shelf, or constructed by the athletic trainer.
- In the event of an emergency, athletic trainers should have the skills and proper tools for removing protective equipment.
- Equipment removal should be addressed in the EAP and practiced at least annually.
- EMS and other stakeholders should be involved in creating the EAP and practicing equipment removal.
- Athletic trainers should review the NATA position statements and other relevant documents related to the use of protective equipment.

 Go to HK*Propel* to complete the activities and case studies for this chapter.

Go to HK*Propel* to (1) view videos of fitting protective equipment and (2) download foundational skill check sheets for fitting and removing various protective equipment.

CHAPTER 12

Taping and Bracing

David A. Wilkenfeld, EdD, LAT, ATC

CHAPTER OBJECTIVES

After reading this chapter, you will be able to do the following:

- Identify the scientific principles that guide the application of common prophylactic procedures for the lower extremity, upper extremity, and spine

- Understand the indications, contraindications, and precautions of protective prophylactic procedures

- Understand evidence on the efficacy of protective prophylactic procedures

- Discuss legal issues concerning the application of protective prophylactic procedures

- Discuss application guidelines for kinesiology taping

- Apply common nonelastic taping techniques for the lower extremity and upper extremity

- Apply common rigid strap taping techniques for the lower extremity and upper extremity

- Apply common elastic taping and wrapping techniques for the lower extremity, upper extremity, and spine

- Apply common bracing and splinting techniques for the lower extremity, upper extremity, and spine

Select application steps in this chapter are reprinted by permission from D.H. Perrin and I.A. McLeod, *Athletic Taping, Bracing, and Casting* (Champaign, IL: Human Kinetics, 2019).

CAATE STANDARDS

The following CAATE 2020 standards are covered in this chapter:

Standard 62

Standard 78

One of the primary responsibilities of athletic trainers is the development and implementation of strategies to prevent injuries and optimize the overall health and well-being of patients. The application of **protective equipment**, including taping and bracing, is one of the main, and most visible, ways in which athletic trainers can do the following:

- Reduce risk of injury or reinjury
- Promote healthy participation in activity
- Improve a patient's quality of life

Athletic trainers are uniquely qualified as experts in the area of prevention. As such, they have the knowledge and skills to identify and apply the most appropriate protective equipment for a given condition.

In order to master the art and science of taping and bracing, you need to develop the psychomotor skills associated with the techniques and understand the scientific principles that guide their application. Because evidence-based practice is a cornerstone for improving patient care, you should scrutinize the clinical interventions used and look for and try new techniques that are scientifically supported by the literature.[1-3] In regard to taping and bracing, however, limited high-quality research is available to help guide clinical practice. Although many studies examine techniques applied to the foot and ankle, the volume of research becomes limited as we move up the kinetic chain. Therefore, you should be critical when using protective equipment and employ the five-step approach to evidence-based practice outlined by the National Athletic Trainers' Association's book *Athletic Training Education Competencies*, 5th ed.:[4]

1. Create a clinically relevant question.
2. Search for the best available evidence.
3. Critically analyze the evidence.
4. Integrate the appraisal with personal clinical expertise and the patient's preferences.
5. Evaluate the performance or outcomes of the actions.

From nonelastic, rigid strap, and elastic tape to elastic wraps, braces, and splints, it is easy to become overwhelmed by the number of taping and bracing techniques. In this chapter, the focus is on commercially available and commonly used taping, wrapping, and bracing techniques within athletic training practice. This information should complement the material discussed in chapters 11 and 24, and you are encouraged to reference standalone texts on taping and bracing for advanced techniques.[5]

Legal Issues

Use of protective equipment (e.g., tape, wraps, and braces) is beneficial for preventing injury and protecting anatomical structures from further aggravation. Although **product liability** holds manufacturers responsible for product defects in equipment like tape and braces, you have a duty to ensure that the equipment is properly selected, applied, and worn. Failure to do so may result in harm to the patient, the voidance of a product warranty and the manufacturers' liability, and a negligence lawsuit against the athletic trainer for breach of duty. You can mitigate your legal risk related to the use of tape, wraps, braces, and splints by doing the following:

- Understand the injury mechanism and involved structures in order to select the appropriate tape, wrap, brace, or splint.
- Follow manufacturer's guidelines for the application and maintenance of equipment.
- Educate patients and clients on the proper use of the equipment and the potential risks related to its use and misuse.

Regulation

Regulation on the use of taping, bracing, and splinting is common in sports. Most governing athletic associations, such as the NFHS, NCAA, and NFL, provide regulation on the amount of restriction you can provide through taping, bracing, or splinting as well as the materials you can use to protect an injured part.[6-8] Due to the fact that protective equipment can injure other participants, most associations prohibit the use of hard and inflexible materials unless they are covered by foam rubber or a similar soft material. Although regulation of taping, bracing, and splinting is less common outside of sports, athletic trainers who work in nonsport settings should familiarize themselves with any and all rules and regulations related to the use of protective equipment. More information about agencies and organizations that are involved with the regulation of protective equipment can be found in chapter 11.

Documentation

Clinical documentation plays an important role in mitigating risk and is an important aspect of working with protective equipment. For taping, wrapping, bracing, or splinting, do the following:

- List the technique used and the aim of the technique.
- Note any modifications made to the protective equipment.
- Document the distal neurovascular status of the involved limb before and after application of a prophylactic procedure.
- Document all patient education provided on the proper application and use of protective equipment.

More information on documentation for athletic trainers can be found in chapter 5.

Principles of Prophylactic Procedures

Because you will devote many hours to taping, wrapping, and bracing in your practice as an athletic trainer, it is important to perform these tasks in a manner that maximizes your efficiency and effectiveness. In order to optimize your ability to perform these tasks, you, your facility, and your patients should be properly prepared. The following section discusses the basic principles of **prophylactic procedures**, including the types of materials used and general application considerations. More information on facility design for optimizing your effectiveness as an athletic trainer can be found in *Management Strategies in Athletic Training*, 5th ed.[9]

Common Types of Tape and Braces

Taping and bracing play various roles in health care.[5,10] In general, these include the following:

- Limiting excessive or abnormal movement of a joint in order to support ligament and capsular structures

FOUNDATIONAL SKILL

Application Techniques for Taping a Body Part

Prior to Application

1. Check with the patient for allergies to any materials used in the taping procedure.
2. The target area should be clean, dry, and, ideally, free of hair. It is helpful to keep disposable razors or barber's clippers handy in your facility for removing hair.
3. Open wounds should be covered with a sterile dressing. For more information, see chapter 14.
4. Spray a light layer of tape adherent onto the skin.
5. Apply a lubricated pad over sensitive areas, such as the dorsum of the foot, Achilles tendon, or popliteal space.
6. Tape is most effective when applied directly to the skin. For patients who are sensitive or allergic to tape, apply a single layer of foam underwrap before starting your taping procedure.
7. Position the patient for the taping procedure so that the injured or target area is fully accessible. Ask the patient to remain attentive throughout the application process. An inattentive patient will ultimately fail to maintain the appropriate limb positioning, which can compromise the effectiveness of the prophylactic procedure.

During Application

1. Ensure that the patient maintains the appropriate position of function for the taping procedure to ensure the desired result.
2. Unroll only a few inches of tape at a time in order to maintain control of the tape and prevent wrinkles.
3. Guide the tape around the contours of the body while maintaining tension on the tape.
4. Each strip of tape should overlap the previous strip by one-half the width of the tape. Avoid continuous tape application whenever possible.
5. When completed, check for patient comfort and function and for distal circulation and motor and sensory function.

Tape Removal

1. Remove the tape as soon as possible to reduce skin irritation.
2. Using tape cutters or tape scissors, lift the tape away from the skin and cut along the natural contours of the body part.
3. Whenever possible, try to remove the tape in the direction of the hair growth.
4. Cleanse the skin with tape remover, if needed, and soap and water.
5. Educate the patient to inspect the skin regularly for signs of irritation, blisters, or infection.

- Providing compression of anatomical structures
- Improving proprioceptive feedback
- Securing pads, dressings, and splints

A variety of materials are required to address the taping and bracing needs of different structures and injured areas (table 12.1). These include nonelastic and elastic athletic tape, wraps, and braces, as well as rigid strapping and kinesiology tape. Manufacturers produce and market tapes and braces in a variety of colors, textures, sizes, and materials in order to help health care providers meet the needs of their patients.

Nonelastic Tape

Nonelastic tape is used to provide support to joints by limiting abnormal or excessive movement. Although it

TABLE 12.1   **Comparison of Common Tapes**

Materials	Uses
Nonelastic tape 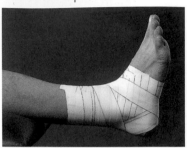	• Limits abnormal or excessive movement • Provides significant support
Elastic tape and wraps 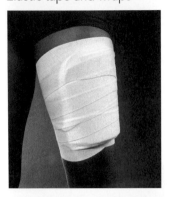	• Provides support to body parts while allowing normal body movement • Secures protective pads, splints, and dressings to the body • Conforms well to body contours, providing multidirectional compression to an area of the body
Rigid strapping tape 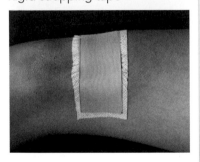	• Restricts motion • Helps correct postural or biomechanical faults • Provides mechanical support and joint stabilization • Limits painful movement
Kinesiology tape 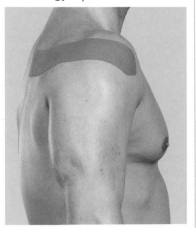	• Provides joint support and unloading • Reduces fascial tightness • Stimulates lymph flow • Facilitates muscle function by decreasing muscle fatigue • Increases proprioceptive input • Increases joint range of motion • Decreases pain

Tearing Tape

1. Hold the roll of tape in one hand. Place the third finger of this hand through the roll of tape to provide stabilization.
2. Place the tape coming off the roll between the tips of the thumb and second fingers of both hands (figure 12.1a).
3. Quickly pull both hands in straight, opposing directions with a slight downward motion to begin tearing the tape (figure 12.1b).
4. As the tape begins to tear, rotate the hands in opposite directions in a tearing motion (figure 12.1c). If the tape becomes crimped or folded, move to a new location on the tape and try again. With practice, these movements become one smooth motion. You can tear some elastic tape with your fingers, but you will need to cut other types with scissors.

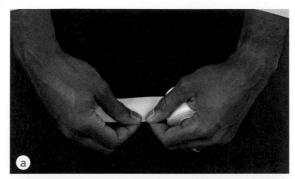

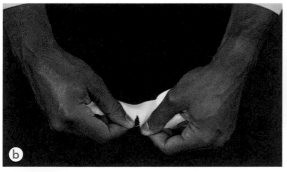

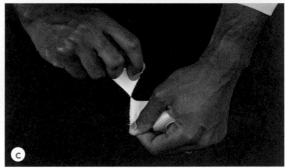

FIGURE 12.1   Tearing tape steps.

provides significant support, nonelastic tape has been shown to loosen with activity, potentially compromising its restraining effect.[11,12] Nonelastic tape is commonly applied to the foot, ankle, knee, elbow, wrist, and hand. An example of a taping technique that uses nonelastic tape is the closed basket weave.

Elastic Tape and Wraps

Elastic tape and wraps are used to do the following:

- Provide support to body parts while allowing for mobility
- Secure protective pads or splints to the body
- Provide compression to an area of the body

For example, when it is necessary to protect the quadriceps muscle group, elastic tape and wraps can be used to secure protective padding while allowing for normal muscle contraction without restricting blood flow. Elastic wraps are also very useful for applying compression combined with ice following an acute lateral ankle sprain.

Rigid Strapping Tape

Rigid strapping tape is commonly used to restrict motion, help correct postural or biomechanical faults, provide mechanical support and joint stabilization, and limit painful movement. Rigid strapping tapes stretch only 30% from the time of initial application[13] and can absorb more total energy before failure compared to nonelastic and elastic tape,[14] making them ideal for creating a bracing type of support to the area. Basic application considerations for rigid strapping tape can be found in the following sidebar. More information on using rigid strapping tape can be found in *Strap Taping for Sports and Rehabilitation*.[13]

Kinesiology Tape

Kinesiology tape is a type of elastic tape that can stretch up to 140% of its original length. Kinesiology tape therefore promotes full joint motion after application rather than restricting it like nonelastic tape. It is applied differently from other types of nonelastic or elastic tape,

Application Techniques for Wrapping a Body Part

Before Application

1. Check with the patient for allergies to any materials used in the wrapping procedure. Most elastic wraps are latex-free.
2. The target area should be clean and dry.
3. Open wounds should be covered with a sterile dressing. For more information, see chapter 14.

During Application

1. When wrapping an injured muscle, place it in a shortened position before starting your wrapping procedure. During the procedure, instruct the patient to maximally contract the muscle.
2. Begin distal to the target area and move in a proximal direction.
3. Overlap each turn of the wrap by one-half the width of the wrap.
4. When applying an elastic wrap, stretch the wrap to approximately one-half of its total elastic capacity.
5. Secure the end of the wrap with elastic tape. All metal clips should be covered with elastic tape.
6. When you have completed the application, check for distal circulation and motor and sensory function.

Wrap Removal

1. Remove the wrap as soon as possible and wash it on delicate cycle. A used wrap should not be reused before being washed.
2. If possible, hang the wrap to dry to prevent loss of elasticity.

Application Guidelines for Rigid Strapping Taping

1. Prepare the skin area to be taped, making sure it is clean and shaven.
2. Position the patient so that you have easy access to the body part you will be taping. Place the limb in the most neutral anatomical position possible.
3. Measure and cut strips of adhesive gauze underwrap, such as Hypafix tape or Cover-Roll, and apply them so that the strapping tape will not contact the skin (some exceptions apply).
4. Measure and cut strips of strapping tape and apply them with adequate tension in the direction of pull desired. Wrinkling of the skin underneath the adhesive gauze under-wrap is desired (figure 12.2*a*).
5. Assess the integrity of the tape by taking the joint through its functional range of motion. You may apply anchor strips of adhesive gauze underwrap to the ends of the tape to secure them (figure 12.2*b*).
6. Assess the completed taping procedure for desired functional outcomes. If tape does not improve symptoms or causes pain in other areas, it should be removed.
7. Give the patient instruction on wear time. Strapping tape can be worn for 2 to 7 days. Swimming, excessive exposure to water, and oily or sweaty skin will decrease wear time. When there is no longer enough tension or symptoms start to return, then it is

time to remove the tape. Tape should be worn only until the muscles have become strong enough to support the area needed for the activity.

8. To remove the tape, start peeling off an edge of the adhesive gauze underwrap. Peel slowly so as not to tear the skin. Removal is easiest when the tape or skin is wet, such as after a shower, bath, or swimming.

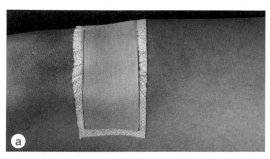
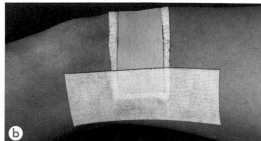

FIGURE 12.2   Applying rigid strapping taping.

often by taking a joint actively through its range of motion while applying the tape over a muscle or muscle group. Despite its popularity, evidence for the effectiveness of kinesiology taping as the only treatment technique for an injury is limited and lacking in quality (see sidebar). General benefits of kinesiology tape may include the following:[13]

- Joint support and unloading
- Reducing fascial tightness
- Stimulating lymph flow
- Facilitating muscle function by decreasing muscle fatigue

- Muscle inhibition to decrease hypertonicity and cramping
- Increasing proprioceptive input
- Increasing joint range of motion
- Decreasing pain

Braces

Braces prevent injuries and support unstable joints and may be used to supplement or replace taping procedures. Braces vary in material, expense, and ease of application, so you should carefully consider the cost–benefit of using braces versus taping in addition to consulting

EVIDENCE-BASED ATHLETIC TRAINING

Use of Kinesiology Tape for the Treatment of Musculoskeletal Injuries

Kinesiology taping has become a very popular treatment for several health conditions over the past two decades. Ten systematic reviews and meta-analyses have evaluated the effect of kinesiology taping on selected outcomes in different populations. These include the use of kinesiology tape for the treatment of sports injuries,[15] musculoskeletal problems,[16-18] chronic low back pain,[19] shoulder pain and disability,[20] and myofascial pain syndrome.[21] In general, kinesiology taping as a standalone treatment or when compared to sham taping either provided no significant benefit or its effect was too small to be clinically meaningful. Zhang and colleagues,[21] however, reported that kinesiology tape could be recommended to relieve pain and improve range of motion for patients with myofascial pain syndrome. Although the evidence in support of kinesiology tape as a standalone treatment is conflicting and not of high quality, limited evidence does exist to support the use of kinesiology tape as a complementary treatment to traditional rehabilitation exercises and therapeutic interventions for decreasing pain associated with musculoskeletal injuries. Despite these findings, health care providers continue to use kinesiology taping in the treatment of various injuries and conditions. Although support for kinesiology taping is limited, clinical decisions should be based on the best available evidence, clinician experience, and patient preferences.

FOUNDATIONAL SKILL

Application Guidelines for Kinesiology Taping

1. To ensure the best adhesion, apply the tape 20 minutes to 1 hour before activity or use tape adherent if applying during activity. Generally, kinesiology tape is water resistant starting 1 hour after application.

2. Cut the ends of the tape in a round shape to prevent rolling of tape corners. Start and end the tape strips without tension, placing them on the skin rather than on another piece of tape. Place the start and end of the tape strips by peeling off 1 to 2 in. (2.5-5 cm) of paper backing. Adhere the tape to the skin, then take the joint through its full range of motion and press the rest of the tape strip to the skin. Avoid excessive stretching of the tape before application.

3. There are four common ways to cut kinesiology tape (figure 12.3):

   • The I-cut is applied directly over the target muscle or to cross a joint for increased stability.

   • The Y-cut is used to surround muscles and relax spasms or facilitate muscle function and increase lymph flow.

   • The X-cut is used to stabilize a joint relative to the target muscle.

   • The fan cut is used to reduce localized edema and increase lymph flow toward the base of the fan.

4. To reduce spasm, apply the tape from muscle insertion to origin with the muscle stretched.

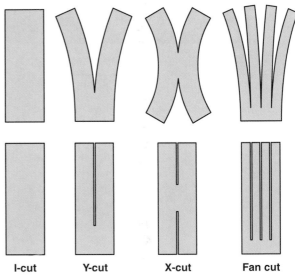

FIGURE 12.3 Common cuts of kinesiology tape.

5. To facilitate muscle function, apply the tape from muscle origin to insertion while elongating the **antagonist muscle**. This type of application will bunch the skin and cause the tape to be convoluted.

6. Tape tension varies depending on the purpose for applying the taping procedure. To assist with bruising, edema, or circulation problems, apply little or no tension. To affect muscle, apply light to moderate tension. To help stabilize joints, apply a large amount of tension.

7. Once applied, rub the tape to activate the adhesive. Educate the patient on general use guidelines and wear time. When the tape gets wet, pat it dry with a towel. Kinesiology tape can usually be worn for 3 to 10 days.

8. To remove the tape, pull it off slowly in the direction of hair growth while holding down the skin around it. Baby oil, vegetable oil, or a tape removal product can be applied to improve patient comfort during tape removal.

---

current literature regarding best practices. A variety of braces are available for every joint in the body; however, a comprehensive review of braces is beyond the scope of this chapter. Examples of common braces for the ankle, knee, shoulder, elbow, and wrist are provided in the following sections. More information can be found in *Athletic Taping, Bracing, and Casting*, 4th ed.[5] When applying any brace, you should follow the man-

ufacturer's instructions included with the braces when purchased.

Common Ankle Braces Bracing techniques for preventing and treating ankle sprains can be classified as lace-up, semirigid, air or gel bladder, and wrap. As highlighted in the Evidence-Based Athletic Training sidebar, bracing can offer several advantages over taping in preventing and treating ankle injuries.

- *Lace-up braces* (figure 12.4*a*) provide moderate support and limit inversion, eversion, plantar flexion, and dorsiflexion. They are available off the shelf in various sizes and can be used with a wide variety of footwear. Many designs have Velcro enclosure straps to anchor the laces, and others include various plastic or steel materials to serve as stirrups and provide additional support.

- *Semirigid braces* (figure 12.4*b*) provide moderate support. They limit inversion, eversion, and rotation, allowing normal dorsiflexion and plantar flexion. These braces consist of a medial and lateral stirrup attached through a hinge to a foot plate. They may be universally manufactured in various sizes or allow for custom molding and fitting. Similar to lace-up braces, these can be used with a wide variety of footwear.

- *Air or gel bladder braces* (figure 12.4*c*) limit inversion and eversion only and are most often used during the acute phase of treatment for an inversion or eversion ankle sprain to provide compression and moderate support. Many preinflated air bladders contain valves that allow for adjustments in the compression and many gel liners can be removed and placed in the freezer to cool, allowing for compression and cryotherapy while wearing the brace.

- *Wrap braces* provide mild support in the prevention of inversion and eversion ankle sprains. These off-the-shelf braces are considered to be either support braces or treatment braces. Support wrap braces have various straps that are applied in a figure-of-eight or heel-lock pattern and are designed to be used during activity. Treatment

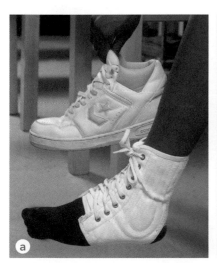 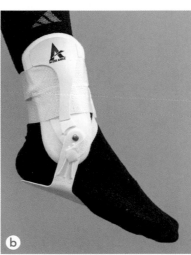 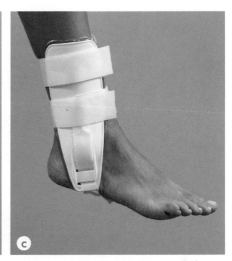

FIGURE 12.4 *(a)* Lace-up ankle brace, *(b)* semirigid ankle brace, and *(c)* air or gel bladder brace.

EVIDENCE-BASED ATHLETIC TRAINING

Comparison of Bracing and Taping for the Functional Treatment of Lateral Ankle Sprains

Functional treatment, which includes the application of supportive bracing or taping, is a commonly accepted method of treating lateral ankle sprains. The question remains, however, whether the use of a supportive brace or taping procedure is more effective in the functional treatment of a lateral ankle sprain. Multiple randomized controlled trials and systematic reviews have attempted to answer this very question.[22-25] Although definitive conclusions cannot be made from these studies regarding the functional treatment of ankle sprains, tape treatments were reported to have more complications, especially in the form of skin irritations, when compared to elastic bandages[22] and semirigid braces.[23] Overall patient satisfaction related to functional outcomes appears to be higher when using braces versus tape.[23] Finally, when considering the use of taping versus bracing procedures for the functional treatment of ankle sprains, you should look at cost. Because braces, unlike tape, are reusable, their relatively low cost along with their higher patient satisfaction and lower incidence of skin irritations may make them the better option for the functional treatment of lateral ankle sprains.

wrap braces are neoprene sleeves that are used for non-weight-bearing activities to provide compression. Some treatment wrap brace designs have removable gel packs attached to the inner liner of the brace, allowing for simultaneous cryotherapy and compression.

When complete support and immobilization of the foot and ankle are required, a walking boot should be used. In some cases, walking boots can even replace a traditional plaster or fiberglass cast because they are lighter and more cost-effective, allow for removal to perform treatment and rehabilitation, and have lower adverse effects on gait and lower extremity kinematics.[26] Walking boots come in a tall design that extends to the proximal lower leg and a short design that extends to the middle of the lower leg.

Additionally, some boot designs contain dials that allow for adjustments in range of motion (figure 12.5).

Common Knee and Patella Braces　Knee braces fall into three categories: prophylactic or preventive, rehabilitative, and functional. Selecting the appropriate knee brace should be based on the short- and long-term goals and objectives, needs of the patient, durability, fit, comfort, and cost-effectiveness.

- *Prophylactic or preventive knee braces* (figure 12.6a) protect the knee from injury during activity by supporting the medial collateral ligament from excessive valgus force. Along with collateral support, these braces also provide resistance against knee hyperextension. Although various designs

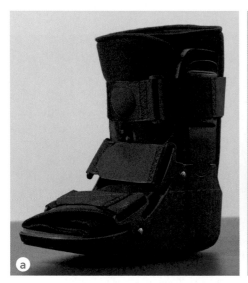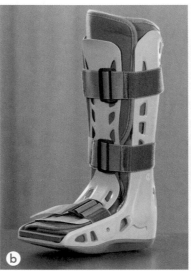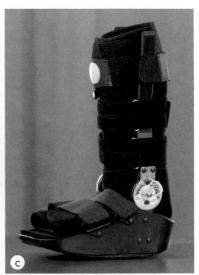

FIGURE 12.5　*(a)* Short and *(b)* tall walking boots; *(c)* walking boot with adjustable range of motion.

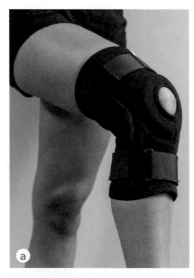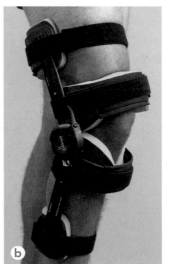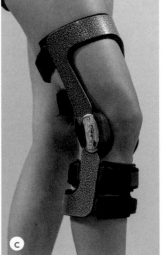

FIGURE 12.6　Examples of knee braces: *(a)* prophylactic or preventive, *(b)* rehabilitative, and *(c)* functional.

exist, they are all applied using some combination of Velcro straps, neoprene wraps, and elastic tape. Although these braces are still used by rehabilitation specialists, scientific evidence to support their use is lacking (see Evidence-Based Athletic Training sidebar).

• *Rehabilitative knee braces* (figure 12.6*b*) protect the knee immediately after injury or surgery by controlling range of motion through predetermined arcs. They use either straight immobilizers made of foam with 2 metal rods running down the sides to prevent all motion or a hinged brace that allows for range of motion to be set using a control dial. Early motion can be important for preventing joint adhesions from forming, enhancing proprioception, and promoting healing of injured tissue. As the patient progresses in their rehabilitation, the allowable range of motion can be adjusted.

• *Functional knee braces* (figure 12.6*c*) are used with patients who experience rotary instability because of injury to the anterior cruciate ligament (ACL) and following reconstructive surgery to reduce strain on ACL grafts. Also known as derotation or ACL braces, they control tibial translation and rotational stress relative to the femur and often provide extension limitations. Similar to with prophylactic or preventive braces, no consensus exists in the literature relative to whether functional knee braces have any beneficial effects on ACL reinjury rates or the function and stability of ACL-reconstructed knees.[30,31]

Patella braces (figure 12.7), also known as patellofemoral braces, maintain patellar alignment, improve patellar tracking, and dissipate force. These braces are often neoprene sleeves with lateral buttresses that prevent

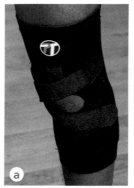
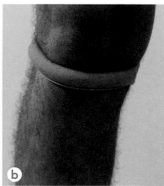

FIGURE 12.7 Examples of patella braces: *(a)* lateral buttress brace and *(b)* patellar tendon strap.

lateral displacement of the patella within the trochlear groove. Because of the pad's shape, these braces are also referred to as J braces. An alternative brace for treating patellofemoral or anterior knee pain is a strap worn over the patellar tendon.

Common Shoulder Braces Shoulder braces provide support, stability, and immobilization and limit range of motion. Although elastic wraps such as the spica wrap (see later in the chapter) provide mild to moderate support and immobilization of the shoulder and arm, several off-the-shelf and custom-made braces are also used to treat sprains, dislocations, subluxations, strains, ruptures, and overuse injuries and conditions. When choosing a shoulder brace, you should consider the needs of the patient and the durability, fit, comfort, and cost-effectiveness of the brace.

• *Slings and immobilizers* (figure 12.8*a*) provide complete support and immobilization of the shoulder, elbow, wrist, and hand following

EVIDENCE-BASED ATHLETIC TRAINING

Use of Prophylactic or Preventive Knee Braces in Sports

Although the use of prophylactic knee braces continues in sports, due to inconsistent findings within the literature, the current evidence regarding the efficacy of prophylactic knee braces remains inconclusive. Since 2008, two systematic reviews[27,28] and one meta-analysis[29] evaluated the evidence pertaining to the effectiveness of prophylactic knee braces in reducing sport-related knee injuries. A consistent lack of high-quality randomized trials makes it difficult to develop an evidence-based recommendation regarding the use of knee braces, and all three studies concluded that the implications of the effectiveness of prophylactic knee bracing cannot be drawn. Data do suggest, however, that in high-risk sport positions such as offensive and defensive line, linebackers, and tight ends, bracing may be effective in preventing medial collateral ligament injuries in college athletes. Therefore, although the evidence may not support the routine use of prophylactic bracing in uninjured knees, athletic trainers should base clinical decisions regarding the use of prophylactic knee braces on the individual needs of the patient.

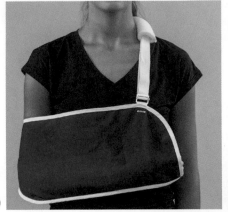
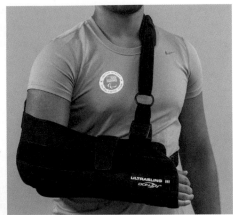
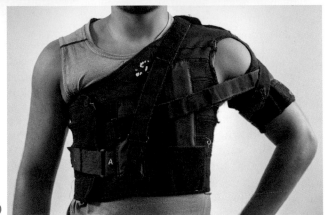

FIGURE 12.8 (a) An off-the-shelf sling and immobilizer, and (b) torso vest stabilizer.

injury or surgery. Immobilizers often come with a pad or inflatable air pillow that allows for immobilization in varying degrees of shoulder abduction. Typically, slings are less expensive than immobilizers.

• *Torso vest stabilizers* (figure 12.8b) provide moderate to maximal support and limit range of motion when preventing and treating various injuries and conditions of the shoulder. Commonly, these limit shoulder abduction and external rotation while allowing for normal flexion, extension, and adduction. Torso vest stabilizers can easily be worn during activities of daily living as well as during sport activity. They are commonly constructed out of neoprene or canvas, which provide varying degrees of stabilization and immobilization.

• *Individual arm cuff stabilizers*, like torso vest stabilizers, provide moderate to maximal support and limit range of motion at the shoulder. These stabilizers must be attached to a fixed surface on the torso of the patient, such as athletic shoulder pads. Before attaching the individual arm cuff stabilizer to any other piece of athletic equipment, you should contact the manufacturer; drilling

holes or otherwise altering the protective equipment may void the warranty.

Common Elbow Braces   Several bracing techniques for the elbow are available to provide immobilization, support, and compression; limit range of motion; and correct structural abnormalities. These include hinged elbow braces and epicondylitis straps.

• *Hinged elbow braces* (figure 12.9a) provide moderate stability to the elbow and are commonly used to control valgus, varus, rotary, and hyperextension stresses following injury or surgery. These braces can be further classified as rehabilitative or functional; rehabilitative braces allow clinicians to adjust the available range of motion and are often used to replace a fiberglass or plaster cast.

• *Epicondylitis straps* (figure 12.9b), also known as counterforce braces, lessen the tension on the wrist extensor or flexor musculature when treating lateral or medial epicondylitis. Several designs are available; however, they all contain a pad or buttress incorporated in the brace that is placed over the wrist flexors or extensors proximally.

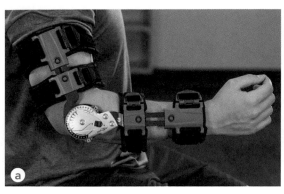
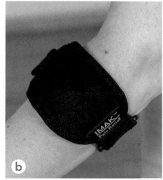

FIGURE 12.9   *(a)* Hinged elbow brace (rehabilitative) and *(b)* epicondylitis strap.

Common Wrist, Hand, and Finger Braces   Off-the-shelf and custom-made braces are available for the wrist, hand, and fingers in a variety of designs. They provide compression, support, and immobilization and limit range of motion.

- *Wrist braces*, like knee braces, are often classified as prophylactic or preventive, rehabilitative, and functional. Prophylactic or preventive and functional wrist braces are commonly used in sports such as biking, skiing, and in-line skating and provide moderate support against sprains, fractures, and dislocations of the wrist. Rehabilitative wrist braces (figure 12.10*a*) can often replace fiberglass or plaster casting in providing compression, immobilization, and support to the wrist and hand, but can also be used during activities of daily living. Many of these braces are also used for hand and thumb injuries (figure 12.10*b*).

- *Finger braces* provide support and immobilization and limit range of motion when treating sprains, fractures, and tendon injuries of the fingers. A wide variety of off-the-shelf and custom-made bracing options exist for the fingers; choose a technique according to available supplies and patient needs. When treating a **mallet finger**

injury, for example, you can apply a commercially available brace (figure 12.11) or fabricate a brace using either malleable aluminum with an open-cell foam pad lining or heat-moldable plastic with a moleskin lining.

Common Thorax and Spine Braces   Injury to the thorax and spine can occur as a result of acute and chronic forces, movements, and stresses. Contusions, sprains, strains, fractures, and costochondral injuries all commonly occur as a result of direct and indirect forces placed on the thorax and spine. Like other areas of the body, it is common to treat these injuries with the application of taping, wrapping, bracing, and padding procedures. A few examples of common braces for the thorax and spine are presented here. For more information related to protective equipment for the spine, please see chapter 11.

- *Rib belts* (figure 12.12*a*) provide compression and mild support for the treatment of rib fractures and contusions, intercostal strains, and costochondral injuries. These off-the-shelf braces come in male and female designs in predetermined sizes based on thorax circumference measurements. They should be applied directly to the skin. When a rib belt is not available, an elastic wrap 4 or 6 in. (10-15 cm) wide can be used to provide compression and support to the thorax. When applying

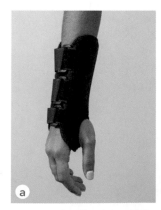
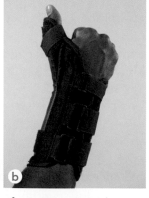

FIGURE 12.10   Examples of common wrist braces: *(a)* rehabilitative and *(b)* wrist brace with thumb spica.

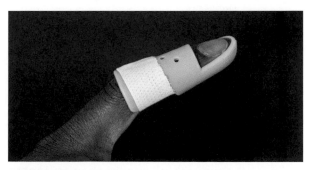

FIGURE 12.11   Commercially available finger brace to treat a mallet finger.

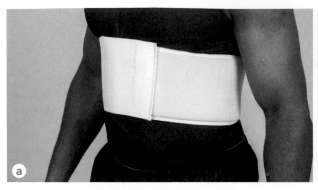 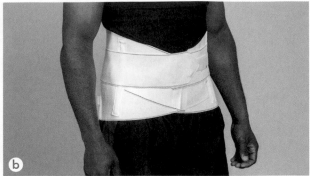

FIGURE 12.12 *(a)* Rib belt and *(b)* lumbar stabilization brace.

either an elastic compression wrap or rib belt, you should have the patient inhale during application to prevent restriction of chest movement and normal breathing.

- *Lumbar stabilization braces* (figure 12.12*b*) are used when preventing and treating abdominal strains, lumbar strains and sprains, spondylolysis, and spondylolisthesis. These braces provide compression and moderate support, limit trunk range of motion, and correct structural abnormalities. Lumbar stabilization braces come in universal fit designs in predetermined sizes based on waist circumference and should be applied directly to the skin. Most of these braces contain a semirigid or rigid stay or insert that can be molded or adjusted for an individual fit, while others contain anterior and posterior rigid panels that are connected with high-tension elastic cords.

- *Cervical collars* are used to provide support and immobilization when preventing and treating sprains, strains, fractures, and disc herniations of the cervical spine. These braces can be used for acute immobilization of the cervical spine (extrication collar; see chapter 14) or extended immobilization during rehabilitative and daily living activities. Most extrication collars are a one-piece design and allow for adjustments in neck circumference and length measurements during application. Extrication collars are manufactured with openings to allow for pulse checks, airway procedures, and visual inspection of the cervical spine. The Foundational Skills sidebar outlines general application guidelines that can be used for most rigid and semirigid acute and extended wear designs. Specific instructions for application of cervical collars are included with each design, and you should follow the manufacturer's recommended step-by-step procedure. Appropriate care of suspected cervical spine injuries is vital to prevent further trauma. For more information, see *Acute and Emergency Care in Athletic Training*.[32]

FOUNDATIONAL SKILL

Construction of an Acromioclavicular Joint Pad

1. Gather necessary materials: paper, felt-tip pen, thermoplastic (heat-moldable) material, 1/8- or 1/4-in. (0.3- or 0.6-cm) foam or felt padding, a heating source, 2- or 3-in. (5- or 8-cm) elastic tape, an elastic wrap, soft open-cell foam, rubber cement, and taping scissors.

2. Cover the area to be padded with paper and draw and cut the pattern (figure 12.13*a*). The acromioclavicular joint, tip of the shoulder, lateral aspect of the upper trapezius muscle, and proximal deltoid should be covered.

3. Lay the paper on the thermoplastic material and outline the pattern with a felt-tip pen.

4. Cut a piece of 1/2-in. (1.3-cm) felt slightly larger than the injured area and attach it to the skin (figure 12.13*b*).

5. Using the paper pattern, cut a piece of thermoplastic material that is partially heated. Completely heat the material following the manufacturer's guidelines.

6. Apply the pliable thermoplastic material to the shoulder over the felt pad and lightly mold it with your hands (figure 12.13*c*). You can apply an elastic wrap over the thermoplastic material to assist with the molding.

7. Continue molding the material to the patient. Follow the manufacturer's guidelines for the recommended amount of time before the material cools. Apply a bag of ice over the material to decrease the cooling time.

8. Once cooled, inspect the thermoplastic material to ensure proper shape and contour. Trim as needed to remove sharp edges and ensure a proper fit.

9. Completely dry the thermoplastic material. Place it on soft open-cell foam and outline an area 1/2 to 1 in. (1.3-2.5 cm) larger than the thermoplastic material (figure 12.13*d*). Cut the foam and adhere it to the thermoplastic material.

10. Using taping scissors, cut out the foam over the raised area of the thermoplastic material shaped by the felt pad (figure 12.13*e*). This will disperse the impact force away from the injured area.

11. Apply strips of elastic tape along the edges of the pad in a square pattern (figure 12.13*f*). The tape strips should extend beyond the open-cell foam. Trim the excess tape around the pad to create a uniform edge.

12. Attach the finished pad to the patient using a shoulder-spica wrapping technique (figure 12.13*g*).

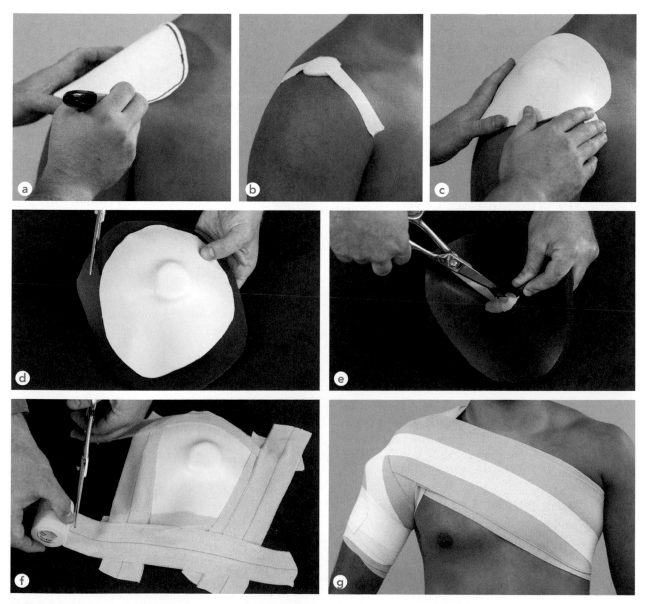

FIGURE 12.13   Construction of an acromioclavicular joint pad.

Construction of a Custom-Made Thumb Brace

1. Gather necessary materials: paper, felt-tip pen, thermoplastic (heat-moldable) material, 1/8-in. (0.3-cm) foam or 2-in. moleskin, a heating source, elastic wrap, 2- or 3-in. (5- or 8-cm) elastic tape, and taping scissors.
2. Position the patient seated with the hand and thumb in a neutral position.
3. Cover the area to be protected with paper and draw and cut the pattern. The brace should encompass the IP, MCP, and CMC joints of the thumb, and should partially incorporate the wrist.
4. Lay the paper on the thermoplastic material and outline the pattern with a felt-tip pen.
5. Partially heat the thermoplastic material and cut out the paper pattern. Completely heat the material following the manufacturer's guidelines.
6. Apply the pliable thermoplastic material to the thumb and lightly mold it with your hands. You can apply an elastic wrap over the thermoplastic material to assist with the molding.
7. Continue molding the material to the patient. Follow the manufacturer's guidelines for the recommended amount of time before the material cools. Apply a bag of ice over the material to decrease the cooling time.
8. Once cooled, inspect the thermoplastic material to ensure proper shape and contour. Trim as needed to remove sharp edges and ensure a proper fit.
9. Apply 1/8-in. foam or 2-in. moleskin to the inside surface of the brace to prevent skin irritation.
10. Apply the brace directly to the skin and secure using the basic thumb figure-eight pattern (see Thumb Taping technique on page 220) with 2- or 3-in. elastic tape.

Common Types of Protective Padding

Numerous padding products are commercially available; however, in certain situations, you might need to manufacture your own pads. Not all commercially available pads work for every situation, so you must be aware of the materials available for use in your specific situation. These protective padding materials (table 12.2) may be used alone, in combination with other padding materials, or in combination with taping and bracing procedures to meet the specific needs of the patient. When developing protective padding, consider **density**, **tensile strength**, **rigidity**, conformability, durability, ease of fabrication, and cost of materials. Although several examples of protective padding application are provided in this chapter, additional application techniques can be found in *Athletic Taping, Bracing, and Casting*, 4th ed.[5]

Common Types of Assistive Devices

Following a lower extremity injury, athletic trainers often use an assistive device so that patients may continue activities of daily living while promoting healing of injured tissue. Many factors are involved in determining whether a patient is an appropriate candidate for an assistive device. These include the patient's cognitive function, vision, vestibular function, upper body strength, physical endurance, and living environment. Impairments in any of these functions could make it impossible for a patient to safely use a device. Therefore, you should complete a thorough assessment of your patient to determine which assistive device is appropriate, if any. Two assistive devices commonly used by athletic trainers are axillary crutches and canes.

Axillary Crutches

Axillary crutches increase the base of support, thereby improving lateral stability. They can be used for non-weight-bearing, partial weight-bearing, or full weight-bearing. Axillary crutches are inexpensive and typically used to provide weight-bearing ambulation support to people with temporarily restricted ambulatory status. Because of the wide base needed for ambulation and the considerable strength needed to use axillary crutches, they can be cumbersome and difficult to use for some patients.

Canes

Canes are commonly used for partial weight-bearing and when a patient has minor problems with balance or

TABLE 12.2 **Protective Padding**

Type	Description
Open-cell foam 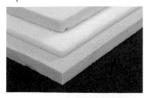	• Provides better protection at lower levels of impact • Regains its original shape quickly after deformation • Often lighter and more comfortable to wear than closed-cell foam • May be combined with closed-cell foam to provide maximum protection
Closed-cell foam 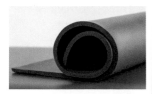	• Provides better protection at higher levels of impact • Regains its original shape quickly after deformation • Usually stiffer than open-cell foam, which can make it more difficult to mold around a specific body part
Felt 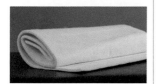	• Varying thicknesses and shapes • Does not readily deform under pressure • May be used to block or limit range of motion at the wrist, neck, elbow, and knee • Often used in combination with other padding materials or braces to improve patient comfort and improve protection provided
Gel 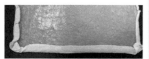	• Typically made of silicone • Effective in dispersing various levels of impact • Often used in combination with other padding materials or braces to improve patient comfort and improve protection provided • Due to its texture, may present some adherence problems
Heat-moldable plastics or fiberglass 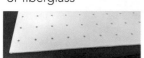	• Activated by heat (e.g., heat gun or hot water) • Once activated, can be easily molded to a specific body part • Provides a hard covering over other padding materials to increase the absorption of high-level impacts • May be used for immobilization or to restrict range of motion

stability. The use of a cane may help a patient to walk more comfortably and safely. In some cases, use of a cane may make it easier for a patient to continue living independently. Canes can be constructed of wood or metal and may have either a single point of contact or multiple points of contact with the ground.

FOUNDATIONAL SKILL

Crutch Fitting

1. Inspect the rubber tips, hand grips, and axillary pads of the crutches and replace any worn or missing pads. Check the integrity of wing nuts and button locks on the crutches for safety.
2. Ask the patient to stand erect in flat shoes with his feet shoulder-width apart. Place the crutch tips 2 in. (5 cm) in front of his feet. Adjust crutch length, allowing for 2 or 3 fingers width between the axillary pads and the patient's axilla. Adjust the hand grip height so that there is 20 to 30 degrees of elbow flexion (figure 12.14).
3. Educate the patient about placing his weight through his hands and the hand grips rather than leaning on the crutches through his axillae, which can cause neurovascular symptoms distally. When standing with crutches, patients should use the tripod stance.

>continued

>continued

The following is an example of language for patient education.

- "Keep the uninvolved foot firmly on the ground and place the crutches in front of your body at a 45-degree angle to that foot. Be careful not to move the crutches too far away or too close to your body since this will not provide the support you need. An ideal position for the crutches is approximately 6 inches to the side and 2 inches in front of your feet."

4. Educate the patient on the appropriate crutch gait.

- Three-point partial weight-bearing gait is used when the patient's injured limb can bear some weight, but he will still need the assistance of crutches. To do this, the patient should put both crutches in front of the body at a 45-degree angle, just like the tripod stance. Instruct the patient to step with the foot of his injured limb up to the crutches, using the crutches to help support his body weight. The patient should then step forward, moving the uninvolved foot in line with the crutches and involved limb.

- Three-point swing-to gait is used to keep all pressure off the injured limb. Starting from the tripod stance, instruct the patient to swing both feet in line with the crutches. Generally, no weight is placed on the injured limb with this gait pattern.

- Three-point swing-through gait is the fastest gait pattern but also the least stable and requires significant upper body strength to maintain balance. This gait pattern is like the swing-to gait, but the legs move past and land ahead of the crutches. Generally, no weight is placed on the injured limb with this gait pattern.

5. Educate the patient on going up and down stairs while using crutches.

- The patient should place both crutches under the arm opposite the handrail.

- To go up stairs, the patient steps up with the uninvolved leg while leaning on the handrail.

- To go down stairs, the patient places the crutches down on the next step and steps down with the involved leg.

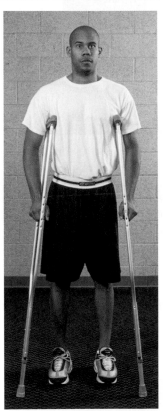

FIGURE 12.14 A patient who is properly fitted with crutches. The hands, not the axillae, should bear most of the weight.

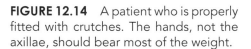
FOUNDATIONAL SKILL

Cane Fitting

1. Inspect the rubber tip and hand grip of the cane and replace any worn or missing pads. Check the integrity of the button locks on the cane, if applicable, for safety.

2. Ask the patient to stand erect in flat shoes with her feet shoulder-width apart.

3. Adjust the length of the cane so that there is 20 to 30 degrees of elbow flexion. The hand grip of the cane should be at the level of the greater trochanter of the femur (figure 12.15).

4. Educate the patient on the proper use of a cane:
   - The patient should place the cane on the uninvolved side and move it forward with the involved leg.
   - The patient should not lean heavily on the cane.
   - To go up stairs, the patient will place the cane in the hand opposite the injured limb. She will step up with the uninvolved leg first, then step up on the injured leg.
   - To go down stairs, the patient should put the cane on the next step first, step down with the involved limb, and then finally step down with the uninvolved limb, which carries her body weight.

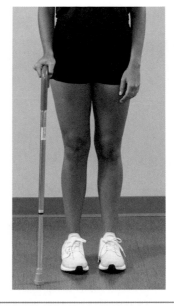

FIGURE 12.15 A patient demonstrating the proper use of a single-point cane.

Taping and Wrapping Techniques for the Lower Extremity

The following taping and wrapping techniques are provided as a guide to application. When taping or wrapping a body part, it is appropriate to modify the technique to the patient's needs. For detailed information and photos on these and other taping and wrapping techniques, see *Athletic Taping, Bracing, and Casting*, 4th ed.[5] When applying any taping or wrapping technique, you should consider the general application guidelines discussed in the Foundational Skills sidebars Application Techniques for Taping a Body Part and Application Techniques for Wrapping a Body Part on pages 191 and 194.

Great Toe Taping

This taping limits motion at the first metatarsophalangeal joint. Most often applied with nonelastic tape, this procedure can be used to prevent hyperflexion, hyperextension, or both. You should apply this procedure directly to the skin. You may also apply a felt pad across the metatarsal heads, which decreases stress on the first metatarsophalangeal joint by redistributing pressure over the second through fifth metatarsophalangeal joints. A steel-plate shoe insert may also be used with this tape to provide additional support to the first metatarsophalangeal joint.

Supplies
- 1″ and 1.5″ (2.5 and 4 cm) nonelastic tape
- Tape adherent

Patient Positioning
Have the patient sit with the foot and ankle in a relaxed position and place the great toe in a neutral position.

Application
1. Begin the procedure by applying anchor strips around the toe and foot using 1- and 1.5-in. nonelastic tape, respectively (figure 12.16*a*).
2. Using 1-in. nonelastic tape, apply strips to the plantar surface of the foot to prevent hyperextension or to both the plantar and dorsal surfaces of the foot to prevent hyperextension and hyperflexion.
3. Apply additional strips to provide extra support (figure 12.16*b*).
4. Complete the procedure by securing anchor strips around the toe and foot (figure 12.16*c*).

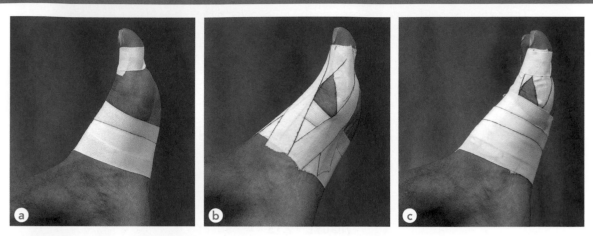

FIGURE 12.16   Taping for great toe sprains.

Arch Support Taping

Patients who run or jump excessively or have pes cavus or pes planus feet frequently develop plantar fasciitis and strains to the longitudinal arches or plantar fascia. Some of these patients will experience relief by applying a simple taping procedure (figure 12.17) or a more complex teardrop or X-arch taping procedure (figure 12.18).

Simple Taping Procedure

Supplies
- 1.5″ nonelastic or rigid strap tape
- Felt pad (optional to provide additional support to medial longitudinal arch)
- Tape adherent

Patient Positioning
Seated with the foot in full dorsiflexion and subtalar neutral

Application
1. Using 1.5-in. nonelastic tape, apply strips by starting on the dorsum of the foot and then moving in a lateral direction to lift, ultimately, the medial longitudinal arch (figure 12.17a, b).
2. Three or four strips will normally be adequate to support the medial longitudinal arch (figure 12.17c).

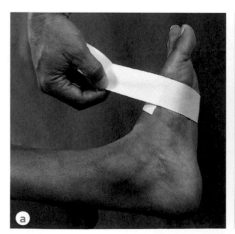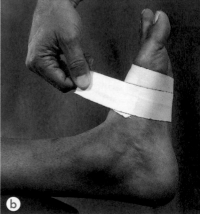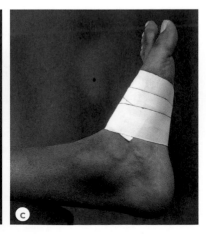

FIGURE 12.17   Simple taping to support the longitudinal arch.

Teardrop or X-Arch Taping Procedure

Supplies
- 1″ and 1.5″ nonelastic or rigid strap tape
- Felt pad (optional to provide additional support to medial longitudinal arch)
- Tape adherent

Patient Positioning
Seated with the foot in full dorsiflexion and subtalar neutral

Application
1. Place an anchor strip along the metatarsal heads with 1.5-in. nonelastic tape (figure 12.18*a*).
2. Next, apply 1-in. nonelastic tape strips from the head of the first metatarsal, around the heel, and back to the starting point (figure 12.18*b*). Place subsequent teardrop or X-strips from the medial to lateral aspect of the plantar surface of the foot (figure 12.18*c*).
3. Apply a horseshoe strip using 1-in. nonelastic tape from the lateral anchor to the medial anchor (figure 12.18*d*).
4. Complete the procedure (figure 12.18*e*) with strips that mimic the simple arch taping procedure described in figure 12.17.

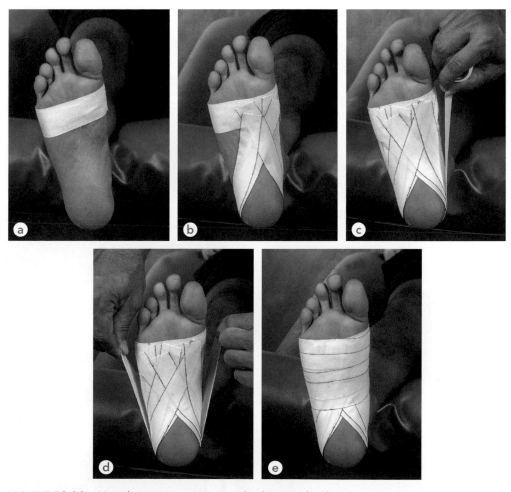

FIGURE 12.18   X-arch taping to support the longitudinal arch.

Closed Basket Weave Ankle Taping

This taping procedure is used to provide external support to the lateral ankle ligaments in the prevention and treatment of lateral ankle sprains. Although the procedure described here is for an inversion ankle sprain, modifications can be made for eversion ankle sprains by neutralizing the pull of the stirrups. Ideally, you should use 1.5-in. nonelastic tape and foam pads with lubricant. Place the foam pads over the Achilles tendon and dorsum of the ankle before beginning the procedure to reduce skin irritation and blistering caused by friction.

Supplies
- 1.5″ nonelastic tape
- Foam pads (For ease of illustration, these photos do not show the use of foam pads.)
- Foam underwrap (if not applying tape directly to the skin)
- Tape adherent

Patient Positioning

The patient holds his ankle in full dorsiflexion with neutral inversion or eversion.

Application
1. Place 2 anchor strips on the lower leg just below the musculotendinous junction of the gastrocnemius and, possibly, around the foot (figure 12.19a). Because the foot anchors frequently cause constriction and discomfort, consider them optional.

2. To prevent or protect inversion sprains, apply a stirrup strip from the medial aspect of the leg and pull under the heel to the lateral aspect of the leg (figure 12.19b).

3. Place a horizontal horseshoe strip from the medial to lateral aspect of the foot followed by another stirrup in a weaving fashion. Continue this process until you have applied 3 stirrups. Completely enclose the leg with horizontal strips (figure 12.19c).

4. Apply heel locks to the medial and lateral aspects of the ankle one at a time (application to the lateral side of the ankle is shown here). Note how to apply the lateral heel lock by pulling in an upward direction (figure 12.19d).

5. The final product supports the ankle without constricting the distal aspect of the foot (12.19e).

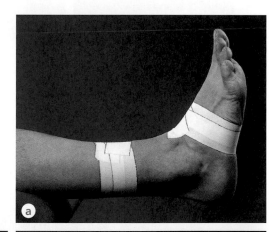

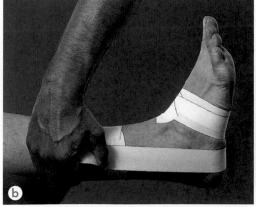

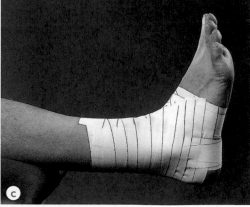

FIGURE 12.19 Closed basket weave taping procedure for the ankle.

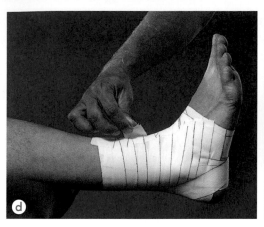
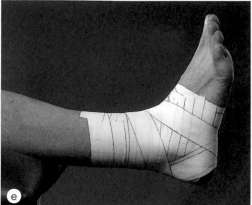

FIGURE 12.19   *>continued*

Achilles Tendon Taping

Taping the Achilles tendon limits excessive dorsiflexion and, in doing so, reduces the tension placed on the tendon. The taping consists of applying anchors around the leg and foot and a series of strips to limit dorsiflexion while the patient maintains her ankle in slight plantar flexion.

Supplies
- 1.5″ nonelastic tape
- 2″ or 3″ elastic tape
- Foam pad
- Tape adherent

Patient Positioning
  Prone with foot in a relaxed position off the edge of the table

Application
1. Apply anchor strips using 1.5-in. nonelastic tape proximally and distally with a friction pad to protect the Achilles tendon (figure 12.20*a*).
2. Apply 2 or 3 strips of tape in an X fashion across the posterior aspect of the ankle to limit dorsiflexion (figure 12.20*b*).

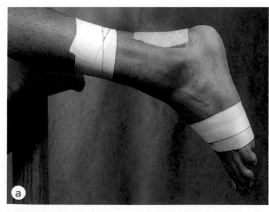
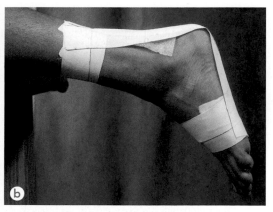

FIGURE 12.20   Taping procedure to protect a strained or inflamed Achilles tendon.

>continued

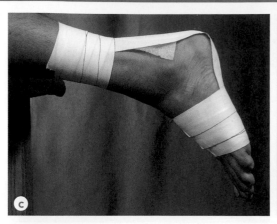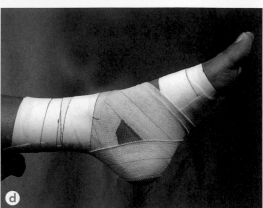

FIGURE 12.20   >*continued*

3. Apply proximal and distal anchors (figure 12.20c). Vary this procedure by using elastic tape to limit dorsiflexion. This would create a softer end point for limiting dorsiflexion.

4. Secure the entire procedure by applying both a figure eight and heel locks with elastic tape (figure 12.20d).

Patellofemoral Taping: McConnell Technique

Patellofemoral (pain) syndrome is a collection of biomechanical dysfunctions that cause pain at the patellofemoral articulation. Used to realign the patella within the trochlear groove and decrease symptoms associated with patellofemoral (pain) syndrome, this McConnell taping technique requires you to evaluate both the position of the patella (e.g., tilt, glide, rotation) and the patient's response to your treatment. This technique is also used in conjunction with a comprehensive rehabilitation program. Successful application of this taping technique should relieve the patient's pain during functional activities.

Supplies
- Rigid strapping tape
- Adhesive gauze underwrap
- Tape adherent

Patient Positioning
Seated with the knee in full extension

Application
1. Assess the patella for tilt and rotation positioning.
2. After shaving the knee, cover the patella with adhesive gauze underwrap.
3. Reassess for position.
   - Correct the tilt of the patella by applying a piece of strapping tape from the middle of the patella to the medial femoral condyle (figure 12.21a).
   - Correct the glide of the patella by applying the strapping tape from the lateral border of the patella and pulling medially to the medial femoral condyle (figure 12.21b).
   - Correct external rotation by applying strapping tape from the inferior pole (border) of the patella, pulling toward the opposite shoulder (figure 12.21c).
   - If the tilt of the patella is not correct, apply an additional tilt strip (figure 12.21d).
4. Reassess the patient for pain while he performs the functional activities that cause discomfort.

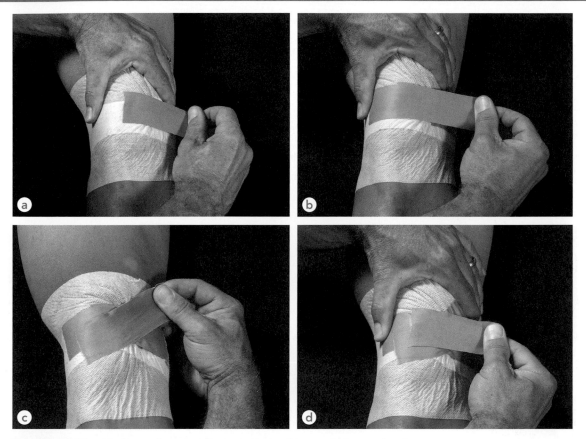

FIGURE 12.21 McConnell taping for a patient with patellofemoral pain.

Hip Flexor Strain Elastic Wrap

A hip strain commonly involves the muscles that either flex or adduct the hip. When applying an elastic wrap to support one of these muscle groups, commonly known as a hip spica, it is important to pull the wrap in the same direction as the movement that is being supported. This wrapping technique should be applied over compression shorts; as such, you may want to instruct your patient to void her bladder prior to having the wrap applied.

Supplies
- Elastic wrap 4″ or 6″ wide
- 2″ or 3″ elastic tape

Patient Positioning
Have the patient stand with the heel of the injured leg on a 2-in. taping block to help ensure your taping procedure does not limit range of motion or restrict blood flow. Place the patient's involved hip in external rotation.

Strain of the Adductor Muscles

Application
1. Have the patient place the hip in an internally rotated position.
2. Apply an elastic wrap by pulling the thigh into internal rotation. Note how the elastic wrap folds over itself to lock it in place (figure 12.22a).

3. The wrap continues around the waist to complete the spica (figure 12.22*b*).

4. Use elastic tape to trace the elastic wrap in the appropriate direction based on the presence of a hip adductor or flexor strain (figure 12.22*c*).

Strain of the Flexor Muscles

Application

1. Apply an elastic wrap by pulling the thigh into external rotation and flexion (figure 12.22*d*).

2. The wrap continues around the waist to complete the spica (figure 12.22*e*).

3. Use elastic tape to trace the elastic wrap, applying it in the same direction as the elastic wrap (figure 12.22*f*).

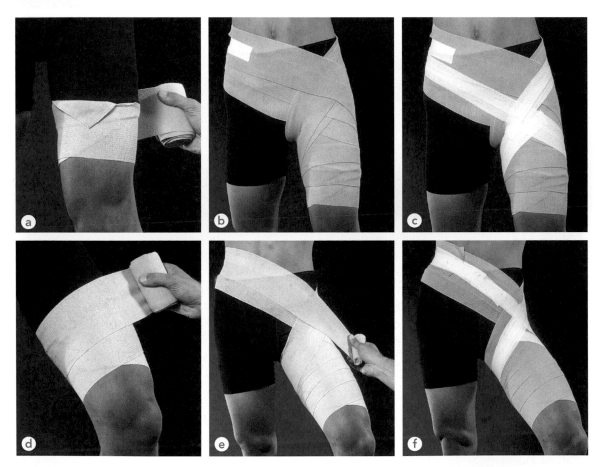

FIGURE 12.22   Hip spica wrap for supporting both the hip adductors *(a-c)* and hip flexors *(d-f)*.

Thigh Strain Elastic Wrap

A thigh strain may involve either the quadriceps or the hamstrings muscle group. Application of an elastic wrap to encircle the thigh can provide compression and support for either muscle group. This wrapping technique should be applied directly to the skin, if possible, or over compression shorts. As such, you may want to instruct your patient to void his bladder prior to having the wrap applied. If you need to support the hamstrings, apply the elastic wrap in a manner similar to the quadriceps wrap and combine it with a hip spica (see figure 12.22) in order to support the proximal attachment site of the muscle group.

Supplies
- Elastic wrap 4″ or 6″ wide
- 2″ or 3″ elastic tape
- Tape adherent

Patient Positioning
Have the patient stand with the heel of the injured leg on a 2-in. taping block to help ensure your taping procedure does not limit range of motion or restrict blood flow.

Application
1. To prevent slipping of the wrap, apply tape adherent or roll tape into a small strip and apply the roll to the thigh before applying the wrap (figure 12.23*a*).
2. Apply the wrap in a circular pattern around the thigh, moving from distal to proximal (figure 12.23*b-c*).

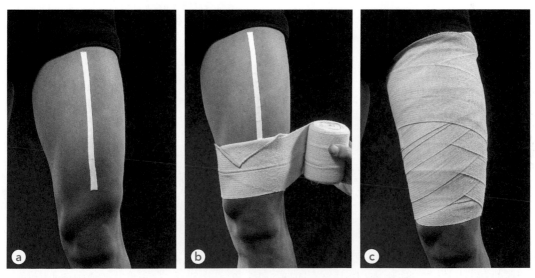

FIGURE 12.23   Elastic wrap to support a strain of the quadriceps muscles.

Taping and Wrapping Techniques for the Upper Extremity

The following taping and wrapping techniques are provided as a guide to application. When taping or wrapping a body part, modify the technique to the patient's needs. For detailed information and photos on these and other taping and wrapping techniques, see *Athletic Taping, Bracing, and Casting*, 4th ed.[5] When applying any taping or wrapping technique, you should consider the general application guidelines discussed in the Foundational Skills sidebars Application Techniques for Taping a Body Part and Application Techniques for Wrapping a Body Part, listed on pages 191 and 194.

Shoulder Spica Elastic Wrap

This technique can be used to provide support and mild stabilization for the glenohumeral joint and prevent excessive abduction and external rotation. The shoulder spica elastic wrap is also commonly used to secure protective padding on the arm and shoulder. Check and monitor the patient's distal pulse, motor function, and sensory function to determine if the wrap is too tight.

Supplies
- Elastic wrap 4″ or 6″ wide
- 2″ or 3″ elastic tape

Patient Positioning
  Standing with the involved shoulder placed in internal rotation and the hand on the hip

Application
1. Start the wrap on the arm and pull medially across the anterior chest (figure 12.24a).
2. Place the wrap, continuing around the arm and again proceeding around the chest (figure 12.24b).
3. Use elastic tape to trace the elastic wrap (figure 12.24c).

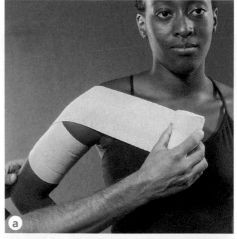

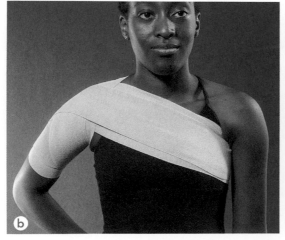

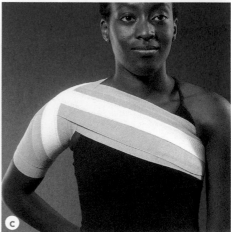

FIGURE 12.24   An elastic-wrap shoulder spica.

Acromioclavicular Joint Taping: McConnell Technique

Sprains to the acromioclavicular joint (known colloquially as a separated shoulder) commonly occur when a person falls on the hand, elbow, or shoulder. Used to help reapproximate the acromioclavicular joint, this rigid strap taping procedure does not restrict shoulder movement and can be left in place for an extended period of time.

Supplies
- Adhesive gauze underwrap
- Rigid strapping tape
- Tape adherent

Patient Positioning
Standing with the involved arm resting by his side

Application
1. Apply the first adhesive gauze underwrap strip vertically from the deltoid tuberosity past the acromioclavicular joint by 3/4 to 1-1/4 in. (2-3 cm). Apply the second strip from the coracoid process to the spine of the scapula (figure 12.25*a*).
2. Apply the first strip of strapping tape vertically over the underwrap strip while approximating the acromioclavicular joint (figure 12.25*b*).
3. Apply the second strip of strapping tape anterior to posterior. The point of the crossing strips should center over the acromioclavicular joint (figure 12.25*c*).
4. An additional layer of strapping tape strips may be necessary.

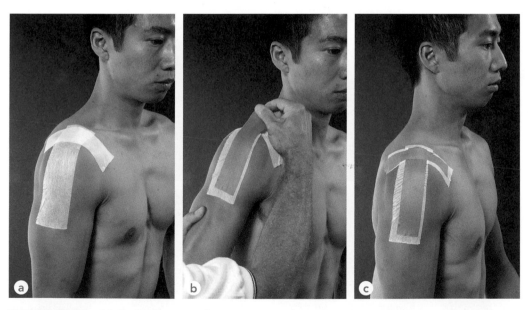

FIGURE 12.25   McConnell taping for an acromioclavicular joint sprain.

Elbow Hyperextension Taping

Following a hyperextension injury, soft tissue and bony structures on the anterior aspect of the elbow suffer trauma. In order to restrict painful motion while permitting functional movement, you can apply this taping technique using nonelastic and elastic tape. Check and monitor the patient's distal pulse, motor function, and sensory function to determine if the wrap is too tight.

Supplies
- 1.5″ nonelastic tape
- 2″ or 3″ elastic tape or 4″ elastic wrap
- Tape adherent

Patient Positioning
Standing or seated with the involved elbow in a position of function

Application
1. Begin the procedure on a shaved arm and apply proximal and distal anchor strips (figure 12.26*a*).
2. Form an X with 3 strips of tape over the anterior aspect of the elbow.
3. Apply proximal and distal anchor strips to secure the tape (figure 12.26*b*).
4. Crimp the strips on the anterior aspect (figure 12.26*c*).
5. The bridge created over the anterior elbow can be problematic for some sports, such as wrestling. Eliminate this problem by enclosing the taping procedure with elastic tape or an elastic wrap (figure 12.26*d*).

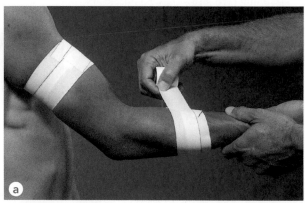

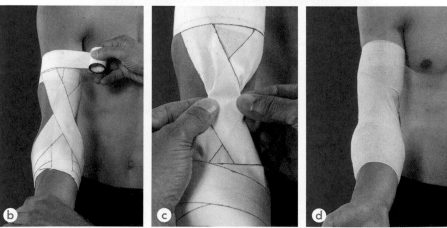

FIGURE 12.26 Elbow hyperextension taping procedure.

Basic Wrist Taping Technique

Wrist injuries often occur following a hyperflexion or hyperextension mechanism of injury. For mild symptoms, use a basic wrist taping technique.

Supplies
- 1.5″ nonelastic tape
- Tape adherent

Patient Positioning
Seated or standing with the involved wrist in a neutral position

Application
1. Apply 3 or 4 strips of nonelastic tape around the wrist (figure 12.27).
2. Apply the strips from distal to proximal, overlapping the previous underlying strip by one-half the width of the tape.

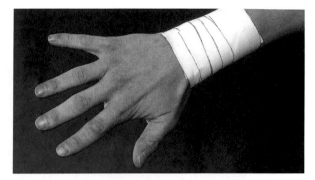

FIGURE 12.27   Basic wrist taping technique.

Wrist Hyperextension or Hyperflexion Taping Technique

To further limit range of motion and provide additional support to the wrist, include the hand in your procedure. To improve patient comfort, have your patient spread her fingers during tape application so that the tape is not applied too tightly and crimp the tape when bringing it through the web space of the thumb and index finger to reduce skin irritation.

Supplies
- 1.5″ nonelastic tape
- Tape adherent

Patient Positioning
Seated or standing with the involved wrist in a neutral position

Application
1. Begin by placing anchor strips around the wrist and hand (figure 12.28*a*).
2. To limit hyperflexion, place 3 strips and an X over the dorsum of the hand (figure 12.28*b*).
3. Limit hyperextension by placing 3 strips and an X over the palmar aspect of the hand (figure 12.28*c*).
4. Complete the procedure with 2 figure eights around the wrist and hand (figure 12.28*d-e*).

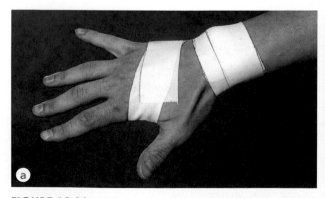

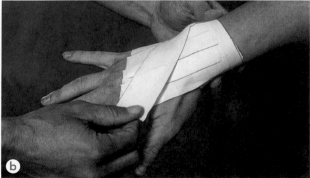

FIGURE 12.28   Wrist taping procedure that involves the hand to provide greater limitation of motion.

>*continued*

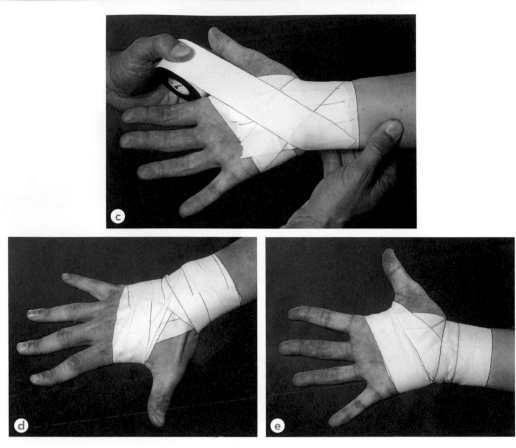

FIGURE 12.28   *>continued*

Thumb Taping

Most thumb sprains result from hyperextension of the first metacarpophalangeal joint and involve injury to the ulnar collateral ligament. Thumb taping provides support and limits thumb extension. Check capillary refill after taping to ensure adequate blood flow to the thumb.

Supplies
- 1″ and 1.5″ nonelastic tape
- Tape adherent

Patient Positioning
  Seated or standing with the involved thumb positioned in slight flexion and adduction

Application
1. Apply anchor strips around the wrist using 1.5-in. nonelastic tape. Next, begin a strip of 1-in. tape from the palmar surface of the wrist and proceed around the thumb. Adduct the thumb as the strip passes toward the dorsal surface of the wrist (figure 12.29*a*).
2. To prevent the bulk that will result from continuous strips around the wrist, individually apply the figure-eight strips.
3. As you apply the figure eights, successively overlap the preceding strips in a staircase fashion (figure 12.29*b*).
4. Place anchor strips around the wrist to complete the procedure (figure 12.29*c*).

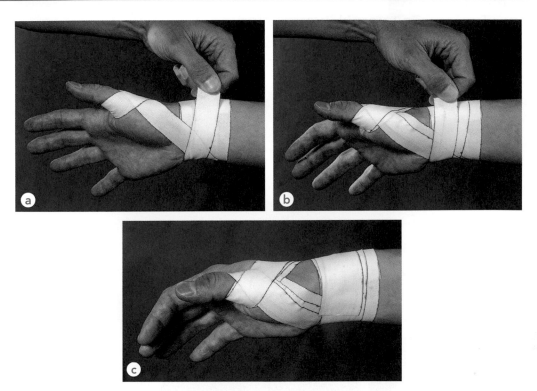

FIGURE 12.29   Figure-eight taping to support the metacarpophalangeal joint of the thumb.

Finger Taping: Buddy Taping

This taping technique involves using adjacent fingers to support injured fingers. Check capillary refill after taping to ensure adequate blood flow to the finger.

Supplies
   1/2″ or 1″ nonelastic tape

Patient Positioning
   Have the patient sit or stand with the fingers you wish to tape in full extension. Please note that, if at all possible, the 5th finger should not be left alone (e.g., tape the 4th and 5th fingers together or tape the 3rd, 4th, and 5th fingers together).

Application
   1. Apply strips on the proximal and middle phalanges.
   2. Note how the proximal interphalangeal (PIP) and distal interphalangeal (DIP) joints are left open to permit some motion of the fingers while providing support (figure 12.30).

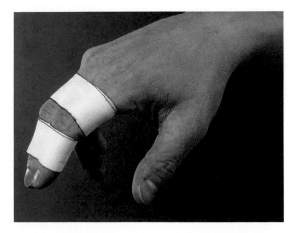

FIGURE 12.30   Buddy taping for the fingers.

Finger Taping: Collateral Ligament Taping

Use this collateral ligament taping procedure if additional support for the medial and lateral collateral ligaments is needed or if the patient needs to wear gloves. Check capillary refill after taping to ensure adequate blood flow to the finger.

Supplies
1/2″ or 1″ nonelastic tape

Patient Positioning
Seated or standing with the involved finger in full extension

Application
1. Place anchor strips on the proximal and distal parts of the finger (figure 12.31*a*).
2. Create an X over the involved collateral ligament with 3 strips of tape (figure 12.31*b*).
3. Secure the tape with proximal and distal anchors (figure 12.31*c*).

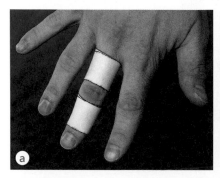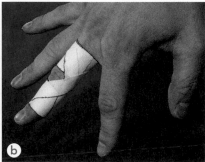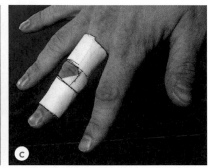

FIGURE 12.31   Taping for the collateral ligament of a finger.

CLINICAL BOTTOM LINE

- Prophylactic procedures provide support and protection to body parts while allowing functional movement.
- Athletic trainers must conduct a comprehensive orthopedic examination in order to identify the needs of the patient. Only then can they select the appropriate prophylactic procedure.
- Prophylactic procedures, such as braces and padding, can be purchased off the shelf or custom-made for the patient.
- Athletic trainers should refer to the manufacturer's guidelines for the fitting, use, and maintenance of braces and assistive devices.
- When using prophylactic procedures, the skin should be inspected regularly for signs of irritation, blisters, or infection. Using an appropriate brace instead of a taping procedure may reduce recurrent skin irritation.
- Although prophylactic procedures are commonly used by clients and clinicians, limited high-quality research is available to help guide their use. Athletic trainers should therefore be critical in their use of prophylactic procedures and employ the principles of evidence-based medicine.

 Go to HK*Propel* to complete the activities and case studies for this chapter.

Go to HK*Propel* to (1) view videos of various taping techniques and (2) download foundational skill check sheets for various taping and bracing techniques.

PART III

Immediate and Emergency Care

The two chapters in part III present entry-level information on emergency planning and acute care procedures. Emergency care begins with planning across the health care system, which includes industry, rehabilitation centers, hospitals, physician's offices, and athletic venues. Chapter 13 provides the critical concepts of emergency planning that athletic trainers need in order to act quickly should an urgent situation occur. Chapter 14 builds on the information in the preceding chapter, providing information on the acute emergency care and procedures essential for working as an entry-level athletic trainer. Injury and illness assessment are also discussed to connect important components and provide a holistic view of emergency planning and immediate care.

CHAPTER 13

Emergency Planning in Health Care

Ellen K. Payne, PhD, LAT, ATC, EMT

CAATE STANDARDS

The following CAATE 2020 standards are covered in this chapter:

Standard 59

Standard 61

Standard 62

Standard 69

Standard 70

Standard 85

Standard 92

CHAPTER OBJECTIVES

After reading this chapter, you will be able to do the following:

- Explain the importance of, and rationale behind, emergency planning

- Summarize the key components of an emergency action plan

- Identify different types of emergencies addressed in emergency action plans

- Describe the process of creating and implementing an emergency action plan

- Discuss the athletic trainer's role in emergency planning

- Discuss the team-based approach to emergency care

- Explain the importance of communication and the appropriate ways to communicate during an emergency

- Discuss the athletic trainer's role in psychological first aid and the referral process

- Summarize various special considerations that factor into emergency planning

Emergency planning is one of the most important aspects of an athletic trainer's duties and responsibilities, regardless of employment setting. Although catastrophic injuries and true emergencies are rare in the traditional athletic training setting, athletic trainers should prepare for extreme situations. Good emergency planning is more than just having a plan of what to do during an emergency situation; it involves the following:

- Helps mitigate risk and prevent injuries through careful planning and education

- Details the actions of the sports medicine team and other stakeholders during an emergency

- Allows for high-quality care for the patient in a minimal amount of time

- Outlines follow-up care and actions needed postevent

If a **catastrophic injury** or **medical emergency** does occur, once activated, the emergency action plan (EAP) is vital to an efficient, integrated response by all stakeholders. When doing emergency planning and activating the EAP, athletic trainers may work with the athletic director; coaches; visiting athletic trainers; athletic training students, residents, or interns; physicians; police; and emergency medical services (EMS) personnel. Prior to reading this chapter, please review the following chapters:

- Chapter 1 Athletic Training and the Health Care Team: Information on the members of the sports medicine team, including their education, scope of practice, and how they contribute to the sports medicine team
- Chapter 6 Management, Planning, and Professional Development: Information on legal liability and risk-management procedures
- Chapter 7 Blood-Borne Pathogens: Information on universal precautions and disease prevention that should be included in the EAP and used in the care of patients
- Chapter 8 Prevention Strategies and Procedures: Information on preventing injuries and illness, including important information on heat-related illnesses and other conditions

This chapter addresses emergency planning in the traditional athletic training setting, including the basics of emergency planning, the components of the EAP, activation and implementation of the EAP, and various special considerations to make when planning and caring for emergencies. Athletic trainers working in nontraditional settings, such as a physician's practice, rehabilitation clinic, or industry, should also follow an EAP specific to their setting.

Components of an Emergency Action Plan

The EAP is a comprehensive document that is specific to an institution's location, resources, facilities, and sports.

The purpose of the EAP is to give stakeholders a response plan when an emergency situation arises. An EAP should thoroughly address all possible emergency situations and how to respond to them. This can also involve planning for both home and away events (competitions, practices, and conditioning sessions) and special events such as tournaments that may be hosted on campus. The EAP "should be comprehensive and practical, yet flexible enough to adapt to any emergency situation."[1] Both the National Collegiate Athletic Association (NCAA) and the National Federation of State High School Associations (NFHS) recommend that every institution have an individualized EAP,[2,3] and the importance of having an EAP is well documented in the literature.[1,4-9] When developing an EAP, you should consult the National Athletic Trainers' Association (NATA) position statement on emergency planning in athletics.[1] This document gives institutions a blueprint for creating an individualized EAP and outlines the minimum components of an EAP.

Personnel

Defining the roles of each person on the sports medicine team and other stakeholders who may assist during an emergency is an important aspect of the EAP. As previously mentioned, involved personnel may include the athletic director; coaches; visiting athletic trainers; athletic training students, residents, or interns; physicians; police; and EMS personnel. All members of the sports medicine team must work together, promote interprofessional practice concepts, and be aware of the expertise and skills of other team members. Although the skills of many EAP team members may overlap, other roles are uniquely defined. For example, although both physicians and **paramedics** can start an intravenous (IV) line, paramedics perform the skill routinely in the prehospital

EVIDENCE-BASED ATHLETIC TRAINING

Minimum Components Included in an EAP

The NATA position statement on emergency planning lists the minimum components to include in an EAP:[1]

- The responsibilities of all personnel involved with the plan
- The type and location of emergency medical equipment
- Chain of command and communication between the sports medicine team and other personnel
- Policies and procedures for protective equipment removal, if needed
- Locations and types of receiving medical facilities
- Means of transportation to appropriate medical facilities
- Specific EAP for every venue or site on campus
- Review of the EAP by legal counsel and administrators of the institution
- Annual review and rehearsal of the EAP

setting, unlike most team physicians. In many locations, this skill is beyond the scope of practice for **emergency medical technicians (EMTs)**. A team-based, interprofessional approach to care can be facilitated by detailing roles and responsibilities in the EAP, practicing the EAP at least annually, and maintaining good communication among members of the sports medicine team before, during, and after an incident.

All personnel included in the EAP should be trained, at a minimum, to recognize an emergency, provide basic life support (BLS) and first aid, and prevent disease transmission.[1,2,6,8] Emergency recognition is especially important for members of the coaching staff, who could be acting alone as the first responder on the scene of a potential emergency until additional help arrives. As first responders, coaches must be able to recognize a potential emergency, activate the EAP, and provide basic lifesaving care until the athletic trainer or EMS arrives. Athletic trainers should work with the institution's administration to require and offer basic CPR and AED training for all members of the coaching staff.

When an emergency situation occurs, follow the **chain of command**, which starts with the most highly trained person on staff, usually the institution's team physician or medical director if that person is present at the event.[9] At most colleges and secondary schools, the team physician is usually present during football games or other high-risk or high-profile events. During most day-to-day activities in the athletics department, one of the athletic trainers on staff will be in charge of the situation. The athletic training staff will always act as primary medical providers at the site (when present) and should manage the situation according to the following rank:

1. Team physician
2. Head athletic trainer
3. Assistant athletic trainer

When an athletic trainer is not present at an event or practice, the head coach should activate the EAP and manage the situation until additional help arrives. If the head coach is not present, then one of the assistant coaches should be prepared to take on this role. The welfare of the injured or ill patient is always the priority; therefore, immediate care in some form should be provided until an athletic trainer or EMS arrives on the scene. This means that if no members of the athletic training or coaching staff are present, then another trained person, such as a team manager or member of the athletic department administration, should step in and help the patient until help arrives.

Athletic trainers acting as a preceptor for a CAATE-accredited athletic training program should work closely with the college or university's clinical education coordinator to find the best way to incorporate athletic training students into the EAP. All athletic training students must have a current BLS certification so that they can be a valuable asset during an emergency. Athletic training students should not fill the role of a certified staff member and must be appropriately supervised, so they should not be placed in a situation where they are the only members of the athletic training staff present. If an athletic training student does find herself alone when an emergency occurs, she should activate the EAP and provide care within the scope of her BLS certification.

The arriving EMS personnel should be briefed on the status of the patient (e.g., name, age, **chief complaint**, vital signs), the patient's medical history, if known, and any care already provided to the patient. At this point, care can be transferred from the athletic training staff to the EMS personnel responding. EMS personnel are always in charge of transportation of the patient and advanced skills beyond those that athletic trainers can do (e.g., IV medication administration). EMS protocols vary greatly by region, so you should be aware of the staffing and policies of the local EMS. For example, the nature of the call may determine if an advanced life support (ALS) ambulance staffed by paramedics or a BLS ambulance staffed by EMTs responds to the call. In other locations, one paramedic and one EMT may staff the ambulance. They will determine who is in charge of the call based on their organization's protocols. All EMS personnel must follow their organization's protocol and work on the direction of their **medical control**. Work with your local EMS agencies to learn who (paramedics or EMTs) will be responding and what their protocol is for calls. The chain of command and good communication between members of the sports medicine team will help prevent turf wars and promote collaborative interprofessional practice.

Emergency Medical Equipment

Another important component of the EAP is planning for potentially needed emergency medical equipment. A detailed inventory of equipment should be available, along with the locations of the equipment. All emergency medical equipment should be kept in good working order and updated and tested per the manufacturer's guidelines. All members of the sports medicine team should be trained on the use of the equipment, and that training should be documented. Emergency medical equipment should be provided for the visiting team if needed. If the visiting athletic trainer is unfamiliar with its use, he should be instructed on how to call for help.

At a minimum, you should have access to the following equipment:

• Spine board and associated equipment (e.g., cervical collars, cervical immobilization device, and straps)

- Automated external defibrillators (AEDs) and associated equipment (e.g., CPR mask or bag valve mask)
- Personal protective equipment (e.g., masks, eye protection, gloves) and biohazard bag
- Various splinting equipment
- Tourniquet and various dressings for wound care
- Diagnostic tools (e.g., penlight, pulse oximeter, blood pressure cuff, stethoscope, rectal thermometer)
- Patient or athlete's emergency medical information
- Protective equipment removal tools (e.g., screwdrivers, FM extractor, Trainers Angels) if needed
- Emergency cooling equipment (e.g., large tub, tarp, ice water) if needed
- Communication devices (e.g., radios, cell phones)

Additional equipment can include the following:

- Approved emergency medication (e.g., EpiPens, aspirin, naloxone, glucose)
- Oxygen, appropriate delivery devices (e.g., non-rebreather mask, bag valve mask), and airway maintenance devices (e.g., oral and nasal airways, suction)
- Rescue ring or other devices for pool rescue

Emergency medical equipment should be strategically located within each facility and across campus. When possible, equipment should be brought to events to have on hand on the bench. If not on the bench, equipment should be centrally located for easy access. Items like an AED should be placed in strategic locations within the facility and around campus so they can be retrieved within 3 minutes from all venues.

Communication

Good communication is key during an emergency situation. A communication plan needs to be determined before an actual emergency occurs. Although cell phones have become the standard for most communication, during some situations, they may not be the best option. For example, during severe weather, cell phone service may be interrupted and a landline may be the only option for outgoing calls. Also, cell phones work only when charged and there is adequate service to the location. When possible, landline phones should be available in the athletic training facility and other locations (e.g., field houses). Emergency phone numbers should be posted next to all phones and distributed to those using their personal cell phones. In some locations, a "9" or different number must be dialed to get an outside line; this should be clearly noted by every phone. If another emergency number should be called instead of 911, that should also be clearly noted by every phone. For example, some institutions require staff to call campus police or another local emergency number.

Other communication devices, such as two-way radios and walkie-talkies, may also be used during events. EMS personnel providing stand-by coverage at a football game should receive a walkie-talkie to allow for easy communication if they are needed. For some situations, hand signals or devices such as whistles and horns may be used for emergency communications. If nonverbal communication is going to be used to communicate with members of the sports medicine team, even as a back-up method if technology fails, then all parties need to know the meaning of these signals. This is something that should be addressed during the medical time out prior to the event starting (see the section Prior to the Event later in this chapter).[10]

Also outlined in the communication plan is what happens after the emergency (after the 911 call). The

FOUNDATIONAL SKILL

Activating EMS: Calling 911

1. To activate EMS, use a cellphone or landline telephone from the athletic training facility (or easiest accessed location) to dial 911 or the local emergency number (emergency numbers should be posted by all phones).
2. Be prepared to give the following information:
   a. Your name, title, and callback number
   b. Name and age of injured or ill patient
   c. Injury or illness the patient has suffered, current status, and any care being given
   d. Location of patient
   e. Best place to enter the venue or site
3. Do not hang up before the dispatcher does.

communication plan should cover who contacts others not present at the time of the event. The patient's parents or guardians or other identified emergency contact people will need to be notified. Key personnel not on site, such as administrators and mental health providers, will need also to be notified after the incident has been stabilized and the patient transported to the hospital. A list of important contacts should be created during the EAP planning process to aid in communication after an event.

Transportation Plan

The EAP should outline the logistics of any patient transportation in case the situation requires the patient to be moved to a medical facility. This process usually begins with activating EMS by calling 911 or the local emergency number. If an ambulance is on standby at the event, the EMS personnel can be notified via radio or hand signals as outlined in the communication plan. Whenever possible, an ambulance should be on site for events, not just high-risk sports such as football, ice hockey, and men's lacrosse. If the dedicated ambulance providing standby coverage for an event does transport a patient to the hospital, a second ambulance will need to come to the site to resume coverage before play can resume. The ambulance company should prearrange these details prior to the event.

The venue- or site-specific EAP should detail the optimal method for the ambulance to gain access to the site. This should include who will meet the ambulance and help escort it to the scene and who has access to

unlock any gates leading to the site. Detailed maps from the main access road to each site on campus should be included in the EAP. The EAP should also include who will travel to the hospital with the patient if her parents or guardians are not on site at the time of the incident. This is usually delegated to a member of the coaching staff such as an assistant coach.

The transportation plan should also include directions to the local medical facilities in case the patient is not going to be transported by ambulance or to allow the patient's parents or guardians to drive to the facility. Directions to the local medical facilities, along with information about the services provided at different medical facilities, will help visiting athletic trainers or other people not familiar with the local area.

Maps

Maps are an important component of the EAP. The EAP should include maps to each venue or site for transportation purposes and the floor plan for each venue. The maps should include identification of the following items (figure 13.1):

- Entrances and exits
- Elevators
- Phones
- Emergency medical equipment
- AEDs
- Fire extinguishers

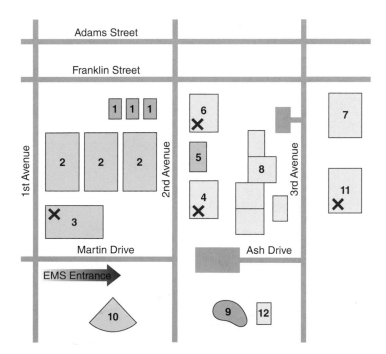
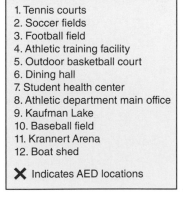

1. Tennis courts
2. Soccer fields
3. Football field
4. Athletic training facility
5. Outdoor basketball court
6. Dining hall
7. Student health center
8. Athletic department main office
9. Kaufman Lake
10. Baseball field
11. Krannert Arena
12. Boat shed

✗ Indicates AED locations

FIGURE 13.1   Example of a labeled EAP map.

Trauma Center Levels

Level I

- Capable of providing total care for every aspect of injury, from prevention through rehabilitation
- Provides 24-hour in-house coverage by general surgeons and prompt availability of care in specialties, such as orthopedic surgery, neurosurgery, anesthesiology, emergency medicine, radiology, internal medicine, plastic surgery, oral and maxillofacial surgery, pediatrics, and critical care
- Provides leadership in prevention and public education to surrounding communities
- Operates an organized teaching and research effort to help direct new innovations in trauma care

Level II

- Provides prompt assessment, resuscitation, surgery, intensive care, and stabilization of injured patients and emergency operations
- Provides 24-hour immediate coverage by general surgeons as well specialists in orthopedic surgery, neurosurgery, anesthesiology, emergency medicine, radiology, and critical care
- Can refer tertiary care needs, such as cardiac surgery, hemodialysis, and microvascular surgery, to a level I trauma center

Level III

- Demonstrates an ability to provide prompt assessment, resuscitation, surgery, intensive care, and stabilization of injured patients and emergency operations
- Provides 24-hour immediate coverage by emergency medicine physicians and the prompt availability of general surgeons and anesthesiologists
- Has developed transfer agreements for patients requiring more comprehensive care at a level I or level II trauma center

Level IV

- Demonstrates an ability to provide advanced trauma life support (ATLS) prior to transferring patients to a higher-level trauma center
- Provides evaluation, stabilization, and diagnostic capabilities for injured patients
- Has basic emergency department facilities for implementing ATLS protocols
- Has trauma nurses and physicians available on patient arrival
- May provide surgery and critical-care services if available
- Has developed transfer agreements for patients requiring more comprehensive care at a level I or level II trauma center

Level V

- Provides initial evaluation, stabilization, and diagnostic capabilities and prepares patients for transfer to higher levels of care
- Has basic emergency department facilities for implementing ATLS protocols
- Has trauma nurses and physicians available on patient arrival
- Has after-hours activation protocols if facility is not open 24 hours a day
- May provide surgery and critical-care services if available
- Has developed transfer agreements for patients requiring more comprehensive care at level I through III trauma centers
- Has medical facilities designated as adult or pediatric trauma centers

Adapted from American Trauma Society, *Trauma Center Levels Explained* (2018). www.amtrauma.org/?page=traumalevels. Accessed April 7, 2018.

Step-By-Step Instructions

The EAP should include step-by-step instructions for different emergencies at each venue or site. These are usually presented in a flowchart or bulleted format to make them easier to use in the field (figure 13.2). Instructions should be applicable to many situations and no longer than one page in length. They are useful to give to visiting athletic trainers, coaching staff, and even staff athletic trainers for review. These sheets can be posted on office walls or other easily accessible locations.

Types of Emergencies Covered in an Emergency Action Plan

Emergency action plans should address what to do in the event of a catastrophic injury or a trauma, medical, weather-related, or psychological emergency. Catastrophic injuries include the following:

- Fatalities
- Nonfatalities that result in permanent functional disability
- Nonfatal, serious injuries that are recoverable and do not result in permanent disability

The EAP should include a step-by-step plan to follow in the event of an emergency at all venues, home and away events, and games and practices. All necessary components of the EAP, as addressed previously, should be fully developed in the plan.

Trauma- and Medical-Related EAPs

This type of EAP covers protocols to follow in the event of a catastrophic or traumatic injury or medical emergency. When creating institution-specific protocols for trauma- and medical-related emergencies, you should consult the best available evidence and the latest published guidelines and recommendations from the NATA and other organizations.[1,2,4-6,9,12,13]

FIGURE 13.2 Example EAP for a secondary school.

In case of an emergency, follow this plan:

1. Contact the athletic trainer for situations that are not life threatening.
   a. Keep the patient calm until the athletic trainer arrives.
2. If the athletic trainer is not present or a life-threatening or true medical emergency situation is taking place:
   a. Provide emergency care if certified (CPR/AED/first aid).
   b. Contact EMS.
      1. Dial 911.
      2. Provide your name, the exact location, the phone number you are calling from, the number of injured people, the condition of the injured or ill, and care being provided. Stay on the line!
      3. Landlines are located in the coach's office in the field house and the athletic director's office across from the gym.
   c. Send someone to meet EMS.
      1. Refer to a venue-specific plan for where someone should meet EMS and where to direct the ambulance.
   d. Retrieve emergency medical equipment as necessary for MD, AT, or EMT.
      1. AEDs are located in the lobby of the gym, the football locker room in the field house, and the athletic training room.
   e. Provide appropriate crowd control until the situation is resolved.
   f. Contact the athletic trainer and athletic director ASAP.

The athletic trainer or designated coach will contact the parents or guardian if they are not present. If a parent or guardian is not present, a member of the coaching staff will accompany the patient to the hospital and remain with him until a parent or guardian arrives.

Protocols should be created for the following traumatic injuries:

- Catastrophic head or neck injuries
- Severe bleeding
- Fractures and dislocations
- Other potential traumas

Protocols should be created for the following medical emergencies:

- Sudden cardiac arrest
- Diabetic emergencies
- Asthma, anaphylaxis, and respiratory emergencies
- Exertional sickling
- Exertional heat illness
- Exertional hyponatremia
- Other potential medical emergencies

The acute care skills required to manage many of these conditions are addressed in chapter 14.

Weather-Related EAPs

Prevention strategies and the education of athletes, coaches, and other stakeholders are the keys to planning for weather-related emergencies. See chapter 8 for strategies for preventing environmental emergencies. Even with the best prevention plan, not all weather-related emergencies can be prevented. You must develop policies for addressing these types of emergencies if they do occur. When creating institution-specific protocols for weather-related emergencies, consult the best available evidence and the latest published guidelines and recommendations from the NATA and other organizations.[1,2,4,5,19-23]

An EAP for weather-related emergencies should address all possible types of weather for your location, including (but not limited to) the following:

- Lightning and thunderstorms
- Severe wind and tornadoes
- Extreme cold
- Extreme heat
- Extreme humidity

Specific to weather-related emergencies, the EAP should address the following:

- Who can suspend and resume activities based on the weather
- Who is in charge of monitoring the weather
- How the weather will be monitored
- Chain of communication during a weather-related emergency

EVIDENCE-BASED ATHLETIC TRAINING

Evolution in Spinal Immobilization Protocols

In the July 2014 issue of the *NATA News*, Goffnett and Pickett discussed the evolution of spine boarding protocols for athletic trainers.[14] They addressed some of the known adverse effects of prolonged immobilization on the board and lack of evidence to the benefits. The authors refer to both the NEXUS criteria[15] and Canadian C-Spine Rules[16] for evidence-based approaches to determining if immobilization is necessary. Both clinical prediction rules have been validated in the prehospital setting. The NATA released the position statement *EMS Changes to Prehospital Care of the Athlete with Acute Cervical Spine Injury* in reaction to changes in EMS spinal immobilization protocols nationwide.[17] In 2015, the NATA also released *Appropriate Prehospital Management of the Spine-Injured Athlete*, which was an update to previous, outdated recommendations on prehospital management of potential cervical spine injuries and equipment removal.[18] In 2020 two documents were published related to the current evidence in spinal motion restriction (SMR).[34,35] It is now recommended, when adequate help is available, to remove all (helmet and shoulder pads) protective equipment prior to transport to the hospital since athletic trainers are the most qualified members of the health care team to do so. The minimal equipment removal recommendation (when adequate personnel are not available) is the removal of the facemask on all patients whether or not the airway is compromised. This allows for access to the airway if needed during transport to the hospital. The documents also discuss the various options for SMR beyond just the use of the long spine board. These changes to the recommendations are not the end of the line. As new research becomes available and the evidence about best practices for spinal motion restriction evolves, athletic training protocols must evolve too.

- Specific protocols for each possible weather emergency based on the best available evidence
  - Acute care to be provided (see chapter 14 for the emergency care of various weather-related medical emergencies)
  - Additional equipment needed (e.g., cooling tub, rectal thermometer, lightning monitor)
- Plan for the evacuation of both the athletes and spectators from the venue if needed

Psychological Emergencies

In your role, you need to be prepared for more than just physical injuries and illness. You must also help athletes suffering from various mental health concerns. One resource is to become trained in mental health first aid.[24] This course helps athletic trainers learn the risk factors and warning signs for mental health concerns, strategies for how to help someone in both crisis and noncrisis situations, and how to help refer the patient for additional help. You should be aware of the mental health resources available in your institution and local community.

Like physical medical emergencies, psychological emergencies are rare, but you need to have a plan in case an emergency does occur. The following signs indicate a situation that may warrant an emergency mental health referral:[25,26]

- The patient demonstrates or voices an imminent threat to herself (suicidal thoughts or behaviors)
- The patient demonstrates or voices an imminent threat to others
- The patient reports feeling out of control
- The patient is incoherent or confused
- The patient expresses delusional thoughts
- Other serious signs of a mental health emergency

You should work with their institution's counseling centers or other mental health care providers to create an EAP specific to psychological emergencies as part of the interprofessional team.[2,25,26] When developing a mental health EAP, consider the following items specific to this type of emergency:[25,26]

- Respond with care and empathy.
- If the patient appears violent or acts violently, call 911 or the local emergency number and act to protect others from harm.
- If the patient is potentially suicidal and not violent, do not leave him alone.
- Align with the institution's policies and procedures for mental health emergencies and have the plan reviewed by the institution's mental health professionals, administrators, and legal counsel.

Developing an Emergency Action Plan

The institution's primary medical personnel (e.g., head athletic trainer, team physician) should work together to develop a comprehensive EAP for each venue or site and type of emergency.[9] All necessary components of the EAP should be fully developed and reviewed with the institution's legal counsel and administration or board. Development of an EAP can be completed in the following steps:

1. Gather the necessary information:
   - List all practice and game sites.
   - List the types of events at the sites (competitions, practices, and conditioning sessions).
   - List available personnel working at each of these sites.
   - Review venue entrances and exits for transporting the patient to the ambulance and medical facility.
   - List the location of the nearest receiving medical facility.
   - List available emergency medical supplies and equipment and their location.
   - Obtain local EMS protocols for cervical-spine management and other injuries or medical emergencies.
2. Create a detailed plan for each venue or site:
   - Address all necessary components specific to the site.
   - If sites have similar locations or other commonalities, the EAP can be duplicated, but be sure to address any differences within the plan.
   - Test the feasibility of the plan.
3. Review the EAP with the following people:
   - Local EMS and hospital personnel
   - Institution's legal counsel
   - Institution's administration or board
4. Post and share the EAP with all stakeholders.
5. Review and practice the EAP annually.

Implementing the EAP

Every institution should review and rehearse its EAP at least annually. Special attention should be paid to changes that have occurred since the last review of the document in personnel, available equipment, facilities, and best practices in athletic training and prehospital care. The team physician and local EMS agencies should be consulted on any proposed changes to an EAP. For

National Athletic Trainers' Association's Statements Related to Emergency Planning

The NATA currently has many published position and consensus statements related to emergency planning, weather-related emergencies, patient care, and protective equipment use and removal.[1,4, 6,7,12,18-22,25,26,34,35] These official position statements are created by a panel of experts in the specific areas who review the evidence-based literature related to each topic and make recommendations. Review these statements and incorporate the recommendations into your facility's EAP when feasible. The recommendations made in the position statements do not dictate care, but they should be independently evaluated for their applicability to each institution's unique situation. As changes in the recommendations are released, you must stay abreast of them to ensure the best possible patient care is being provided by your organization. In today's litigious society, failure to stay up to date on best practice recommendation could open you up to a lawsuit. These position statements are found on the NATA website and are referenced throughout this chapter.

example, the current best practices in bleeding control call for the use of a tourniquet when severe bleeding will not stop with direct pressure.[13] With this information, the athletic training staff should purchase tourniquets to be placed in every staff athletic trainer's medical kit or other appropriate location and train the staff on tourniquet use. The EAP should be updated to show where the tourniquets are located and list the policies and procedures for their use. After the EAP has been updated, it needs to be redistributed to stakeholders so they are aware of the changes and how the changes can affect their roles in an emergency.

As stated previously, the EAP should be reviewed and rehearsed at least annually. If possible, it should also be rehearsed at the beginning of each sports season and whenever there are changes in personnel. This rehearsal allows for each member of the sports medicine team to review their roles and responsibilities during an emergency. If possible, various mock scenarios could be part of the interprofessional trainings with EMS personnel and other members of the sports medicine team.[34,35]

Prior to the Event

Whenever possible, both local EMS and receiving medical facilities should be made aware of athletic events on campus. This could involve providing both with copies of the home game schedules prior to each sports season and altering them in advance of hosting tournaments, championships, and other special events. Notifying both EMS and hospital personnel of events will allow each to have proper staffing and other resources in place in the event of an emergency.

Immediately prior to each athletic event, the sports medicine team should hold a medical time out.[10,34,35] The purpose of this meeting is to review the key components of the venue's EAP and make sure that all those involved

with the health care of the athletes are on the same page if an emergency occurs. This meeting should include the athletic trainers, EMS personnel, team physician, and any other medical personnel in attendance. Both the home and the visiting team's medical staff should take part in this meeting. The meeting should address the following items:[10]

- Each person's role and location during the event
- Procedures during an emergency
- Communication procedures
- Ambulance location and exit route, if present at the event
- Ambulance notification procedures and entrance route, if not present at the event
- Emergency equipment available on site and its location
- Potential issues that could affect the event and the EAP (e.g., weather, event size)

During the Event

Although true emergency situations are rare in most traditional athletic training settings, you need to be prepared for the worst. Good planning and prevention strategies help accomplish that, but not all emergencies can be prevented. When something does occur, athletic trainers and other members of the sports medicine team need to be prepared for action. Chapter 14 addresses the on-the-field assessment and acute care skills possibly needed in these situations. In case of an emergency situation, all members of the sports medicine team need to perform their outlined role and work together to accomplish the goals of maintaining life, decreasing further injury, and rapidly transporting the patient to the receiving medical facility.

Postevent or Follow-Up

The work does not end after the patient has been transported to the hospital. After the event, key personnel who were not present will need to be notified. This may include administrators and mental health providers. Before an emergency happens (specifically, a catastrophic event), you should identify local resources that are available to assist with the mental health care of the people involved in the situation and the teammates, friends, and family of the patient.[25,26] EMS agencies work with critical incident stress management teams to debrief personnel involved with catastrophic incidents and other potentially stressful calls.[27] You should be included in those debriefings when possible. Another resource is ATs Care, a peer-to-peer support program provided thought the NATA, offering education, training, and support after a critical incident.[28] Mental health care of athletic trainers and other members of the sports medicine team should not be overlooked.

After patient care has been completed and the situation has been wrapped up, incident reports and other documentation must be completed. The incident report should include all the details of the situation, including patient information, the care provided and by whom, the timeline of the incident, the equipment sent to the hospital, and so on. A standard athletic training SOAP note will also need to be completed for the patient's medical records. At a later date, key stakeholders in the incident should debrief about the situation and update the EAP if needed. Many lessons can be learned after an incident that can help improve the EAP for future incidents.

Special Considerations

Whenever possible, you should prepare for all possible emergencies at your institution, including catastrophic injuries or trauma, medical emergencies, weather-related emergencies, and psychological emergencies. Depending on where you are working, the structure of the organization, sports offered, and other variables, you should consider additional situations when planning for emergencies. This section details considerations for protective equipment removal, emergencies involving nonathletes, championships and other large events, and emergency planning in nontraditional settings.

Protective Equipment Removal

Depending on the sports offered by the institution, emergency removal of protective equipment will likely be part of the EAP. Equipment must be removed when a patient has a potential head or spine injury or requires CPR.[12,29,34] It also needs to be completed prior to or during emergency cooling of a patient with heat stroke.[21,30] All protective equipment (e.g., helmet, face mask, and shoulder pads) should be removed prior to transport to the hospital if there are an adequate number of trained providers on scene.[18,34,35] This change allows for improved patient care on the field and during transport. It also allows for those most familiar with the workings of the protective equipment to do the actual removal.[18] At minimum, the patient's facemask should be removed prior to transport.[34,35] Athletic trainers and other stakeholders (e.g., EMS personnel) who will be involved with equipment removal need to practice these skills at least annually.[1,5,12,21,30-32,34,35] This is another opportunity for interprofessional trainings with EMS personnel and other members of the sports medicine team. The EAP should clearly outline when protective equipment should be removed, by whom, and how. The steps for removing various types of protective equipment, along with the tools needed for removal, are outlined in chapter 11.

Emergencies Involving Nonathletes

You should also be prepared to provide basic life support to nonathletes if the need arises. This could include coaches, officials, parents, and other spectators who develop an acute condition while attending an event the athletic trainer is covering. Although they are rare, you should also be prepared to assist in multivictim emergencies that may occur during an event you are covering (e.g., bleacher collapse, lightning strike). Knowing the basics of **triage** is an important step in being prepared for potential larger-scale emergencies. Work with your local EMS providers to learn the method of triage used by your agency (e.g., START, SALT) and be prepared to assist EMS if a **mass casualty incident** occurs. The EAP should outline how these situations are handled, since they are likely different from those involving an athlete (e.g., unknown medical history, attending alone, multiple patients).

Championships and Other Large-Scale Events

Athletic trainers hosting or attending large-scale events, such as conference championship events, should be aware of league or conference policies and procedures. Planning for these events goes beyond the typical athletic department EAP and must include heightened levels of security in case of acts of violence or terrorism. These types of events are typically planned months in advance in coordination with the host site staff, local police and EMS, and other stakeholders. The NCAA's website outlines the best practices for planning these types of events.[33] Although most athletic trainers will have a limited role in planning for these events unless they are hosting one at their facilities, they will have a role in the plan if something goes wrong.

EAPs for Nontraditional Settings

Athletic trainers working in nontraditional settings, including clinics, hospitals, and industrial settings, should be aware that they will have less of a decision-making role in creating their organization's EAP. In these settings, you will likely have a role within a preestablished plan for the larger organization. Also, the types of emergencies encountered in these settings can be very different than those that occur in the traditional athletic training setting because of the difference in patient population and activities.

FOUNDATIONAL SKILL

START Triage

Figure 13.3 shows the steps for when to start adult triage.

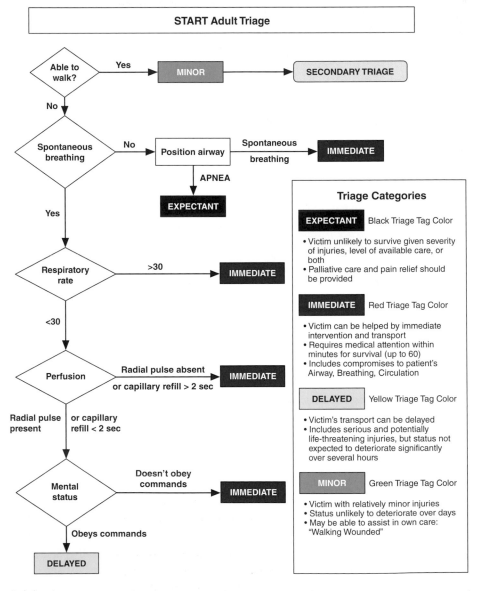

FIGURE 13.3   Adult triage.

Reprinted by permission from U.S. Department of Health & Human Services (2020). https://chemm.nlm.nih.gov/startadult.htm

CLINICAL BOTTOM LINE

- Emergency planning is one of the most important aspects of an athletic trainer's job.

- An institution's EAP should address the members of the sports medicine team and their roles during an emergency, the type and location of emergency medical equipment to be used, the communication plan, the transportation plan, maps of the venue or sites, and step-by-step instructions for different emergencies.

- An institution's EAP should address what to do in the event of catastrophic or trauma emergencies, medical emergencies, weather-related emergencies, and psychological emergencies.

- The development of an EAP is a team approach. The EAP should be carefully created and tested to ensure that all aspects of the plan are fully developed.

- An institution's EAP should be reviewed by the institution's administration and legal counsel, along with local EMS and hospital personnel.

- Athletic trainers should review and practice their institution's EAP at least annually with other key personnel listed in the EAP.

- Athletic trainers should review the NATA position statements and other relevant documents related to emergency planning and the care of acute conditions.

- Athletic trainers must stay up to date on changes to emergency planning, acute care guidelines, and evidence-based practice and integrate changes into the EAP as appropriate.

Go to HK*Propel* to complete the activities and case studies for this chapter.

Go to HK*Propel* to download a foundational skill check sheet for calling 911.

CHAPTER 14

Acute Care and Emergency Procedures

Ellen K. Payne, PhD, LAT, ATC, EMT
David C. Berry, PhD, MHA, AT, ATC

CAATE STANDARDS

The following CAATE 2020 standards are covered in this chapter:

Standard 59

Standard 61

Standard 62

Standard 69

Standard 70

Standard 75

Standard 92

CHAPTER OBJECTIVES

After reading this chapter, you will be able to do the following:

- Describe the steps in the primary assessment of an emergency and know when to intervene

- Explain the components of the secondary assessment for both traumatic and medical emergencies

- Identify various vital signs, how they are obtained, and what the clinical implications suggest

- Understand the importance of monitoring the patient, the ongoing assessment process, and emergency referral

- Describe various ways to safely move a patient during an emergency situation

- Understand various interventions used in the prehospital setting, including airway management, splinting, wound care and bleeding control, shock management, emergency cooling, and emergency medications

Opportunities for athletic trainers to demonstrate many of their acute care skills are infrequent, but the stakes are high when they are needed. Athletic trainers need to practice these lifesaving skills often so they are ready to perform them when the need arises. For example, many athletic trainers will never perform CPR on an actual patient during the course of their professional careers. However, if the need does arise in your work, you must be able to react and perform the skills as trained without thinking. Advanced airway management is another low-frequency skill in athletic training; however, it carries a potential of risk. If this skill is incorrectly performed, it could be detrimental to the outcome of the patient. Prepare to be the master of your own skills proficiency rather than waiting for the annual proficiency testing, if such a protocol exists at your institution. Because of the importance of these skills in the outcome of the patient, practice them frequently and become acquainted with your organization's emergency action plan (EAP).

Prior to reading this chapter, please review the following:

- Chapter 7 Blood-Borne Pathogens: provides information on protecting the athletic trainer from possible exposure to blood-borne pathogens and other potentially infectious materials.

- Chapter 13 Emergency Planning in Health Care: provides information on the basics of emergency planning in traditional athletic training settings.
- Chapter 16 Clinical Diagnosis and Medical Referral: details the complete assessment process along with variations for different settings, including concussion assessment, pertinent clinical prediction rules, and documentation and communication.

This chapter focuses on the assessment of emergent injuries or medical conditions and the prehospital care of seriously injured or ill patients. This text purposely avoids the term "on-the-field assessment" because emergency situations can happen anywhere: in an athletic training clinic, workplace, locker room, or classroom, as well as on the field or court. No matter the location, athletic trainers need to be prepared to respond, assess the situation and the patient, and act accordingly. The goal of this chapter is to present the principles of the emergency assessment process and outline action steps for sizing up the scene and performing a primary assessment, secondary assessment, and ongoing assessment. Various prehospital interventions are introduced, including airway management, splinting, wound care and bleeding control, shock management, emergency cooling, and emergency medications. For a more in-depth look at prehospital intervention for athletic trainers, please refer to *Acute and Emergency Care in Athletic Training*.[1]

Principles of Emergency Assessment

The emergency assessment of a potentially critically injured or ill patient varies from the assessment completed in the athletic training clinic. In this text, the emergency assessment is divided into 4 parts:

1. Scene size-up
2. Primary assessment
3. Secondary assessment
4. Continued patient monitoring (ongoing assessment)

These components are further divided to allow the athletic trainer to perform a rapid and systematic assessment of the patient.

Scene Size-Up

Scene size-up is the first thing an athletic trainer, or any emergency responder, must do during an emergency situation; she assesses the situation and determines if the scene is safe to respond. Although most

situations an athletic trainer finds herself in are not dangerous (unlike a fire or an active shooter), the scene still needs to be assessed. Safety includes the following:

1. Ensuring your own personal safety and the safety of others, including other rescuers, bystanders, and patients (in that order)
2. Determining the mechanism of injury or nature of the illness
3. Identifying the number of patients
4. Determining what additional resources are needed (e.g., equipment, extra help)

Evaluating scene safety on an athletic field may be as simple as making sure play has stopped and the athletic trainer has been officially called onto the field. During a road race, it may mean stopping vehicle traffic. In the athletic training clinic, it may mean moving away from or stabilizing a piece of equipment. No matter the event you are providing coverage for, you need to make sure the scene is safe before approaching the patient so that you will not become injured as well. This can be accomplished with a 360-assessment, which requires you to be aware of the surroundings 360 degrees around you. This awareness is useful all of the time, not just during the situation at hand.

Ensure your own safety and the safety of others during the assessment and treatment of the patient by doing the following:

Personal Safety (Note the Following)
- Location of the emergency
- Extent of the emergency
- Apparent scene dangers
- Apparent number of injured or ill patients
- Behavior of the patients and any bystanders

Personal and Bystander Safety
- Thoroughly evaluate the scene.
- Use **personal protective equipment (PPE)** appropriate to the situation (see chapter 7 for a complete review of PPE).
- Change gloves between patients if caring for multiple patients.
- Do not attempt to do anything that you are not trained to do.
- Communicate effectively and appropriately to secure additional personnel and community resources.
- Frequently wash your hands or use hand sanitizers to reduce the spread of germs.

Safety of Others

- Never move a critical patient unless there is an immediate danger.
- Continue to scan the area for possible dangers while approaching the patient.
- Use appropriate emergency moves if the patient is in immediate danger.
- Look for others who may be in potential danger or interfering with the care of the patient (i.e., teammates) and have them move to safety.
- If the scene is safe and additional assistance is needed, enlist the aid of bystanders (i.e., coaches).

Next, you will determine the possible **mechanism of injury (MOI)** or **nature of illness (NOI)** and the number of patients injured. The MOI refers to the method by which damage (trauma) to skin, muscles, organs, and bones happens and helps determine how likely it is that a serious injury has occurred. Some examples of MOI are the following:

- Impact, blunt, or penetrating injuries
- Rotational, acceleration, or deceleration injuries
- Falls from a significant height
- Contact with equipment, balls, or the ground

The NOI describes the medical condition that resulted in the need for emergency medical care. Examples include fever, difficulty breathing, chest pain, headache, and vomiting. Scan the scene for clues to the NOI. Observing the patient can tell you a great deal about the situation:

- Presence of a metered-dose inhaler, epinephrine autoinjector, partially eaten sandwich, or insulin
- Medical alert bracelet or necklace (figure 14.1)
- Strong smell emanating from the patient

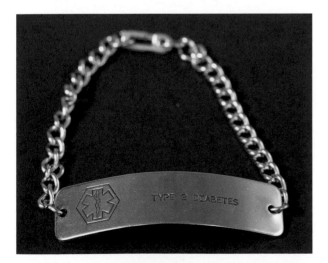

FIGURE 14.1   An example of a medical alert bracelet.

Conscious patients may be able to describe their symptoms, yet in some situations, there may be no evidence of trauma. Coaches, teammates, bystanders, or family members may provide additional information. Recognizing the MOI or NOI and the number of patients injured will help you plan the steps for providing immediate care and securing additional resources.

After determining the number of patients and the MOI or NOI, you should call 911 and activate the EAP, as discussed in chapter 13. This is also the time to identify the need for other additional resources (e.g., ambulance or rescue squad, fire department, or law enforcement). Of course, if the need for additional resources arises later in the assessment or during patient care, do not hesitate to call for additional help.

After you have assessed the scene and deemed it safe, take the proper precautions against blood-borne pathogens (use of PPEs), as addressed in chapter 7. This important step should never be overlooked when providing care for patients. At this time, if the patient is conscious, you should obtain consent prior to helping him. If the patient is unconscious, consent is implied.

Primary Assessment

The ability to properly assess a patient is one of the most important skills an athletic trainer can master. To work efficiently, you must approach patient assessments systematically to evaluate and manage patients with acute conditions, including **triaging** conditions that are life threatening or otherwise urgent. The emergency care provided to the patient will be based on assessment findings. The purpose of the primary assessment is to identify and treat any life-threatening conditions. It allows you to discover the signs and symptoms of immediate threats to life (i.e., compromised airway, breathing, cardiac function, and severe bleeding).

The primary assessment is divided into the following steps (figure 14.2):

1. General impression
2. Assessing level of consciousness
3. Assessing the ABCs

Be aware that it may be necessary to expose pertinent areas of the patient's body for examination. Factors to consider when exposing the patient include the following: (1) type of athletic equipment, if applicable, (2) protecting the patient's modesty, (3) presence of teammates, coaches, and bystanders, and (4) environment or weather conditions.

General Impression

A general impression is an across-the-room assessment. As you approach the patient, you will form a general

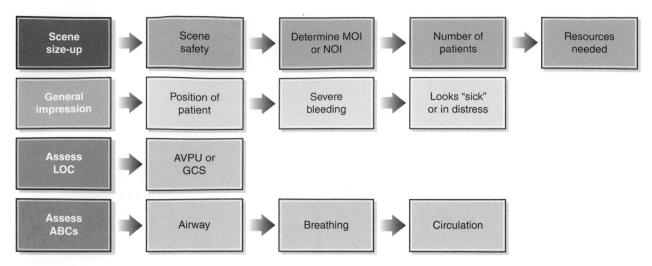

FIGURE 14.2 Steps to the scene size-up and primary assessment.

impression before he tells you his complaint. You can form a general impression in 60 seconds or less. The purpose of forming a general impression is to note serious problems, such as severe, life-threatening bleeding that requires additional resources, or minor problems that can be treated easily and added to the patient's oral history. The general impression allows you to further decide if the patient looks sick or in distress as opposed to his normal self. If the patient looks sick or in distress, you must act quickly. As you gain experience, you will develop an instinct for quickly recognizing when a patient is sick or injured.

Assessing Level of Consciousness

The next step in the primary assessment is determining the patient's level of consciousness (LOC). Assessing a patient's airway and determining LOC often occur at the same time. Level of consciousness is also called level of responsiveness or mental status. **Altered mental status (AMS)** suggests a change in a patient's level of awareness. A patient's mental status can be graded using several different scales, but the most common is the **AVPU scale**:

- A = alert (e.g., patient can answer questions and respond to commands)
  - Alert and oriented (A patient who can answer appropriately to questions about person, place, time, and event said to be "alert and oriented times 4," or "A and O times 4")
  - Alert and disoriented
- V = verbal (e.g., patient will squeeze the athletic trainer's hand or respond to other requests)
- P = painful (e.g., patient reacts to painful stimuli such as pinching the inner arm or a sternal rub)
- U = unresponsive (e.g., patient does not respond to any stimuli)

EMS use the **Glasgow Coma Scale (GCS)** during the primary survey to obtain a more detailed assessment of the patient's neurological status (table 14.1). This miniature neurological examination is used to establish a baseline level of responsiveness and note any obvious problem with central nervous system function.

The GCS score can be indicative of illness or injury severity:

- A score of 3 represents coma or death.
- A score of 8 or less indicates severe head injury.
- A score of 9 to 12 indicates moderate head injury.
- A score of 13 to 15 indicates mild head injury.

TABLE 14.1 The Glasgow Coma Scale (GCS)

Eye opening	Spontaneous	4
	To sound	3
	To pressure	2
	None	1
Verbal response	Oriented	5
	Confused	4
	Words	3
	Sounds	2
	None	1
Motor response	Obey commands	6
	Localizing	5
	Normal flexion	4
	Abnormal flexion	3
	Extension	2
	None	1

Forming a General Impression

Many conditions warrant activating the EAP and summoning emergency medical services (EMS):

- Severe, life-threatening bleeding
- Respiratory distress (e.g., **anaphylaxis**) or arrest
- Cardiac distress or prolonged chest pain
- Seizures
- Suspected head, neck, or spinal injuries

Assess for immediate life-threatening conditions by determining whether the patient:

- Is conscious
- Has an open and clear airway
- Is breathing
- Has a pulse

Observe and listen for signs and symptoms:

- Signs are evidence of injury or illness that are observed (e.g., bleeding, open wounds, deformity, body positioning [**decerebrate** versus **decorticate**; see figure 14.3]).
- Patient experience (e.g., pain, nausea, headache, **dyspnea**).

Decorticate Positioning

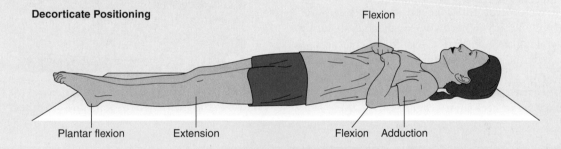

Flexion

Plantar flexion   Extension   Flexion   Adduction

Decerebrate Positioning

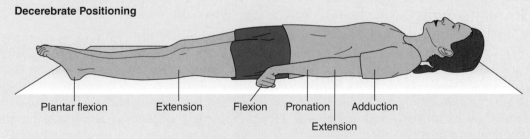

Plantar flexion   Extension   Flexion   Pronation   Adduction
Extension

FIGURE 14.3   Decerebrate and decorticate body positioning.

During this time, scan for and immediately control severe, life-threatening bleeding with any available resources if it is safe to do so. You may delegate the responsibility to another responder in order to begin the primary assessment. If severe bleeding is present, apply a tourniquet or pressure bandage per the institution's EAP.

Determine if spinal precautions are necessary based on your general impression and likely MOI.

A declining GCS is concerning in any setting and should prompt reassessment of the patient and possible airway intervention. Although a GCS of 15 is known as "fully awake," it does not mean that a patient is healthy or uninjured; she may still be critically ill or injured. Critical decision making based on the clinical presentation is necessary to ensure aggressive and proper management of the patient.[2]

If the patient is conscious, you can determine mental status by establishing her orientation to person, place, time, and event. Obtain consent prior to helping the patient if you have not already done so. Additionally, for trauma patients or unresponsive patients with an unknown MOI or NOI, be sure to take spinal precautions. **Spinal motion restriction (SMR)** is necessary to minimize movement that could cause injury to the spinal cord. Never use smelling salts to arouse an unconscious patient (see the following sidebar).

Assessing the ABCs

After determining the patient's LOC, assess the patient's airway (A), breathing (B), and circulation (C), or ABCs. Although the ABCs are taught in basic first aid and life support courses, different organizations recommend variations to the process. First, quickly scan the patient for severe bleeding, if you have not already done so during the general impression. Next, assess the patient's airway. If he is conscious and talking, then his airway is open and clear. If not, open the airway, using either the **head-tilt/chin-lift maneuver** or a **jaw-thrust technique** if you suspect a head or neck injury (figure 14.4).

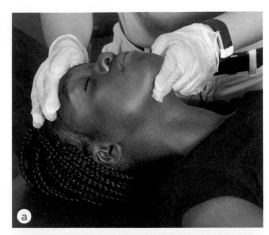
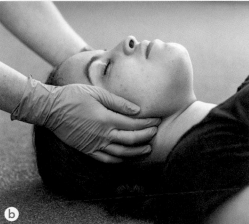

FIGURE 14.4   Opening the patient's airway via (a) the head-tilt/chin-lift maneuver or (b) jaw-thrust technique.

EVIDENCE-BASED ATHLETIC TRAINING

Smelling Salts

Smelling salts are a preparation of ammonium carbonate ($(NH_4)_2CO_3H_2O$) and perfume that were traditionally sniffed as a stimulant to relieve faintness. Although smelling salts have experienced a resurgence in popularity among athletes as a pregame stimulant or a pick-me-up when performance is lacking, little is really known or understood about these agents. Unfortunately, some people and organizations are still recommending the use of smelling salts to revive injured patients. However, current evidence-based research and recommendations categorically state that smelling salts are contraindicated because they cause a withdrawal reaction that has the potential to cause or exacerbate a spinal injury. Although there are numerous case reports of their toxicity when ingested in large doses or inhaled in high concentration for prolonged periods, there are no reports of complications related to the use of smelling salts in sport. The real danger in using smelling salts for sport-related concussions is the potential for a lack of careful and complete neurological assessment. Serious head injuries often present in the early stages as less serious than they really are, and an initial improvement, thought to be due to the beneficial effects of smelling salts, may mask the development of a more serious condition, particularly if the practitioner is inexperienced. In the sports setting, the real danger is that the ill-advised use of smelling salts may delay a thorough assessment and appropriate treatment.[3]

EVIDENCE-BASED ATHLETIC TRAINING

Acute Care Skill Retention

Regular rehearsal and practice of acute care clinical skills is necessary in order to maintain proficiency in these critical areas. Popp and Berry[7] evaluated retention of airway management knowledge and skills, specifically oropharyngeal airway (OPA) and nasopharyngeal airway (NPA) use, in athletic training students. The study provides evidence that skill decay occurs in clinical skills associated with the acute care competencies, specifically airway adjunct devices. However, the study also showed that knowledge might not decay as rapidly as skill. Therefore, athletic training programs should provide students with opportunities to practice these competencies to maintain their clinical skills, especially because these skills are not frequently used in the clinical setting.

If you find fluid in the airway, immediately clear the airway (i.e., with a manual finger sweep or suction) and insert either a basic airway device or an advanced airway per the institution's standing protocol for airway management. After opening the airway, assess the patient's breathing (table 14.2). Look for no breathing or only gasping and simultaneously check the patient's carotid pulse. If the patient is not breathing, perform ventilation with a bag valve mask (BVM) or pocket mask. If the patient is breathing inadequately, this may need to be addressed at this time by providing oxygen or some form of ventilatory support. In an unconscious adult, you may detect isolated or infrequent gasping (**agonal breathing**), which can occur after the heart has stopped beating. Agonal breathing is an abnormal pattern of breathing and

brainstem reflex characterized by gasping and labored breathing that is accompanied by strange vocalizations and **myoclonus**. If agonal breathing occurs, care for the patient as if he is not breathing at all and begin CPR.[4]

The last step (however, note that breathing and circulation are often assessed simultaneously) in the ABCs is assessing the patient's pulse.[4] Can you definitely feel the pulse within 10 seconds? (Assess for at least 5 seconds, but not for more than 10 seconds.) This is typically done at the carotid artery for unconscious or critical patients (adults and children) or at the radial artery for less critical patients. If the patient does not have a pulse, initiate CPR as the AED is prepared (an AED should be readily available within 3 minutes for all athletic venues).[5,6] As part of this step, you should assess skin color, temperature, condition, and **capillary refill** as you look for signs of significant external bleeding and the resulting beginning stages of **shock**.

Timing of Primary Assessment

The primary assessment should be completed in approximately 2 minutes or less, depending on the interventions preformed, but it is important to address any significant findings during the ABCs. If there are any deficits to the ABCs, activate the EAP and call EMS. See figure 14.5

TABLE 14.2 Breathing Rates

	Normal	Abnormal
Adult	12 to 20 breaths per minute	<8 or >20 breaths per minute
Child	15 to 30 breaths per minute	<10 or >30 breaths per minute
Infant	25 to 50 breaths per minute	<20 or >60 breaths per minute

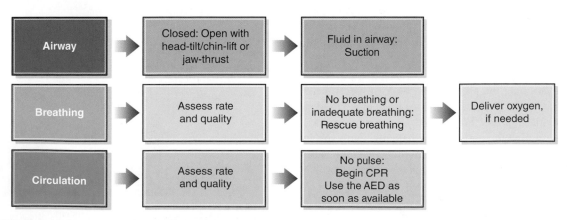

FIGURE 14.5 Primary assessment flowchart.

for a flowchart of the primary assessment. If the patient's condition is not life threatening, you should continue on to the secondary assessment after completing the primary assessment and managing any pertinent issues. Finally, determine if the patient requires on-scene stabilization or immediate transport (load-and-go situations) with additional emergency care en route to a hospital.

Secondary Assessment

After you have completed the primary assessment and addressed any deficiencies to the ABCs, you should move on to the secondary assessment if the patient is not already en route to the hospital with EMS. If you have not yet obtained consent from the patient, do so prior to starting the secondary survey. The goal of this assessment is to identify any conditions or injuries that you may not have identified during the primary assessment and to dive deeper into the patient's condition. The secondary survey depends on the patient, situation, and time available. For instance, a patient with an isolated injury, such as a painful ankle, would typically not require a head-to-toe physical examination. The procedure for performing a secondary survey is the same for trauma and medical patients. However, the physical findings may have a different meaning depending on whether the patient is a trauma or medical patient. The secondary assessment can include a physical examination (head to toe or focused), assessment of vital signs, assessment of the **chief complaints**, and SAMPLE history:

S = signs and symptoms

A = allergies

M = medications

P = past pertinent history

L = last meal

E = events leading up to this incident

If you identify any life-threatening or serious conditions during the secondary assessment, activate the EAP.

The exact order of secondary assessment varies depending on whether the patient is conscious or unconscious or has a medical- or trauma-related emergency.

Physical Examination

When examining the patient, first look (inspect), listen (auscultate), and then feel (palpate) body areas to identify potential injuries. For a rapid assessment, you will need to examine the patient systematically, with special emphasis on areas suggested by the chief complaint, when provided. Here is the order in which the rapid assessment should be conducted:

1. Head and Face

- Palpate for depression and soft areas.

- Inspect for blood or clear fluid from the ears, nose, or mouth; discoloration around the eyes; or vomit.
- Clear fluid, called **cerebrospinal fluid (CSF)**, may indicate brain damage or skull fracture. Do not attempt to stop the drainage. Rather, apply dressings to absorb the fluid and slow down the bleeding. Stopping the drainage may increase the pressure within the skull and cause an increase in intracranial pressure, further damaging the brain.

2. Neck

- Palpate for step deformities of the cervical spine.
- Consider applying a cervical collar and evaluate the need for SMR.
- Examine the anterior neck for deformity of the trachea and **jugular vein distention** (figure 14.6).

3. Clavicle and Shoulders

- Palpate for pain, tenderness, and deformity.

4. Chest

- Expose the chest and inspect the chest wall anteriorly and laterally, feeling for crepitus, deformities, tenderness, movement, and any asymmetries.
- Auscultate (midclavicular and lateral) the lungs bilaterally.
- Palpate the sternum and ribs for pain, tenderness, and deformity.

5. Abdomen

- Expose the abdomen and inspect the area for discoloration and bleeding.
- Gently palpate the quadrants (using the umbilicus as a reference guide, divide the abdomen into

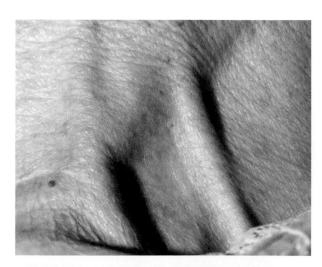

FIGURE 14.6 Jugular vein distension.
Dr P. Marazzi / Science Source

four quadrants: upper, lower, left, and right). The abdomen should be soft and nondistended.

- Guarding of the abdomen and rebound tenderness could indicate internal bleeding or significant abdominal trauma.

6. Pelvis and Hips

- Inspect for deformity and discoloration.
- Palpate for physical signs of injury.
- Compress the iliac crest to assess for instability and reaction to pain.[8]
- If a pelvic fracture is suspected, be sure to avoid excessive movement.

7. Extremities

- Start on one side of the body (either left or right) and examine the left arm, then the right. Follow the same procedures for the lower extremity.
- Palpate beginning at the proximal end (at the shoulder for the upper extremity and inguinal area for the lower extremity).
- Once at the distal end, assess circulation, movement, and sensation (CMS).
- Locate the radial and pedal arteries to assess for a pulse bilaterally.
- Palpate for bilateral sensation within the upper and lower extremities and assess for movement of the fingers and toes.

8. Back

- Palpate along the accessible spine when the patient is supine.
- Palpate and observe the whole spine when log-rolling the patient.
- Assess for tenderness and pain.

While performing the physical exam, compare each body part on one side of the body to the corresponding body part on the other side. A helpful memory aid for remembering what to look and feel for during the physical exam is DCAP-BTLS:

D = deformities and discoloration

C = contusions

A = abrasions and avulsions

P = penetrations and punctures

B = burns

T = tenderness and temperature

L = lacerations

S = swelling and symmetry

You may also conduct a more detailed physical exam once you have completed the focused history and initial physical exam and applied interventions. However, this exam is not carried out on every patient. The detailed physical exam is a more systematic head-to-toe exam that helps the practitioner acquire information about injuries or conditions that may need additional care. It also involves inspection, auscultation, and palpation, but you can spend more time gathering and processing the findings. Avoid touching any painful areas or having the patient move an area that causes discomfort.

Patients with an acute trauma are usually easier to assess and manage. The athletic trainer, who possibly witnessed the event, will do a thorough assessment and then manage the injury with or without the assistance of EMS.

Specifics of the Medical Assessment

Medical conditions pose additional challenges for many athletic trainers, especially if they are not familiar with the patient's medical history or did not witness the event. Signs and symptoms of a medical condition may not be as specific as a trauma; the patient may simply feel sick or may be unconscious and unable to provide any information. Many different medical conditions can occur in the traditional athletic training setting, but a few of the more common medical emergencies you may have to handle include the following:

- Stroke
- Diabetic emergencies
- Asthma
- Severe allergic reactions
- Drug overdose
- Heat illnesses
- Syncope
- Cardiac distress
- Respiratory distress

If a patient is sick or suffering from a potential medical condition, your secondary assessment may focus on a medical assessment as opposed to a physical examination. A medical assessment involves an evaluation of the chief complaint, vital signs, and SAMPLE history. The physical examination (head to toe or focused) may be less of a priority depending on how the patient presents. The mnemonic OPQRST can be used here to assess the patient's pain and other symptoms:

O = onset

P = provocation or palliation

Q = quality

R = region or radiation

S = severity

T = time (history)

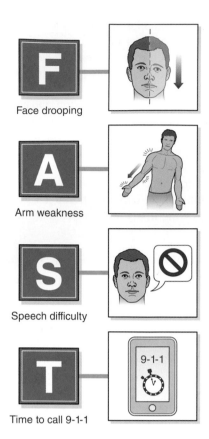

FIGURE 14.7 FAST stroke assessment.

If a patient is unconscious, you can obtain information from family members, coaches, teammates, and bystanders. Complete a head-to-toe survey on all unconscious patients; this may be also warranted on a conscious patient depending on how he presents and the time available. Some medical conditions, like a stroke, have special assessment tools (figure 14.7). Additional information about specific conditions are found in chapters 15 and 18.

Vital Signs

An important aspect of the secondary assessment is obtaining baseline vital signs. Vital signs are measurements of the body's most basic functions. Once obtained, they are used to help determine the patient's condition and, after the medical interventions and care have been given, whether the patient is improving or deteriorating. You should take two or more sets of vital signs so that you can note changes (trends) in the patient's condition and her response to any interventions. Reassess and record vital signs at least every 5 minutes in an unstable patient and at least every 10-15 minutes in a stable patient, both before and after any interventions.[8] Note any changes to the vital signs. If the patient is deteriorating, emergency transport may be warranted.

The following four main vital signs are routinely monitored by athletic trainers in the prehospital setting:

1. Pulse
2. Respiration
3. Temperature
4. Blood pressure

In addition, athletic trainers often assess skin condition, capillary refill, pupil reaction, pulse oximetry, and blood glucose levels while taking the patient's vital signs. These vital signs are also addressed in this section.

Pulse Pulse assessment includes checking for the rate, quality, and rhythm. Pulse rate is a measurement of the heart rate, or the number of times the heart beats per minute. As the heart pushes blood through the arteries, the arteries expand and contract with the flow of the blood. Assessment of the pulse rate requires the identification of pulse points. Pulse points are areas where the major arteries travel close to the skin's surface and lie directly over a bone, allowing for easier palpation of the pressure wave created by the heartbeat. The following are common pulse point sites (figure 14.8):

Upper Extremity

- Radial
- Brachial

Lower Extremity

- Femoral
- Popliteal
- Posterior tibial
- Dorsalis pedis

To determine pulse rate, record the number of beats for 15, 30, or 60 seconds. At the end of the counting interval, multiply the number of heartbeats by 4, 2, or 1, respectively. In adults, the normal pulse rate is between 60 and 100 bpm (beats per minute; table 14.3). The pulse rate may fluctuate and increase with medications, exercise, illness, injury, and emotions. People who participate in regular vigorous or strenuous physical activity will normally present with markedly lower pulse rates at rest due to the morphological, functional, and electrophysiological changes in cardiac structure and function that result from training. Known as the athletic heart syndrome, the patient may present with bradycardia and pulse rates ranging from 35 to 50 bpm.[9,10] **Bradycardia** is a heart rate less than 60 bpm while **tachycardia** is a heart rate greater than 100 bpm.

Checking a pulse also allows the athletic trainer to assess the quality of the pulse.

- *Rhythm:* examines the evenness of the pulse; can be either regular or irregular.
  - In a regular pulse, the interval between each contraction of the heart's ventricle remains constant.

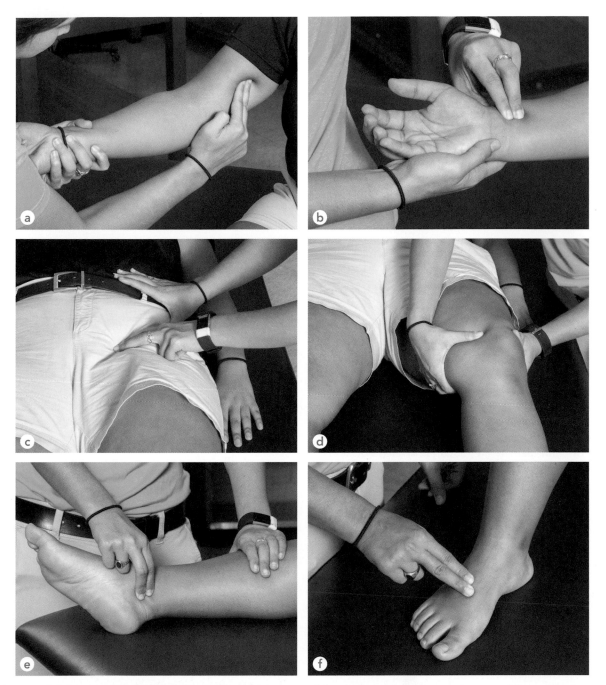

FIGURE 14.8 Common pulse points: *(a)* brachial artery, *(b)* radial artery, *(c)* femoral artery, *(d)* popliteal artery, *(e)* posterior tibial artery, and *(f)* dorsalis pedis artery.

- In an irregular pulse, the beats are unsteady or uneven. An irregular pulse and signs and symptoms of a cardiovascular disorder require immediate referral to advanced medical care.
- *Quality:* examines the force of the pulse as the blood moves into the artery during a heartbeat.
  - Normally regular or strong
  - An abnormal finding is a pulse that is either bounding, weak (e.g., **thready pulse**), or absent.

When quality and rhythm are paired, the athletic trainer may recognize a pulse that is one of the following:

- Rapid and strong, resulting from early stages of shock, overexertion, fright, anxiety, heat illness, diabetic emergency (e.g., **hyperglycemia**), or fever
- Rapid and weak, resulting from internal bleeding, later stages of shock, heat illness, diabetic emergency (e.g., **hypoglycemia**), or a failing circulatory system

TABLE 14.3 **Normative Values for Pulse and Respiratory Rate by Age Group**

Age (in years)	Pulse range	Respiratory range
Birth to 1	120-160	25-50
1-3	80-130	20-30
4-5	80-120	20-30
6-12	70-110	20-30
13-18	55-105	12-20
19-40	60-100	12-20
41-60	70-100	16-20
>60	Based on health status	Based on health status

- Slow and strong, resulting from a stroke, skull fracture, or brain trauma
- Absent pulse, normally suggesting cardiac arrest

Respiration When assessing respiration, check for both the rate and quality. Respiration rate is the number of breaths a patient takes and is measured by counting the number of breaths for 1 minute by noting how many times the chest rises. When checking respiration, you should also note whether the patient has any difficulty breathing.

Respirations can be measured by visual inspection, palpation, or listening to lung sounds. In a responsive adult or child, palpate the radial pulse and relocate the patient's arm up to the lower rib cage, near the xiphoid process (figure 14.9). This position works well because you can feel each breath cycle (rise in the chest and belly) and the patient will typically remain unaware of what is occurring.

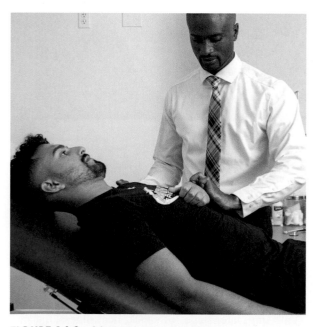

FIGURE 14.9 Measuring respirations.

In adults, the normal respiratory rate is between 12 and 20 breaths per minute (see table 14.3). Factors affecting respiration rate include age, physical conditioning, degree of exercise recently completed, history of illness and medical conditions, rise in body temperature, and fear or anxiety.

Assessing respiration not only measures rate of breathing, but also can indicate the following qualities of respiration:

- *Rhythm.* Here, you will examine the evenness of the breaths. Rhythm can be either regular or irregular.
  - In a regular respiratory rate, the interval between each breath (inhalation and exhalation) remains constant.
  - In an irregular respiratory pattern, each breath (inhalation and exhalation) may be unsteady or uneven.

    In a responsive patient, rhythm will be affected by such things as speech (i.e., talking), movement, and anxiety; therefore, this measure may not be entirely reliable.

- *Depth.* This is assessed by observing the degree of movement in the chest wall. It indicates the amount of air inhaled or exhaled during breathing. Depth is generally described as normal, deep, or shallow.
  - Normal inspiration and expiration, or the volume of air exchanged with each breath in an adult, is approximately 500 mL of air (i.e., tidal volume).
  - Deep respirations occur when large volumes of air are inhaled and exhaled with full lung expansion. Deep breathing can occur in patients with a fever, heat illness, anxiety, allergies, or other medical conditions or illnesses.
  - Shallow respirations occur when small volumes of air are inhaled and exhaled, often with

minimal use of the lungs. Shallow respirations can occur in patients with anxiety, asthma, infection, brain injury, or other conditions or illnesses.

- *Effort.* Normal respiratory ventilation should be effortless, with normal, symmetrical expansion of the chest with each inspiration. Respiratory effort can be broken down into three categories:

  - *Normal.* The patient can speak and carry on a conversation without pausing and presents with normal or average, equal movements of the chest without the use of accessory muscles (e.g., the sternocleidomastoid and scalenes).

  - *Labored.* This constitutes a medical emergency, often resulting from airway obstructions, heart attack, chest trauma, lung disease, or other medical illnesses. The patient often presents with increased breathing effort, use of accessory muscles, nasal flaring, retractions, and noisy breathing.

  - *Noisy.* Noisy or abnormal breathing usually indicates the presence of a respiratory disorder or illness. Noisy breathing can be assessed with or without a stethoscope (auscultation), depending on the severity of the condition.

Temperature A person's normal body temperature can vary based on a number of factors, including recent activity, time of day, and food intake. A patient's temperature can also vary based on the method used to measure it.[11] In general, normal body temperature ranges from 97.8°F (36.5°C) to 99°F (37.2°C). Temperature at or above 100.4°F (38°C) is considered abnormal. You can quickly assess temperature while getting the general impression of the patient during the primary survey by touching the back of your (gloved) hand to the patient's forehead. Temperature should be assessed more thoroughly during the secondary assessment. Temperature can be assessed by the following means:

- Oral
- Rectal
- Axillary
- Tympanic
- Temporal

The method you select to measure temperature depends on the patient and how she presents. In most medical situations (i.e., suspected fever), you will assess the patient's temperature via the oral, tympanic, or temporal methods, depending on the type of thermometer available. Fever can be caused by a variety of conditions, most commonly infection (either viral or bacterial). Fever alone is rarely a medical emergency, but when presented in conjunction with other signs and symptoms, it could indicate something more serious.

For suspected exertional heat stroke and hypothermia, rectal temperature is the clinical gold standard for assessing core temperature.[12-15] Other methods are not valid or reliable in these situations. For the most valid estimate of core temperature, use a flexible rectal thermistor and insert it 15 cm (6 in.) into the rectum.[16]

Blood Pressure Blood pressure is a measurement of the amount of pressure exerted against the arterial walls, both during contraction of the heart (**systolic**) and relaxation (**diastolic**). Taking blood pressure requires the use of a sphygmomanometer (blood pressure cuff; figure 14.10) and a stethoscope, although blood pressure can be taken by palpation if there is no stethoscope available or it is too noisy to hear.

FOUNDATIONAL SKILL

Assessing Rectal Temperature

1. Follow standard precautions and wear PPE.
2. Prepare the thermistor with probe cover (if needed) and lubrication.
3. Drape the patient as appropriate.
4. Hold the thermistor at the premarked line (15 cm) with one hand.
5. Use the other hand to shift one gluteal cheek to the side.
6. Insert the thermistor to the premarked line (15 cm).
7. Position the cord and pull the patient's clothing back into position or drape appropriately.
8. Plug the thermistor into the thermometer receiver.
9. Do not remove the thermistor until the athlete recovers and his temperature returns to normal ranges. (The thermistor can be transported to the hospital.)
10. Wash your hands.

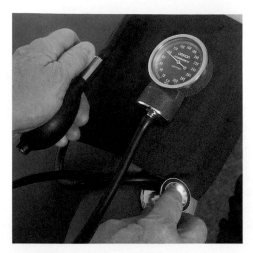

FIGURE 14.10 Sphygmomanometer.

Blood pressure can be affected by numerous factors:

- Sex
- Age
- Race
- Patient positioning
- Medications
- Stress
- Exercise
- Caffeine
- Dehydration
- Smoking
- Health status
- Decreased blood volume

FOUNDATIONAL SKILL

Steps to Assessing Blood Pressure

Blood Pressure Using a Stethoscope

1. Have the patient rest in a seated or supine position. (If she is seated, make sure the patient's legs are not crossed and her feet are flat on the floor.)
2. Locate the patient's brachial artery in the cubital fossa.
3. Place the (appropriately sized) blood cuff approximately 1 in. (2.5 cm) above the antecubital space.
4. The patient's arm should be supported at chest level with the palm facing up.
5. Place the stethoscope over the brachial artery.
6. Grasp the ball pump in your dominant hand and close the valve.
7. Inflate the blood pressure cuff to 20 to 30 mmHg above where you stop hearing a pulse.
8. Slowly release the pressure at the rate of approximately 2 to 3 mmHg per second.
9. The first sound heard is the systolic pressure.
10. The last sound heard is the diastolic pressure.
11. Record the patient's blood pressure as systolic/diastolic.

Blood Pressure by Palpation

1. Have the patient rest in a seated or supine position. (If he is seated, make sure the patient's legs are not crossed and his feet are flat on the floor.)
2. Place the (appropriately sized) blood cuff approximately 1 in. above the antecubital space.
3. The patient's arm should be supported at chest level with the palm facing up.
4. Using your nondominant hand, locate the patient's radial pulse on the same arm as the cuff. Once you have located the pulse, do not move your fingers until you complete taking the blood pressure.
5. Grasp the ball pump in your dominant hand and close the valve.
6. Inflate the blood pressure cuff to 20 to 30 mmHg above where you stop feeling a pulse.
7. Slowly release the pressure at the rate of approximately 2 to 3 mmHg per second.
8. When you feel the pulse again, that is the systolic pressure.
9. Release the remaining pressure in the cuff.
10. Record the patient's blood pressure as systolic/palpation.

TABLE 14.4 Normative Values for Blood Pressure by Age Group*

Age (in years)	Blood pressure range (systolic)
Birth to 1	70-90/50 mmHg
1-3	70-100/<80 mmHg
3-5	80-110/<80 mmHg
6-18	80-119/<80 mmHg
19-60	<120/80 mmHg
>60	Based on health status, optimal <120/80 mmHg

*Note – the blood pressure of females tends to be 8-10 mmHg less than males of the same age.

- Decreased capacity of the blood vessels
- Decreased ability of the heart to pump blood

A patient has **hypotension** when her blood pressure is lower than the normal range and **hypertension** when her blood pressure is higher than the normal range (table 14.4). Hypotension is common among athletes with lower heart rates. Hypotension-associated trauma, severe bleeding, the later stages of shock, or serious illness can be life threatening. Hypertension is commonly seen in older people and is associated with atherosclerosis, arteriolosclerosis, obesity, smoking, diabetes, a family history of hypertension, and other factors. In the emergency care setting, hypertension can be associated with heart attacks, strokes, head trauma, and emotional distress.

Skin Condition The patient's skin condition can provide you with valuable information on his status,

during both a trauma and medical emergency. Assessing the patient's skin condition provides information on circulation and **perfusion**. Skin condition includes color, temperature, and moisture. You should evaluate all three together because they are often related, especially in patients with hypoperfusion.

Skin color checks can be performed for all patients, regardless of skin pigmentation. For patients with darker pigmentation, skin color changes may be easier to assess in areas like the fingernail beds, palms of the hands, or mucous membranes in the mouth, among other areas. Skin color in these areas is normally pinkish due to the underlying oxygenated blood flow. Poor peripheral circulation will cause the skin to appear pale, ashen, or gray. The skin appears bluish when there is an inadequate air exchange and low oxygen levels; this condition is called **cyanosis**. Flushed or red skin can indicate high blood pressure, fever, carbon monoxide poisoning, sunburn, or other conditions where the body is unable to dissipate heat. **Jaundice**, or yellowing of the skin and sclera of the eyes, can be an indicator of liver disease.

Skin temperature is different than body temperature, discussed previously. Normal skin temperature is warm to the touch. Abnormal skin temperatures are hot, cool, cold, or clammy (cool and moist). Skin temperature can quickly be assessed by placing the back of a gloved hand on the patient's forehead. The patient's skin will feel hot to the touch if she has a significant fever, sunburn, or hyperthermia. The skin will feel cool if the patient has hypothermia, inadequate perfusion, or is in the early stage of shock. Cool, pale, clammy skin is a good indicator of shock. This occurs when the body shunts blood away from the extremities and skin in order to supply blood to

FOUNDATIONAL SKILL

Capillary Refill Assessment

1. Apply pressure to the patient's nail bed until it is blanched (figure 14.11).
2. Release the pressure.
3. Record the amount of time until the patient's nail bed returns to its normal color.

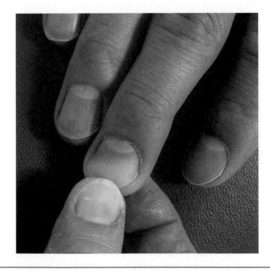

FIGURE 14.11 Capillary refill test.

the vital organs. The skin will feel cold is the patient is experiencing profound shock, hypothermia, or frostbite.

Lastly, skin is normally dry. Skin that is wet, moist, or excessively dry can indicate a problem. In the early stages of shock, the patient's skin will become moist (but not excessively sweaty) and could be described as clammy or damp. A patient with excessive sweating that is not due to exercise can be described as **diaphoretic**.

Capillary Refill   Like skin condition, capillary refill is also used to assess peripheral circulation in patients. Skin condition is more reliable and commonly used with pediatric patients than with adults.[8] As with other assessment techniques, capillary refill is just one tool in the athletic trainer's toolbox. It should be used with other signs and symptoms, like AMS and cyanosis, to help determine the proper intervention for a patient. Capillary refill is not a good assessment tool for respiratory function, but delayed or absent capillary refill can be indicative of conditions like hypovolemic shock or hypothermia, where the body is shunting the blood from the periphery to maintain the blood supply to vital organs. For example, in the athletic population, a patient whose MOI is a blow to the abdomen (e.g., as in football, ice hockey, or baseball) may present with an absent or delayed capillary refill. A delayed capillary refill, along with other signs and symptoms, could indicate internal bleeding (e.g., possible liver laceration). Capillary refill can be delayed because of other conditions like hypothermia and frostbite. Normal capillary refill time is less than 2 seconds, or the time it takes to say "capillary refill."

Pupil Reaction   The patient's pupil size and reaction should also be assessed. Pupils should be PEARRL (Pupils Equal And Round, Reactive to Light; many other similar acronyms are used). Both pupils should be the same size and shape and react the same way when exposed to light (using a pen light). Note any abnormal findings (figure 14.12) and whether they are unilateral or bilateral, such as the following:

- *Dilated pupil:* could be indicative of brain stem dysfunction, oculomotor nerve damage, shock, blood loss, or drug use
- *Constricted pupils:* could be indicative of disease, drug use, or brain stem dysfunction
- *Bilateral fixed pupils:* could be indicative of serious brain injury with a poor prognosis

Abnormal findings provide valuable information about the patient's status and possible cause of his condition.

Pulse Oximetry   Pulse oximetry is the estimate of peripheral oxygen saturation in the blood (SpO2; figure 14.13). Normal pulse oximetry is 95% to 100%, and anything under 95% is considered **hypoxic** (table 14.5). The

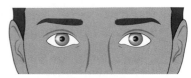

Normal pupils

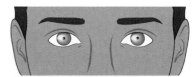

Constricted pupils

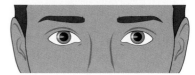

Dilated pupils

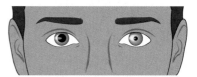

Unilateral dilated pupils

FIGURE 14.12   Examples of pupil reactions.

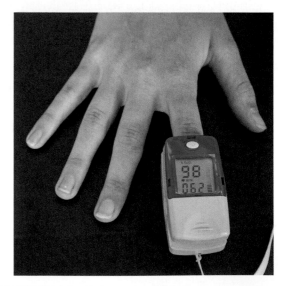

FIGURE 14.13   Pulse oximeter.

accuracy of the pulse oximetry reading can be affected by patient movement, dark nail polish, placement of the blood pressure cuff, vasoconstriction (e.g., hypothermia, shock), or loss of red blood cells (e.g., due to blood loss, anemia). Because of the potential for an inaccurate reading with a pulse oximeter, you should interpret the results with caution and use them as part of a compressive

TABLE 14.5 **Pulse Oximetry Values**

Normal	95% to 100%
Mild hypoxia	91% to 94%
Moderate hypoxia	86% to 90%
Severe hypoxia	<85%

patient assessment.[17] Pulse oximetry should not drive patient care. The device is useful for monitoring oxygen therapy, artificial ventilations, and other interventions. Most pulse oximeters also display the patient's heart rate.

Blood Glucometry Monitoring the blood glucose of any patient with an AMS, whether or not she is known to have diabetes, is important. You should assess blood glucose levels on patients who are known diabetics, unresponsive for unknown reasons, and complaining of **malaise** or generalized weakness. Perform an assessment

for any other patient for whom you form a poor general impression during your primary assessment. The information obtained can help you identify the reason a patient is unresponsive or has any change in mental status; both hypoglycemia and hyperglycemia can cause AMS. The normal range for blood sugar is 80 to 120 mg/dL.

Patient Monitoring and Ongoing Assessment

Ongoing assessment of the patient and his vital signs helps you determine if the patient is improving or deteriorating, especially after care has been provided. Reassess SAMPLE history, OPQRST, pain scale, and vital signs and additional measures as you wait for EMS to arrive or determine if you need to call EMS. You can repeat a head-to-toe or focused physical assessment of the patient if time allows or if the patient's condition requires it. Reassess vitals every 5 minutes for critical patients and every 10-15 minutes for stable patients.[8]

FOUNDATIONAL SKILL

Assessing Blood Glucose Level

1. Follow standard precautions and wear PPE.
2. Insert a new test strip into the meter, then clean the skin (typically the side of the finger) with an alcohol wipe.
3. Puncture the site with the lancet needle.
4. Dispose of the needle in the sharps container.
5. Wipe away the first drop of blood with gauze.
6. Obtain a drop of blood on the test strip (figure 14.14), per the manufacturer's instructions.
7. Obtain the reading and record it.
8. Place a bandage over the puncture site.

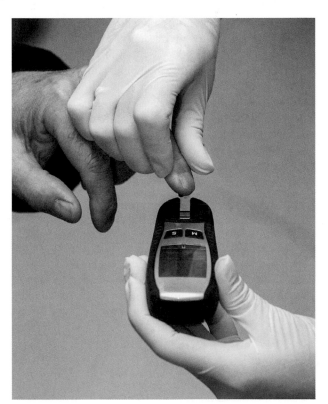

FIGURE 14.14 Measuring blood sugar.
picsfive - Fotolia

Patient Referral

For many situations discussed in this chapter (and many more not discussed), referral to advanced medical care begins with activating the site's EAP and calling for EMS assistance and transport. Depending on your local EMS protocols and the condition of the patient, that may mean either a basic life support (BLS) or advanced life support (ALS) ambulance. You do not get to determine which sort of ambulance responds when someone calls 911, but you should know the difference in the care each can provide (addressed in chapter 13). Activation of the EAP can occur immediately after the incident or later in the assessment if your findings warrant it. You may also activate the EAP if the patient's status begins to deteriorate or the patient does not respond to standard care, such as a patient with asthma not responding to a rescue inhaler. Depending on the findings of the secondary assessment, the patient may also simply need to go to urgent care or another sort of walk-in clinic (e.g., if the patient needs stitches or an X-ray). Many patients may just need a nonurgent follow-up with their personal physician or the team physician. For example, a patient who has asthma may need medication changes if he is having frequent asthma attacks with the current medication. Of course, not all patients who receive an emergency assessment will even need a referral; not everyone has to go to the hospital or see the doctor. The best course of action for the patient depends on the institution's policies and procedures and your judgment as the athletic trainer. Remember the adage "when in doubt, refer them out."

As addressed in chapter 11, protective equipment removal should be completed prior to transport via ambulance if adequately trained personnel are available and it can be done safely.[18,19] Emergency equipment removal is warranted when a patient has a potential head or spine injury or requires CPR.[20,21] The patient's face mask should always be removed prior to transport even if no other equipment is removed to allow for access to the airway should it become necessary during transport.[18] When possible, equipment should also be removed prior to or during emergency cooling of a patient with heat stroke.[13,22] Emergency equipment removal policies and steps should be outlined in the site-specific EAP.[5,13,18-20,23,24]

Moving and Transporting the Injured or Ill Patient

During both emergency and nonemergency situations, you may be required to move an injured or sick patient. You can use a variety of techniques to move a patient depending on her condition (e.g., conscious vs. unconscious, severity of injury), the equipment and amount of help available, and the distance or terrain that the patient is being moved. Critical patients should be moved only if absolutely necessary, such as if the scene is unsafe or the patient must be moved to provide the appropriate care. Noncritical patients should be moved or assisted out of the area in the safest way possible. When deciding to move a patient, consider the following:

- Can the patient be moved without causing harm?
- Should the patient be moved now?
- How many people do I need to help me safely move the patient?
- Can the patient walk (with or without assistance)?
- Does the patient require SMR or other precautions prior to being moved?

Here are some lifting and moving basics:

- Lift with your legs, not your back.
- Use a power grip (figure 14.15).
- Do not twist or jerk.
- Try not to reach.
- Try to minimize the number of times the patient is moved.
- Have a lifting and moving plan and coordinate every move in advance.
- Communicate with your patient.
- Communicate with your assistants and use clear instructions and a count before performing moves.
- Ask for help when needed.

You may be called on to move patients in a variety of situations and scenarios, so you should become familiar with the available resources and equipment prior to an actual emergency. Familiarity occurs by practicing the EAP. Depending on your work setting, you may need to move a patient from special situations like foam pits, trampolines, pole vault mats, and other equipment. Familiarize yourself with these potential hazards.

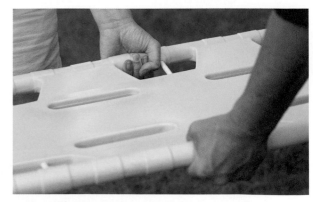

FIGURE 14.15 Power grip.

Lifts and Drags

Lifts and drags are typically used for moving patients over short distances and during emergent situations. They are not used for moves over longer distances. Figure 14.16 shows some of the many common lifts and drags used in prehospital care.

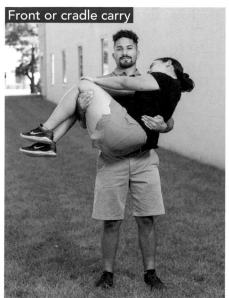

Front or cradle carry

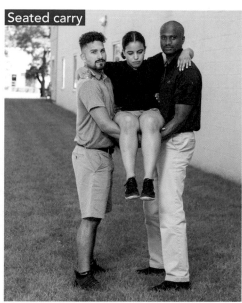

Seated carry

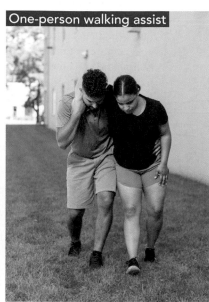

One-person walking assist

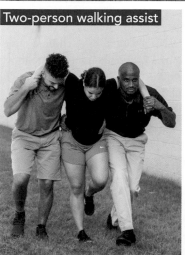

Two-person walking assist

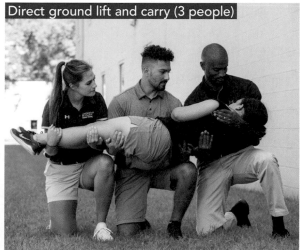

Direct ground lift and carry (3 people)

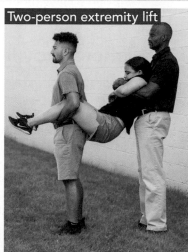

Two-person extremity lift

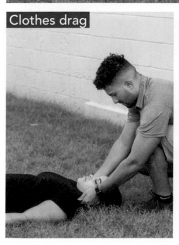

Clothes drag

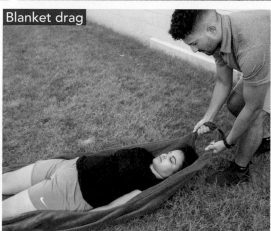

Blanket drag

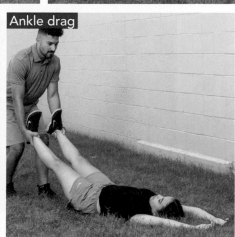

Ankle drag

FIGURES 14.16   Common lifts and drags.

Transporting a Patient

An injured or ill patient can be moved for short distances with one of the lifts or drag methods shown in figure 14.16. For longer distances, use equipment for easier patient transportation. These include the scoop stretcher, CombiCarrier II, long spine board, vacuum mattress, and ambulance stretcher. The equipment and method selected are determined based on the patient's injuries, equipment and amount of help available, and distance or terrain that the patient is being moved. Remember that the rule for moving patients in EMS is "don't carry what you can roll." If the patient can safely stay where he is until EMS arrives, the ambulance stretcher may be the easiest method that creates the least amount of movement of the patient.

Recovery Position

If you must leave an unconscious patient for any reason, place her in the recovery position to help maintain the airway. This position helps prevent **aspiration** if the patient vomits. This lateral, side-lying position is for an unresponsive patient who is breathing (does not require any interventions) with no suspected injury to spine or pelvis, including no major trauma (figure 14.17).

Emergency Interventions

Although the emergency interventions presented in this chapter are usually performed after the patient assessment is complete, you must be prepared to intervene earlier if the patient's condition warrants it. As discussed previously, for conditions such as severe bleeding, unopened airway, or cardiac arrest, stop the assessment and address the problem immediately. Other conditions, such as a potential fracture or dislocation, can be addressed after the secondary assessment is complete. This section provides an overview of some of the interventions you may have to use in an acute or emergency situation.

Emergency Cardiac Care

Although certifications for emergency cardiac care (ECC), including CPR and AED use, must be maintained by every athletic trainer, this chapter does not address the specific steps for providing CPR. The exact procedures and steps for performing CPR vary slightly by certifying organization and change periodically as new evidence is published related to prehospital cardiac care. All ECC-certifying organizations recognized by the Board of Certification (BOC) must adhere to the most current international guidelines for cardiopulmonary resuscitation and emergency cardiac care.[25]

In accordance with the BOC,[26] ECC certification must include the following:

- Adult CPR
- Pediatric CPR
- 2-rescuer CPR
- AED
- Airway obstruction
- Barrier devices (e.g., pocket mask, BVM)

Refer to your ECC-certifying agency for the steps to perform CPR, use an AED, perform rescue breaths, and clear an obstructed airway. Although most ECC certifications last 2 years, reviewing the cardiac chain of survival and practicing ECC skills is a recommended part of the athletic trainer's annual EAP review to help improve patient outcomes if a sudden cardiac arrest or a myocardial infarction does occur.[6]

Airway Management and Supplemental Oxygen

Airway management and supplemental oxygen delivery are interventions that may need to occur at any time during the assessment, depending on how the patient presents. These interventions go beyond opening the airway,

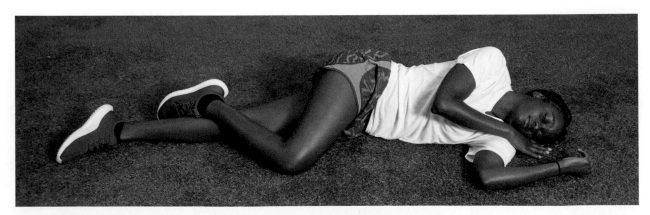

FIGURE 14.17 The recovery position.

which is discussed during the primary assessment. For athletic trainers, airway management typically involves suction, basic or advanced airway adjunct placement, and supplemental oxygen delivery.

Suction

Suction is used to remove blood, vomit, secretions, other fluids, and small food particles from an unconscious patient's airway to help prevent aspiration. Suction uses negative pressure, just like a vacuum cleaner, to remove the fluids or small particles. After placing the patient in the recovery position, remove large items with a finger sweep. Suction can be either mechanical or manual, and the tip of the suction device can be either hard or soft, depending on the equipment. Suction is indicated when a gurgling sound can be heard during respirations, ventilations are impeded by the fluids or particles, or the recovery position and finger sweep are ineffective.

Airway Adjuncts

Airway adjuncts (blind insertion airway devices) are used when a patient's airway is already open (via the head-tilt/chin-lift maneuver or a jaw thrust) to maintain its integrity. They work by keeping the tongue in place or the nasal passage open. Airway adjuncts include basic airways (e.g., OPA [oropharyngeal airway] or NPA [nasopharyngeal airway]) and advanced airways or supraglottic airways (e.g., King airway, Combitube, i-gel). Although **endotracheal intubation** remains the gold standard for airway management, it does not use a blind insertion airway device and is beyond the scope

of practice for athletic trainers. See table 14.6 for a brief summary of airway adjuncts. Airway adjuncts should be used as soon as possible, but should not delay the start of CPR if needed.

Supplemental Oxygen

Although it is technically a drug, supplemental oxygen is covered here because it can be an important component in airway management. Supplemental oxygen can be used on patients with either injury or illness to help prevent hypoxia and shock. It can and should be used in conjunction with an airway adjunct (discussed previously). That said, supplemental oxygen is not indicated for every patient. You must use the patient's present signs and symptoms, history, vital signs, and pulse oximetry reading to determine if and how you administer oxygen. In general, supplemental oxygen is indicated for patients with the following:

- Altered mental status (AMS)
- Cardiac arrest or distress
- Respiratory arrest or distress
- Signs or symptoms of hypoxia
- Stroke
- Signs or symptoms of shock
- Pulse oximetry reading below 95%
- Significant trauma (e.g., fractures, head trauma)

Supplemental oxygen can be delivered through different devices (figure 14.18) and at various flow rates. Table

---

FOUNDATIONAL SKILL

Suctioning a Patient

1. Open the patient's airway.
2. Remove any large items with a finger sweep.
3. Turn on the suction machine and make sure it provides suction against your hand.
4. Measure the distance of insertion of the suction tip, using the distance from the corner of the mouth to the earlobe.
5. Insert the suction tip into the back of the patient's mouth and begin suctioning, moving the device out of the patient's mouth from back to front with a sweeping or circular motion (avoid using a jabbing motion).
6. Suction should last no longer than 15 seconds for adults, 10 seconds for children, and 5 seconds for infants.
7. After completing the suctioning, monitor the patient and be prepared to provide ventilations with a BVM or oxygen therapy.
8. Suction again if needed.
9. Detach tubing, properly dispose of fluids, and clean up the equipment.
10. Document the intervention.

TABLE 14.6   **Summary of Airway Adjuncts**

		Indications	Contraindications
OPAs		Unconscious patient	Orofacial trauma, gag reflex
NPAs		Can be used with either a conscious or unconscious patient Clenched jaw When an OPA is contraindicated[27]	Epistaxis
Advanced airways (e.g., King, Combitube, i-gel)		Unconscious patient	Orofacial trauma, gag reflex, ingested caustic substances

14.7 summarizes these options. The process and skills associated with delivering oxygen to a patient should be covered in either an athletic training emergency course or as part of additional certification within many ECC training courses.

Splinting

Splinting is one of the most commonly used acute care skills for athletic trainers. Splinting is required to immobilize the injured area for possible fractures, dislocations,

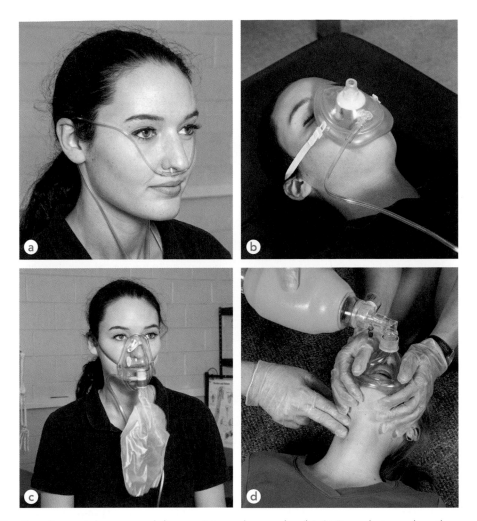

FIGURE 14.18 Supplemental oxygen delivery: *(a)* nasal cannula, *(b)* CPR pocket mask with oxygen intake, *(c)* non-rebreather mask, and *(d)* bag valve mask.

TABLE 14.7 **Supplemental Oxygen Delivery Devices**

Device	Flow rate (L/min or lpm)	Oxygen concentration (%)	Indication
CPR pocket mask with an oxygen intake	10-15	30-60	Not breathing, inadequate breathing, breathing
Nasal cannula	1-6	24-44	Breathing
Non-rebreather mask	10-15	90-100	Breathing
Bag valve mask with reservoir	15	Nearly 100	Not breathing, inadequate breathing, breathing

Based on Cleary and Walsh Flanagan (2020); Pollak et al. (2011).

and some sprains and strains. A variety of equipment can be used for splinting: SAM splints, vacuum splints, soft splints (e.g., pillow), rigid splints (e.g., padded boards), and different specialty splints (e.g., traction splint). No matter the type of splint used, the basic concepts remain the same:

- Address any open wounds first.
- Check distal CMS before applying the splint.
- Measure and form the splint to the uninjured side or body part.
- Apply the splint to the injured body part.

- Immobilize the joint above and below the injury site.
- Fill any voids between the splint and the body part, if needed.
- Secure the splint in place.
- Leave the area of the injury uncovered to allow for inspection and monitoring.
- Recheck distal CMS and check patient comfort.
- Refer the patient to the appropriate medical professional.
- Document the intervention.

Not all injuries that need splinting require activation of the EAP. If referral is necessary, it is up to the athletic trainer to decide the best course of action for the patient.

Wound Care and Bleeding Control

Wound care is an acute care skill frequently practiced by athletic trainers in a variety of settings. The proper management of hemorrhaging in the prehospital setting is essential to maintaining the circulating blood volume in an acute trauma.[28] Although not all wounds constitute a true medical emergency, it is important for athletic trainers to manage acute skin trauma efficiently and effectively. Wounds should be cleaned, **debrided**, and dressed based on the best available evidence to prevent infection and promote healing.[29]

When caring for any wound, follow these steps:

1. Follow standard precautions and wear PPE.
2. Control the bleeding.
3. Clean and, if needed, debride the wound.
4. Dress the wound.
5. Refer the patient to the appropriate medical professional, if needed.
6. Document the intervention.

Controlling bleeding is an important acute care skill and one of the few actions in which initial emergent care can critically influence a patient's outcome. The first step in controlling bleeding is to apply direct pressure. The use of pulse pressure points and elevation of injured extremities to control external bleeding is discouraged due to the lack of evidence indicating effectiveness.[30] You may firmly apply a pressure bandage (figure 14.19) over the dressing for continuous pressure while you continue your assessment and patient care. You must perform ongoing monitoring to ensure the bleeding remains controlled.

When direct pressure fails to control external bleeding, consider applying a tourniquet.[28,30,31]

When dressing a wound after bleeding has been controlled, athletic trainers have a variety of options:

- Hemostatic gauze
- Wound closure strips (i.e., Steri-Strips)
- Dermal adhesive
- Stitches
- Occlusive dressings
- Sterile gauze
- Nonadherent pads

Avoid using medicated ointments and dressings if the patient is going to be referred for stitches or advanced treatment. Not all wounds are simple to manage, and more complex wounds require special consideration.

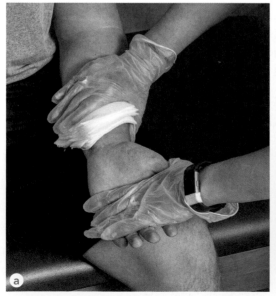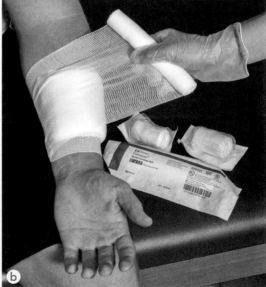

FIGURE 14.19 *(a)* Direct pressure and *(b)* pressure dressing.

FOUNDATION SKILL

Tourniquet Application

1. Follow standard precautions, wear PPE, and activate the emergency action plan.
2. Attempt to apply direct pressure to control bleeding.
3. If you cannot quickly control the bleeding, proceed to tourniquet application.
4. Position the tourniquet just proximal (2 in., or 5 cm) to the source of the bleeding, but not directly on a joint (figure 14.20a).
5. Secure the tourniquet in place and apply circumferential pressure as described by the manufacturer.
6. Tighten the tourniquet until the bleeding stops (figure 14.20b).
7. Secure the tightened tourniquet in place and mark the time and date of application on the patient's skin (next to the tourniquet) or the tourniquet.
8. Do not cover the tourniquet.
9. Frequently reevaluate the injury site for active bleeding, increasing tourniquet pressure as needed. Consider applying additional tourniquets proximal to the initial placement.

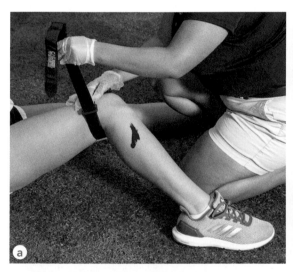 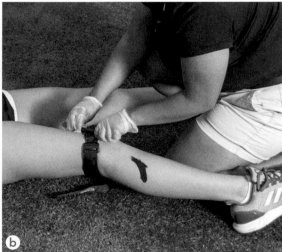

FIGURE 14.20   Tourniquet application.

Refer the patient to the proper medical professional for any of the following:

- Severe bleeding
- Wounds that need heavy debridement
- Wounds that need stitches (if they cannot be done by the athletic trainer in house)
- Wounds involving the eyes, ears, lips, tendon, bones, nerves, or genitals
- Punctures
- Burns
- Patients who need an updated tetanus shot
- Wounds displaying signs of infection

Possible complications if wounds are not treated properly include the following:

- Infection (including MRSA)
- Delayed healing
- Shock
- Death

Sutures and Staples

Sutures and staples are advanced wound closure techniques commonly used by athletic trainers working in the physician's practice. In the traditional setting, patients with deep wounds that require sutures or staples for tissue **approximation** may need to be referred out to the team

---

FOUNDATIONAL SKILL

Management of Epistaxis

1. Follow standard precautions and wear PPE.
2. Apply direct pressure to the septal area.
3. Have the patient tilt his head forward.
4. Place ice over the bridge of the patient's nose.
5. Consider the use of nasal packing (nose plug) to control the bleeding, if needed.
6. If the bleeding does not stop, continue the preceding management practices and refer the patient to the appropriate medical professional.
7. Document the intervention.

---

physician, urgent care, or emergency department.[29] With that said, some athletic trainers may do sutures and staples in the athletic training clinic as part of prehospital care. Consult your state practice act and standing orders before integrating these skills in the prehospital setting since they are invasive in nature and carry risk. Proper suture and staple procedures require considerable training and should be done maintaining **aseptic technique**.

Shock Management

Shock occurs due to inadequate perfusion of blood and oxygen entering the body (**hypoperfusion**). Shock is produced by an increase in cardiovascular system size (e.g., anaphylaxis), decreases in cardiac output (cardiogenic), decreases in respiration (respiratory), and decrease in intravascular volume (**hypovolemic**). Hypovolemic shock may be caused by dehydration from vomiting or diarrhea, exertional heat illnesses, or rapid and substantial loss of blood (i.e., hemorrhagic shock).[32] When hypoperfusion occurs, the body begins to compensate by decreasing blood flow to the extremities and concentrating on supplying blood to the vital organs and maintaining blood pressure. Vasoconstriction causes blood flow to be shunted from the extremities to the vital organs. This process maintains adequate blood pressure, supplying organs with the oxygen needed to survive. Thus, skin blood flow is decreased, resulting in cyanosis; the skin will be a pale or ashen color, cool to the touch, and moist. If the body is unable to compensate and no interventions are done to stop the progression, the body is said to be in decompensated stage of shock. The patient's systolic blood pressure will be less than 90 mmHg and distal pulses will be difficult to obtain. When the body can no longer adjust for blood loss and perfusion to the major organs cannot be maintained, the patient is said to be in irreversible shock; tissue death, organ damage, and even death are possible in this stage.

In general, management of shock includes the following:

- Controlling any bleeding
- Positioning the patient supine
- Keeping the patient warm
- Maintaining an open airway
- Administering high-flow oxygen (15 lpm)
- Monitoring vitals
- Rapid transport to hospital
- Giving the patient nothing by mouth (even if the patient is complaining about thirst)

Spinal Motion Restriction

Spinal motion restriction (SMR), also known as spinal immobilization, is one of the most important prehospital emergency procedures performed in the athletic setting following a trauma. Understanding when SMR is warranted is of paramount importance to the care of the patient during these potentially catastrophic events. Failure to provide immediate and appropriate care due to a lack of knowledge or emergency equipment on scene may be cause for negligence. Although full spinal immobilization with the long spine board (LSB) was for many years the traditional management strategy for all potential head, neck, and back injuries, advances in technology, a wider array of equipment, and evidence related to the use of the LSB have prompted clinicians to increasingly use selective spinal immobilization.[18,24,33,34] Selective spinal immobilization can be performed based on the results of a focused spinal assessment that uses objective criteria to determine whether a patient requires full spinal immobilization or variations in SMR. It is well known that selecting appropriate padding, which minimizes movement due to discomfort from a rigid LSB, is beneficial for the well-being of the patient. Even when used properly, the LSB is not without potential complications. LSB use can cause pain, pressure sores, and respiratory compromise.[35] Because of this shift in views, EMS personnel and athletic trainers should focus on performing selective spinal immobilization while paying attention to patient comfort.

Selective spinal immobilization involves using valid and reliable criteria to determine which patients need SMR. Two criteria are frequently used in the prehospital setting: NEXUS and Canadian C-Spine Rules. Both were originally developed to help emergency department staff to determine which patients needed cervical spine imaging.[36,37] They have been adapted for use in the prehospital setting by EMS personnel and athletic trainers to determine the need for SMR. The NEXUS guidelines are easier to use and remember; the process begins with establishing the patient's MOI. With this protocol, trauma patients do *not* require cervical spine immobilization if they exhibit the following characteristics:

- Alert, stable, and reliable (e.g., show no signs of intoxication or drug use, can communicate appropriately)
- No focal neurologic deficit
- No altered level of consciousness
- Not intoxicated
- No midline spinal tenderness
- No distracting injury

Figure 14.21 provides a flowchart to determine if SMR is warranted per the NEXUS guidelines.

Alternative devices, such as the CombiCarrier II or the vacuum mattress, have grown in popularity due to the evidence against the use of the LSB with all trauma patients. Additionally, the option of SMR with a cervical collar and a soft padded stretcher placed at a 30- to 45-degree angle makes the use of a transfer device (from the position the patient is found in onto the stretcher) a much better option; the CombiCarrier II is a great choice in this situation. The vacuum mattress also allows for a more comfortable position with adequate padding of the voids and a more molded position around the patient. This is particularly beneficial in patients with anatomical deformities or who are in a nontraditional in-line supine position. Just like with the LSB, proper use of alternative equipment requires substantial practice by clinicians to reach skill competency. If you are planning to incorporate one of these into your sports medicine program, you should train pertinent stakeholders (including local EMS personnel) on their use, including their advantages and disadvantages. Training emergency department staff on the proper removal of patients from these devices is also important to consider. Make sure your EAP allows for options, since a singular option may not work in all emergency situations.[18]

Management of Heat-Related Conditions and Emergency Cooling

Preventing heat-related emergencies is covered in chapter 8. But even the best-laid plans can go awry; the management of heat-related conditions must be in the institution's

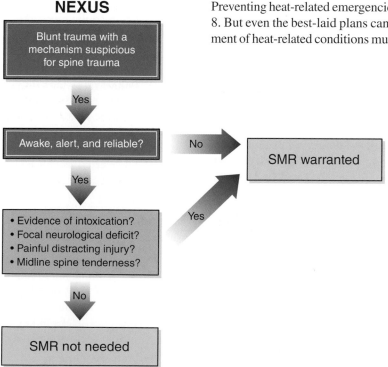

FIGURE 14.21 Flowchart for SMR.

FOUNDATION SKILL

Applying a Cervical Collar

1. Remove any jewelry in the area and keep the patient's hair away from her neck; cut off excessive clothing (e.g., a hooded sweatshirt) if needed.
2. Place the patient's head in a neutral position and maintain head support.
3. Measure the distance between the top of the shoulders to the jawline with your fingers.
4. Select the appropriate cervical collar (adjust the collar to the correct size).
5. Place the cervical collar to the side of the patient's neck. Slide the back portion of the collar under the patient's neck.
6. Align the chinpiece with the patient's chin.
7. Fasten the Velcro securely.

EAP.[13] During environmental conditions that could lead to heat illness, you must constantly monitor athletes for the signs and symptoms of heat stress. Heat-related illnesses include heat syncope, heat cramps, heat exhaustion, and heat stroke.

- Heat syncope typically occurs after a person has been standing for a long period of time or during sudden changes in posture. This occurs because of vasodilation. The patient could present with tachycardia, hypotension, possibly an elevated respiratory rate, and fainting.
- A patient with heat cramps has severe cramping during exercise in the heat. Most commonly, the cramping occurs in the patient's calves, but it could occur in other places such as the abdomen.
- Exertional heat exhaustion occurs when the patient is unable to sustain adequate cardiac output. The signs and symptoms include profuse sweating, pale skin, mildly elevated temperature, dizziness, nausea, vomiting or diarrhea, hyperventilation, persistent muscle cramps, loss of coordination, faintness or dizziness, and decreased performance. The patient's core temperature (measured rectally) will be less than 105°F (40.5°C).
- Exertional heat stroke can happen to anyone, but is most common in military recruits, distance runners, cyclists, and American football athletes. This is a serious, life-threatening condition. The specific cause is unknown, but it involves a breakdown of the thermoregulatory mechanism. The patient can present with a sudden collapse; loss of consciousness; central nervous system dysfunction; flushed, hot skin; minimal sweating (which may not be true with athletes); shallow breathing; strong, rapid pulse; and a core temperature (measured rectally) greater than 105°F (40.5°C). If

you are unable to measure core temperature, use central nervous system dysfunction as the main indicator of exertional heat stroke.

Treatment for heat syncope, heat cramps, and heat exhaustion all begin with moving the patient out of the hot environment and sun and into a cooler place (e.g., climate-controlled environment).

- For heat cramps, the patient may simply need to drink cool fluids and stretch the area before returning to activity. After return to play, monitor the patient closely.
- For heat syncope and heat exhaustion, position the patient supine with her legs elevated and begin cooling measures (e.g., apply ice pack or ice towels, remove excessive clothing). Ice packs should be placed on the back of the neck, armpits, and groin area, where there is a large superficial blood supply. Give the patient cool fluids to drink. You should assess and monitor the patient's vitals over the course of treatment. A patient who has had heat syncope or exertional heat exhaustion should not return to play the same day and should be referred to physician for follow-up care and clearance for return to play.

For a patient with exertional heat stroke, you must take drastic measures to cool the patient to prevent irreversible tissue damage or death.

- The current best-practice guidelines call for cold water immersion (bath or tub filled with water 35°F to 58°F, or 3°C to 14°C) and patient monitoring. If cold water immersion is not possible, place ice packs in key locations (e.g., the neck, armpits, and groin area).
- Active cooling should continue until the patient's core temperature is approximately 101°F (38.5°C), measured rectally.

- During this process, closely monitor the patient's ABCs and vitals and give IV fluid, if available.

- If you have not yet activated the EAP, do so as soon as possible. This patient will require EMS transport to the hospital for additional care, *but cooling should take place prior to transport.* It is especially important that this be outlined in the EAP. The institution should communicate with EMS about this policy before an incident because their protocols will likely differ for this treatment.

- Any patient experiencing exertional heat stroke should not return to play until she receives clearance from a physician. The return to play process should be gradual. You should monitor the patient's status throughout.

Emergency Medications

The legal use of emergency medicines in athletic training is regulated on both the state and federal levels and can vary greatly state to state.[38] You must work with the supervising physician to make sure your institution's policies, procedures, and EAP related to emergency medication storage, dispensing, and administration align with requirements of your state practice act and state and federal laws. Additional, athletic trainers working in the secondary school setting must work closely with the school nurse to make sure they follow state laws and school policies related to medications.

Prior to assisting any patient with a medication, verify the following information (also known as the 6 rights of medicine administration):

1. Right patient
2. Right medication
3. Right dose
4. Right time
5. Right route
6. Right documentation

Take a complete set of vitals both before and after assisting with medications. This information will help you determine if a medication can safely be administered and if the medication has helped improve the patient's condition. Document all this information. Only after verifying all information can you assist with the medication. You also must decide if and when you need to activate the EAP and call EMS. The following sections highlight some common medications used by athletic trainers during a medical emergency.

Aspirin

In the prehospital setting, aspirin (acetylsalicylic acid, or ASA) is used for chest pain of cardiac origin. This is because aspirin is an antiplatelet drug that inhibits platelet clumping, preventing a clot in the coronary arteries from getting worse. It should not be administered for headaches since the headache may be associated with head injuries or medical conditions such as strokes. For these conditions, aspirin is contraindicated.

For a potential cardiac-related event, encourage the patient to chew an aspirin as long as he has no allergy or other contraindications (e.g., head injury) to taking aspirin. The patient must be able to follow instructors and chew the pill. You may administer 4 noncoated baby aspirins (4 × 81 mg each = 324 mg) or 1 noncoated adult aspirin (325 mg) to the patient. These must be chewed to allow for the fastest absorption rate. (Remember that in cardiac-related chest pain, time is muscle.) Activate the EAP if EMS have not already been requested.

Nitroglycerin

Nitroglycerin (or "nitro") is also used for cardiac events. It works as a vasodilator to help increase the amount of blood that is able to flow to the heart muscles; therefore, the heart does not have to work as hard. This helps reduce the chest pain associated with cardiac events. Nitroglycerin should be used in conjunction with aspirin with cardiac patients. Have the patient chew the aspirin before administering nitroglycerin.

Prior to administering nitroglycerin, ask the patient if he is taking any sexual enhancement drugs, both prescribed medications and herbal supplements. If the patient is on any of these medications, nitroglycerin is contraindicated. Nitroglycerin is also contraindicated for patients with a head injury. Lastly, the patient must have a systolic blood pressure of at least 100 mmHg prior to administration. This is one of the reasons you must assess a patient's blood pressure prior to administering any medications.

The standard dosage of nitroglycerin is 0.4 mg given under the tongue through tablet or meter-dosed spray. Tablets usually take 30 seconds to 1 minute to dissolve; note that it will take longer for them to dissolve if the patient has a dry mouth. You must use a gloved hand when touching nitroglycerin tablets. The side effects of nitroglycerin include dizziness, lightheadedness, headache, and a burning sensation under the tongue. The patient's pain should lessen within approximately 1 to 5 minutes of administration. A second dose can be given 5 minutes after the first dose. Activate the EAP if EMS have not already been requested.

Inhalers and Nebulizers

Fast-acting meter-dosed inhalers (MDI), or rescue inhalers, are commonly prescribed to patients with asthma, emphysema, allergies, and other respiratory conditions. The use of the inhaler is indicated at the onset of acute respiratory distress (e.g., trouble breathing with wheezing). A rescue inhaler is contraindicated for patients with tachycardia due to cardiac complications. When possible, measure a peak flow reading just before and a few minutes after each dose. The inhaler takes approximately 5 minutes to work. Be prepared to give additional doses. Some possible side effects of rescue inhalers include tachycardia, hypertension, anxiety, and restlessness. Activate the EAP and request EMS if the patient's breathing does not improve with the use of the rescue inhaler. See chapter 23 for the steps for using an inhaler.

You may also need to assist patients who are prescribed a nebulizer for delivering their medications. These are used both preventively and in the emergency setting. If you are working in the secondary school setting, work closely with the school nurse to establish a plan for assisting this patient when needed.

Glucose

Oral glucose should be provided to patients with hypoglycemia. When it is absorbed by the body, it provides glucose for the cells to use. Emergency oral glucose is in a gel form to allow for easier absorption. Some patients may also have glucose tablets that can be chewed. If glucose gel or tablets are unavailable, other forms of sugar found in common foods, such as orange juice, soda, and jelly beans, are acceptable.[4] Oral glucose is indicated for patients with hypoglycemia who are conscious, have control over their airway, can follow commands, and can swallow. Oral glucose gel comes in a 15 g tube. Administer the gel slowly and monitor the patient to ensure she is swallowing the gel. Glucose tablets come in 15 to 20 g tablets. Instruct the patient to chew the tablet completely and swallow. After 5 to 10 minutes, reassess the patient's blood glucose and vitals. You can deliver a second dose if the patient's blood glucose is still low. Call EMS if the patient does not improve.

If a glucometer is unavailable, oral glucose can be given to patients with diabetes who are presenting with AMS. If the patient has hypoglycemia, the dose of oral glucose can have a positive effect on the patient's condition. If the dose of oral glucose does not improve the patient's condition, consider if the patient is having a stroke or another medical condition unrelated to blood glucose. Activate the EAP at this time.

If the patient is unconscious, you cannot give oral glucose. Activate the EAP. Some patients with diabetes may have an emergency glucagon kit for use when unconscious or if oral glucose treatment fails. Athletic trainers need additional training to give emergency glucagon to a patient. If you are working in a secondary school setting, work with the school nurse to receive training and to make sure school policies and procedures are followed. Glucagon comes in a prepackaged kit that includes 1 mg of powder and 1 mL of fluid that are mixed together to activate. If glucagon is administered to a patient, EMS must be called because the effects of the treatment are not long lasting and additional, advanced interventions are required.

Epinephrine

In the prehospital setting, anaphylaxis is treated with oxygen and epinephrine (EpiPen). Epinephrine stimulates the nervous system and causes bronchodilation to help open the constricted airways. Epinephrine is contraindicated in patients with chest pain of cardiac origin and hypertension. The dosing of epinephrine is 0.3 mg for adults and 0.15 mg for children. This is premeasured in the autoinjector pens. The side effects of epinephrine include hypertension, tachycardia, anxiety, and restlessness. Many patients are now prescribed two dose packs. Be prepared to administer the second pack if symptoms do not resolve or if it will take longer than 5 to 10 minutes for EMS to arrive.

FOUNDATIONAL SKILL

Administering Epinephrine Autoinjector

1. Remove the autoinjector from the packaging.
2. Open the cap and grasp the autoinjector with your fist.
3. Remove the safety release.
4. Hold the tip of the autoinjector on the lateral aspect of the patient's thigh.
5. Push the autoinjector firmly against the patient's thigh at a 90-degree angle until it activates.
6. Hold the autoinjector in place for 10 seconds.
7. Massage the injected site for approximately 10 seconds.
8. Monitor the patient's vital signs and response to the medication.
9. Consider giving a second dose in 5 to 10 minutes after administering the first dose.

Naloxone

Naloxone (Narcan) is used to reverse respiratory depression associated with opioid overdose (figure 14.22). It is recommended for use in all unresponsive patients with either a confirmed or suspected opioid overdose.[4] Note that giving naloxone to a patient who has not overdosed has few negative effects, so if the signs and symptoms of an overdose (unconscious, respiratory distress, bilateral pinpoint pupils) are present, you should administer the medication to the patient.

Naloxone can be delivered through intravenous, intramuscular, or intranasal routes, but you are more likely to see the intranasal delivery route. Intranasal naloxone is a 2 mg dose that should be administered according to the manufacturer's directions. This typically involves delivering half the dose in one nostril and half in the other (a nasal airway must be removed prior to administration). After administering the medication, give a few breaths with a BVM to help the medication enter the body (since the patient is likely to have shallow breathing). Be prepared to remove the oral airway if the patient begins to vomit, manage the airway with suction if needed, and assist with ventilations. You need to be prepared if the patient becomes violent when he becomes conscious, so activate the EAP and notify both EMS and the police before giving the medication. If the first dose of naloxone does not increase respiratory drive in the patient, you can give a second dose after 2 to 5 minutes.

Intravenous Access

Intravenous (IV) access is a skill that is used in the management of many emergent conditions (both trauma and illness). You should consult your state practice act and standing orders before integrating this skill in the prehospital setting because it is invasive in nature and risky. IV placement requires considerable training and should be done maintaining aseptic procedures.

Obtaining IV access involves using a needle to place a catheter in the patient's vein to allow direct access to the circulatory system. IVs are commonly placed through a vein in the hand, forearm, or antecubital fossa, but placement can be done anywhere a superficial vein is present. The IV is then used for medicine administration, fluid delivery, and blood sample collection. Sometimes the IV is placed in the patient without delivery fluids to maintain the open vein for easy access by emergency department personnel. For example, in the prehospital setting, IV access can allow for fluid and electrolyte delivery in patients who are moderately to severely dehydrated or suffering heat illness.[5,39] IV access also allows the team physician or paramedic to administer certain medications, including pain medication and naloxone. Lastly, IV access allows for the collection of blood samples in the prehospital setting. This may be done to help hospital staff diagnose a stroke in a patient. With the increased research on biomarkers in patients with concussions, in the future, athletic trainers may be on the frontline of collecting blood samples for analysis related to concussion diagnosis and prognosis.[40,41]

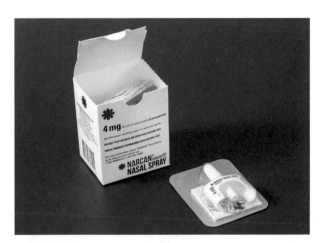

FIGURE 14.22   Intranasal Naloxone.

CLINICAL BOTTOM LINE

- Emergency care assessment and skills are some of the most critical for athletic trainers to learn and be confident performing. Although some skills are used more frequently in the traditional athletic training setting than in other settings, all are important and can have a significant effect on the patient's outcome. Athletic trainers should practice these skills frequently and be prepared for any potential situation that arises. They must stay up to date on changes in the evidence and best practices related to emergency care skills.

- For the safety of all people involved in an emergency situation, the athletic trainer must thoroughly size up the scene before starting care. This step should never be skipped.

- The athletic trainer must assess the patient quickly and efficiently, stopping to provide lifesaving interventions when warranted. Both the primary assessment and secondary assessment should be thorough and complete to make sure injuries or illness are not overlooked and important information is obtained to make clinical decisions and determine the proper interventions.

- Athletic trainers can provide a variety of interventions in the prehospital setting, including CPR or AED, spinal motion restriction, airway management, splinting, wound care and bleeding control, shock management, emergency cooling, and emergency medications, among others.
- The patient's condition should be monitored until EMS arrives, a referral is determined, or the patient is deemed no longer in distress and can safely leave the care of the athletic trainer.
- Athletic trainers should prepare for all potential emergencies at their institution. This includes having a detailed EAP, the necessary equipment to treat the patient, and a good working relationship with EMS.

 Go to HK*Propel* to complete the activities and case studies for this chapter.

Go to HKPropel to (1) view videos of various vital sign assessments and (2) download foundational skill check sheets for various acute care and emergency procedures.

PART IV

Injury and Illness Evaluation

Knowledge of injuries, illness, and evaluation and referral processes is essential for athletic trainers. Chapters 15 and 16 focus on competency in evaluation and diagnosis. Chapter 15 presents foundational information on the pathophysiology, biomechanics, and pathomechanics needed to understand musculoskeletal and nerve injuries and sudden illness. Chapter 16 builds on this further with information on practicing clinical diagnosis and identifying how, when, and to whom to refer patients after initial assessment. The subsequent chapters in part IV provide a broader understanding of the whole patient, focusing on psychosocial interventions, special populations, and life-span care. They present information on a range of illnesses and methods for evaluation to address the increasing diversity athletic trainers encounter in client populations and professional settings. Unique to this section is information about medical imaging (chapter 17), an expanding area of responsibility for athletic trainers. In order to provide patient-centered, holistic care during medical interventions that they might encounter in a diversifying employment setting, athletic trainers must understand the medical conditions that patients experience across the life span (chapter 18). Clinical practice requires athletic trainers to identify physical and psychological injury and illness and then either provide appropriate care or make a referral (chapter 19). Chapter 20 covers the unique challenges and opportunities of working with clients in special populations.

CHAPTER 15

Pathophysiology of Musculoskeletal and Nerve Injury

James R. Scifers, DScPT, PT, LAT, ATC

CHAPTER OBJECTIVES

After reading this chapter, you will be able to do the following:

- Describe normal anatomy and physiology of soft tissue, bone, and nerve

- Describe normal bony changes that occur during aging

- Classify various injuries to soft tissue, bone, and nerve

- Identify various types of soft tissue injuries and their common mechanisms of injury

- Determine signs and symptoms of various grades of ligament sprains and muscle strains

- Differentiate the conditions of tendinopathy, tendinitis, tendinosis, tenosynovitis, and bursitis

- Describe the normal processes of bone healing, soft tissue healing, and nerve healing

- Predict normal healing times for various types and grades of soft tissue injury, various bone injuries, and classifications of nerve injury

- Understand the most appropriate diagnostic imaging modalities for identifying soft tissue pathology, bone injury, and nerve injury

CAATE STANDARDS

The following CAATE 2020 standards are covered in this chapter:

Standard 55

Standard 70

Standard 71

Standard 72

Standard 73

Pathophysiology is the disordered physiological processes associated with disease or injury. Athletic trainers must understand pathophysiology because altered physiologic processes often contribute to musculoskeletal and nervous system pathologies seen in physically active people. Biomechanics is the study of mechanical laws related to normal (nonpathological) movement and structure of the human body. By contrast, pathomechanics refers to the abnormal or pathological mechanics that occur in the presence of altered anatomy, physiology, or pathology within the human body. You must learn about the normal and abnormal mechanics of the human body in order to better understand various mechanisms of injury associated with injuries to soft tissue, bone, and nerves. Knowledge of normal mechanics and pathomechanics will further assist you in preventing injury in patients completing athletic activity, work-related activity, and activities of daily living. This chapter focuses on the pathophysiology, biomechanics, and pathomechanics associated with bony, soft tissue, and nerve injury in physically active people. Additionally, tissue healing, diagnostic techniques, and treatment are discussed for a variety of common pathologies associated with physical activity.

Soft Tissue Injury

The most commonly injured soft tissues are muscles, tendons, and ligaments. These injuries can be associated with athletic participation, work-related trauma, or activities of daily living. Soft tissue injuries can be classified as traumatic or overuse based on their **mechanism of injury**. Traumatic injuries include sprains, strains, and muscular contusions. Overuse injuries include tendinopathies, also referred to as tendinitis, and bursitis.

Sprains

Ligaments connect bone to bone and provide static support to joints. Traumatic injuries to ligaments are called sprains. Commonly sprained joints include the ankle, knee, shoulder, elbow, and wrist. Ankle sprains are among the most common musculoskeletal injuries in both athletes and the general population.[1-2] Sprain severity is classified using a scale that defines the injury as either grade I, II, or III. Table 15.1 outlines the grading of sprains.

Strains

Strains involve injury to muscle or tendon. Common strains related to sport activity include injury to the quadriceps, hamstrings, gastrocnemius, adductors, and lumbar spine. Similar to sprains, strains are graded based on the severity and the degree of tissue damage using a scale of I to III. Table 15.2 outlines the grading of strains.

Contusions

Muscle contusions typically result from direct trauma to tissue. These injuries may also be referred to as a hematoma or bruise. This mechanism of injury results in local damage to the muscle and associated bleeding due to injury to capillaries in the area of trauma. Signs and symptoms of muscle contusion include the following:

- Pain
- Point tenderness
- Muscle spasm
- Muscle inhibition

TABLE 15.1 Grading of Sprains

Sprain grade	Signs and symptoms	Ligamentous stress testing results
Grade I	Pain Mild inflammation Minimal swelling No to mild discoloration Minimal loss of function	Pain only
Grade II	Pain Joint instability Moderate inflammation Moderate swelling Some discoloration More marked loss of function	Pain and laxity
Grade III	Pain Joint instability Significant inflammation Swelling Discoloration Significant loss of function	Laxity only*

*The reason pain is not present with ligamentous testing is because 100% of the ligament is torn, meaning no nervous input is intact to transmit pain messages to the brain.

FOUNDATIONAL SKILL

Suspected Ligament Injury

When examining a patient with a suspected ligament injury, the athletic trainer may choose to apply ligamentous stress tests to the involved joint. When performing these tests, the athletic trainer must assess for both pain and laxity in order to identify the presence or absence of ligament injury, as well as to fully understand the degree to which the ligament is damaged.

TABLE 15.2 **Grading of Strains**

Strain grade	Signs and symptoms	Strength testing findings
Grade I (mild)	Minimal, well-localized pain Muscle spasm Mild muscle weakness Minor disability	Pain and mild weakness
Grade II (moderate)	Moderate and poorly localized pain Loss of range of motion Mild discoloration Swelling and inflammation Muscle spasm Moderate muscle weakness Moderate disability	Pain and weakness
Grade III (severe)	Diffuse pain Swelling Inflammation Discoloration Muscle spasm Significant muscle weakness Deformity in muscle belly Significant loss of range of motion Significant disability[3-4]	Pain and significant weakness

- Swelling
- Inflammation
- Discoloration
- Loss of range of motion
- Loss of function

Common areas of muscle contusion include the quadriceps (figure 15.1), the hamstrings, and the biceps brachii. Although contusions are generally considered minor injuries, a significant complication that could arise from improperly treated contusions is **heterotopic ossification**.[5]

Overuse Injuries

Overuse injuries can occur due to repeated activities associated with physical activity, work-related activity, or activities of daily living. Commonly observed musculo-skeletal overuse injuries are **tendinopathies** and bursitis. Tendinopathies include the following:

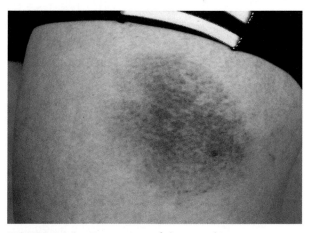

FIGURE 15.1 Contusion of the quadriceps.
Cordelia Molloy / Science Source

- *Tendinitis:* an inflammation of the tendon or the tendon sheath that is typically caused by repeated microtrauma or stress to the tendon

FOUNDATIONAL SKILL

Contusion Care

Contusions require appropriate care to prevent reinjury and the possibility of heterotopic ossification from occurring. When returning people to activity, athletic trainers should appropriately pad contusions to prevent secondary injury to the tissue.

- *Tendinosis:* a degeneration of collagen tissue making up the tendon as a result of chronic overuse
- *Tenosynovitis:* inflammation of the tendon sheath or synovium that is associated with trauma, overuse, or infection

These conditions are frequently confused with one another. As a result, clinicians often misdiagnose patients with tendon injuries. The clinical implications of such misdiagnosis are important in developing effective treatment plans for patients suffering from tendon injuries. For example, in the case of tendinitis, anti-inflammatory medications can assist in reducing pain and inflammation; however, in the presence of a tendinosis, the same anti-inflammatory medications can delay tissue healing and increase the risk of reinjury. Table 15.3 outlines the differences between overuse injuries.

Bursitis is an inflammation of the bursa, a small, fluid-filled sac that cushions and protects the bone, tendon, and muscle adjacent to the joint. Bursitis is the result of a single traumatic event or, more commonly, repeated trauma to the bursa. It often results from repeated micro-trauma associated with repetitive movements done during physical activity, work-related activity, or activities of daily living. A bursa can become inflamed as a result of friction or compression. Common locations for bursitis include the ankle, knee, hip, shoulder, and elbow.

Soft Tissue Healing

An understanding of soft tissue healing is necessary in order to develop appropriate treatment, rehabilitation, and return to activity programs for patients suffering from soft tissue injuries. Soft tissue healing involves three phases: the inflammatory phase, the repair phase, and the remodeling phase (figure 15.2).

Inflammatory Phase

- The acute inflammatory stage occurs within hours to several days after injury.
- The inflammatory process involves containing, neutralizing, or diluting the injury-causing agent or lesion.
- The inflammatory process is consistent regardless of the type of soft tissue that is injured.

TABLE 15.3 Comparison of Overuse Injuries

Overuse injury	Definition	Signs and symptoms	Treatment goal
Tendinitis	Inflammation of the tendon or tendon sheath that is typically caused by repeated micro-trauma or stress to the tendon	Pain Inflammation Swelling that worsens with physical activity	Reducing inflammation
Tendinosis	Degeneration of collagen tissue making up the tendon as a result of chronic overuse; result of repeated trauma to the tendon that occurs when the tissue is not allowed to rest or properly heal[6-7]	Pain Weakness Loss of function	Strengthening and realigning collagen tissue within the injured tendon
Tenosynovitis	Inflammation of the tendon sheath or synovium that is associated trauma, overuse, or infection	Pain Inflammation Swelling Stiffness Loss of function[8-9]	Reducing inflammation

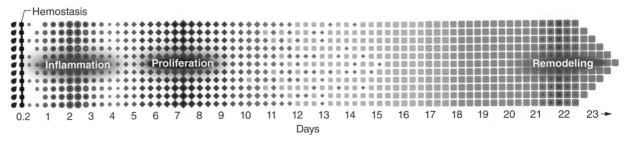

FIGURE 15.2 Overview of the tissue healing process.

- Typical treatment interventions employed by the athletic trainer during the acute inflammatory stage of soft tissue healing include partial immobilization, cryotherapy, compression, and elevation.

Repair Phase

- The repair phase of healing occurs within days or weeks of the injury.
- Tissue repair is characterized by cell proliferation, capillary proliferation, and wound closure.
- During this stage of soft tissue healing, **fibroblastic proliferation** is essential for tissue repair and wound closure.
- The time frame for tissue repair varies based on the type of tissue injured and the severity of injury.

Remodeling Phase

- The remodeling phase of tissue healing may last for weeks, months, or even years.
- During this phase of healing, the repaired tissue is realigned and strengthened based on the activity of the patient.
- Ideally, tissue remodeling takes place under the supervision of a rehabilitation professional who specifically designs a treatment and rehabilitation program aimed at remodeling the repaired tissue based on anticipated tissue stresses to allow for safe return to functional activity.
- Failure to properly model tissue prior to the client's return to functional activity may result in repeated injury.
- As with the repair phase, the time frame required for tissue remodeling varies greatly based on the type of tissue injured and the severity of injury.

Tissue healing following ligament sprain is determined primarily by the severity of ligament injury, but may also be affected by the specific ligament injured.

- Grade I ligament injuries typically repair within 10 days of the injury.
- Grade II ligament sprains typically repair within 4 weeks of the injury.
- Grade III ligament sprains may or may not undergo repair without surgical intervention. This decision depends on the specific ligament injured. In cases of grade III lateral ankle sprains or medial collateral ligament sprains at the knee, tissue repair will typically occur within 6 weeks of the date of injury. However, other ligaments, such as the anterior cruciate ligament (ACL) of the knee will not heal on their own following grade

III sprains and will require surgical repair. Tissue remodeling following ligament graft placement is prolonged and may last more than 12 months.

Tissue healing times for muscle strains generally mimic those for ligament sprains.

- Grade I muscle strains require approximately 7 to 10 days for healing.
- Grade II muscle strains require 2 to 4 weeks for tissue healing.
- Grade III muscle strains require 4 to 6 weeks for tissue healing. Like grade III ligament sprains of the ACL of the knee and the ulnar collateral ligament (UCL) of the elbow, grade III tendon ruptures do not heal and will typically require surgical repair. In some cases, patients suffering from tendon ruptures are able to function without surgery; injury to the long head of the biceps tendon is an example of an injury that may not require surgical repair for return to normal function. Common examples of tendon ruptures requiring surgical repair for return to function include injuries to the Achilles' tendon, the patellar tendon, the distal biceps tendon, and the supraspinatus tendon.

In general, treatment and rehabilitation time, or the time required to return to unrestricted activity following ligament sprain or muscle strain, can be predicted by doubling the time required for tissue repair.

Soft tissue contusions generally require a few days to several weeks to heal based on the severity of the injury. In these injuries, you should treat the initial inflammatory stage using rest, ice, compression, and elevation to prevent heterotopic ossification and accelerate return to activity. Inflammatory injuries such as tendinitis, tenosynovitis, and bursitis typically require 2 to 3 weeks for tissue healing and 4 to 6 weeks for return to normal activity. Overuse injuries that involve degeneration of collagen tissue, such as tendinosis, require longer tissue healing times in the range of 2 to 3 months.

Soft Tissue Treatment

Basic treatment of soft tissue injury during the acute, inflammatory stage of tissue healing should involve the use of rest, ice, compression, and elevation (RICE) to control pain and inflammation.[10-11] During the repair phase of tissue healing, treatment should include the use of therapeutic modalities aimed at promoting tissue healing. These include superficial and deep heating modalities, pulsed ultrasound, and LASER. Rehabilitation during the repair phase of tissue healing should slowly progress through range of motion, stretching, strengthening, and proprioceptive exercises that protect newly healed or healing tissue without compromising it. During the repair stage of tissue healing, you should begin the process of realigning collagen tissue according to the anticipated direction of stress by applying transverse friction massage, end-range range of motion exercises, and gentle soft tissue stretching.[12-13] During the tissue remodeling stage of tissue healing, progress all aspects of the rehabilitation process to fully realign and strengthen healed tissue and promote a full return to preinjury activity.[10-11]

Tendinitis and tenosynovitis should be treated with the same general guidelines that are used to address ligament sprains and muscle strains. During the initial treatment of bursitis, avoid compression if the mechanism of injury to the bursa involved compressive forces. Furthermore, patients suffering from bursitis may benefit from one or more corticosteroid injections to reduce soft tissue inflammation.[14]

Diagnostic Imaging for Soft Tissue Injury

The most effective diagnostic imaging tools for identifying soft tissue lesions are musculoskeletal ultrasound (MSKUS) and magnetic resonance imaging (MRI).[16-17] Musculoskeletal ultrasound provides real-time visualization of soft tissue pathology and allows clinicians to perform dynamic evaluations (such as ligament stress testing) during imaging. Furthermore, MSKUS is less expensive than other forms of diagnostic imaging and provides no radiation to the patient during assessment.[18] In cases where musculoskeletal ultrasound is inconclusive, magnetic resonance imaging can provide additional details for diagnosing various soft tissue pathologies.[16-18] See chapter 17 for more information on medical imaging.

Bone Injury

Bones function to provide the rigid framework needed to support and protect tissue. Additionally, long bones provide anatomical attachment sites for muscles that become a system of levers allowing for bone movement, also known as **osteokinematics**. Bone injury typically involves acute trauma or repeated trauma. The most common injury to bone is fracture; however, numerous other pathologies, such as bone contusions, stress fractures, and growth plate injuries, are commonly observed in orthopedic medicine. Both short bones and long bones are susceptible to injury, but the pathomechanics of injury to each are unique.

Anatomical Properties of Bone

Bone is primarily made up of collagen and **hydroxyapatite**.

- Type I collagen makes up approximately 90% of the organic content of bone and provides for approximately 40% of bone's weight. This collagen tissue allows bone to be somewhat **viscoelastic**, which decreases bony injury.

- Hydroxyapatite (HA) is the main inorganic constituent of bone. HA is a calcium and phosphate–based mineral found between collagen tissue. HA makes up approximately 60% of bone's weight and provides the rigidity bones need for structure and movement.

The combination of collagen and hydroxyapatite make up bone's **stress tolerance**, which describes how tissue (in this case, bone) responds to various stresses. Collagen's viscoelasticity and hydroxyapatite's rigidity allow bone to respond favorably to a variety of stresses throughout weight-bearing, activities of daily living, and athletic activity.

Bone is the strongest tissue in terms of resisting compression. **Wolff's law** states that bone growth and remodeling occur in direct response to forces that are placed on the tissue. Compression provides the greatest example of this law. As bone undergoes compression through weight-bearing activities such as walking, running, and jumping, it becomes thicker and stronger. Wolff's law can be applied to both bone growth and development in healthy tissue and bone healing after injury.

Although Wolff's law demonstrates methods in which bone grows and heals after injury, continued excessive

---

EVIDENCE-BASED ATHLETIC TRAINING

Treating Tendinosis

Significant research has been conducted in order to determine the best treatment approach for patients with a diagnosis of tendinosis. Tendinosis should be treated with a combination of eccentric strengthening exercises, stretching exercises, extracorporeal shockwave therapy treatment, and platelet-rich plasma injections. Anti-inflammatory medications (both corticosteroid and nonsteroidal anti-inflammatory medications) and therapeutic modalities (including ultrasound, phonophoresis, iontophoresis, and LASER) have all been shown to be ineffective in the treatment of tendinosis.[7,15]

loads lead to **bone stress response**, or weakening of the bone. Bone stress response occurs over time with repeated, excessive loading of bone. This stress response leads to bony injuries like **stress fractures** and **stress syndromes**.

Compression is the force most easily resisted by healthy bone. Additionally, bone resists tensile or tensioning and traction forces fairly well. However, in the presence of shear forces (i.e., those perpendicular to the bone) and torsional (i.e., twisting) forces, bone is more susceptible to injury. Figure 15.3 shows how these common forces impact bone.

Bony Anatomy

Two types of bone are found in the body.

1. **Cortical bone**, also known as compact bone, is dense, stiff, and hard. It forms the outer layer of bone and can withstand a large amount of stress. Cortical bone is found primarily in the shafts of the long bones. This type of bone provides the rigidity needed for structure. Cortical bone makes up about 80% of the skeletal system.
2. **Trabecular bone**, also known as cancellous or spongy bone, has a honeycomb-like structure. It makes up the inner layer of bone and is found in the ends of long bones, the scapula, and in the vertebrae of the spine. This tissue provides the elasticity needed for the bone to withstand stress and not break. Trabecular bone makes up the remaining 20% of the skeletal system.

Long bones, those which make up the appendicular skeleton, have a common anatomical makeup.

1. The ends of the long bones are primarily made up of trabecular bone and are known as the **epiphysis**.

- The shaft of long bones is primarily made up of cortical bone and is called the **diaphysis**.
- The area between the epiphysis and the diaphysis is known as the **metaphysis**. The metaphysis contains the growth plate, or **epiphyseal plate**, that allows for long bone growth during childhood and adolescence.

Figure 15.4 shows the relationship of these three portions of long bone.

The epiphysis is covered by articular cartilage, a thin layer of specialized connective tissue that provides for protection and viscoelasticity where joints are formed between two bones. Articular cartilage functions to provide a smooth, lubricated surface for joint articulation and protection of the **subchondral** cancellous bone found just beneath the articular cartilage. The medullary cavity is found inside the shaft of the long bone. This central cavity, sometimes referred to as the marrow cavity, is where bone marrow is stored. Figure 15.4 shows the anatomy of the long bone, including the location of articular cartilage and the medullary cavity.

Bony Physiology

Bone formation, also known as **ossification**, is the process by which new bone is formed. Bone growth and development are determined by osteoclast and osteoblast activity.

- **Osteoclasts** are responsible for bone reabsorption associated with bone breakdown. This function is critical in maintenance, repair, and remodeling of bones.
- **Osteoblasts** synthesize dense, cross-linked collagen and proteins (HA) that allow for bone formation and development.

When osteoblast activity exceeds osteoclast activity, bone formation occurs and bone density increases. In

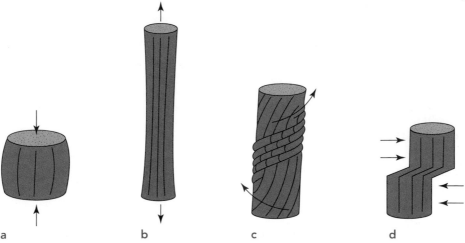

FIGURE 15.3 Types and mechanisms of injury forces: *(a)* compression, *(b)* tensioning, *(c)* torsional/twisting, and *(d)* shearing.

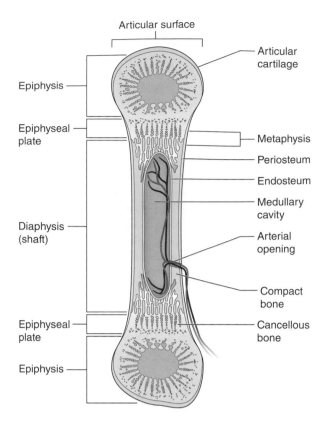

Labels around figure:
- Articular surface
- Articular cartilage
- Epiphysis
- Epiphyseal plate
- Metaphysis
- Periosteum
- Endosteum
- Medullary cavity
- Diaphysis (shaft)
- Arterial opening
- Compact bone
- Cancellous bone
- Epiphyseal plate
- Epiphysis

FIGURE 15.4 Anatomy of the long bone.

cases where osteoclast activity exceeds osteoblast activity, bone breakdown occurs and bone density decreases.

Bony Changes During Aging

Bone characteristics change from childhood to adulthood. In young children, bone is described as being woven with randomly interspersed cartilage. This allows for equal strength of bone in all directions, which is important as young children develop basic motor skills such as standing, walking, running, and jumping. Woven bone is not as strong as adult bone but is more flexible and better able to tolerate falls without injury.

During childhood and into the teenage years, new bone is added to the skeleton faster than old bone is removed. This results in bone growth and formation of larger, heavier, more dense bone. This bone growth typically occurs until the mid-20s. The teens and early 20s are often described as the **bone-building years** because of their significant importance in preventing future bone disease.

During the late 20s and 30s, bone growth and bone loss tend to be fairly equal, resulting in a status quo in terms of bone strength and density. Around age 40, for most people, bone loss may begin to exceed bone growth, resulting in weaker, less dense bones that are more prone to injury. This bone density loss continues throughout the remainder of life, leading to poor spinal posture, increased fall risk, and increased fracture risk.

Women are at greater risk of bone density loss than men. This is primarily due to the fact that women have smaller, thinner bones than men do. Also, following menopause, women lose bone density more rapidly due to a sharp decline in the production of estrogen. Bone loss in women greatly exceeds bone loss in men between the ages of 45 and 65 years due to the loss of estrogen associated with menopause. However, after age 65, bone loss is roughly equal between women and men because men typically suffer a drop in testosterone after age 65. Loss of bone density is more prevalent in White and Asian populations (approximately 33%) than in Hispanic (approximately 25%) and Black (approximately 19%) populations.[19]

Bone density loss can be retarded by the ingestion of calcium and vitamin D and regular weight-bearing exercise. Bone density losses are accelerated by inactivity, tobacco use, and excessive use of alcohol.

EVIDENCE-BASED ATHLETIC TRAINING

Measuring Bone Density

Bone density can be measured using a test known as dual-energy X-ray absorptiometry (DEXA) to determine if it is normal, slightly decreased (osteopenia), or greatly decreased (osteoporosis). DEXA measures the mineral content of bone, known as a T-score. Bone density and fracture risk have an inverse relationship, with fracture risk increasing as bone density decreases. Research has shown that a 50-year-old White woman with a T-score of −1 was at a 16% greater risk of hip fracture than the same patient with a T-score greater than −1. This injury risk increases to 27% with a T-score of −2 and to 33% with a T-score of −2.5. Patients with T-scores between −1 and −2.4 are considered to have osteopenia, while those with T-scores of −2.5 and greater are considered to have osteoporosis.[47] According to the National Osteoporosis Foundation (NOF), DEXA testing is recommended for women older than 65 years, postmenopausal women younger than 65 years who have one or more risk factors, and postmenopausal women who have had a recent fracture.

When bone loss exceeds bone growth, **osteopenia** and **osteoporosis** can develop. Osteopenia is a less severe form of bone loss than osteoporosis. It is estimated that osteopenia occurs in 50% of American adults over age 50.[19] Osteopenia, if untreated, serves as a precursor to osteoporosis, with both conditions leading to an increased prevalence of fracture. Both osteopenia and osteoporosis are more likely to occur if patients did not achieve maximum peak bone mass during the bone-building years.

Periostitis

Periostitis, also known as periostalgia, is a condition that results in inflammation of the outer layer of bone known as the periosteum. A common example of periostitis is shin splints. Periostitis can be acute, usually resulting from infection to the bone, or chronic, resulting from repeated trauma and stress to the bone. This condition is common in athletes who place repetitive stress on bones through running and jumping. Common signs of periostitis include swelling and tenderness of bone at the site of injury.

Fractures

Fractures are the most common bone injury, with over 1 million occurring each year in the United States.[20] A fracture is an injury that breaks or changes the contour or shape of the bone. Fractures occur due to high force or impact to the bone. Most fractures are the result of trauma associated with sports injuries, accidents, and falls. There are several types of fractures:

- *Complete fracture:* complete break in bone, causing separation into two or more pieces
- *Closed fracture:* fracture where skin is not broken
- *Displaced fracture:* fracture resulting in a space or gap between two ends of bone
- *Open or compound:* fracture where bone protrudes through the skin

- *Partial fracture:* incomplete break in bone
- *Pathological fracture:* fracture caused by disease such as osteoporosis
- *Stress fracture:* small crack in bone due to overuse or repetitive microtrauma

Table 15.4 provides additional information on the classification of common fractures.

Epiphyseal Injury

Epiphyseal injuries or growth plate injuries are traumatic injuries that occur to open epiphyseal plates within the metaphysis of long bones. These injuries are seen in children and adolescents who have not yet experienced closure of the epiphyseal plates and are still growing. These injuries are particularly concerning because trauma to an open growth plate can lead to premature closure, resulting in altered bone length. Epiphyseal injuries are common in children, making up 15% to 30% of all bone injuries in this population. **Salter-Harris fractures** are another name for this type of injury. Dr. Robert Salter and Dr. William Harris first described these growth plate fractures in the *Journal of Bone and Joint Surgery* in 1963. The authors initially described the fractures as types I to V (table 15.5). Later, types VI to IX were added to the literature.

Stress Fracture

Stress fractures, also referred to as hairline fractures, are common injuries in sport. These fractures occur due to overuse and repetitive trauma to bone associated with activities such as running and jumping. Stress fractures are most common in the weight-bearing bones of the lower extremity, but can occur in the spine and upper extremity as well. In general, for lower extremity injury, as ground reaction forces increase, so does the risk of stress fracture. Stress fractures are commonly associated with training errors where the amount or intensity of an

---

FOUNDATIONAL SKILL

Weight-Bearing With Lower Extremity Fractures

Patients suffering fractures of the lower extremity are often limited in weight-bearing during the inflammation and repair phases of bony healing. Athletic trainers are responsible for progressing weight-bearing in these patients as bone healing occurs in order to ensure appropriate bone remodeling. In doing so, athletic trainers often progress patients from non-weight-bearing during the initial weeks after injury to partial weight-bearing as bony healing begins occurring to full weight-bearing as bone healing is complete. This progression in weight-bearing status allows the newly healed bone to remodel as a result of progressively more aggressive compressive forces that occur as the patient places more weight on the involved lower extremity.

TABLE 15.4   **Classification of Common Fractures**

Classification	Illustration	Description
Transverse		Fracture splits perpendicular to the shaft of the bone.
Linear (longitudinal)		Fracture splits down the length of the bone.
Oblique		Fractures have a spiral shape, but they occur when one end of the bone is twisting while the other end of the bone is in a fixed position. Oblique fractures can be displaced or nondisplaced.
Spiral		Fractures have an S-shaped separation and occur when the ends of the bones are twisted in opposite directions.
Greenstick		Fracture is an incomplete break of a bone that has not fully ossified. The fracture resembles a break in a green twig of a tree.
Comminuted		Fracture consists of more than 3 fragments at the fracture site and can be caused by a hard blow or a fall in an awkward position.
Avulsion		Fractures occur when a ligament or tendon pulls off a piece of bone from its attachment site.
Impacted (compression)		Fracture results from a fall from a height that causes the bone to be compressed.
Blow out		Fracture occurs at the orbital wall of the eye.
Serrated		In this fracture, the bony fragments have a sawtooth fracture line.
Stress		Fracture is caused by repetitive microtraumas that exceed the stress-bearing capacity of the bone, leading to a vibratory summation point in the bone.

TABLE 15.5   **Salter-Harris Classifications of Epiphyseal Fractures**

Classification	Illustration	Description
Type I		Complete separation of the physis occurs in relation to the metaphysis, with no fracture to the bone.
Type II		Separation of the growth plate occurs along with a small portion of the metaphysis.
Type III		The physis fractures.
Type IV		Portions of both the physis and metaphysis fracture.
Type V		A crushing force causes a growth deformity without displacing the physis.

activity is increased too rapidly. However, these injuries can also be the result of increased stress on bones due to changes in playing surface, improper footwear, or increased physical activity. Finally, stress fractures have also been linked to the **relative energy deficiency in sports (RED-S)** in female athletes, especially endurance athletes, gymnasts, and performing artists. RED-S includes energy deficiency due to disordered eating, low bone mass, and menstrual disturbances, including amenorrhea and oligomenorrhea.

Signs and symptoms of stress fractures are as follows:

- Pain with activity or weight-bearing
- Pain that diminishes with rest or non-weight-bearing
- Night pain
- Localized point tenderness over bone
- Localized swelling

Apophyseal Injury

Apophyseal injury is unique to adolescent athletes, most commonly occurring between the ages of 8 and 15 years. This overuse injury results in inflammation at the site of tendon insertion onto a growing bony prominence. Apophyseal injuries are most common in highly active, skeletally immature people. This condition most commonly presents as pain and deformity at the origin or insertion of large tendons. Common sites of injury include the following:

- Tibial tuberosity, known as Osgood-Schlatter disease
- Posterior calcaneal tubercle, known as Sever's disease
- Inferior pole of the patella, known as Sinding-Larsen-Johansson syndrome

Causes of apophyseal injury include skeletal immaturity, repetitive microtrauma, muscle–tendon imbalances, improper training programs, and overuse.[21]

Bone Tissue Healing

Bone healing following fracture can involve **primary healing** or **secondary healing**. Primary healing, also known as direct healing, requires anatomical reduction of the fracture site without any gap formation between the injured bone. In primary healing, lamellar bone remodeling occurs, along with formation of the Haversian canal and blood vessels without bony callus. When no gap exists at the fracture site, **contact healing** can occur within 4 weeks of injury or can require years to occur.[22] During contact healing, lamellar bone is oriented longitudinally to the long bone axis, creating a strong repair. If a gap exists, as little as 1 mm in size, at the fracture site, **gap healing** occurs through osteoclasts filling in the gap and lamellar bone orienting perpendicular to the axis of the bone. This repair is much weaker than contact healing and may require up to 8 weeks to occur.[22]

Secondary healing, also known as indirect fracture healing, is the most common type of bone healing. Secondary healing occurs through the use of casting, immobilization, and internal or external fixation of the fracture site (see chapter 24 for casting information). The phases of secondary bone healing are reaction, repair, and remodeling. Table 15.6 describes these phases.

Bone healing can be promoted through the following:

- Proper nutrition
- Meeting dietary recommendations for calcium intake
- Cessation of smoking
- Using augmentation devices for fracture healing, such as electrical stimulation or therapeutic ultrasound[24]

Obstructions (i.e., issues that delay healing) or complications (i.e., abnormal healing) may affect bone healing.

Obstructions
- Poor blood supply, leading to **osteocyte** death
- Poor nutrition that can reduce healing rates
- Infection

TABLE 15.6   Stages of Secondary Healing

	Reaction phase	Repair phase	Remodeling
Description	Inflammation occurs and granulation tissue formation begins.	Cartilage callus formation occurs and lamellar bone deposition takes place.	Original bone contour is regained through remodeling of the fracture site, based on Wolff's law.[23]
Timing	Occurs immediately after fracture and requires approximately 7 days to complete	Occurs during days 7 to 14 after fracture, with callus formation peaking approximately 14 days after fracture	Occurs during week 3 after fracture and may require up to 5 years to complete[22]

- Age, with older adults demonstrating a slower healing rate
- Malalignment of fracture site, disrupting callus formation[25]

Complications

- Infection
- Nonunion, defined as no progression of healing 6 months after fracture
- Malunion
- Improper healing of fracture
- Delayed union[26-28]

Bone Injury Diagnosis

When seeking to identify fractures through clinical examination, you have multiple options available during the assessment process, such as physical examination techniques and clinical imaging tools. Research suggests that a combination of clinical examination techniques and diagnostic imaging tools is the best method for identifying bony injury and assessing healing.[29]

Common signs and symptoms of fracture include the following:

- Pain
- Swelling
- Discoloration
- Deformity
- Crepitus
- Inability to bear weight (for lower extremity injury)
- Loss of function

Although any of these signs or symptoms may lead you to correctly rule in or rule out fracture, evidence suggests that using these examination findings in combination will further improve your diagnostic accuracy.[30,31]

Special tests for fracture include examination techniques that compress or bump or tap injured tissue in order to reproduce pain at the injury site. Additional testing options include using therapeutic ultrasound or tuning forks to vibrate fractured bone, again reproducing pain at the fracture site. Research data regarding these techniques does not support their valid use in diagnosing fracture in patients.[32] The combination of a tuning fork test with a stethoscope placed proximally on the involved bone proved better at ruling in and ruling out long bone fracture, demonstrating a sensitivity of 83%, a specificity of 80%, and a diagnostic accuracy of 81%.[33]

Diagnostic Imaging for Bone Injury

Numerous diagnostic imaging tools are available for identifying bony fractures. Plain radiographs, or X-rays, are most commonly used as the first imaging technique when fracture is suspected. (See chapter 17 for more information on medical imaging.) In cases where fractures are not obvious on X-ray, MRI, computed tomography (CT) scan, and bone scan may be used to make a diagnosis. This is commonly observed in the presence of stress fractures, which often are not observed on X-ray during the first 2 weeks of healing. Musculoskeletal ultrasound, also known as diagnostic ultrasound, is an accurate diagnostic tool for ruling extremity fractures in and out.[34]

When selecting diagnostic imaging for identifying lower extremity stress fracture, conventional radiography is likely to result in false negative findings, especially during the early stages of stress fracture. MRI has been

EVIDENCE-BASED ATHLETIC TRAINING

Forearm Fracture Clinical Prediction Rule

Research suggests that in the presence of a forearm fracture, pain with wrist extension was the most sensitive finding (96%) and ecchymosis was the most specific finding (98%). The authors created a clinical prediction rule for forearm fracture that included the combination of edema, deformity, and pain with forearm pronation. The sensitivity of these three findings in combination was 94%, and the specificity was 51%. These findings suggest that athletic trainers can diagnose forearm fracture without the use of diagnostic imaging in 34% of cases.[31]

EVIDENCE-BASED ATHLETIC TRAINING

Value of the Clinical Examination

Although clinical examination techniques yield appropriate referral for imaging modalities, spine research suggests that clinical examination alone successfully identifies the actual site of fracture in only 62% of cases. Furthermore, clinical examination alone demonstrates a sensitivity of 48% and a specificity of 85% for all fractures of the thoracic and lumbar spine and a sensitivity of 79% and a specificity of 83% for clinically significant fractures.[30]

found to be the most sensitive and specific imaging modality for identifying lower extremity stress fracture.[35]

Bone Injury Management

Fracture management can be either conservative or surgical. Conservative care of fracture consists of closed reduction and either casting or splinting. Closed reduction is necessary in the presence of significantly displaced or angulated fracture. When closed reduction is inadequate, surgical intervention may be required.[36] In cases where healing is delayed or a high risk of **avascular necrosis** is suspected, electrical stimulation may be used as an adjunct to promote fracture healing.[37]

Indications for open reduction and internal fixation of fractures include open fractures, displaced fractures, fractures associated with neurovascular compromise, irreducible fractures, and **pathologic fractures**.[38] Pediatric patients are much more likely to be treated conservatively due to the excellent remodeling potential of pediatric bone.

Nerve Injury

The nerve is the primary structure of the **peripheral nervous system (PNS)**. The nerve is an enclosed bundle of nerve fibers known as an axon. The function of the nerve is to provide sensory and motor input to and from the **central nervous system (CNS)** to the periphery.

Neurons are composed of three main parts (figure 15.5):

1. Dendrites
2. Cell body
3. Axon

Signals are received by the dendrites, travel to the cell body, and are relayed by way of the axon-to-axon

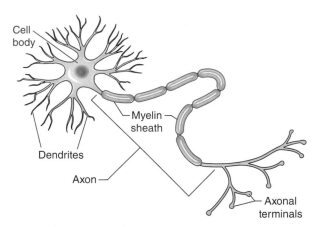

FIGURE 15.5   Structure of a typical neuron.

terminals at the synapse. The synapse is the communication point between two neurons. Neurotransmitters are chemical substances released at the axon terminals when a nerve impulse arrives. Neurotransmitters diffuse across the synapse, causing the transfer of the nerve impulse to another nerve fiber.

Electrochemical nerve impulses are called action potentials and are transmitted along the axon to either peripheral organs or the CNS. Axons are **myelinated** by **Schwann cells** to allow for more rapid transmission of impulses. Within the nerve, each axon is surrounded by a layer of connective tissue called the endoneurium. Axons are bundled together in fascicles. Each fascicle is covered in a layer of connective tissue known as the perineurium. The entire nerve is then covered in a layer of connective tissue known as the epineurium (figure 15.6).

Classification of Nerve Injury

Peripheral nerve injury is classified into three types (table 15.7):

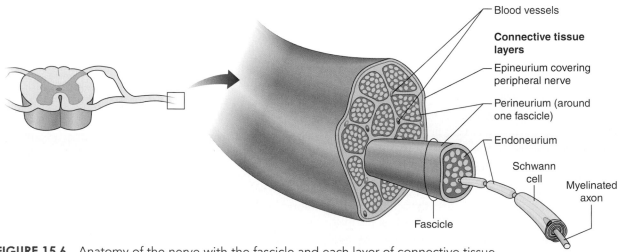

FIGURE 15.6   Anatomy of the nerve with the fascicle and each layer of connective tissue.

TABLE 15.7 **Classes of Nerve Injury**

Class	Description	Recovery time
Neuropraxia	A temporary interruption of conduction within the nerve without Wallerian degeneration	Full recovery within days or weeks[36]
Axonotmesis	Loss of continuity of the axon and its myelin covering or endoneurium	Weeks or months via axonal regeneration without surgical intervention
Neurotmesis	Entire nerve is disrupted or severed.	Recovery requires surgical intervention.

1. *Neuropraxia.* This condition involves a temporary interruption of conduction within the nerve without **Wallerian degeneration**, or loss of axonal continuity. With this condition, there is a physiologic block of nerve conduction within the affected axon. In this injury, all connective tissue coverings of the nerve are intact and conduction proximal to and distal to the injured area is intact. With neuropraxia, no conduction can occur across the injured area. Full recovery from neuropraxia typically occurs within days or weeks.[39] Entrapment injuries, such as carpal tunnel syndrome or tarsal tunnel syndrome, are common examples of neuropraxias.

2. *Axonotmesis.* This condition involves the loss of continuity of the axon and its myelin covering or endoneurium. With axonotmesis, the epineurium and perineurium are both preserved. Wallerian degeneration and sensory and motor deficits occur distal to the site of injury. Recovery typically occurs within weeks or months via axonal regeneration without surgical intervention. Scar tissue formation may interfere with axon regeneration.[39] Axonotmesis commonly occurs due to stretching of the nerve; for example, this is seen in the median or ulnar nerves as a result of posterior elbow dislocation.

3. *Neurotmesis.* With this condition, the entire nerve is disrupted or severed. With neurotmesis, Wallerian degeneration occurs distal to the site of injury. No nerve conduction occurs distal to the lesion. Recovery requires surgical intervention.[39] A clinical example of a neurotmesis is the severing of the brachial plexus secondary to severe trauma to the cervical spine and shoulder.

Nerve Tissue Healing

Nerve regeneration, in the case of neuropraxia and axonotmesis, will occur at a rate of approximately 1 mm per day beginning about 4 weeks after injury occurs. Sensory nerves are more resilient and have better recovery rates than motor nerves. Motor nerves that fail to heal within 24 months are unlikely to heal without surgical intervention.

In cases of neurotmesis, healing will not occur and surgery is needed to repair the severely damaged nerve. With or without surgical intervention, several factors affect nerve repair, including the following:[37,40]

- Regeneration potential of the injured nerve
- Local vascularization
- Scarring at injury site
- Degree of nerve lesion
- Length of nerve defect
- Time to surgical repair (if applicable)
- Patient's age

Nerve Tissue Management

Management following peripheral nerve injury may include nonsurgical or surgical approaches. The key to nonsurgical approaches is to create the ideal environment for nerve healing. This may require reducing edema around the nerve, promoting blood supply to the injured nerve, and preventing or reducing neuroma formation in the area of healing. In the acute stages of nerve injury, therapeutic modalities and medications that reduce inflammation may aid in the creation of these ideal healing environments.[41] In later stages of nerve healing and repair, therapeutic modalities that promote increased blood flow to the injured tissue can be beneficial. The use of iontophoresis to deliver gabapentin, a medication used to treat nerve pathologies, may be useful in prevention or reduction of neuromas at the site of nerve injury.[42]

Diagnostic Testing and Imaging for Nerve Injury

Diagnostic testing for nerve injury can involve nerve conduction velocity (NCV) testing or electromyography (EMG). Nerve conduction velocity assesses abnormal nerve conduction by determining the time required to send a signal along the injured nerve. Decreased nerve conduction velocity indicates nerve injury. Electromyography assesses nerve health by measuring muscular response to nerve stimulation. EMG testing, which can be performed using surface electrodes or needle electrodes, is used to assess for neuromuscular conditions, such as carpal tunnel syndrome, sciatica, **muscular dystrophy**, or **myasthenia gravis**.[43] See chapter 17 for more information on medical imaging.

Diagnostic imaging following nerve injury may include MRI, MSKUS, or CT.[44-46] Research has determined that MSKUS is more sensitive than MRI and just as specific as MRI for detecting peripheral nerve lesions; therefore, it is the preferred diagnostic imaging tool to use in the presence of a suspected peripheral nerve injury.[46]

CLINICAL BOTTOM LINE

- Athletic trainers must have a thorough knowledge of the normal anatomy and physiology of tissue in order to understand pathophysiology and tissue healing following injury.

- Tissue healing times vary based on the type of tissue injured and the severity of the injury.

- Signs and symptoms of various tissue injuries will determine the appropriate treatment interventions employed by the athletic trainer.

- Tissue healing can be accelerated or impeded by a variety of factors. Athletic trainers should provide the ideal state for tissue healing by using appropriate therapeutic interventions throughout the healing and rehabilitation process.

 Go to HK*Propel* to complete the activities and case studies for this chapter.

CHAPTER 16

Clinical Diagnosis and Medical Referral

Ellen K. Payne, PhD, LAT, ATC, EMT

CHAPTER OBJECTIVES

After reading this chapter, you will be able to do the following:

- Define the key terminology used by athletic trainers and other health care providers during the assessment process

- Describe the steps used in the assessment of athletic injuries

- Differentiate the key variances in the assessment process between on-the-field, off-the-field, and medical evaluations

- Describe the need for, and process of, an ongoing assessment for injuries

- Describe the steps in a sideline concussion assessment and the ongoing concussion assessment procedures

- Identify published clinical prediction rules and how they apply to patient assessment

- Recognize the need for referring patients to team physicians and other members of the sports medicine team

- Describe the purpose of patient-based outcome measures and identify measures frequently used in the outpatient orthopedic setting

- Summarize key aspects of both written and oral communication with patients, physicians, and other stakeholders during the assessment process

CAATE STANDARDS

The following CAATE 2020 standards are covered in this chapter:

Standard 39
Standard 40
Standard 45
Standard 50

Athletic trainers are called to complete many different tasks in clinical practice, but the most prevalent are assessment, evaluation, and clinical diagnosis. You must be able to evaluate a multitude of acute and chronic injuries and medical conditions in your day-to-day practice. The **assessment** process varies depending on where the **evaluation** occurs (e.g., on the field, sideline, or athletic training clinic), the nature of the condition (e.g., acute or chronic injury, medical condition, concussion), and what diagnostic equipment is available (e.g., diagnostic imaging, cardiac monitors, glucometers). Accurate clinical diagnosis is key to developing a proper treatment plan and identifying the need for timely referral to other members of the sports medicine team. After completing the initial evaluation, you should perform ongoing assessments to monitor the patient's progress, modify the treatment if necessary, and document outcomes.

The success of the assessment process and accuracy of the evaluation rely on strong foundational knowledge in human anatomy and physiology. This chapter is presented with the assumption that you have had foundational coursework in these areas and understand anatomical and medical terminology. For a more in-depth look at the orthopedic examination process, including region-specific assessments, please refer to *Examination of Musculoskeletal Injuries*.[1]

Clinical Assessment and Diagnosis

Clinical assessment and diagnosis are the cornerstone to athletic training clinical practice. Although there is some variation to the assessment process for on-the-field, off-the-field, orthopedic, and medical evaluations, the same framework can be used to guide the process for each. The general steps for assessment and diagnosis are commonly outlined with the acronym HOPS:

- History
- Observation
- Palpation
- Special tests

This chapter provides a thorough explanation of the HOPS process.

Sometimes the acronyms

- HIT (history, inspection, testing),
- HIPS (history, inspection, palpation, special tests), or
- HOPE (history, observation, palpation, evaluate function)

are also used when describing the process. Whichever acronym is used, the goal is the same: a systematic assessment of the patient to help determine a clinical diagnosis.

During the assessment process, you should gather objective data related to the patient's conditions; this can include goniometer measurements, vital signs, and orthopedic special tests. This information, which is reproducible and independent of the examiner preforming the **examination**, allows you to document patient outcomes from the initial evaluation (**baseline**) until discharge from care and return to activity. Objective data and **outcome measures** are important for reimbursement for services, monitoring patient and clinician goals, and demonstrating the effectiveness of the treatment plan.

Your goal in the assessment process is to do the following:

1. Gather information about a patient's condition or injury.
2. Formulate a **clinical diagnosis**.
3. Identify impairment and functional limitations.
4. Use that information to select the appropriate interventions.

The clinical diagnosis is what you believe the condition or injury to be based on the information obtained during the assessment. Only a physician can use the term *medical diagnosis* when determining a patient's condition or injury, but the clinical diagnosis is similar.

During the assessment process, many conditions and injuries present with similar **signs** and **symptoms**. As you work through the process of determining the clinical diagnosis, you will develop a differential diagnosis. The **differential diagnosis** is all the possible pathologies based on the information provided at that point in the assessment. Often, to proceed from the differential diagnosis to the clinical diagnosis, additional diagnostic tests are needed. The results of these tests (e.g., blood work, radiography, diagnostic ultrasound) will rule out injuries or conditions and allow the athletic trainer and ordering physician to come to the diagnosis.

History

The history component of the assessment is often the most important part for formulating the initial differential

EVIDENCE-BASED ATHLETIC TRAINING

Agreement Between Physicians and Athletic Trainers on Diagnoses

A study published in the journal *Orthopedics* examined the level of agreement on diagnosis between secondary school athletic trainers and physicians.[2] For each case, the athletic trainer's clinical diagnosis was compared with the physician's medical diagnosis. In this study, they agreed on the diagnosis of their patients 92% of the time. Athletic trainers and physicians agreed 100% when it came to evaluating patients with dislocations and 98% of the time when evaluating patients with a concussion. The largest disparity came with the evaluation of meniscal and labral injuries, with agreement on only 71% of the cases. Another area of frequent disagreement in diagnosis between the athletic trainers and physicians was related to fractures, which require radiography for diagnosis. If the athletic trainers in the study had had direct access to imaging, the athletic trainers and physicians may have agreed more frequently on the diagnosis.

diagnosis. Prior to beginning the assessment, you should obtain consent from the patient or the patient's parents or guardians, if available (chapter 5 addresses types of consent). Also consider the sociocultural differences between patients, which are addressed in chapter 4. The information obtained while taking a history will provide a reference to what is normal for that patient and the changes that occurred to bring the patient in for evaluation at this time.

Some key aspects to obtaining a thorough history include the following:

- Ask open-ended questions whenever possible.
- Use active listening skills when the patient responds.
- Document exactly what the patient says, using quotes if possible.

The questions asked during the history component of the assessment will vary depending on the type of condition being assessed (e.g., orthopedic injury, illness, medical condition), the timing of the injury (e.g., **chronic** or **acute**), and the location of the injury (e.g., shoulder, wrist, knee, chest). No matter what is being assessed, you should always ascertain the following:

- **Chief complaint**
- **Mechanism of injury (MOI)** or **nature of illness (NOI)**
- Effect on **activities of daily living (ADLs)**
- Relevant past medical history (PMH or PMHx)
- General health (e.g., family history, medications, general medical conditions that could influence healing)
- Current symptoms
- Onset of symptoms (chronic versus acute)
- Location of the symptoms
- Comparison to the opposite side where applicable

The mnemonic SAMPLE is often used to help obtain basic patient history:

S = signs and symptoms

A = allergies

M = medications

P = past pertinent history

L = last meal

E = events leading up to this

When assessing a possible injury, more specific questions can be asked:

- Relevant sounds or sensations (e.g., snapping or popping sound, feeling of a joint or limb giving out, numbness or tingling, **instability**, weakness)
- Pain scale (0-10; see figure 16.1)
- Referred pain
- Type of pain (e.g., sharp, dull, burning)
- Changes in the signs and symptoms over time
- **Provocation** or **alleviation** of symptoms
- Any treatments already provided (self-treatments or treatments by another health care provider)

The mnemonic OPQRST is often used when assessing a patient's pain:

O = onset

P = provocation or **palliation**

Q = quality of the pain

R = region or radiation

S = severity

T = time (history)

Answers to the questions asked during the history portion of the assessment may lead to additional follow-up questions that are more specific. After taking a complete history, you should be able to develop a list of

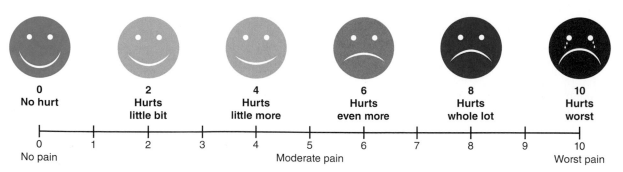

FIGURE 16.1 Example of a pain scale.

potential differential diagnoses to help guide the rest of the assessment.

Observation

The next step in the assessment is observation of the patient and the injured area. Experienced athletic trainers often conduct this step during the history component. Observation of the patient begins as you approach the patient on the field or as the patient walks off the field or enters the clinic. During the initial observations, you will form a general impression of the patient and the situation. Initial observations will often help you determine if you are dealing with a potential emergency. During nonemergent situations, observation continues as the patient removes equipment or clothing to prepare for the examination. In general, watch the patient's gait (e.g., **antalgic gait**) and extremities for **bilateral**, symmetrical movements. You should observe the patient's facial expressions during movement and any muscle guarding or abnormal positioning of the patient. As the observation process continues, look for the following:

- Deformity
- Swelling
- **Ecchymosis**
- Wounds (e.g., abrasion, laceration, avulsion)
- Signs of infection
- Signs of previous surgery (e.g., scars)
- Bilateral symmetry

The mnemonic DCAP-BTLS, used in EMS during the rapid trauma assessment, can also be helpful during the observation process:

D = deformities and discolorations

C = contusions

A = abrasion and avulsions

P = penetrations and punctures

B = burns

T = tenderness and temperature

L = lacerations

S = swelling and symmetry

Findings from the observation process may lead to additional follow-up questions for the patient. For example, you should follow up on any scars you observe that the patient did not mention during the history component.

Palpation

The third step in the assessment is palpation, which is not as stressed in the evaluation process as history and

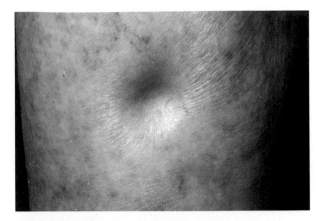

FIGURE 16.2 Pitting edema.
Dr P. Marazzi / Science Source

special tests, but is still a very important component of the process.[3] If you have not already obtained consent to touch the patient, ask permission now. Palpation is a systematic process and should always be conducted bilaterally. Developing a routine for palpations is important so that no structures are missed. While becoming more comfortable with the palpation process, you may want to start with the bony structures or prominences and then move on to the soft tissue in the area so as not to miss any structures. Palpation of internal organs of the abdomen and thorax are also completed during some injuries, but the technique to palpate them is addressed in chapter 18 with the general medical conditions. During the palpation process, you will be identifying pertinent anatomical structures and feeling for the following:

- **Point tenderness**
- **Trigger points**
- Changes in tissue density (e.g., **pitting edema** [figure 16.2], **hemorrhage**)
- **Crepitus**
- Temperature change
- Bilateral symmetry

Observe the patient's facial expressions during palpations for signs of pain or discomfort. Findings during the palpation process may lead to additional follow-up questions for the patient. For example, you should ask follow-up questions about any painful responses elicited during palpation.

Special Tests

In the HOPS acronym, the *S* means "special tests." This category is broken down into several components:

- Range of motion
- Joint stability and ligamentous tests

FOUNDATIONAL SKILL

General Procedures for Palpation

1. Obtain consent to touch the patient and explain to him what is going to happen.
2. Remove equipment or bulky clothing to expose the area, but make sure to drape the patient to protect his privacy as needed.
3. Palpate the uninjured side first so the patient can become accustomed to the palpation process.
4. Start with soft pressure and gradually increase as needed.
5. Make all contact deliberate.
6. When palpating the injured side, start away from the painful site and injured structures and move toward the injured area last.
7. Approach palpation systematically.
8. While palpating the patient, watch his face for any signs of pain or discomfort.

- Selective tissue tests
- Neurovascular assessment

At this point in the assessment, you should have a general idea of the possible injury or injuries present and should be able to formulate a differential diagnosis. This allows you to select the pertinent tests and tailor the tests performed to help rule in or out a possible diagnosis. Orthopedic special tests are unique to each joint or area. There are many to choose from when completing an assessment. The selection of a special test should be based on the test's accuracy and reliability.

Range of Motion

In some patients, a range of motion (ROM) baseline is established during their preparticipation examination. If this information is available, you can refer to it during the injury assessment. If measurements have not been assessed prior to injury, you can compare assessment results of the injured area with those from the opposite extremity or with published normative data for the population. Examine any abnormal findings from ROM assessment further. For example, if pain is produced during ROM, ask the patient to describe the pain felt. Observe the patient's facial expressions during ROM testing for signs of pain or discomfort. ROM is typically assessed during the initial evaluation of the injury, throughout the rehabilitation process, and prior to return to play (RTP) to help determine the patient's readiness to return to activity.

Three types of ROM assessment are done during the assessment:

1. Active ROM (AROM)
2. Passive ROM (PROM)
3. Resistive ROM (RROM)

Active Range of Motion (AROM)

AROM is completed first when assessing a patient's ability to move. During this step in the assessment, the patient moves the area being evaluated of her own accord and without assistance. This allows you to assess the **osteokinematics** of the joint. AROM should be assessed throughout the full ROM whenever possible. AROM allows you to assess the patient's willingness to move, coordination, and general muscle trength.[4] Obvious fracture or dislocations are **contraindications** for performing AROM. If the patient cannot complete AROM, she should not be asked to do RROM. If a patient cannot complete the full ROM, it may be due to pain, muscle weakness, or a structural problem within the joint blocking the range of motion.

Passive Range of Motion (PROM)

During PROM, you will move the patient through the full ROM with no effort from the patient during movement. Pay special attention to the quality of the **end feel**, or resistance at the end range of motion. Normal end feels occur at the anticipated end ROM. They are often described as soft, firm, or hard and are dependent on the type of tissue involved. Identifying end feel allows you to assess the **arthrokinematics** of the joint. For example, passive knee flexion ends in a soft end feel since the muscles of the hamstrings and gastrocsoleus complex are contacting each other and preventing further ROM. An abnormal end feel can indicate pathology to the tissue or joint. Table 16.1 provides examples of normal and abnormal end feels.

During PROM (and sometimes AROM), you can use a **goniometer** (figure 16.3) to obtain objective measurements (in degrees), which are more accurate than visual estimates.[5] Table 16.2 provides normal range of motion

TABLE 16.1 **Joint End Feels**

	Description	Example
Normal end feels		
Hard	An unyielding, abrupt sensation that is painless; bone to bone	Elbow extension
Soft	Soft, painless compression at the end ROM	Elbow flexion, knee flexion
Firm	Elastic with a slight give, stretch; abrupt	Forearm supination
Abnormal end feels		
Hard or bony	Hard, unyielding, possibly painful end feel when not expected (sooner or later in ROM than usual or when soft or firm end feel is normal); bony grating or bony block	Malunion fracture, osteophytes
Firm	Firm stretch when not expected (sooner or later in ROM than usual or when soft or hard end feel is normal)	Capsular, muscular, ligamentous, or fascial shortening
Soft or boggy	Soft or boggy end feel when not expected (sooner or later in ROM than usual or when firm or hard end feel is normal)	Edema, synovitis
Empty	No physical restriction in movement; movement beyond anatomical limit; pain prevents full ROM	Inflammation, bursitis, fracture, complete ligament rupture

Based on Shultz, Houglum, and Perrin (2016); Norkin and White (2009).

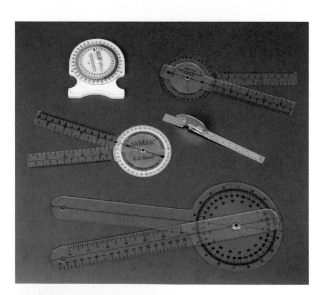

FIGURE 16.3 Goniometers.

information for select joints. During this time, you can determine if the patient has **hypomobility** or **hypermobility** when compared bilaterally or with the normative values for patients of the same age and gender.

Resistive Range of Motion (RROM)

The final step in ROM assessment is RROM, or strength testing. Here, you will provide resistance against a certain movement in order to assess the strength of the muscle or muscle group. Again, RROM is contraindicated if the patient cannot perform AROM or if a fracture or dislocation is suspected. Pain, or the fear of pain, can influence the results of strength testing, so you should document if either occurs during the assessment. The purposes for assessing muscle strength are the following:

- Assess strength, power, or endurance of the muscle or muscle group
- Identify functional impairment within specific muscles or muscle groups
- Provide feedback to aid in the rehabilitation plan or intervention selection
- Determining a patient's readiness to RTP

Depending on the patient and the goals of the assessment, RROM can be completed in various ways:

- Isolating individual muscles
- Assessing gross strength within a single plane

TABLE 16.2 **Range of Motion**

	Degrees		Degrees
Shoulder movement			
Flexion	150-180	Extension	50-60
Abduction	170-180	Adduction	45
Horizontal abduction	30-45	Horizontal adduction	90-135
Internal rotation	70-90	External rotation	60-90
Elbow movement			
Flexion	135-160	Extension	−5-0
Forearm movement			
Supination	75-90	Pronation	75-90
Wrist movement			
Flexion	60-80	Extension	60-70
Ulnar deviation	30	Radial deviation	20
Metacarpophalangeal movement			
Flexion	90	Extension	30-45
Abduction (fingers)	20	Adduction (thumb)	70
Hip movement			
Flexion	90-135	Extension	10-30
Abduction	25-50	Adduction	10-30
Internal rotation	20-45	External rotation	30-45
Knee movement			
Flexion	110-145	Extension	−10-0
Internal rotation	10	External rotation	10
Ankle movement			
Dorsiflexion	10-20	Plantarflexion	30-50
Inversion	10-30	Eversion	10-30
First metatarsophalangeal movement			
Flexion	45	Extension	70-90
Neck or cervical spine movement			
Flexion	45-60	Extension	45-75
Lateral flexion	45	Rotation	60-80
Trunk movement			
Flexion	120-150	Extension	20-45
Lateral flexion	10-35	Rotation	20-45

Based on Pescatello (2014); Norkin and White (2009): Hoppenfeld (1976); Comana (2010).

- Taking objective measurements with additional equipment
- Completing functional activity assessment

When assessing RROM, the uninvolved side should be assessed first and can be used as a comparison. However, in some instances, doing both limbs simultaneously will allow for a side-by-side strength comparison. RROM is traditionally graded on a scale of 0 to 5 (table 16.3).

Strength can be assessed through the entire ROM or as a **break test** (i.e., **isometric contraction**). Break tests are often used to quickly assess gross strength or during the neurological assessment. Break tests are usually completed with the joint being tested in the mid-range.

FOUNDATIONAL SKILL

General Procedures for Taking Goniometric Measurements

1. The patient should be in a position as close to **anatomical position** (figure 16.4) as possible to allow for the correct starting position at zero. This may involve the patient lying supine or prone, along with various seated positions. Use the same patient positioning each time you take a measurement to allow for reliable results (as documented in the patient's chart).

2. Explain the procedure and demonstrate the motion that is going to be measured. Whenever possible, the same athletic trainer should assess the patient's movement to increase the reliability of the results.

3. Ask the patient to actively complete the motion so you can gauge the amount of movement.

4. Because motion should be isolated to the joint that is being measured, stabilize the proximal segment of the joint to prevent accessory motion.

5. Proper alignment of the goniometer is key. Carefully position the goniometer to accurately measure the joint motion. Align the fulcrum with the joint axis and place the arms in the correct position with the corresponding landmarks for each measurement.

6. Do not press the goniometer against the body during the measurement.

7. When reading the goniometer, move to take the reading at eye level.

8. Take the first reading at the starting position and record it.

9. Remove the goniometer and assess range motion (either actively or passively).

10. Realign the goniometer with the landmarks and retake the measurement.

11. Repeat this process three times and calculate the average.

12. Record the average measurement.

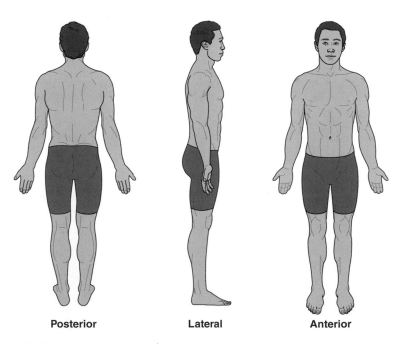

Posterior   Lateral   Anterior

FIGURE 16.4 Anatomical position.

TABLE 16.3 **Muscle Strength Grading Scale**

Grade	Contraction strength	Description
0	None	No visible or palpable contraction
1	Trace	Visible or palpable contraction with no motion
2	Poor	Full ROM gravity eliminated
3	Fair	Full ROM against gravity
4	Good	Full ROM against gravity, moderate resistance
5	Normal	Full ROM against gravity, maximal resistance

Instruct the patient not to move, then position her and stabilize the proximal segment. Next, you will progressively increase the resistance applied in an attempt to break the patient's position. The patient must receive at least a 3 out of 5 on the muscle strength grading scale (be able to hold the test position) to complete a break test.

Strength can also be assessed through the full ROM. This involves asking the patient to move the joint against resistance in one plane. You will apply resistance as the patient completes the full ROM, adjusting the amount of force used to meet the strength of the patient. During this type of strength testing, apply the maximum amount of resistance that still allows the patient to move. This type of strength assessment may be of increased importance if the patient is unable to hold a break test and further assessment of strength is needed. The term *manual muscle test (MMT)* is also used when discussing strength assessment. MMTs are generally done to assess specific muscles or muscle groups within their functional plane of motion, with an attempt to isolate accessory muscles that help perform the motion. Specific attention is paid to patient positioning, stabilization of the area, and movement patterns. The terms *MMT* and *RROM* are often used synonymously, and both are graded on the 0 to 5 muscle strength grading scale.

All of the assessment techniques presented allow for subjective measurement and grading of the patient's strength, which can vary greatly by examiner. To obtain objective measurements of strength, you can use a variety of devices. These devices are typically limited to use in the clinic and are not readily available during on-field evaluations. These devices can assess **isotonic, isometric**, or **isokinetic** strength or contractions (**concentric** and **eccentric contractions**), depending on the device selected.

- The measurement of isotonic strength is done with a dumbbell, barbells, and other equipment to test the patient's strength through the ROM. This allows for a more functional strength test than isometric or isokinetic testing. Examples of this type of test include 1-repetition max or 10-repetition max tests.

- An example of an isometric strength device is a grip dynamometer (figure 16.5), which measures grip strength.
- Isokinetic testing measures maximal force against a fixed velocity. This type of assessment is frequently used when assessing quadriceps and hamstring strength when determining a patient's readiness to RTP after ACL surgery. The Biodex machine (figure 16.6) is an example of an isokinetic machine.

Joint Stability and Ligamentous Tests

During this portion of the assessment, you will be assessing noncontractile tissue, including ligaments and the joint capsule for **laxity** and instability. You can also assess joint play. This involves assessing the joint motion while providing a gliding or distraction force and then

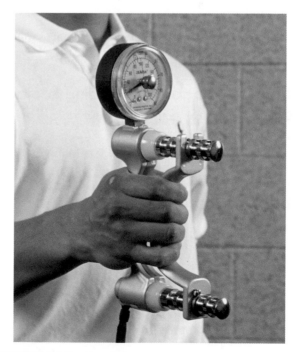

FIGURE 16.5 Hand dynamometer.

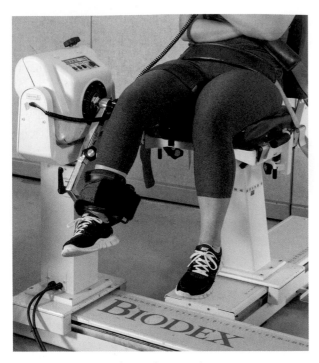

FIGURE 16.6   Biodex isokinetic dynamometer.

comparing the results bilaterally. A joint can be described as hypomobile or hypermobile, which does not always mean the joint is unstable.

During the ligamentous stress tests, you will be assessing the end feel of the joint and attempting to stress the ligament and capsule. Pain may or may not present with a positive test. Ligamentous end feels can be described as the following:

• *Firm.* A normal, nonpathological finding would be a firm end feel. This signifies that the capsule

or ligament stabilizing the joint is intact and preventing additional motion.

• *Soft.* A soft end feel can mean stretching of the tissue being tested. This is laxity, the positive sign for a ligament sprain.

• *Empty.* An empty end feel indicates a complete rupture of the ligament or a third degree sprain.

Ligamentous stress tests are compared bilaterally and are graded based on the severity of the tissue damaged (table 16.4).

Selective Tissue Tests

Tests done in this portion of the examination are specific and unique to the joint, body region, or structures being assessed. At this point in the assessment, you should have the differential diagnosis narrowed down and be able to select the pertinent test that will either help rule in or out a specific diagnosis. As stated previously, you should select which tests to perform based on their accuracy and reliability. No test is perfect, and often multiple tests need to be performed to best determine the pathology.[9] Compare tests bilaterally. Depending on the test, a positive finding could be provocation of the symptoms or alleviation of the symptoms. These tests include those for fractures, meniscus and labral tears, and disc injury, among others. If there is a possibility of injuring it, there is probably a special test for it.

Neurovascular Assessment

Neurovascular assessment helps identify nerve and vascular damage from injury and various diseases and conditions. It can be further divided into a neurological assessment and a vascular assessment. This portion of the

TABLE 16.4   **Ligament Grading Scale**

Grade	Physical examination findings	Pathophysiology	Impairment
1	Minimal swelling Minimal tenderness to palpation Firm end feel No laxity	Microscopic collagen fiber tears, stretch of ligament	Minimal
2	Moderate swelling Moderate tenderness to palpation Decreased ROM Soft end feel Laxity Possible instability	Tear of some, but not all, of the ligament	Moderate
3	Significant swelling Significant pain with palpation Empty end feel Laxity Instability	Complete tear or rupture of the ligament	Severe

assessment may be done earlier in the process, depending on how the patient presents. For example, if a possible fracture is suspected, distal circulation, movement, and sensation are assessed very early in the process to determine the severity of the injury and the need to activate the emergency action plan (EAP).

Neurological Assessment

The neurological assessment identifies nerve root impingement, peripheral nerve damage, central nervous system (CNS) damage, and other pathology. You do not need to perform a complete neurological assessment on every patient, but you should do one whenever the patient complains of radiating pain, burning pain, numbness, tingling, weakness, paralysis, or other symptoms that are associated with neurological conditions. Pay special attention to bilateral symptoms, which may be the result of CNS damage. The neurological assessment can include upper and lower quarter screens, cranial nerves, and peripheral nerve sensory distribution patterns.

The upper and lower quarter screens are further divided into sensory testing, motor testing, and reflexes. Sensory testing is completed by assessing dermatomes. **Dermatomes** (figure 16.7) involve an area of skin inner-

vated by a spinal nerve root. These follow a specific sensory pattern on the body. This should be assessed bilaterally, starting with the uninjured side. While assessing dermatomes, instruct the patient to look away from the area being assessed. There are different ways to assess sensation within a dermatome, including two-point discrimination, sharp and dull discrimination, and general sensation (e.g., "Can you feel this?"). Abnormal findings include **hyperesthesia**, **hypoesthesia**, **paresthesia**, or **anesthesia**.

Motor testing is the next component of the upper and lower quarter screens. It tests the strength of a muscle innervated by a specific nerve root or **myotome** (table 16.5). This is done with a break test (isometric contraction) held for 6 to 8 seconds. If you note muscle weakness during this portion of the assessment, test another muscle innervated by the same nerve root. If one muscle is weak, peripheral nerve pathology or muscle pathology should be suspected. If both muscles are weak, nerve root or peripheral nerve pathology should be suspected.

The last component of the quarter screens is deep tendon reflex testing, which involves an involuntary response to stimuli. **Reflexes** should be conducted with the patient looking away from the area and must

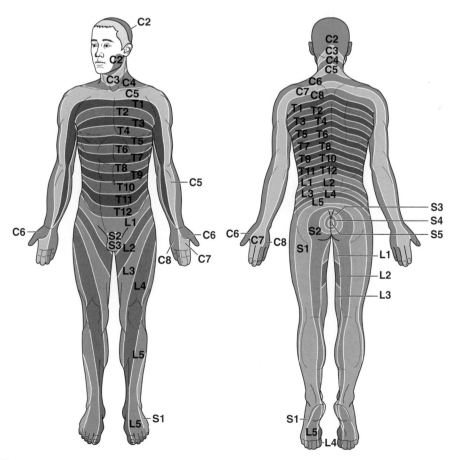

FIGURE 16.7 Dermatome map.

TABLE 16.5 **Myotomes**

Upper extremity myotomes	Nerve root	Lower extremity myotomes	Nerve root
Shoulder shrug	C4	Hip flexion	L1, L2
Shoulder abduction	C5	Knee extension	L3
Elbow flexion Wrist extension	C6	Ankle dorsiflexion	L4
Elbow extension Wrist flexion	C7	Great toe extension	L5
Opposition	C8	Ankle plantarflexion Ankle eversion Hip extension	S1
Finger abduction	T1	Knee flexion	S2

be compared bilaterally. If a patient is unable to relax during this portion of the screen, you can perform the Jendrassik maneuver to help elicit a response.[10] When testing a lower extremity reflex with the Jendrassik maneuver, ask the patient to pull apart her clasped hands (figure 16.8). During an upper extremity reflex test, ask the patient to press her feet together. Alternatively, you can ask the patient to clench her jaw. Reflexes are graded on a 4-point scale (table 16.6). Commonly assessed deep tendon reflexes are presented in table 16.7.

TABLE 16.6 **Reflex Grading Scale**

Grade	Description
0	No response
1+	Hyporeflexia: diminished response, low normal
2+	Average: normal response
3+	Hyperreflexia: brisker than average
4+	Hyperactive: very brisk, with **clonus**

TABLE 16.7 **Commonly Assessed Deep Tendon Reflexes**

Upper extremity reflexes	Nerve root	Lower extremity reflexes	Nerve root
Biceps	C5, C6	Patellar	L2-L4
Brachioradialis	C6	Achilles	S1
Triceps	C7		

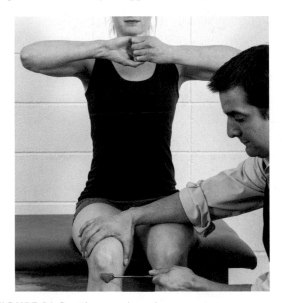

FIGURE 16.8 The Jendrassik maneuver.

FOUNDATIONAL SKILL

How to Assess a Deep Tendon Reflex

1. Make sure the limb is in the correct position and relaxed.
2. Locate the tendon through palpation (ask the patient to contract the associated muscle if needed to help locate the tendon, but make sure he is relaxed when assessing the reflex).
3. Tap the tendon lightly.
4. If you have not already obtained an adequate response, have the patient perform the associated Jendrassik maneuver and try again.
5. Perform reflex testing bilaterally.
6. Document the grade of the reflex.

Cranial nerves are frequently assessed when the patient has potential head, eye, or facial injuries, such as concussion or facial fracture. Table 16.8 outlines the 12 cranial nerves and their functions. If a deficiency is found, it could be a sign of a serious head injury, so the EAP should be activated and the patient should be immediately referred.

Peripheral nerve sensory distribution patterns should also be assessed if the patient presents with neurological symptoms. Figure 16.9 shows the anterior and posterior views of the nerve distributions.

Vascular Assessment

Vascular assessment includes both systemic (e.g., carotid, femoral) and peripheral (e.g., radial, posterior tibialis) pulses and capillary refill. This assessment may be completed much earlier in the overall process, when symptoms warrant (e.g., fractures, dislocations) or the patient's pulse may not be assessed at all. Chapter 14 addresses how to take a pulse and capillary refill with the emergency assessment and vital signs. If pulses are absent or weak, you may need to activate the EAP. A slow or delayed capillary refill can indicate poor circulation to the distal aspect of the extremity.

Additional Assessment Components

The previously mentioned components outline the steps conducted during the majority of patient evaluations. Other components are often added to the assessment to help determine the clinical diagnosis and treatment plan. This includes assessment of related areas, vital signs, gait analysis, posture screening, and functional testing. The following sections outline these components.

Assessment of Related Areas

Frequently, you will need to assess the area above or below the injured site to rule out injuries or conditions that are part of the differential diagnosis. This is because pain in one area is often actually referred from another place. For example, a patient who presents with shoulder pain with no MOI and no findings on the physical examination should be questioned about general health, medications, and other signs and symptoms because the shoulder is a referred pain area for cardiac-related events. Another less serious example is patella femoral pain. In this case, the patient should also have her ankles, hips, and posture and

TABLE 16.8 Cranial Nerves

Number	Name	Composition	Function
I	Olfactory	Sensory	Smell
II	Optic	Sensory	Vision
III	Oculomotor	Motor	Pupil reaction and size Elevation of upper eyelid Eye adduction and downward rolling
IV	Trochlear	Motor	Upward eye rolling
V	Trigeminal	Mixed	Motor: mastication Sensory: areas of the face, including the forehead, temple, nose, lips, tongue, and jaw
VI	Abducens	Motor	Lateral eye movement
VII	Facial	Mixed	Motor: facial muscles Sensory: taste
VIII	Vestibulocochlear	Sensory	Hearing and equilibrium
IX	Glossopharyngeal	Mixed	Motor: pharyngeal muscles (swallowing) Sensory: taste
X	Vagus	Mixed	Motor: muscles of the pharynx and larynx; parasympathetic control of the heart, lungs, and digestive tract Sensory: gag reflex, internal organs
XI	Accessory	Motor	Trapezius and sternocleidomastoid muscles
XII	Hypoglossal	Motor	Tongue movement

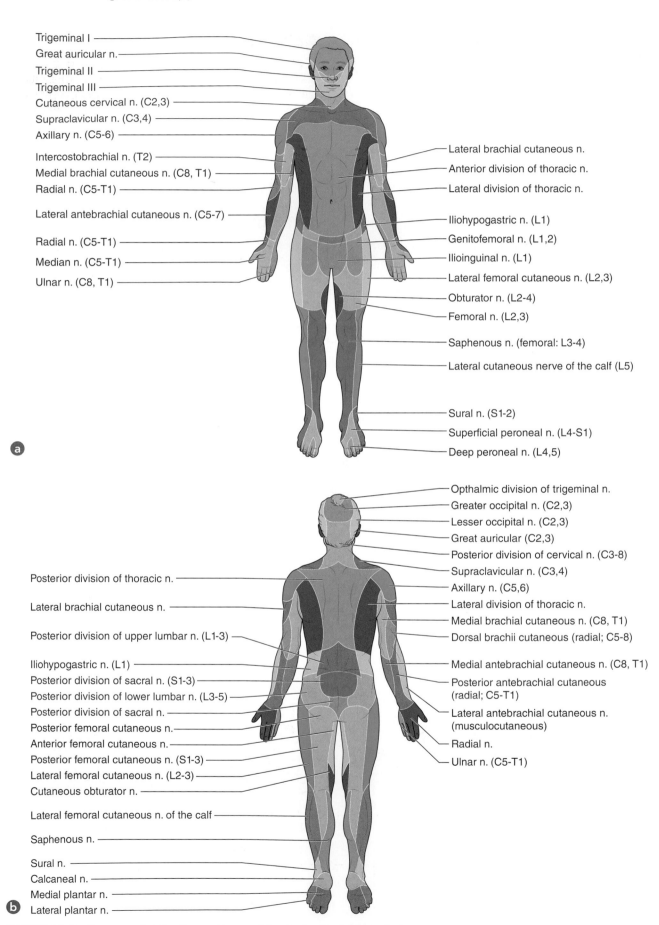

Trigeminal I
Great auricular n.
Trigeminal II
Trigeminal III
Cutaneous cervical n. (C2,3)
Supraclavicular n. (C3,4)
Axillary n. (C5-6)
Intercostobrachial n. (T2)
Medial brachial cutaneous n. (C8, T1)
Radial n. (C5-T1)
Lateral antebrachial cutaneous n. (C5-7)
Radial n. (C5-T1)
Median n. (C5-T1)
Ulnar n. (C8, T1)

Lateral brachial cutaneous n.
Anterior division of thoracic n.
Lateral division of thoracic n.
Iliohypogastric n. (L1)
Genitofemoral n. (L1,2)
Ilioinguinal n. (L1)
Lateral femoral cutaneous n. (L2,3)
Obturator n. (L2-4)
Femoral n. (L2,3)
Saphenous n. (femoral: L3-4)
Lateral cutaneous nerve of the calf (L5)
Sural n. (S1-2)
Superficial peroneal n. (L4-S1)
Deep peroneal n. (L4,5)

a

Posterior division of thoracic n.
Lateral brachial cutaneous n.
Posterior division of upper lumbar n. (L1-3)
Iliohypogastric n. (L1)
Posterior division of sacral n. (S1-3)
Posterior division of lower lumbar n. (L3-5)
Posterior division of sacral n.
Posterior femoral cutaneous n.
Anterior femoral cutaneous n.
Posterior femoral cutaneous n. (S1-3)
Lateral femoral cutaneous n. (L2-3)
Cutaneous obturator n.
Lateral femoral cutaneous n. of the calf
Saphenous n.
Sural n.
Calcaneal n.
Medial plantar n.
b Lateral plantar n.

Opthalmic division of trigeminal n.
Greater occipital n. (C2,3)
Lesser occipital n. (C2,3)
Great auricular (C2,3)
Posterior division of cervical n. (C3-8)
Supraclavicular n. (C3,4)
Axillary n. (C5,6)
Lateral division of thoracic n.
Medial brachial cutaneous n. (C8, T1)
Dorsal brachii cutaneous (radial; C5-8)
Medial antebrachial cutaneous n. (C8, T1)
Posterior antebrachial cutaneous (radial; C5-T1)
Lateral antebrachial cutaneous n. (musculocutaneous)
Radial n.
Ulnar n. (C5-T1)

FIGURE 16.9 Sensory distribution patterns: *(a)* anterior and *(b)* posterior.

gait assessed due to the many factors that can contribute to patella femoral pain.

Vital Signs

Vital signs (also addressed in chapter 14 for emergency assessments) are also often part of the standard assessment. This is beyond the assessment of neurovascular status addressed previously, especially during the assessment of medical conditions. Vitals signs include pulse, respiration, blood pressure, temperature, skin color, pupil reaction, and pulse oximetry.

Gait Analysis

The patient's gait is observed informally during most potential lower extremity or low back injuries where the patient can still walk. As stated before, observation of the patient begins as he walks into the clinic. Other times a more systematic assessment of the patient's gait may be warranted. You need to be familiar with both the walking and running gait cycles, what occurs during each phase of the cycle, and commonly observed variations. The details of each phase are beyond the scope of this text, but figure 16.10 reviews the phases.

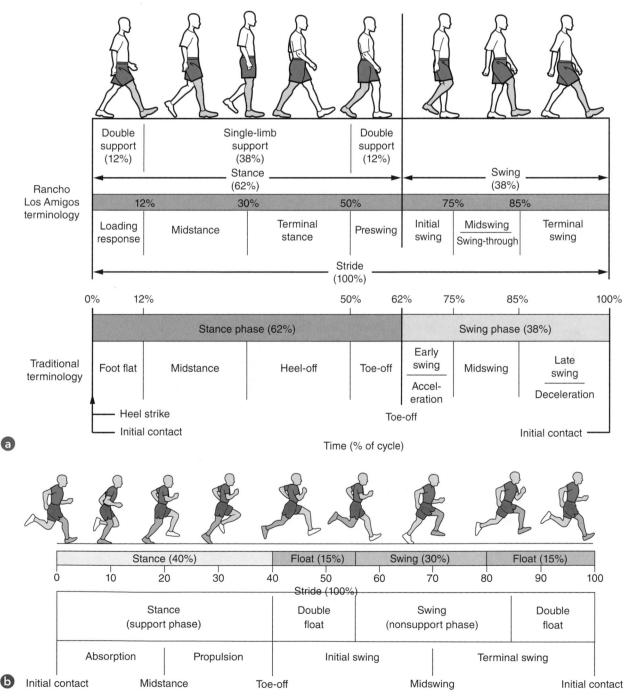

FIGURE 16.10 The phases of gait: (a) walking and (b) running.

When a detailed assessment of a patient's gait is warranted, it should be done systematically. It is helpful to use a gait analysis tool, or check sheet, such as the one in figure 16.11. Start with a general, overall observation of the patient's gait from anterior, posterior, and lateral aspects of the patient. You should observe for bilateral

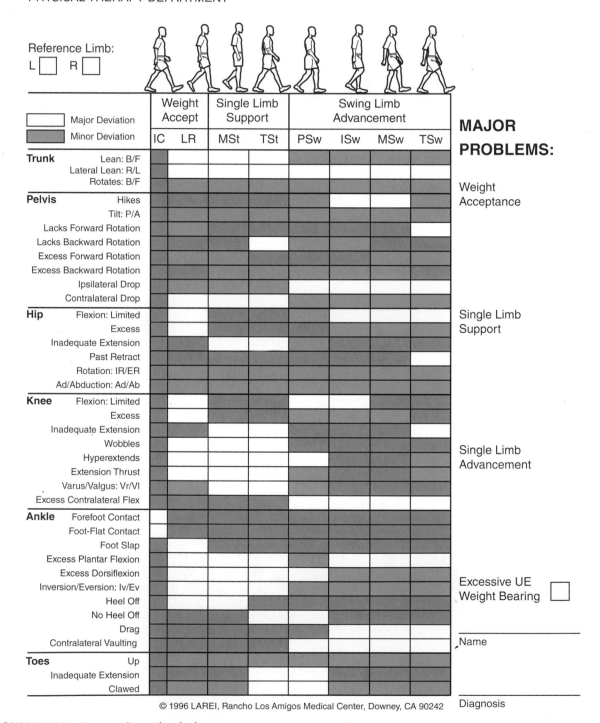

FIGURE 16.11 Gait analysis check sheet.

Reprinted by permission from Rancho Research Institute, *Observational Gait Analysis* (Downey, CA: Rancho Research Institute).

symmetry, rhythm and rate of gait, and stride length. Also observe the trunk and upper extremities for movement patterns. After the general observation of the patient's gait, focus on one leg at a time and one joint at a time, systematically working down the extremity. Again, do this from all three aspects to allow for a complete view of the patient's gait. You should document your findings on the check sheet.

Postural Screening

A postural screening is completed with the patient standing and wearing as few items of clothing as possible to allow for a better view of important landmarks. Assess posture from the anterior, posterior, and lateral aspects to get a full view of the patient and any abnormal aspects of her posture. When possible, use a plumb line (figure 16.12) for a reference point during an assessment. You should record postural deviations as mild, moderate, severe, or within normal limits (WNL) and compare deviation bilaterally. Postural screening is important after an injury that could alter the patient's posture (e.g., knee injury) or when assessing chronic conditions where poor posture could be the reason for the patient's pain and dysfunction (e.g., low back pain). Figure 16.13 provides a checklist of normal posture.

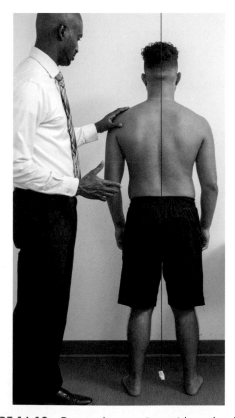

FIGURE 16.12   Postural screening with a plumb line.

Functional Testing

Functional testing determines if a patient is ready to return to activity. During the initial assessment of minor injuries where return to activity the same day is possible, this is an important step that should not be overlooked. For more severe injuries, functional exercises become part of the later stage of the rehabilitation process and are ultimately used to see if the patient is ready to return to sport, activity, or work. These activities should be progressive in nature, starting with generalized tests and progressing to those that are more specific. These tests should mimic activities and movements required in that patient's sport or activity whenever possible. This type of testing is very individualized to the patient and the injury he is returning from. This is one of the reasons you need to have a good working knowledge of different sports (and position requirements within the sport), activities, and job requirements. Functional tests should assess the patient's ability to move through the full ROM, strength to protect himself, confidence, and general readiness to return to activity. Chapter 19 explores the psychosocial aspect of return to play.

Examples of functional tests for the lower extremity include the following:

- Running forward and backward
- Dribbling a soccer ball
- Running a play pattern
- Doing other sport-specific drills

Examples of functional tests for the upper extremity include the following:

- Throwing a ball
- Catching a ball
- Pushing and pulling exercises
- Doing other sport-specific drills

Variations in the Assessment Process

The previous information outlines the components of the assessment process for most injuries or conditions presented in the athletic training setting. That said, every assessment is different and should be individualized to the patient's needs. The order of the process can vary based on how the patient initially presents or as findings warrant additional investigation. The assessment process will also be different based on where the assessment is occurring (e.g., on the field, on the sideline, or in the athletic training clinic). The following sections address common variations to the assessment process.

FIGURE 16.13 Postural assessment checklist.

Anterior View

☐ Overall body symmetry: symmetrical alignment of the left and right sides

☐ Feet and ankles: The medial malleoli should be level. The feet should turn out slightly from midline.

☐ Knees: There should be equal distance between the knees, and the tibias should be straight with no signs of rotation. The patella should face forward and be level.

☐ Thighs: There should be equal distance between the thighs, and the femurs should be straight with no signs of rotation. The muscle bulk should be equal on both sides.

☐ Torso: The plumb line should be through the center of the sternum, umbilicus, and bisect the pelvis and pubic symphysis. The ASIS should be level.

☐ Shoulders: Shoulders should be approximately level (although the dominate side may be lower) and the clavicles should be level.

☐ Head: The head should face forward with no rotation or lateral flexion.

Posterior View

☐ Overall body symmetry: symmetrical alignment of the left and right sides.

☐ Feet and ankles: The medial and lateral malleoli should be level. The Achilles tendons should be straight. The calcaneus should be vertical.

☐ Knees: The legs should be straight with no genu varum or genu valgum.

☐ Thighs: The greater trochanters and the gluteal folds should be level.

☐ Torso: The plumb line should be midline on all vertebrae with no curvature to the left or right. The rib cage should be symmetrical. The PSIS should be equal distance from the center and be level.

☐ Shoulders: There should be equal distance between the borders of the scapula with no signs of winging. The shoulders should be approximately level (although the dominate side may be lower).

☐ Head and neck: The head should face forward with no rotation or lateral flexion.

Lateral View

☐ Overall body symmetry: symmetrical alignment of load-bearing joint landmarks with the plumb line.

☐ Knees: There should be no flexion or hyperextension.

☐ Pelvis: The ASIS and PSIS should be on the same plane. The gluteal muscle bulk should be equal on both sides.

☐ Spinal curves: The cervical spine should have a lordotic curve, the thoracic spine should have a kyphotic curve, and the lumbar spine should have a lordotic curve. None of these should be overly exaggerated.

☐ Shoulders: The plumb line should go through the AC joint. The shoulders should not be rounded forward.

☐ Head: The head should be positioned over the body, not forward or back.

On-the-Field Injury Assessment

When assessing a potential injury on the field, court, or anywhere the injury occurred, you must start with a primary survey including the ABCs (airway, breathing, circulation), followed by the treatment of any life-threatening conditions. You may decide to activate the EAP and call EMS at this point or at any point in the assessment deemed necessary based on the severity of the injury and if the patient is presenting with signs of shock. After the primary survey, move on to the secondary assessment, which can include a head-to-toe examination and the taking of vital signs, if warranted. Chapter 14 addresses primary and secondary assessments, moving and transporting the patient, and the immediate management of life-threatening conditions in detail.

If the patient is conscious and the injury is not life threatening, you will likely modify the assessment to allow for a quick yet thorough on-field examination of the injury prior to making decisions about moving the patient for further assessment or transport from the current location. This is determined based on the severity of the injury. You may check the neurovascular status of the patient, palpate for additional injuries, assess the patient's ability to move, and perform a quick, abbreviated history (e.g., MOI, pain scale, relevant medical information). Again, this is to determine if the patient should be transported as is or allowed to move off the field for a more detailed assessment.

Sideline Assessment

The sideline assessment is completed after the patient is escorted off the field or if the patient comes to the athletic trainer of her own accord. This is not the assessment of life-threatening injuries (addressed in chapter 14). The main purpose of this type of assessment is to gather initial information about the injury and determine if the patient can RTP, with or without any interventions.

This assessment is similar to the general assessment outlined previously with the one key difference: You know it is an acute injury and likely saw the injury occur. You may already be developing potential differential diagnoses from the information you gathered watching the injury occur and the patient come off the field or court. Because of this, you may abbreviate the history portion to pertinent questions only and complete the palpation earlier in the process. You may limit ROM testing to AROM and break tests to assess overall strength. You will then conduct ligamentous and special tests to rule in or out potential diagnoses. The results of initial ligamentous and special tests are important because they may be completed prior to muscle guarding or swelling, which can alter the results. Some important differences with this type of assessment compared to those done in the athletic training clinic is that you will likely have less access to various equipment, many objective measurements will not be completed at this time, and, while not as rushed as during an on-the-field assessment, time is still an important factor.

At this point in the assessment, you should have a potential clinical diagnosis. If there is a possibility of the patient returning to play, you should complete functional testing (see previous) to determine the patient's physical and psychological readiness and ability to protect herself during activity. Often an intervention, such as taping,

bracing, stretching, or wound care, is needed prior to RTP. If the patient is not going to return to activity, she should begin the appropriate initial treatment, such as icing, wrapping, splinting, or using crutches, and be told the follow-up plan for after the event.

Athletic Training Clinic Assessment

Most of the assessments an athletic trainer completes will not be on the field or sideline but will occur in the athletic training clinic. These patients can present with acute or chronic injuries or other nonorthopedic conditions. The initial assessment will follow most of the steps outlined previously but may deviate based on findings. For example, a chronic condition may require a more thorough history to help determine the nature of the condition. In the clinic, you should have access to more equipment and should not be rushed. Objective measurements will be taken, unlike in the on-the-field or sideline assessment where you may not have the equipment or time. Also, outcome measures should be given to help objectify interventions (see Outcome Measures later in the chapter).

In the athletic training clinic, the patient often presents with medical and other conditions, not an injury. Although the assessment of medical conditions follows a similar process, some aspects (e.g., ROM) may not be completed. Internal organs will be assessed through **auscultation** and palpation. Chapter 18 presents the details of medical assessment and chapter 19 outlines the psychosocial evaluation process. Finally, chapter 20 addresses details pertaining to special populations.

Ongoing Assessment

The assessment does not end with the diagnosis and subsequent **referral**, if warranted. Athletic trainers must provide an ongoing assessment of the injury to determine if the treatment plan has been effective or if additional intervention is needed. The ongoing assessment can be a formal or informal process, depending on the status of the patient and the information needed. Conducting an informal ongoing assessment can be as easy as asking the patient how he is doing that day and if there have been any changes in his symptoms or function. The more formal ongoing assessment involves repeating many of the steps outlined previously and providing objective measurements to document changes in the condition based on the interventions applied. Assessment data obtained during this process can be compared with baseline measurements. Outcome measures should also be repeated as part of the ongoing assessment to objectively document changes (see Outcome Measures later in this chapter). Unanticipated changes, or a worsening condition, should be referred to the proper physician for follow-up.

Part of the ongoing assessment is determining the patient's readiness to RTP. As stated earlier, sometimes determining a patient's ability to RTP is done immediately after the initial assessment on the sideline. Other times, this can be done after an extensive rehabilitation program lasting weeks or months. No matter the injury or condition the patient is returning from, he should pass objective tests prior to being released. The patient should be pain free and able to protect himself during activity. The assessment should include ROM, strength, ability to perform sport-specific functional tests, and psychological readiness.

Concussion Evaluation

The assessment and evaluation of a **sports-related concussion (SRC)** can be a difficult task, even for a seasoned athletic trainer. New research about concussion seems to come out daily, and recommendations for assessment and treatment are updated as new information becomes available. Currently, there are many different objective measures available to help with SRC assessment, diagnosis, and return-to-play decisions, but the experts agree that those tools only aid the clinical judgment of the practitioner.[11-16]

Concussion evaluations in traditional athletic training settings usually begin with an on-the-field or sideline assessment. Traumatic, acute conditions (e.g., cervical spine injury, severe traumatic brain injury, skull fracture) should be ruled out immediately. If a more serious injury is identified, you should activate the venue's EAP, as addressed in chapter 13. Clinical prediction rules, such as the Canadian CT head rule or NEXUS II CT head rule, can be used to help determine if referral and subsequent imaging are warranted.[17,18] The primary goal of the assessment on the field or sideline is to rule out more serious injuries and determine if an SRC has occurred.[11,13,15,16,19] If a concussion is suspected, the organization's concussion management protocols should be followed.

Any athlete with a suspected concussion should be removed from participation and screened using a standardized, objective assessment tool (e.g., the Sport Concussion Assessment Tool 5, or SCAT5).[11,13,15,16,19,20] When possible, this assessment should be done in a distraction-free environment. The SCAT5 takes approximately 10 minutes to administer and includes assessment of signs and symptoms, cognitive function, and balance. More specifically, this includes orientation questions, symptoms checklist, the Standardized Assessment of Concussion (SAC), and modified Balance Error Scoring System (BESS) testing. Additional sideline testing can include saccadic eye movements through the King-Devick test to help determine if the patient has a concussion.[19,21-25]

Concussion assessment should be serial in nature when a concussion is suspected, even when the initial sideline assessment is negative due to the possibility of delayed onset of new symptoms or deterioration of initial symptoms. Ongoing assessment should include a symptom checklist and daily monitoring, among other tests, although some tests will not be conducted again until the patient is asymptomatic.[16] The results of concussion tests should be compared to baseline testing when available,[16] although baseline testing is not required for diagnosing a concussion.[11] Frequently, baseline testing will be administered before the competitive season as part of preparticipation examinations. Baseline testing includes the following:

- Concussion and related history
- Physical and neurological evaluation

EVIDENCE-BASED ATHLETIC TRAINING

Athletic Training Position Statement: Management of Sport Concussion

The National Athletic Trainers' Association (NATA) currently has a published position statement on the management of sport concussions.[16] This official position statement provides best-practice recommendations for clinical practice related to concussions, including prevention, evaluation, and return to play, among other areas. This statement was created by a panel of experts who reviewed the related literature and then made recommendations based on a systematic review of the evidence available. You must review this statement and make sure the recommendations are incorporated into your facilities' policies and procedures manual and EAP when feasible. The recommendations made in the position statements do not dictate care, but they should be independently evaluated for their applicability to each institution's unique situation. You must stay abreast of any changes in the recommendations as released to ensure you provide the best possible patient care. In today's litigious society, failure to stay up to date on best-practice recommendations could open you up to lawsuits. This position statement is found on the NATA website.

- Balance assessment
- Neurocognitive function

Baseline testing can be performed using the SAC, SCAT5, or ImPACT (Immediate Post-Concussion Assessment and Cognitive Test) tests or other neurocognitive assessment tools.

Concussions have been recognized as a special circumstance that may affect a patient's psychological well-being and mental health.[11,26] Patients diagnosed with a concussion should be monitored for changes in behavior and psychological well-being while being treated and as they return to activity.[26,27] Refer patients to the appropriate specialist and use a team-based approach to care.

Clinical Prediction Rule

Clinical prediction rules (or clinical decision rules) are clinical decision-making tools that factor in patient history, physical examination, laboratory tests, and diagnostic imaging to inform the diagnosis, prognosis, or treatment or intervention of a patient.[28] The use of clinical prediction rules is just one way athletic trainers can incorporate evidence-based practice into their evaluation of a patient. Clinical prediction rules are developed with a rigorous three-step process:

1. *Derivation.* Possible predictive factors are identified and tested, and then the clinical prediction rule is created. It is compared with the current gold standard during this step.

2. *Validation.* The accuracy and reliability of the predictive factors are assessed in various settings and with various populations to validate their use.

3. *Impact analysis.* This step involves an investigation of how the clinical prediction rule affects patient outcomes, clinician practice, costs, and other factors.

Although many clinical prediction rules are available for use in different aspects of health care, not all have been thoroughly evaluated.[29-31] For example, one study found 434 unique rules available for use in the primary care setting, but only 54.8% of them had been validated and just 2.8% had completed the impact analysis step.[30] Athletic trainers using clinical prediction rules during the evaluation process should be aware of the evidence supporting their use and possible limitations.

In the sports medicine setting, clinical prediction rules are regularly used to help determine if diagnostic imaging is warranted. The goal of this type of clinical prediction rules is to decrease costs and patient wait time in the emergency department and improve patient outcomes. Although they are currently underutilized in the sports medicine setting,[31,32] there has been an increasing amount of research published on clinical prediction rules as the use of evidence-based practice in athletic training increases. Clinical prediction rules commonly used during the evaluation process in the sports medicine setting, which have gone through impact analysis, are listed in the following sidebar.

Medical Referral

Common sense and experience help significantly with the referral process.[41] The old adage "When in doubt, refer it out" definitely still holds true, but you need to find the correct balance of when to refer patients out and when to assess and treat in house. If you refer every patient to the team physician, your employer may question what role you are playing beyond that of a first aid provider. If every patient is being sent out, then why is the athletic trainer there? That said, some patients do need to be referred out to other members of the health care team. This is especially true in potential emergency situations, which are addressed in chapter 14.

Examples of Clinical Prediction Rules

Canadian C-Spine Rule: imaging for patients at risk for cervical-spine fracture[33]

Canadian CT Head Rule: imaging for patients with blunt head injury[17]

Cantor Score: likelihood of strep throat[34]

NEXUS C-Spine Rule: imaging for patients at risk for cervical-spine fracture[35]

NEXUS II CT Head Rule: imaging for patients with blunt head injury[18]

Ottawa Ankle Rules: imaging for patients with ankle trauma[36,37]

Ottawa Knee Rules: imaging for patients with knee trauma[37,38]

Pittsburgh Knee Rules: imaging for patients with knee trauma[37,39]

Wells Score: likelihood of lower-extremity deep vein thrombosis[40]

In many situations, whether emergent or nonemergent, you will need to rely on members of the sports medicine team and the expertise they bring to the table. During a standard orthopedic assessment, referral is often needed to allow the physician to order additional testing that is not directly available to most athletic trainers. This helps the physician rule in or out potential diagnoses that could not be made without the testing. Chapter 17 covers imaging commonly ordered by physicians. Imaging includes tests such as bone scans, radiographs, and magnetic resonance imaging. Other diagnostic tests the physician may order include electrocardiography, nerve conduction studies, and blood testing. Chapter 18 addresses these diagnostic tests. Refer patients out when their injuries or conditions are outside the athletic training scope of practice or beyond state practice acts. You must also know your own strengths and weaknesses so that you can recognize when a patient's injury or condition is outside of your comfort zone. It is okay to ask for help when evaluating or treating a patient.

In most cases, you will refer patients to the team physician overseeing your practice. You should develop this important relationship through good communication and mutual trust. The team physician and athletic trainers should work together to develop a network of specialists for referrals in all aspects of care. In some situations, you will directly refer a patient to other specialists. This is especially true when working with a patient with a potential psychosocial condition. Patients with a complicated concussion may also be referred directly to a specialist such as a neuropsychologist or another member of the sports medicine team. Develop a referral plan based on the recommendations presented in the related NATA position statements.[16, 26,27]

Documentation and Communication of the Injury Evaluation

The final step in the injury evaluation process is documenting and communicating the clinical diagnosis, patient limitations, treatment plan, and other pertinent information. Written and oral communication skills are important for athletic trainers working in every setting.[42] Athletic trainers communicate frequently with physicians, nurses, physical therapists, and other health care providers; patients; parents or guardians; coaches and administrators; insurance companies; and other stakeholders in the patient's care.

Chapter 5 provides detailed information about the importance of documentation and medical records in athletic training. There are many ways to document an injury. How you approach this process varies based on the specific setting you work in. No matter what method you use (e.g., electronic medical records, paper), injury documentation is an important aspect of your responsibilities. Although barriers to documentation have been identified in the literature,[43] you need to prioritize documentation to meet the standards of professional practice.[44] Documentation of injuries allows for the following:[43-48]

- Improved communication with patients, parents, physicians and other health care providers, and stakeholders
- Monitoring of patient care and outcome assessments
- Insurance reimbursement
- Compliance with state practice acts and industry standards
- Legal protection for the patient and athletic trainer

The following sections focus on the practical aspects of documenting injury evaluations, outcome measures, and patient communication.

SOAP Notes

One common way injury evaluations are documented in athletic training and other health care fields is the SOAP (subjective, objective, assessment, plan) note method. This method provides a simple, clear, and organized way to document all aspects of the initial evaluation, any subsequent reevaluations, and interventions provided. SOAP notes are typically written using standard medical terminology and abbreviations (see appendix A for a detailed list). Table 16.9 describes the components of a SOAP note, and figure 16.14 provides an example of a SOAP note form.

Outcome Measures

With the drive to increase the use of evidence-based practice in athletic training and the need for objective data to meet reimbursement requirements, the use of outcome measures is increasing in athletic training practice. Outcome measures can be either clinician-based or patient-based instruments.

- Clinician-based measures tend to be disease oriented and focus on the evidence related to the disease, condition, or injury (e.g., ROM, girth measurements) rather than outcomes meaningful to the patient. Many of these measures are addressed in the objective portion of the injury evaluation.
- Patient-based measures tend to assess patient-oriented evidence that matters, including goals and expectations the patient has for her care and treat-

TABLE 16.9   **SOAP Note Components**

Component	Description	Examples
S = subjective	Patient history Chief complaint How the injury occurred (in the patient's own words, if possible) Symptoms the patient tells the athletic trainer Pertinent information that cannot be observed or measured	"I stepped in a hole and rolled my ankle." Type of pain (e.g., dull, burning, sharp) Pain scale (0-10) Symptoms (e.g., nausea, headache, dizziness, confusion)
O = objective	Signs observed by the athletic trainer and any objective measurements taken Results of special tests and diagnostic tests	Vital sign measurements Signs (e.g., vomiting, swelling, discoloration, temperature increase) Special test results, such as (+) Lachman's test, mBESS 27/30, (-) X-ray
A = assessment	Clinical diagnosis Differential diagnosis, if additional testing is required	1st degree lateral ankle sprain
P = plan	Treatment plan Current interventions Orders for additional testing or referrals, if needed Home care instructions given to the patient	RICE Revaluate in 24 hours Refer for X-ray

ment (e.g., symptom improvement, health-related quality of life, satisfaction).[49,50]

Although both types of assessments are meant to be used together to better understand the disease, condition, or injury, the focus in this section is on patient-based outcome measures.

"'Patient-based outcome measure' is a short-hand term referring to the array of questionnaires, interview schedules and other related methods of assessing health, illness and benefits of health care interventions from the patient's perspective."[51] A variety of outcome measures are available for use depending on your work setting and the types of injuries or conditions you are assessing. In general, outcome assessment instruments can be classified as the following:

- Disease specific
- Site specific
- Dimension specific
- Generic
- Summary item
- Individualized
- Utility

SOAP notes can also be used to research outcomes of interventions and progression of an injury or condition.[46] Outcome measures are derived from the framework of

one of the available disablement models (addressed in chapter 2).[49] The goal of outcome measures is to evaluate the efficiency and effectiveness of care and help drive clinical practice guidelines. Using outcome measures will also help you improve communication with patients and other health care professionals.[52]

The process of selecting an outcome assessment instrument is "similar to those steps necessary to selecting clinical tools to measure range of motion, strength, swelling, or diagnostic tests based on their accuracy."[53] Consider the following criteria:[51]

- Appropriateness
- Reliability
- Validity
- Responsiveness
- Precision
- Interpretability
- Acceptability
- Feasibility

One barrier to using outcome assessment instruments is that they are time consuming for patients to complete and for clinicians to score and interpret.[52] Even so, outcome measures need to be integrated into clinical practice in all athletic training settings in response to changes in the health care system.

FIGURE 16.14   Example of a SOAP note form.

SOAP Notes Form

Patient's name: Record/ID#: _____

Injury date: _____   Record date: _____

Sport: _____

Subjective (history): _____

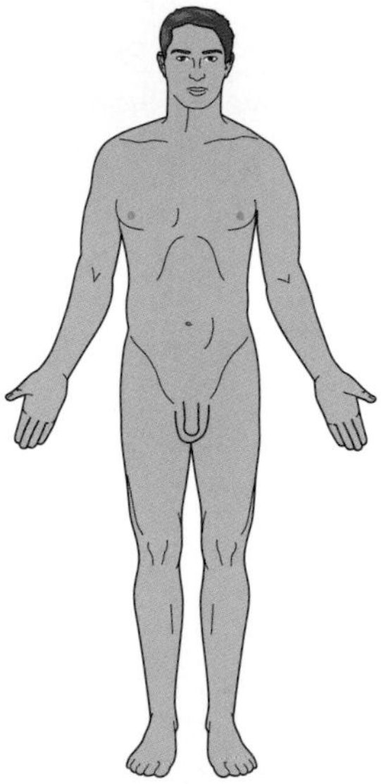

_____

_____

_____

_____

_____

_____

Objective (observation, palpation, ROM, strength, neurological
    tests, special tests):

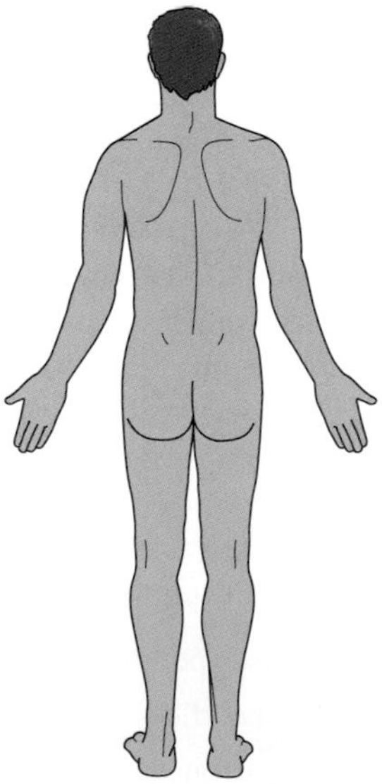

_____

_____

_____

_____

_____

_____

_____

_____

_____

_____

_____

_____

_____

_____

_____

_____

Assessment (impression): _____

_____

_____

Plan (treatment and disposition): _____

_____

_____

_____

Reprinted by permission from S.J. Shultz, P.A. Houglum, and D.H. Perrin. *Examination of Musculoskeletal Injuries*, 4th ed. (Champaign, IL: Human Kinetics, 2016), 33.

Once the outcome measure has been selected, the patient should complete the assessment at the beginning of the evaluation. This will be considered the baseline assessment for the patient. The instrument should be completed throughout the treatment period as needed. This process helps quantify changes in the patient, individualize care, and assess the outcome of the treatment plan at discharge. Patient-based outcome measures ultimately help you integrate evidence-based practice into your clinical practice, support research and advocacy efforts, and improve patient care.[50]

Patient Communication

Successful patient encounters require effective communication.[42,54] This implies that the patient and athletic trainer have developed a partnership and the patient has been fully educated in the nature of his condition and the different methods for addressing the problem. This allows the patient to be actively involved in the decision-making process and establishes agreed-upon expectations and goals. Many models exist to help health care providers improve their ability to communicate with and educate their patients.[54,55] These models focus on the quality of the encounter rather than its length. These approaches have been demonstrated to improve patient satisfaction and allow the provider to demonstrate empathy and concern. Learning and practicing good communication skills allows you to build trust, improve the quality of care provided, and ultimately improve outcomes.

Use patient-focused communication skills during direct patient encounters:[54]

- Sit down during patient encounters.
- Develop an understanding of the patient as a person, not as a disease or a musculoskeletal condition.
- Show empathy and respect.
- Listen attentively and work to create a partnership.
- Elicit the patient's concerns and calm any fears.
- Use humor when appropriate.
- Answer questions honestly.
- Inform and educate patients about treatment options and the course of care.
- Involve patients in decisions concerning their medical care.
- Demonstrate sensitivity to patients' cultural and ethnic diversity.

Patients often measure quality of care by how well the athletic trainer listens, validates their complaints, and acknowledges concerns. Quality is also measured by how thoroughly the athletic trainer explains the diagnosis and treatment options and how well she involves the patient in decisions concerning care. Thus, communication plays an important part in the way patients perceive, recall, and evaluate their interaction with the athletic trainer. Finally, patients who have filed malpractice suits against their athletic trainer often cite poor communication and lack of empathy as a factor in pursuing legal action.[56]

CLINICAL BOTTOM LINE

- In general, the HOPS acronym is used to guide the assessment of patients. Athletic trainers should use this systematic process to ensure a complete assessment occurs and an accurate clinical diagnosis is determined.
- Athletic trainers should realize that many times, the assessment process is altered based on the location of the assessment, the type of injury or condition being assessed, and the severity of the injury or condition. Athletic trainers must be able to adapt to the situation.
- The assessment does not end after the initial evaluation, but rather continues until the patient returns to activity.
- Concussion evaluations are one of the most complicated and important assessments that athletic trainers perform. Athletic trainers should stay up to date on the continuing changes in the field related to concussion assessments and use best practices based on the current literature.
- Clinical prediction rules and patient-based outcome measures are two tools athletic trainers can use to incorporate evidence-based practice into their clinical practice.
- Recognizing the need to refer patients to the team physician and other members of the sports medicine team is an important aspect of providing patient-centered care.

- Both written and oral communication with patients, physicians, and other stakeholders are important aspects of the assessment process.
- Athletic trainers should review the NATA position statements and other relevant documents related to the assessment of various injuries and conditions.

 Go to HK*Propel* to complete the activities and case studies for this chapter.

Go to HK*Propel* to download a foundational skill check sheet about the steps of the evaluation process.

CHAPTER 17

Medical Imaging

Leamor Kahanov, EdD, ATC, LAT
Loraine Zelna, MS, RT (R)(MR)

CAATE STANDARDS
The following CAATE 2020 standard is covered in this chapter:

Standard 72

CHAPTER OBJECTIVES

After reading this chapter, you will be able to do the following:

- Define medical imaging
- Recognize foundational concepts of medical imaging
- Comprehend the interprofessional aspect of medical imaging in athletic training
- Distinguish the different types of medical imaging
- Identify appropriateness of imaging for diagnosis

Medical imaging is an important component in the diagnosis and treatment of patients. Although ordering a medical image is relegated to licensed practitioners, athletic trainers should understand the diagnostic process and know how to evaluate images to best manage patients' treatment and rehabilitation. Although certified athletic trainers do not receive the state-required licenses to order or read medical images, they should participate in conversations with practitioners regarding their patients' medical images.

Medical imaging serves five primary areas in the continuum of care for patients:

1. Diagnosis
2. Preparticipation screening, when indicated
3. Informing a treatment or rehabilitation plan
4. Diagnostic procedures
5. Return to participation or activities of daily living

Activity-related injuries may be divided into acute injuries, traumatic injuries, and chronic overuse injuries, all of which may require imaging as a component of diagnosis and management. During medical imaging for diagnosis, coordination is required between the practitioner, patient, and insurance carriers. Athletic trainers, particularly practitioners who bear some responsibility for insurance oversight, should understand that insurance reimbursements often dictate the order in which imaging procedures are conducted.

This chapter provides an overview of the medical imaging modality options available for the diagnosis of injury, abnormality, or pathology. It discusses the imaging options most likely to be encountered by athletic trainers: diagnostic radiography (X-ray), computed tomography (CT), magnetic resonance imaging (MRI), nuclear medicine, and diagnostic medical sonography (DMS), also known as ultrasound. Additionally, the chapter addresses the imaging life cycle, from the order to the report. Athletic trainers are often the first to evaluate a patient in acute circumstances. Recognizing and recommending the most appropriate medical imaging procedure, based on the American College of Radiology appropriateness criteria,[1] to the primary health care provider will expedite diagnosis and treatment for the patient.

Radiologic Science and Its Roles in Imaging

Medical imaging and *radiologic technology* are all-encompassing terms relative to diagnostic imaging and therapeutic procedures. In this chapter, the term *medical imaging* is used to describe the various imaging options for diagnostic purposes. The diagnostic imaging options, usually noted as modalities, are largely dependent on the nature of the injury or illness.

Understanding the different health care professions and their roles is paramount for the athletic trainer, who must navigate the health care system with and for patients.

Likewise, facilitating interprofessional care to improve patient outcomes may require interaction and collaboration with radiologic science technologists to assist patients and procure imaging. Each of the modalities is unique and useful in the diagnosis of differing pathologies and requires differing certifications to qualify in the performance of the examinations (table 17.1).

Medical Imaging

Radiography is useful in the diagnosis of disease, trauma, or abnormality. Wilhelm Conrad Röntgen discovered X-rays in 1895. The initial radiographic images were made onto glass photographic plates. George Eastman, founder of the Kodak company, first introduced radiographic film in 1918. Most recently, the digital revolution has allowed radiographic images to be recorded and stored digitally.

A **radiographic image** is obtained through the use of ionizing radiation (X-rays) in combination with an image receptor (either film or digital; see figure 17.1). The proper term for images that are acquired using X-rays is *radiograph*. Many health care providers use the lay-term *X-ray* when viewing the image, yet X-rays are invisible ionizing radiation that are used in combination with an image receptor to produce a visual image (radiograph).

TABLE 17.1 **Radiologic and Diagnostic Technologies: General Uses and Practitioner Certification**

Radiologic technology	Use	Required practitioner certification
Diagnostic radiography (X ray)	First step in the diagnosis of fracture or soft-tissue injury Not as discriminating for soft-tissue injuries	Registered radiologic technologist (R) from the American Registry of Radiologic Technologists (ARRT)
Diagnostic medical sonography (DMS; also known as *ultrasound*)	Imaging using sound waves to help diagnose sprains, strains, tears, trapped nerves, arthritis, and other musculoskeletal conditions	American Registry for Diagnostic Medical Sonography (ARDMS) or primary or post-primary education from the ARRT (S)
Computed tomography (CT)	Acute trauma to bony structures Imaging of the nervous and gastrointestinal systems	Registered radiologic technologist with post-primary certification in computed tomography (R)(CT)
Magnetic resonance imaging (MRI)	Valuable in the assessment of structures with high water content, such as joints and the nervous system	Registered radiologic technologist with post-primary certification in magnetic resonance (R)(MR) or ARRT primary certification in magnetic resonance (MR)
Nuclear medicine	Demonstrate anatomic and physiological information of the body Provide therapy for certain cancers	Registered nuclear medicine technologist (N) from the ARRT or Nuclear Medicine Technology Certification Board (NMTCB)

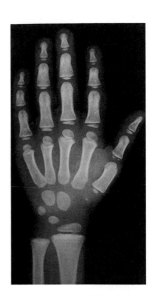

FIGURE 17.1 Radiograph ("X-ray").

Radiographic images of the genitourinary, cardiac, peripheral vascular, and nervous systems often require the injection of a contrast agent to visualize the organs. The patient may be required to ingest a barium-based contrast agent for evaluation of the gastrointestinal system. Patients must be screened for potential contraindications when any contrast agent is required. Although radiographic images are often the first ones required for diagnosis, because of their limitations, additional images often need to be ordered from a licensed health care practitioner.

Computed Tomography

Computed tomography (CT) is a radiographic study that uses ionizing radiation and the principles of tomography to make a series of three-dimensional cross-sectional images that are stored and reconstructed

Understanding Role Definitions and Credentialing

- Radiologic science technologists typically perform imaging procedures.
- The American Registry of Radiologic Technologists (ARRT) provides the national credentialing examination for most of the radiologic sciences and specialty areas, such as diagnostic radiography, computed tomography, and MRI.
- Diagnostic medical sonography is an exception to the credentialing because sonography practitioners must receive a separate credential through the American Registry for Diagnostic Medical Sonography (ARDMS) or the ARRT.
- Two nationally recognized paths to becoming certified to perform nuclear medicine exist: Registered nuclear medicine technologists are credentialed by either the Nuclear Medicine Technology Certification Board (NMTCB) or the ARRT.

Uses of Radiographic Images

Radiographs can be obtained of the following systems:

- Skeletal
- Gastrointestinal
- Genitourinary
- Cardiac
- Peripheral
- Vasculature
- Nervous

EVIDENCE-BASED ATHLETIC TRAINING

Diagnostic Acuity of Conventional Radiographs

The following is the diagnostic acuity of conventional radiographs:[2-7]

- Radiography uses ionizing radiation (X-rays) to produce an image.
- Body structures exposed to X-ray beam are superimposed on each other to produce a flat image. Radiography measures the structure, size, and position of anatomy.
- Radiography is limited in its ability to distinguish types of tissues. It can distinguish only air, bone, fat, and metal. Ligaments and tendons are not fully visualized, and various contrast media are needed to visualize internal organs and vessels.
- Radiography is sensitive to voluntary and involuntary movement. Imaging of the chest, abdomen, and pelvis requires the patient to hold his breath.

by a computer. Two investigators, Allan Cormack and Godfrey Hounsfield, shared the Nobel Prize for their work on devising computed tomography in 1979.[8] The cross-sectional images are acquired in multiple planes, such as sagittal, coronal, and transverse (figure 17.2).

CT may require the ingestion of an iodine- or barium-based contrast medium to demonstrate the gastrointestinal system and the injection of an iodinated contrast medium to enhance vessels, tumors, or other abnormal-ities. Patients must be screened for sensitivity to the contrast agent prior to the examination. CT is useful in the diagnosis of disease, trauma, and abnormality and also assists in planning and guiding interventional procedures such as biopsy. It is also used for planning and monitoring the effectiveness of radiation therapy treatments.

Magnetic Resonance Imaging

Magnetic resonance imaging (MRI) is an imaging technique that uses a strong magnetic field and radio waves, rather than ionizing radiation, to produce cross-sectional images of the body (figure 17.3). Contrast agents such as a gadolinium-based medium (metal with paramagnetic effects) can be used in conjunction with MRI to enhance imaging of systems or organs; however, contrast agents can be difficult for patients with comorbidities to process. In 1952, Bloch and Purcell were awarded the Nobel Prize in physics for their development of nuclear magnetic precision measurements. Although there is discrepancy over who first discovered this imaging, Lauterbur and Mansfield were jointly awarded the Nobel Prize in physiology or medicine in 2003 for their discoveries in MRI.[12]

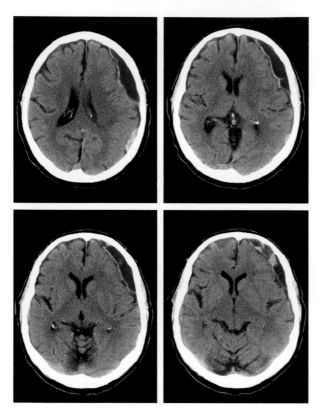

FIGURE 17.2 CT scan.
Callista Images/Image Source/Getty Images

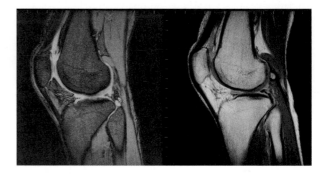

FIGURE 17.3 MRI.
NICK VEASEY/SCIENCE PHOTO LIBRARY/Getty Images

EVIDENCE-BASED ATHLETIC TRAINING

Diagnostic Acuity of Computed Tomography

The following is the diagnostic acuity of computed tomography:[9-11]

- Uses ionizing radiation directed from many angles to create images
- Cross-sectional images: Body organs are separated by using multiple slices that are acquired a single slice at a time. CT creates three-dimensional images through reconstruction of digital data and measures the structure, size, and position of anatomy.
- Sensitive to distinguishing subtle differences in various tissues (i.e., CNS, abdomen, pelvis, bony anatomy)
- Sensitive to voluntary and involuntary movement; requires cessation of respiration for imaging the chest, abdomen, and pelvis
- Resolution: 1 to 1.5 mm

EVIDENCE-BASED ATHLETIC TRAINING

Diagnostic Acuity of Medical Resonance Imaging

The following is the diagnostic acuity of medical resonance imaging:[12-15]

- MRI uses magnetic waves and radiofrequency pulses to create volumetric images.
- Cross-sectional images: Body organs are separated by using multiple slices that are acquired by volume. MRI creates three-dimensional images through reconstruction of digital data and measures the structure, size, and position of anatomy. Physiological evaluation is possible in the area of research.
- MRI is sensitive to distinguishing very small differences in tissue composition. Body structures with high water content are well visualized (i.e., CNS and joints).
- Volumetric image acquisition: This method is sensitive to voluntary and involuntary motion artifacts. Therefore, chest, abdomen and pelvis are challenging procedures.
- Resolution: 0.5 to 1 mm

MRI is useful in the diagnosis of disease, pathologies, and abnormalities of the nervous, cardiac, gastrointestinal, and genitourinary systems and joints of the body. Due to the use of a very strong magnetic field that is always functioning, anyone entering into the magnetic field must be carefully screened for contraindications, including technologists, patients, caregivers, and other health care workers. Safety is a serious concern for MRI technologists. According to the American College of Radiology (ACR), all facilities with MRI units are required to designate four distinct safety zones:

- Zone I is the general public area located outside of the MR environment.
- Zone II is where the patient is likely screened for the MR examination and is located between the general public area and the stricter zones III and IV.
- Zone III is restricted to designated MR personnel or those non-MR personnel who are accompanied and supervised by a designated MR staff person. It should be physically restricted from the general public.
- Zone IV is the MR scanner room itself. Only qualified MR personnel and thoroughly screened patients may enter this area.

Another consideration is related to thermal load from focal RF-related discomfort or injury. The ACR provides guidance for facilities to assist in limiting the possibilities of focal RF-related potentials.[22] Although MRI is considered an excellent modality in the evaluation of any body part with high water content, such as joints and the nervous system, several conditions may prohibit a patient from qualifying for this procedure:

- MR-unsafe metal implants
- Metal fragments in the eyes
- Prior surgical procedures that may be contraindications for a magnetic field

The athletic trainer may provide relevant history and contraindications during discussions with the health care provider and medical technologists as part of an interprofessional health care model.

Functional MRI (fMRI) is a diagnostic tool often used in sports medicine to assess cerebral blood flow and neural activity, particularly associated with brain injury. The same MR safety considerations are required for fMRI as identified previously for MRI. MRI and fMRI use the same basic principles of physics to scan anatomical images, but rather than providing images of anatomical tissues (MRI), the fMRI provides images of metabolic activity. Therefore, fMRI is a good diagnostic tool for identifying changes in the brain.

Ultrasound or Diagnostic Medical Sonography

Diagnostic medical sonography (DMS) is also known as *ultrasound* or *sonography*. DMS is an imaging and therapeutic modality that images or treats deep structures of the body by measuring and recording the reflection of high-frequency sound waves. DMS for evaluation of the heart, fetus, cardiac, musculoskeletal tissue, and tumors versus normal tissue began in the 1950s with the first moving pictures of the heart[16] and gained popularity in the 1960s. Real-time ultrasonic units were introduced in the 1970s and provided visualization and recording of moving images (figure 17.4).[16]

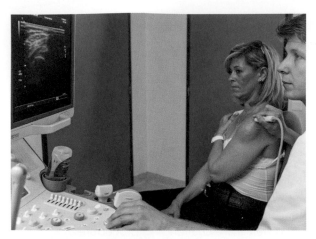

FIGURE 17.4 DMS imaging.

BSIP/Universal Images Group via Getty Images

DMS does not require the use of ionizing radiation and is, for the most part, noninvasive. DMS is useful for visualizing organs, vessels, and musculoskeletal tissue in real time and examining a fetus in pregnant women and the brain and hips in infants. It may aid in diagnosing the causes of pain, swelling, and infection in the body's internal organs. DMS is also used to help guide biopsies and diagnose heart conditions, problems with vascular and musculoskeletal tissue, and damage after a heart attack.

DMS is emerging as a valuable method for assessing musculoskeletal issues, primarily for superficial structures (limited to one quadrant of a joint with high resolution). Advantages over other methods include lower cost, ability to perform dynamic examinations, higher spatial resolution of superficial structures, better patient comfort, and essentially no contraindications.

Several different types of DMS machines are used for various purposes. Selecting the correct DMS unit is key to appropriate tissue assessment (table 17.2). Practitioners and technologists must have additional certifications to order and evaluate imaging produced from DMS.

Nuclear Medicine

Nuclear medicine is a discipline that uses radioactive isotopes in the diagnosis and treatment of disease, including many types of cancers; heart disease; gastrointestinal, endocrine, and neurological disorders; and other abnormalities within the body. More commonly in athletic training, bone scans are used to assess bone diseases and conditions, including fractures, infection, and cancer.[17,18] Nuclear medicine tests use small amounts of radioactive materials (tracers) that are injected, swallowed, or inhaled to identify diseases and conditions in the body. Cells and tissues that are in the process of cell repair most actively take up the largest amounts of tracer, thus identifying an issue. A gamma camera is used to record the radioactive isotope emissions that are tagged to the affected cells. Reactions to the radioisotope are rare; therefore, nuclear medicine is a relatively safe diagnostic tool.

The tracer principles were discovered in 1923 by de Hevsy, often called the father of nuclear medicine, and expanded in the 1930s.[8,12] During the mid-1960s, the use of nuclear medicine for human evaluation grew with

TABLE 17.2 **Diagnostic Medical Sonography**

DMS machine type	Machine qualities	Use
Basic ultrasound machine	Commonly used machine High-frequency sound waves Transabdominal transducer head Two-dimensional images Can record sound	Primarily internal organs Fetus Musculoskeletal
Doppler ultrasound	Changing frequencies to assess moving objects Measures movement and speed of objects in the body	Musculoskeletal Fetus Heart Blood flow
3D and 4D ultrasound	Multiple images of objects are meshed together through computer programs to create 3D and 4D images. Images are clearer than 2D.	Deep soft-tissue structures Nerves Blood flow
Breast ultrasound and echocardiogram ultrasound	Sensitive to small abnormalities Monitors blood flow in and out of the breast area	Breast Cardiac (may also be used for cardiac screenings)
Transvaginal or transrectal scanner	Transducer scanner used internally	Vaginal abnormalities Fetus

EVIDENCE-BASED ATHLETIC TRAINING

Diagnostic Acuity of Medical Sonography (Ultrasound)

The following is the diagnostic acuity of medical sonography (ultrasound):[15-17]

- Ultrasound uses sound waves to create images. Transducers convert electrical energy into acoustic energy for transmission and acoustic energy into electrical energy for reception.

- Cross-sectional images: Body organs, vessels, and fetus are visualized. Ultrasound can create three-dimensional images through reconstruction of digital data and measures the structure, size, and position of anatomy and the hemodynamics and anatomy of vascular structures.

- Volumetric image acquisition: This modality is sensitive to imaging artifacts caused by reflections.

advances in technology. The 1970s brought the visualization of additional organs with nuclear medicine, including liver and spleen scanning, brain tumor localization, and studies of the gastrointestinal tract. In the 1980s, nuclear medicine began to be used for diagnosing heart disease; the integration of digital computers added additional power to the technique. The 2000s brought hybrid imaging techniques for functional evaluation (PET, or position emission tomography) and superb imaging capabilities of CT and bone scans.[8,12] Additionally, in some facilities, nuclear medicine images are fused with CT or MRI to provide a more precise diagnosis. Nuclear medicine can also be used as a therapeutic modality to treat some cancers.

Imaging Life Cycle

Following clinical evaluation of an injury, the typical ordering cycle for imaging begins with identifying the specific anatomical area desired for imaging. This information, provided as a component of an image order, is helpful to the radiologic technologist who performs the imaging procedures and the radiologists who interpret the examination.

Typically, when the patient checks in at the Department of Imaging, she should present an order. The order must include the following:

- Patient's name
- Date of birth
- Specific body part to be imaged
- Severity of injury or illness
- Symptoms
- Patient history

For example, for a patient who injured her right elbow and wrist, the order must indicate the following information: "Right forearm including elbow and wrist; patient fell two days ago; severe pain toward the elbow when extending; history of prior fracture of the radial head."

EVIDENCE-BASED ATHLETIC TRAINING

Diagnostic Acuity of Nuclear Medicine

The following is the diagnostic acuity of nuclear medicine:[19-21]

- Nuclear medicine requires radiopharmaceuticals for diagnosis, therapy, and medical research.

- It determines the cause of a medical condition based on the physiological function of organs and tissues and is primarily used to measure human cellular, organ, or system function.

- CT and positron emission tomography (PET) systems are matched in size and position and combined to evaluate both anatomy and physiology. Single photon emission computed tomography (SPECT) and PET provide more differentiation of body densities (i.e., metastatic disease). MRI and PET merge to assess metabolic and anatomic information (i.e., neurological, oncologic, cardiologic)

- Resolution: PET: 3 to 5 mm; SPECT: 8 to 10 mm

FOUNDATIONAL SKILL

Imaging Order Guidelines

- Identify the body part to be examined. Be specific: List the side of the body (i.e., right or left) and organ (e.g., quadrant, upper, lower).
- Note the severity of the injury or illness (i.e., acute or chronic, trauma or nontrauma).
  - Provide all signs and symptoms relative to the ordered procedure.
  - Include a detailed history of what resulted in the need for an imaging procedure.
- Identify whether the patient experienced trauma resulting in acute pain or has chronic pain in the anatomical area without trauma.
- Identify signs and symptoms experienced by the patient. Provide signs and symptoms relevant to the examination ordered and prior procedures or underlying conditions related to the imaging study.
- Provide any information from the patient's history related to the procedure ordered: history of _____ (what happened, when did it happen, where are the symptoms, how did it happen?) and reason for the imaging (e.g., to rule out fracture, rule out internal bleeding).
  - Identify a timeline of the injury or illness.
  - Include the answers to the following: What happened, when did it happen, where are the symptoms, and how did it happen? All this information leads to the purpose and reason for the imaging examination.

ACR Appropriateness Criteria

The ACR appropriateness criteria are evidence-based guidelines to assist referring physicians and other providers in making the most appropriate imaging or treatment decision for a specific clinical condition. Employing these guidelines helps providers enhance the quality of care and contribute to the most efficacious use of radiology.

From the time of clinical evaluation, health care professionals work to choose the most appropriate imaging modality for the best patient diagnosis. The imaging modalities of choice vary depending on the anatomical area of interest. Although radiography is the first step in the evaluation of anatomical areas in many injuries, you should understand the typical sequencing of imaging procedures based on anatomical area (figure 17.5).

Reviewing the Imaging Report

There are several key items to consider when reviewing an imaging report:

- Identification of the procedure examined
- Patient history
- Comparison procedures, if available
- Projections that were performed by the radiologic technologist
- Detailed findings of the images performed

- Final outcome of the images read by the radiologist
- Significant information regarding the patient diagnosis

With the digital era of imaging, radiographic images are reviewed and reports are dictated in a timely fashion. Health care providers can access the results of imaging procedures through desktop, laptop, or mobile devices within hours of their performance. Mobile devices give providers, primarily radiologists, remote access through a DICOM viewer (Digital Imaging and Communications in Medicine), which provides digital screen sharing with physicians. Picture archiving and communication systems (PACS) are used in nearly all facilities that have imaging capabilities. Health care providers may gain access to PACS through articulation agreements between imaging facilities and individual health care providers. This access provides flexibility and ease of viewing images and reports, which facilitates the care of the patient and therefore improves the treatment timeline.

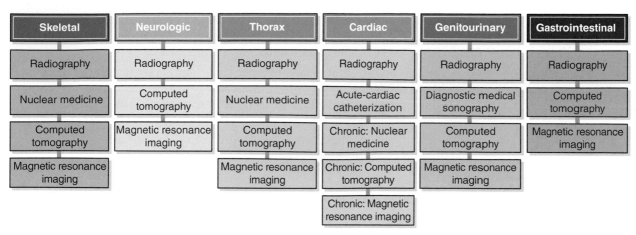

FIGURE 17.5 Image ordering sequence.

Evaluating Radiographic Images

In order to recognize an abnormality in imaging, athletic trainers should have basic knowledge of the normal appearance of radiographic anatomy. Diagnosing injuries and conditions is outside the scope of practice for medical imaging technologists and athletic trainers. The diagnosis is made by a radiologist, who is a medical doctor specialized in the field of radiology (medical imaging). However, you should be able to recognize what is normal and abnormal in order to assist in a favorable patient outcome. You must be familiar with basic anatomical structure, including the normal appearance of bony structures, soft tissue, and organs.

Patient outcomes depend on quality images to promote an accurate diagnosis. High-quality imaging is critical for allowing the radiologist to properly view the soft tissue. Any changes from a normal baseline assist the evaluation of the bony anatomy close to the proximity of the soft-tissue abnormality. The ability to detect quality images and globally identify normal and abnormal images is an asset for athletic trainers. Your role in assisting health care providers with medical images often depends on the relationship between the professionals. You may provide assistance with ordering images, facilitating insurance billing, obtaining images, reviewing and educating patients, or performing imaging enhanced treatments. Athletic trainers who want to enhance their ability to discriminate medical images should seek continuing education in these areas.

Medical Imaging and Administration

Although radiographs are not the best choice for joint and ligament damage, they may lead to a probable diagnosis. The cost for diagnostic radiographs is much less than for an MRI.

The **radiologist**, a physician specifically trained to supervise and interpret radiology examinations, analyzes the diagnostic radiographs and often suggests additional modalities, such as MRI, that will detect and confirm diagnosis of ligaments and tendons.

The athletic trainer who is responsible for obtaining insurance approvals for physician- or practitioner-ordered medical imaging should understand the approval process. Aside from the varying costs associated with medical imaging procedures, each imaging modality provides a unique diagnostic capability.

CLINICAL BOTTOM LINE

- Understanding foundational concepts of medical imaging within the context of interprofessional collaboration is essential to facilitating diagnosis, treatment or rehabilitation, and return to sport participation or activities of daily living.

- Athletic trainers often have an integral role in patient-centered care by educating clients on injuries. Medical imaging can assist patients in understanding their injury diagnosis process or technical procedures where imaging is required to facilitate medical care.

- Athletic trainers who facilitate administration functions in the oversight and coordination of budget, services, and operations should have an understanding of the interplay between patient needs and insurance requirements.

- Medical imaging describes the various imaging options for diagnostic purposes and therapeutic interventions, including, but not limited to, radiographic images, nuclear radiology, computed tomography (CT), magnetic resonance imaging (MRI), and diagnostic ultrasound.

- Medical imaging serves five primary areas of athletic training in the continuum of care for patients based on interactions with radiologists, primary care practitioners, and medical imaging technologists. Athletic trainers should participate in discussions about medical imaging in diagnosis, preparticipation screenings, treatment and rehabilitation, and return to activity or participation.

- Athletic trainers are responsible for facilitating the following aspects of medical imaging and patient care:

  - The procedure for ordering and reviewing an imaging report, including the identification of the image or procedure examined

  - Working in conjunction with a medical professional for a shared patient

  - Patient history, comparison procedures, the projections that were performed by the radiologic technologist, the detailed findings of the images performed, and the impression providing the final outcome of the images read by the radiologist

  - Reviewing the radiologist findings with the practitioner and the patient

  - Providing the patient with an educational overview on the next steps in treatment, management, or rehabilitation

- Athletic trainers need to understand the appropriateness of imaging for diagnosis and discussion with other health care providers.

 Go to HK*Propel* to complete the activities and case studies for this chapter.

CHAPTER 18

Commonly Encountered Medical Conditions in Athletic Training

Tim Braun, PhD, LAT, ATC, CSCS

CAATE STANDARDS

The following CAATE 2020 standards are covered in this chapter:

Standard 71

Standard 72

CHAPTER OBJECTIVES

After reading this chapter, you will be able to do the following:

- Explain steps to the medical examination done with orthopedic injuries, including auscultations, percussion, and palpation

- Describe and differentiate between common medical diagnostic tests

- Recognize specific general medical conditions

- Identify applicable differential diagnosis for each condition

- Describe appropriate management for each condition

- Categorize each condition by type of disease or infection

Athletic trainers often work in interdisciplinary teams with other health care professionals to ensure optimal patient care. Rather than focusing solely on athletic injuries, you must be able to understand and evaluate a range of acute and chronic medical conditions and refer patients to the appropriate specialists for treatment when needed. This chapter provides an introductory overview of general medical conditions encountered across the life span. In your role, you will have to understand ways to mitigate risk factors, associated signs and symptoms, and disease progressions for clients as they age. Athletic trainers interested in evidence-based practice should further investigate the information in each section. This chapter provides essential evaluation information on applicable auscultations, palpations, and diagnostic testing.

Examination Process

Athletic trainers must be able to proficiently complete thorough evaluations during preparticipation examinations and if clients show signs of illness. As part of the preparticipation examination, you may identify disqualifying conditions or symptoms that warrant referral. Throughout the year, patients will present with acute or chronic injuries or illnesses that require evaluation. You must understand and be able to apply all aspects of the examination process. An incomplete evaluation decreases the diagnostic accuracy. By accurately diagnosing the condition, you may facilitate timely referrals to the appropriate specialists for further evaluation and treatment. Chapter 14 details how to take vital signs and chapter 16 describes how to take a medical history and complete an observation. Refer to those chapters for discussion about those stages of the examination process.

Auscultations

As part of the physical examination, auscultations of the heart, lungs, and abdomen assess for the presence or absence of normal or inaccurate sounds. Auscultation should precede any palpations. A stethoscope is required for the examination. The stethoscope head should be applied directly to the skin. You should maintain firm pressure over the specific area for a maximum of 3 minutes.

Lung Auscultations

Breath sounds should be noted over all the lobes of the lungs in various locations in a fixed sequence (figure 18.1). You should evaluate pitch, intensity, quality, and duration of inspirations and exhalations.

- Normal sounds: equal dry, smooth, and unobstructed over each lobe

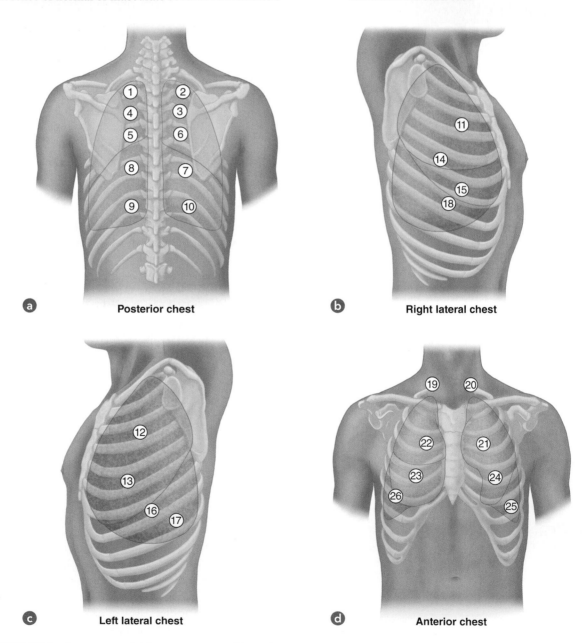

(a) Posterior chest

(b) Right lateral chest

(c) Left lateral chest

(d) Anterior chest

FIGURE 18.1 Lung auscultation sequence of locations.

- Abnormal sounds:
  - Stridor: wheezelike sounds; potential airway narrowing or tonsillitis
  - Crackles: clicking or rattling sounds; potential pneumonia or bronchitis
  - Wheeze: high-pitched sounds; potential asthma or chronic obstructive pulmonary disease (COPD)
  - Rhonchi: resemble snoring sounds; potential pneumonia or chronic bronchitis

Heart Auscultations

Heart sounds should be noted over the locations associated with each heart valve (figure 18.2). Any deviation warrants referral to a physician.

- Normal sounds: The heart makes "lub" and "dub" sounds as the valves close. The "lub" sound indicates the closing of the valves between the atria and the ventricles. As the ventricles contract,

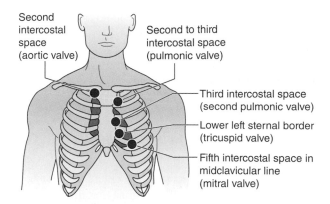

FIGURE 18.2 Heart auscultation locations.

blood flows toward the aorta and lungs. The "dub" sound occurs as the ventricles finish contracting and the aortic and pulmonary valves close.

- Abnormal sounds:
  - Soft, blowing "lub": potential COPD or pleural effusion

FOUNDATIONAL SKILL

Abdominal Palpation Technique

- Place patient in a relaxed hook-lying position, with knees flexed for comfort.
- Perform palpations with palmar aspect of several fingers moving in small circular motions.
- Palpate each abdominal quadrant (figure 18.3).
- Assess for rigidity, pain location, tenderness, masses, density, and swelling.

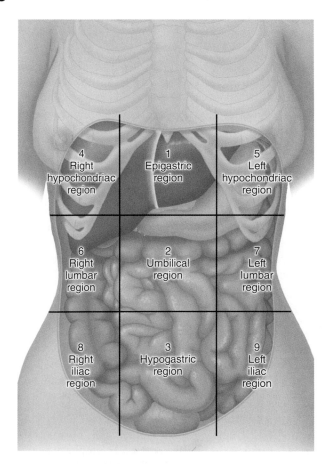

FIGURE 18.3 The nine regions of the abdomen.

- Loud, blooming "lub": potential mitral valve stenosis
- Sloshing "dub": potential heart murmur or aortic stenosis
- Friction sound: potential pericarditis or ventricular fibrillation

Stomach and Bowel Auscultations

Unlike with heart and lung auscultations, the exact placement of the stethoscope is not crucial for stomach and bowel examinations. Perform auscultations before palpations. Any palpations may produce false abnormal sounds.

- Normal sounds: Occasional gurgling indicates **peristalsis**.
- Abnormal sounds: Absence of sound may indicate obstruction, injury, or internal hemorrhage.

Percussion

Percussion over the chest and abdomen may reveal internal damage. Place your nondominant hand over the affected area.[4] Next, use the second and third fingers on your dominant hand to tap the DIP joint of the third finger on your nondominant hand. The tapping should be rapid.

Chest Percussion

Percussion should be performed over the auscultation sites. Normal percussion produces resonance. Hyperresonance may denote COPD, pneumothorax, or asthmatic attack. Dullness indicates the presence of fluid or solid tissue in the hollow cavity. Dull or thudlike sounds may occur with pneumonia, pleural effusions, or tumors.

Abdominal Percussion

Anatomical knowledge is essential for differentiating between usually hollow and solid organs. Tone indicates whether the organ is hollow or solid. Percussion of hollow organs produces **resonance**. Solid organs produce a dull thump. Any differentiation from normal denotes potential internal complications.

Palpations

Because accurate clinical special tests are limited, you must have anatomical knowledge and palpation skills to conduct effective evaluations of abdominal illnesses or injuries. A combination of thorough history taking and accurate palpations increases diagnostic accuracy.

- Abdominal palpations may reveal underlying infections, internal hemorrhage, obstruction, ruptures, or injuries. Abnormal lymphatic palpations may indicate a malignant or inflammatory process.

- Pulse palpations are assessed for rate, rhythm, symmetry, and intensity. Pathological illnesses and injuries may alter all or any of these facets. Peripheral pulse palpations have effectively screened for vascular pathologies, including peripheral arterial disease and vasculitis.

Diagnostic Tests

After establishing working differential diagnoses in the first part of the evaluation, you should use diagnostic tests to confirm or disprove the most likely theory. You must have an understanding of indications and contraindication for each test. As your roles and responsibilities continue to expand, you will likely become responsible for administration and initial interpretation; thus, you must be able to identify normal and abnormal findings. By gaining these skills and knowledge, you will be able to accurately communicate with other members of a patient's medical team.

Electrocardiogram

An electrocardiogram (ECG or EKG) noninvasively measures electrical activity of the heart.[6] The electrical activity corresponds to each heartbeat. It begins with activity in the atria transitioning to the ventricles. A 12-lead ECG takes each individual electrode signal to create the complete ECG waveform.

Indications

- Symptoms including chest palpitations, dizziness, cyanosis, chest pain, **syncope**, and seizure poisoning
- Signs or clinical conditions associated with heart disease, including tachycardia, bradycardia, hypothermia, murmur, shock, hypotension, and hypertension
- Detection of myocardial injury, ischemia, or previous history of either
- Cardiopulmonary resuscitation
- Electrolyte imbalances
- Screening tool for cardiomyopathy

Contraindications
- Patient refusal
- Adhesive allergy

Echocardiogram

An echocardiogram is a noninvasive diagnostic ultrasound that applies sound waves to produce an image of the heart.[7] This test allows assessment of the heart's movements and function of the valves. Echocardiograms are critical in the identification of hypertrophic cardiomyopathy.

Indications

- Chest pain
- Shortness of breath
- Hypotension
- Penetrating or blunt trauma
- Cardiac arrest

Contraindications

- Do not perform during CPR.
- Take care when performing over a wound or incision.

Urinalysis

Urinalysis provides quick general results for specific gravity, pH, and levels of leukocytes, nitrates, protein, glucose, ketones, urobilinogen, bilirubin, and blood (table 18.1).[8] Analysis requires a chemically treated dipstick. For the test, patients are instructed to perform a clean catch, which requires the patient to start the flow of urine into the toilet and then direct it into the cup.

Blood Testing

Blood tests often accompany routine examinations. Complete blood counts detect anemia, infections, clotting disorders, blood-based cancers, or immune system disorders. Immune system disorders include allergy, asthma, immune deficiency disorders, or autoimmune diseases. As part of the exam, blood tests assess red blood cells, white blood cells, platelets, hemoglobin, hematocrit, and mean corpuscular volume (table 18.2).[9]

Nerve Conduction and Electromyography Studies

Nerve conduction and electromyography (EMG) tests examine the electrical activity of the muscles and nerves. In order to contract, muscles must receive electrical

TABLE 18.1   Urinalysis Readings

Specific gravity	1.003-1.030	Low reading: diabetes mellitus, excessive hydration, renal failure High reading: dehydration, diarrhea, urinary tract infection, or renal failure
pH	5.0-9.0	Low reading: COPD, diabetic ketoacidosis High reading: renal failure, urinary tract infections
Glucose	<0.5	Diabetes mellitus, stress
Ketones	0	Diabetes mellitus, alcoholism, anorexia nervosa
Protein	0	Renal disease or injury, hypertension, fever, rhabdomyolysis
Hemoglobin	0	Urinary tract infection, sickle cell anemia, kidney disease or trauma
RBC	0	Kidney stones, vigorous activity, urinary tract infections

TABLE 18.2   Normal Values for Complete Blood Cell Test

Blood contents	Normal	Function
Red blood cells (RBC)	Males: 25-35 mL/kg body weight Females: 20-30 mL/kg body weight	Carry oxygen from lungs to the rest of the body
White blood cells	$4.5\text{-}11 \times 10^3$ cells/mcL	Fight infections and diseases Abnormal levels are signs of infection, blood cancer, or immune system dysfunction.
Platelets	$150\text{-}350 \times 10^3$ cells/mcL	Blood cells that assist in clotting Abnormal levels may be a sign of bleeding or thrombotic disorder.
Hemoglobin	Males: 14-17 g/dL Females: 12-16 g/dL	Iron-rich protein in RBCs that carries oxygen Abnormal levels may be a sign of anemia, thalassemia, or other blood disorders.
Hematocrit	Males: 41-51% Females: 36-47%	Measure of how much space RBCs take up in blood Abnormal levels may be a sign of blood or bone marrow disorders.

impulses via their peripheral nerves.[10] As the muscle reacts, the electrical activity disperses. Often, both studies are completed together.

- Nerve conduction studies measure the speed of electrical impulses down the peripheral nerves. Healthy nerves move faster than damaged ones. Results determine whether the injury is to the myelin sheath or the individual nerve fiber.
- EMG tests examine the electrical signals produced by the muscle at rest and with contractions.

Indications for Both

- *Motor neuropathy:* amyotrophic lateral sclerosis, polio
- *Sensory neuropathy:* paraneoplastic, autoimmune disorders
- *Radiculopathy:* disc herniation, nerve inflammation
- *Plexopathy:* neoplastic, entrapment
- *Entrapment neuropathy:* carpal tunnel syndrom
- *Neuromuscular junction disorders:* myasthenia gravis
- *Myopathy:* polymyositis, muscular dystrophy

Contraindications

- *Coagulopathy.* Patients who take anticoagulation medications or have thrombocytopenia are at a higher risk of bleeding with needle EMG.
- *Electrically sensitive patients.* Patients with central catheters, external or internal pacemakers, and other electrical devices should not undergo an EMG or nerve conduction study.
- *Pneumothorax.* With needle EMG, pneumothorax may occur at the sites of the serratus anterior, supraspinatus, rhomboids, lower cervical paraspinal, and thoracic paraspinal muscles.

Infectious Diseases

Athletic trainers often have a responsibility to teammates and coworkers who are in close quarters or direct skin-to-skin contact with infected patients. You must understand infectious diseases, including routes of transmission, management, and how long conditions are contagious. Without prompt recognition and referral, one patient may quickly infect more. Table 18.3 compares measles, mumps, and rubella (MMR), three increasingly common infectious diseases.

TABLE 18.3 Comparison of Measles, Mumps, and Rubella

Disease	Signs and symptoms	Differential diagnosis
Measles Dr P. Marazzi / Science Source	Fever, cough, conjunctivitis, spotted rash, facial rash, **Koplik's spots, malaise**	Rubella, scarlet fever, enterovirus infections
Mumps Dr P. Marazzi / Science Source	Fever, **parotitis**, headache, earache, jaw pain, malaise, sore throat	Influenza, mononucleosis, bacterial suppurative parotitis
Rubella Dr P. Marazzi / Science Source	Fever, lymphadenopathy, rash, malaise, nausea, sore throat, cough, myalgia	Measles, scarlet fever, mononucleosis, Zika virus

Measles, Mumps, and Rubella

Despite being preventable, measles, mumps, and rubella infections have surged in recent years. In 2019, measles cases in the United States reached the highest level in 25 years.[11] Mumps outbreaks have hit several secondary and higher education U.S. institutions, with some universities reporting hundreds of infected students.[12] The surge in cases has been attributed to the spread of vaccine misinformation, which has prevented many parents from getting their children vaccinated and students from getting necessary boosters.[13] No link exists between the measles, mumps, and rubella (MMR) vaccine and autism spectrum disorders.[13]

The MMR vaccination is approximately 93% effective after one dose and 97% effective after two doses.[13] MMR vaccination recommendations are as follows:

- First dose between 12 and 15 months old
- Second dose between 4 and 6 years
- 18-year-olds with no evidence of immunity: two doses separated by 28 days
- Adults with no evidence of immunity: one dose

Measles

Although the World Health organization declared measles eliminated from **endemic transmission** within the United States, infection rates have risen in recent years.[11] Measles are believed to be one of the most infectious agents known.[14]

- *Transmission.* Patients contract measles from direct contact with respiratory infectious droplets (spread by coughing or sneezing).
- *Treatment.* Treatment is centered on control of symptoms and addressing any secondary bacterial infections. Pain and fever are treated with acetaminophen. Cough is addressed with an over-the-counter suppressant. Vitamin A is recommended for children immediately on diagnostic confirmation.
- *Return to activity.* The incubation period for the infection is 10 to 12 days. Patients are contagious for 8 days, starting 4 days before the first appearance of the rash.

Mumps

As with measles, reports of mumps outbreaks at U.S. universities have increased sharply in recent years.[12] Many of these universities lacked documentation regarding student MMR vaccinations and university-wide policies on communicable diseases. To be effectively immunized, students should have received two doses of the MMR vaccine. In response to these outbreaks, the Advisory Committee on Immunization Practices recommends a third vaccination for college students and members of other high-risk populations.[12]

- *Transmission:* Mumps are contracted by direct contact with respiratory infectious droplets (spread by coughing or sneezing).
- *Diagnostic confirmation:* comes from a blood test
- *Treatment:* Recommendations include a focus on hydration, ice or hot packs for discomfort, and nonaspirin medications, such as acetaminophen or ibuprofen.
- *Return to activity:* Cases are considered infectious from 2 days before the appearance of parotitis to 5 days afterwards.

Rubella

Rubella is a mild, limiting disease in children. However, a pregnant woman can pass the infection to her fetus, with potentially life-altering or deadly consequences for the child.[16]

- *Transmission:* The disease is most likely contracted from inhalation of airborne droplets or direct contact with upper respiratory secretions.
- *Diagnostic confirmation:* comes from a blood test
- *Treatment:* For postnatal infections in adults, treatment is mainly symptomatic, including bed rest, hydration, and the use of nonsteroidal anti-inflammatory drugs for the arthralgia. Congenital-acquired rubella in babies requires a multi-interdisciplinary plan to address the broad range of limitations.
- *Return to activity:* The infectious period is from 7 days before onset of symptoms to 7 days afterwards.

Meningitis

Meningitis is inflammation of the meninges that line the skull and vertebral column.[17] The most likely pathogens are either bacterial or viral. Rare forms have fungal, noninfectious, or unknown etiologies. Severities range from self-limiting to potentially life-threatening.

- *Transmission:* direct contact with respiratory infectious droplets (spread by coughing or sneezing)
- *Symptoms:* neck stiffness, headache, altered mental status, nausea, **photophobia, phonophobia**
- *Signs:* fever, rash, focal neurological deficits, seizures
- *Differential diagnosis:* Meningitis may be diagnosed as vasculitis, West Nile virus, or tuberculosis. Diagnostic confirmation requires blood culture, lumbar puncture, and a computed tomography (CT) scan of the head.
- *Treatment:* Intravenous fluids are recommended for initial treatment. **Empiric** antibiotics should be initiated immediately for suspected bacterial cases, even before culture confirmation. For suspected viral meningitis or encephalitis cases, acyclovir should be added to the treatment. Dexamethasone is traditionally used to assist in inflammation control. Symptomatic control may involve antipyretics, antiepileptics, or analgesics.
- *Return to activity:* The course of treatment is between 7 and 14 days.

Mononucleosis

Mononucleosis is caused by the Epstein-Barr virus.[18,19] While the symptomatic phase lasts 2 to 4 weeks, infected patients actively shed the virus for months after exposure.

- *Transmission:* The chief method is direct salivary contact with an infected patient.
- *Symptoms:* **splenomegaly, myalgia, arthralgia,** chills, sweats, headaches, nausea, and vomiting
- *Signs:* fever, lymphadenopathy, pharyngitis, tonsillar swelling
- *Differential diagnosis:* influenza, rubella, *streptococcus* infection
- *Diagnostic confirmation:* comes from a blood test
- *Treatment:* Symptomatic control is the only recommended treatment course. Control involves getting rest, staying hydrated, and eating well. Over-the-counter pain relievers are optional for treatment of fever and sore throat.

- *Return to activity:* A minimum of 3 weeks of restricted activity is recommended for contact sport athletes to avoid the increased risk of splenic rupture. Athletes must obtain a physician's release to return to activity.[9]

Influenza

Influenza is an acute viral infection.[20,21]

- *Transmission:* inhalation of airborne droplets or direct contact with upper respiratory secretions
- *Symptoms:* nasal congestion, sore throat, body aches, pain, malaise, headaches, and chills
- *Signs:* cough, sweating, and rhinitis
- *Differential diagnosis:* rhinovirus, upper respiratory tract infections
- *Diagnostic confirmation:* involves patient presentation or blood test[20]
- *Treatment:* Seasonal influenza vaccine and antiviral medications are recommended for prevention and treatment for everyone over the age of 6 months.[21] For those suspected of having an active infection, prompt initiation of antiviral treatment reduces morbidity and mortality.[20] Symptomatic control involves ensuring proper hydration and taking over-the-counter medications for pain relief, fever reduction, cough suppression, and nasal decongestion.
- *Return to activity:* Patients are contagious from approximately 24 hours before onset of symptoms to 5 to 10 days following symptoms.

COVID-19

COVID-19 is an infectious disease caused by a newer strain of the coronavirus. The symptomatic phase lasts from 2 to 14 days after contact with the virus. People have varying responses to the virus; some people have mild to moderate respiratory illness, while older people and those with underlying medical conditions (e.g., cardiovascular disease, diabetes, cancer) may develop life threatening symptoms. A concern for athletes is cardiovascular implications, such as myocarditis.[91,96,103] In addition, the psychological, mental, and emotional toll of the quarantine period and loss of athletic participation must be assessed.[92-95,97-102]

- *Transmission:* The chief method is airborne
- *Symptoms:* Fever or chills, cough, shortness of breath or difficulty breathing, fatigue, muscle or body aches, headache, new loss of taste or smell, sore throat, congestion or runny nose, nausea or vomiting, diarrhea

- *Signs:* a range exists from no signs of the virus, to the symptoms indicated above, to only post-virus long-term effects (brain fogginess, breathing difficulties, and other diverse signs currently under investigation)
- *Differential diagnosis:* influenza
- *Diagnostic confirmation:* Two types of testing that can be accomplished through nasal or throat swab and saliva. An antigen test detects proteins of the virus. A PCR (polymerase chain reaction) test, also called a molecular test, detects genetic material of the virus.
- *Treatment:* Symptomatic control is the only recommended treatment course for mild to moderate symptoms. People with symptoms of difficulty breathing, low pulse oximeter reading, confusion, inability to stay awake, or blue or purplish nailbeds or lips should go to the emergency department for immediate care.
- *Return to activity:* Protocol is evolving. Current standards suggest monitoring increased cardiovascular workload over 1 to 2 weeks. Asymptomatic athletes may progress at a faster rate than symptomatic athletes.

Chicken Pox

Infection with the varicella zoster virus causes chicken pox (figure 18.4).[22] Most people contract the virus before 10 years of age, which means the majority of older children and adults harbor the latent varicella zoster virus. Reactivation of the virus leads to replication, which causes zoster (shingles; figure 18.5) in tissues innervated by the involved neurons, leading to inflammation and cell death. This process can lead to persistent radicular pain.

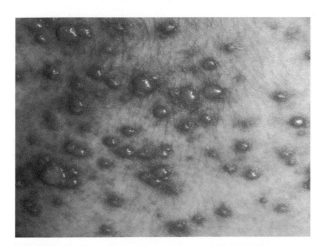

FIGURE 18.4 Chicken pox.

Clinical Photography, Central Manchester University Hospitals NHS Foundation Trust, UK / Science Source

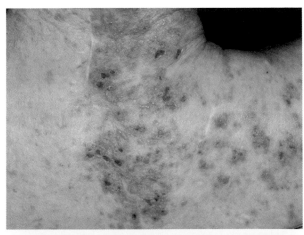

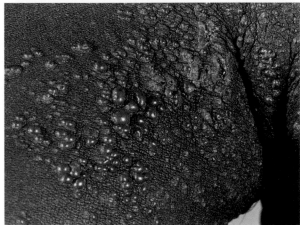

FIGURE 18.5 Shingles.

Dr P. Marazzi / Science Source; Dr M.A. Ansary / Science Source

- *Transmission:* airborne
- *Symptoms:*
  - Varicella (chicken pox) involves malaise, loss of appetite, and pain.
  - Severe varicella is characterized by fever and presence of a complication:
    - Myelitis
    - Cranial nerve palsies
    - Meningitis stroke (vasculopathy)
    - Retinitis
    - Gastroenterological infections (ulcers, pancreatitis, and hepatitis)
    - Neuralgia
- *Signs:* Varicella and zoster present with generalized or unilateral dermatomal vesicular rashes (see figures 18.4 and 18.5). The vesicles are often present on the face and trunk.
- *Differential diagnosis:* measles, rubella encephalitis, enteroviruses, dermatitis

- *Diagnostic confirmation:* involves blood tests and lumbar puncture
- *Treatment:* Varicella (chicken pox) treatment is usually symptomatic relief.
  - Acetaminophen is the preferred antipyretic.
  - Topical antipruritic agents are of anecdotal benefit.
  - Antiviral medications are used only for severe varicella or those patients at greater risk of developing complications based on age, compromised immunity, or chronic diseases to the skin or lung.
- *Treatment:* Treatment recommendations for varicella zoster virus (shingles) are antiviral medications for patients over 50 and those who have lesions around the face or eye, severe rash, or other complications. Antiviral treatment normally lasts for 7 to 10 days. This treatment speeds up formation of new lesions and lesion crusting and reduces pain. Mild zoster pain is treated with NSAIDs or acetaminophen. Lidocaine patches can reduce pain. For severe pain, opioids, anticonvulsants, and antidepressants are recommended.
- *Return to activity:* Varicella and varicella zoster are contagious for 24 to 48 hours before the onset of the rash and until all the lesions are crusted over. Varicella zoster requires a minimum of 5 days of treatment before returning to activity.

Viral Encephalitis

Viral encephalitis, particularly herpes simplex, is a severe neurological infection that may lead to permanent neurological deficits or death.[23] Encephalitis is an inflammation of the brain. Viral encephalitis differs from meningitis in that it disturbs cortical function with subsequent seizures.

- *Transmission:* Viral encephalitis is contracted from inhalation of airborne droplets or direct contact with upper respiratory secretions. Infected animals or insects may transmit the virus via bites.
- *Symptoms:* The clinical triad of symptoms and signs for a neurological infection involve headache, fever, and neck stiffness (elicited by neck flexion).
- *Sign:* new rash presentation, seizures, or other abnormal focal neurological findings
- *Differential diagnosis:* bacterial meningitis, acute disseminated encephalomyelitis, acute ischemic stroke, epilepsy
- *Diagnostic confirmation:* comes from lumbar puncture, CT, or magnetic resonance imaging (MRI)

- *Treatment:* Treatment is essential within the first hour of symptoms. To initiate treatment, the clinician should obtain the patient's vital signs, assess mental status, measure serum glucose level, and start IV fluid resuscitation. When infection is highly suspected, the clinician should start parenteral antimicrobials while waiting for a brain CT. Patients should be started on a combination of ampicillin and vancomycin or vancomycin and trimethoprim-sulfamethoxazole if they have a penicillin allergy. If there is a high suspicion of viral encephalitis, acyclovir should be started at appropriate doses. Antiepileptic medications must be initiated at the first sign of abnormal focal neurologic findings.
- *Return to activity:* Because of the high mortality rate with this illness, patients should complete weeks of therapy before return to activity can be considered.

Hepatitis

Hepatitis can be self-limiting or can lead to the development of fibrosis, cirrhosis, or cancer.[24] Acute infections may occur with limited symptoms, such as jaundice, dark urine, extreme fatigue, nausea, vomiting, and abdominal pain. There are five types of hepatitis: A, B, C, D, and E.

Hepatitis A

Symptoms are normally mild but may progress into severe or potentially life-threatening situations. Unlike hepatitis B and C, hepatitis A does not result in a chronic condition.

- *Transmission:* fecal–oral route or ingestion of contaminated food or water
- *Symptoms:* malaise, loss of appetite, nausea, discomfort
- *Signs:* fever, dark urine, **jaundice**, vomiting
- *Differential diagnosis:* other forms of hepatitis, Epstein-Barr virus, herpes simplex, leptospirosis, **sepsis**
- *Treatment:* Treatment is centered on supportive care of symptoms.
- *Return to activity:* Complete recovery may take several weeks to months. Lab abnormalities return to normal within 1 to 6 weeks.

Hepatitis B

- *Transmission:* Hepatitis B is contracted through **parenteral** contact. The virus lasts outside the body for at least 7 days.
- *Symptoms:* fatigue, nausea, abdominal pain

- *Signs:* jaundice, dark urine, vomiting
- *Differential diagnosis:* other forms of hepatitis, cholangitis, hepatocellular carcinoma, hemochromatosis
- *Treatment:* There is a preventive vaccine. No standard treatment for acute hepatitis B exists. Acute treatment is focused on comfort, adequate nutrition, and hydration. For chronic infections, antivirals are recommended to slow the progression of cirrhosis. Since treatment only slows progression of the disease, patients will need lifelong treatment.
- *Return to activity:* An infected patient will require at least 1 year of treatment.

Hepatitis C

- *Transmission:* Hepatitis C is a blood-borne virus that is transmitted through exposure to an infected sample or source. Mechanisms for transmission include injection misuse, not practicing universal precautions, unscreened blood transfusion, and unsafe sex.
- *Symptoms:* fatigue, decreased appetite, nausea, abdominal pain, joint pain
- *Signs:* fever, vomiting, dark urine, gray-colored feces, jaundice
- *Differential diagnosis:* other forms of hepatitis, cholecystitis, alcoholic liver disease
- *Treatment:* Based on the immune response, new infections of hepatitis C do not always require treatment. For chronic infections, antivirals are the recommended treatment agents. Approximately 30% of patients spontaneously clear the virus within 6 months of treatment.
- *Return to activity:* The usual course of treatment lasts approximately 3 to 6 months.

Hepatitis D

Hepatitis D virus (HDV) requires the hepatitis B virus to replicate. The majority of patients are asymptomatic. A coinfection of HDV in a person with chronic hepatitis B is considered the most severe form of chronic hepatitis, progressing quickly to carcinoma or death.

- *Transmission:* during childbirth or parenteral contact with infected fluids
- *Symptoms:* abdominal pain, nausea, confusion
- *Signs:* fever, vomiting, jaundice, bruising, bleeding
- *Differential diagnosis:* other forms of hepatitis, cholecystitis, pancreatitis, herpes zoster, gastroesophageal reflux disease (GERD), bowel obstruction
- *Treatment:* Current guidelines recommend Pegylated interferon alpha treatment for at least 48 weeks.
- *Return to activity:* Hepatitis D patients may not return to activity for up to a year.

Hepatitis E

This infection is most common among 15- to 40-year-olds. Hepatitis E rarely occurs in the United States or developed countries but is often found in other parts of the world.

- *Transmission:* The disease is contracted through fecaloral routes. Infected people shed the virus via their stools. It is passed in contaminated blood transfusions, food, or water. Less frequently, hepatitis E is ingested in undercooked meat.
- *Symptoms:* reduced appetite, nausea, abdominal pain, itching, joint pain
- *Signs:* mild fever, vomiting, rash, jaundice, hepatomegaly
- *Differential diagnosis:* other forms of hepatitis, hepatic failure, peripheral neuropathy, encephalitis
- *Treatment:* No standardized treatment for hepatitis E exists. Treatment focuses on providing supportive care with vitamins, albumin, plasma, and supplements.
- *Return to activity:* Patients excrete the virus for approximately 3 to 4 weeks following initiation of treatment.

Zika Virus

Although the Zika virus was first identified in 1947, the first major outbreak occurred in 2007, and multiple outbreaks have been reported since.[25] The course of active symptoms is 2 to 7 days, and the majority of people infected do not present symptoms.

- *Transmission:* Zika is most notably transmitted by mosquitoes. Vertical transmission between a mother and her fetus is most likely to result in the development of microcephaly and other neurological deficits in unborn children. The other means of transmission is the exchange of bodily fluids with an infected host.
- *Symptoms:* joint arthralgia, headache
- *Signs:* fever, red eyes, maculopapular rash
- *Differential diagnosis:* Chikungunya, dengue fever

- *Diagnostic confirmation:* comes from blood or urine tests; pregnant women may require a prenatal ultrasound
- *Treatment:* The protocol involves symptomatic care. Bed rest and hydration are encouraged. Pain and fever should be treated with acetaminophen.
- *Return to activity:* Patients may remain contagious for 1 to 2 weeks following symptom presentation. Clinicians must educate patients on how unsafe sex practice leads to transmission of the Zika virus.

Respiratory System Conditions

The respiratory system delivers oxygen through the trachea, down either primary bronchial tube, and into multiple levels of terminal bronchioles. The exchange of O_2 and CO_2 occurs in the alveoli. Diffusion occurs across adjacent capillaries to deliver oxygen back to the heart. Acute or chronic inflammation of the airway will limit oxygen delivery to areas of need, causing subset increases in respiration rate, pulse, and blood pressures. Inability to meet this increased demand will lead to inhibition of athletic and daily activities. As energy demands increase, the system will eventually fail. Clinicians must be able to identify and differentiate risk factors, signs, symptoms, and recommended treatment plans to eliminate inflammatory mediators and thus ensure optimal respiratory function.

Asthma

Asthma is a chronic inflammatory disorder resulting in variable airway obstruction and bronchial hyperresponsiveness.[26] Triggers are allergens, pollutants, infections, aspirin, NSAIDs, inhaled irritants, particulate exposure, and environmental exposure. Athletic trainers should have an emergency action plan (EAP) for asthma. All patients should have a rescue inhaler. See chapter 23 for the steps for using an inhaler.

- *Symptoms:* recurrent episodes of wheezing, inability to catch breath, chest tightness, coughing
- *Signs:* patients with any severity of the following signs of respiratory distress:
  - Significant increase in wheezing or chest tightness
  - Rate of 25 breaths per minute or more
  - Inability to speak in full sentences
  - Uncontrolled cough
  - Prolonged expiration phase
  - Nasal flaring

- For paradoxical abdominal movement, refer patient to the emergency department or his personal physician.
- *Differential diagnosis:* exercise-induced bronchospasm, vocal cord dysfunction, bronchitis, GERD, rhinosinusitis
- *Treatment:* People with exercise-induced asthma should have short- and long-term beta-agonist inhalers. Albuterol, a short-acting beta-agonist, should be taken 10 to 15 minutes before activity. Use of Albuterol more than three times per day should prompt concern and physician referral. Long-acting beta-agonists are meant only for prophylaxis and should be used in combination with a corticosteroid. Leukotriene modifiers, corticosteroids, and chromones are other adjunctive therapies for asthma control.
- *Return to activity:* During an attack, the patient should self-administer rescue medications. After the use of the rescue inhaler, the athlete should be monitored for 15 to 20 minutes. If any of the preceding signs continue or increase, the patient should be referred to a physician for evaluation.

Exercise-Induced Bronchospasm

Exercise-induced bronchospasm (EIB) is a transient narrowing of the airway without acute inflammation in susceptible people.[27] The terms EIB and exercise-induced asthma were used interchangeably in the past, but evidence suggests that they are separate conditions.[27] EIB is associated only with exercise and is mediated by different inflammatory mediators. EIB is most common among athletes who practice cold-weather sports. See chapter 23 for the steps for using an inhaler.

- *Symptoms:* shortness of breath, chest tightness, early fatigue, poor performance
- *Signs:* wheezing, cough
- *Differential diagnosis:* vocal cord dysfunction, chronic lung disease, asthma, general deconditioning, hyperventilation, GERD
- *Treatment:* Reducing symptoms is the center of treatment. Short-acting beta-adrenergic agonists are the treatment of choice. They should be taken 15 to 20 minutes before activity. The treatment duration is 2 to 4 hours. Long-acting beta-agonists should not be used as a monotherapy. Debatable effectiveness of inhaled corticosteroids warrants the addition of the long-acting beta-agonists. Nonpharmaceutical treatment options include improving conditioning and diet, instituting a warm-up period, using nasal strips, and avoiding certain environmental exposures.

- *Return to activity:* Similar to asthma, the patient may administer a prescribed short-acting beta-adrenergic agonist. The symptoms are likely to decrease with the termination of activity within 10 to 15 minutes.

Acute Bronchitis

Patients with acute bronchitis have a heavy cough with inflamed trachea and bronchi but without evidence of pneumonia.[28] Viral infections are most likely responsible. The cough typically lasts 2 to 3 weeks.

- *Symptom:* an acute cough often accompanied by sputum production, nasal congestion, headache, and fever
- *Sign:* wheezes or rhonchi on lung auscultation
- *Differential diagnosis:* Similar conditions include severe asthma, COPD, heart failure, and pneumonia. A temperature over 100°F (38°C) should prompt consideration of influenza or pneumonia.
- *Treatment:* No antibiotics are recommended for viral sinusitis, pharyngitis, and bronchitis. For acute cough, over-the-counter medications are usually recommended, including ibuprofen, acetaminophen, and steam inhalation. Expectorants, like guaifenesin, decrease cough frequency and intensity.
- *Return to activity:* As long as no fever is present, athletes should be allowed to participate as tolerated.

Pneumonia

Pneumonia is an infection of the alveoli and respiratory bronchioles.[29] The predominant cause of community-acquired pneumonia is a viral infection. Bacterial pneumonia is typically caused by *Streptococcus pneumoniae*.

- *Symptoms:* chest pain, confusion
- *Signs:* cough, fever, **tachypnea, dyspnea**, tachycardia
- *Differential diagnosis:* Diagnoses include pulmonary embolism, lymphoma, lupus erythematosus. Chest radiography is indicated in cases with one of the following: fever, tachycardia, tachypnea.
- *Treatment:* Uncomplicated cases of pneumonia are typically treated with narrow-spectrum penicillin alone or in combination with a macrolide antibiotic. Penicillin-resistant strains require broad-spectrum antibiotics, such as cephalosporins.
- *Return to activity:* Patients should be treated for a minimum of 5 days and should be fever free

for 2 or 3 days before discontinuing treatment. Longer recovery time before return to play will be required for cases with extrapulmonary infections.

Rhinovirus

Rhinovirus, or the common cold virus, is a self-limiting illness with durations of 7 to 14 days.[30] It is often found in upper and lower respiratory tract infections. Rhinovirus infections exacerbate asthma reactions.

- *Symptoms:* combination of rhinorrhea, nasal congestion, sore throat, cough, headache, and malaise
- *Signs:* low-grade fever, sneezing
- *Differential diagnosis:* influenza, rhinitis, pertussis, mononucleosis
- *Treatment:* Treatment centers on supportive symptomatic relief, such as decongestants and antihistamine. Development and clinical trials of antiviral medications for prevention and potential treatment are ongoing.
- *Return to activity:* Patients may participate as tolerated.

Rhinosinusitis

Rhinosinusitis is an inflammation of the mucosal lining of the sinuses and the nasal cavity.[31] The majority of acute cases are caused by viral upper respiratory infections. Nearly 80% of patients with asthma display a form of rhinosinusitis. Rhinosinusitis is associated with more severe asthma symptoms. Chronic rhinosinusitis involves sinus inflammation and swelling for 12 weeks or more.[32] It potentially presents with nasal obstruction, olfactory dysfunction, thick mucus drainage, and recurrent bacterial infections.

- *Symptoms:* Symptoms include anterior or posterior drainage, nasal obstruction, **hyposmia** or **anosmia**, and facial pain and pressure. The likelihood of bacterial infection is increased with double sickening, purulent rhinorrhea, and secretions.
- *Signs:* Chronic signs are purulence, edema, nasal polyps, and mucous membrane thickening.
- *Differential diagnosis:* rhinitis, upper respiratory tract infection
- *Treatment:* Consider antibiotics for patients whose symptoms do not resolve within 10 days. Analgesics, intranasal corticosteroids, and nasal irrigation are recommended treatments. Management includes saline irrigation, intranasal or systemic glucocorticoids, antibiotics, and antileu-

kotriene agents. Decongestants, antihistamines, and guaifenesin are not currently recommended because of unproven effectiveness, side effects, and cost.

- *Return to activity:* Athletes may be able to participate as tolerated.

Chronic Obstructive Pulmonary Disease

Chronic obstructive pulmonary disease (COPD) is a common preventable geriatric condition.[33] Regardless of preventability, COPD remains the fourth leading cause of death worldwide.[33] COPD is characterized by chronic airway inflammation that leads to structural repairs, which narrow airways, thicken walls, and lead to loss of alveolar attachments. Emphysema and chronic bronchitis are the two most common contributing factors to COPD.

- *Symptoms:* dyspnea, chest tightness
- *Signs:* cough with or without sputum
- *Differential diagnosis:* asthma, chronic heart failure, tuberculosis
- *Diagnostic confirmation:* pulmonary function test
- *Treatment:* Short-acting beta-agonists are the most commonly prescribed medication. Some patients also receive a long-acting beta-agonist or antimuscarinic agent to supplement the short-acting beta-agonists. The use of an inhaled corticosteroid to supplement bronchotherapy agents is the current standard of care. Despite being useful, home oxygen therapy and pulmonary rehab are used in only 25% of cases.
- *Return to activity:* Exercise training should be a cornerstone of pulmonary rehab.[34] Cardiorespi-

ratory exercise is shown to improve exercise tolerance and reduce dyspnea and fainting. Interval exercise to tolerable levels of dyspnea sensations provides the greatest benefit.

Chronic Bronchitis

Chronic bronchitis is an inflammation of the bronchial tubes leading to mucus production.[35] Diagnosis requires a productive cough for more than 3 months per year for 2 consecutive years. Cough with mucus production increases COPD exacerbations associated with impaired quality of life, deterioration of lung function, increased risk of hospital admissions, and increased mortality.

- *Symptoms:* malaise, chest pain, abdominal pain, dyspnea
- *Signs:* Patients have cough with or without phlegm. Phlegm is clear, yellow, green, or blood tinged. Wheezes or rhonchi heard on lung auscultation. Patients may have hypoxia, hypercapnia, lower leg edema, or cyanotic appearance.
- *Differential diagnosis:* influenza or pneumonia
- *Treatment:* Similar to COPD, medications include chronic bronchodilators and inhaled corticosteroids. Antibiotic therapy and phosphodiesterase-4 inhibitors are used for secondary bacterial infections and anti-inflammatory effects, respectively. Chronic bronchitis, COPD, and emphysema would all benefit from pulmonary rehab.
- *Return to activity:* The introduction to physical activity will provide the same benefits for patients with chronic bronchitis as for those with COPD.[34] Patients should work with a professional to set intensity levels to train at a desirable level of dyspnea.

Pulmonary Rehabilitation

Successful rehabilitation requires an interdisciplinary team that may include physicians, physical therapists, psychosocial therapists, nutritionists, and athletic trainers. Pulmonary rehab entails education, lifestyle modifications, regular physical activity, and avoidance of exposures.[34] These programs have improved function and quality-of-life outcomes for patients with COPD, asthma, pulmonary hypertension, and cystic fibrosis. Patients are also referred after lung surgery.

- *Education.* Effective patient education should include outlining the disease and exacerbating triggers, exposures, and medications.
- *Lifestyle modifications.* Nutrition counseling targets obesity. Therapists may offer behavioral, social, or anxiety-reduction techniques to improve the patient's mental health.
- *Regular physical activity.* Physician clearance and an individualized training format are required for each patient. Exercised-based pulmonary rehabilitation can result in reduced anxiety, depression, cardiovascular disease markers, and episodes of dyspnea and fatigue.

Emphysema

Emphysema is a pathological diagnosis that affects the air spaces distal to the terminal bronchioles. This leads to abnormal permanent enlargement of the lung's air spaces with the destruction of the lung parenchyma and walls without any fibrosis.[35] Damage to bronchioles, alveolar sacs, ducts, and alveoli ultimately decreases the surface area for gas exchange.

- *Symptoms:* shortness of breath, dyspnea, anxiousness
- *Signs:* cough with or without sputum, wheezing, minimal cyanosis, pursed lip breathing, use of accessory muscles to breathe
- *Differential diagnosis:* chronic bronchitis, cystic fibrosis, anemia, heart failure
- *Treatment:* Treatment includes pulmonary function tests (PFT). Blood gases are not usually required in moderate to mild cases. Patients with exacerbations should use beta blockers and anticholinergics with nebulizers and then switch to systemic corticosteroids taken with a metered-dose inhaler. Prevention is smoking cessation and vaccination against pneumococcus and influenza.
- *Return to activity:* The patient should take part in pulmonary rehabilitation. Individualized rehabilitation plans help improve pulmonary function and quality of life in emphysema patients.

Cardiovascular System Conditions

The three main functions of the cardiovascular system are transportation of nutrients, gases, and wastes; pro-tection from infection and blood loss; and maintenance of body temperature. Conditions range from clinically insignificant to potentially catastrophic. Whether as part of a preparticipation examination or initial illness evaluation, you must be able to identify signs and symptoms that warrant referrals. Prompt recognition of conditions and proper management of them decrease the risk of dire complications.

Hypertension

Hypertension is a condition where systolic blood pressure (SBP) values are more than 130 mmHg or diastolic blood pressure (DBP) values are more than 80 mmHg.[36] Uncontrolled hypertension contributes to heart disease, stroke, renal failure, aortic **aneurysm**, and death. Recommendations vary, but consensus suggests that patients with persistent readings over 140/90 mmHg should undergo treatment, with the goal of reducing blood pressure to under 130/80 mmHg.[36]

- *Symptoms:* chest pain, shortness of breath, palpitations, headache
- *Signs:* **diaphoresis**, flushed appearance, heart murmur
- *Differential diagnosis:* coarctation of the aorta, renal artery stenosis, chronic kidney disease, and aortic valve disease
  - Athletic trainers should perform at least two office measurements of blood pressure that should be done on two separate occasions prior to diagnosis. They should take three blood pressure measures at least 1 minute apart, then record the values and average the last two readings.
- *Treatment:* Nonpharmacological treatment requires patient education, weight reduction,

EVIDENCE-BASED ATHLETIC TRAINING

Exercise and Cardiovascular Risk in Patients With Hypertension

As part of a literature review, researchers examined the effects of exercise type, intensity, and duration on patients with hypertension.[38] Regardless of age, exercise session frequency, or baseline body mass index, initiation of cardiorespiratory exercise produces clinically significant reductions in systolic and diastolic blood pressures. Compared to prehypertensive patients, hypertensive patients demonstrate the largest positive effects to cardiorespiratory exercise. Low- to moderate-intensity exercise (50% of estimated $\dot{V}O_2$max) for as little as 30 minutes per week produces significant reductions in hypertension, with the greatest reductions occurring with 60 to 90 minutes of exercise per week. Patients wishing to start a moderate- or vigorous-intensity exercise program should undergo an exercise test. Those with severe hypertension need a clinical evaluation before starting exercise. High-intensity interval training is capable of producing greater improvements in ambulatory blood pressure and $\dot{V}O_2$max. In addition to designing prevention and rehabilitation plans, athletic trainers must have the necessary knowledge to optimize outcomes for hypertensive patients.

smoking cessation, and exercise. Pharmaceuticals should be used with patients who have blood pressure greater than 140/90 mmHg. Prescription choices are angiotensin-converting enzyme inhibitors, angiotensin receptor blockers, diuretics, calcium channel blockers (CCBs), and beta-blockers. A pharmaceutical plan should be tried for 8 to 12 weeks before reassessing the outcome.

- *Return to activity:* Exercise is contraindicated for patients with a blood pressure reading above 200 mmHg or diastolic pressure over 110 mmHg.[37] Clinical evaluations are recommended before initiation of an exercise program.

Hypertrophic Cardiomyopathy

Hypertrophic cardiomyopathy is a genetic disorder characterized by left ventricular hypertrophy and a nondilated left ventricle with preserved or increased ejection fraction.[39] It is the highest cause of sudden death in adolescent athletes. Most are either asymptomatic or mildly symptomatic until the fatal event.

- *Symptoms:* exertional dyspnea, exercise intolerance, chest pain, palpitations, murmur
- *Signs:* orthopnea, peripheral edema, elevated diastolic pressure, syncope, arrhythmia
- *Differential diagnosis:* myocardial hypertrophy (athletic heart)
- *Treatment:* Asymptomatic or mildly symptomatic patients do not require pharmacological treatment. Education regarding genetic information, risk of transmission, and avoiding competitive sports or intense exercise is essential for preventing catastrophic cardiovascular events. Beta-blockers and diuretics may be used for treatment. Atrial fibrillation cases may require cardioversion or pacemaker implantation.
- *Return to activity:* Most patients may participate in low-intensity sports.

Iron Deficiency

Iron deficiency and iron-deficiency anemia result from training stress, insufficient energy, inadequate recovery, and external stressors.[40] Both iron deficiency and iron-deficiency anemia have negative effects on aerobic exercise performance and health. With anemia, the decrease in hemoglobin impairs oxygen delivery, leading to performance decreases. Female athletes are at a greater risk of the condition, with up to 50% of distance runners presenting with low iron and hemoglobin levels.

- *Symptoms:* fatigue, headache
- *Signs:* shortness of breath, cramps, rapid heartbeat, pale skin
- *Differential diagnosis:* thalassemia, sickle cell anemia, rheumatoid arthritis
- *Treatment:* The recommended iron supplement allowance is 18 mg per day for women and 8 mg per day for men, and the upper limit is 45 mg per day. Athletes have shown increases in iron absorption of 40, 80, 160, and 240 mg per day. The highest absorption rate was between 40 and 60 mg on alternate days.
- *Return to activity:* Athletes experiencing symptoms may suffer decreased performance, and athletic trainers may consider restricting their activity. Athletes may participate as tolerated.

Sickle Cell Anemia

Sickle cell anemia is an inherited blood disorder.[41] It is a single-point mutation that leads to the presence of abnormal hemoglobin. When the red blood cells (RBCs) become deoxygenated, the cells **polymerize**, inducing the sickling process and giving rise to sickled RBCs (figure 18.6). Lowered blood pH, RBC dehydration, and hyperthermia also prompt sickling. The resulting stasis causes **hypoxia**. These rigid RBCs are more fragile and prone to **hemolytic** episodes, leading to anemia.

Sickle cell trait is marked by the presence of normal and abnormal hemoglobin. It is prevalent in 20% to 40% of African Americans. The trait is usually considered benign. During athletic participation or under certain circumstances, the vaso-occlusive events (exertional

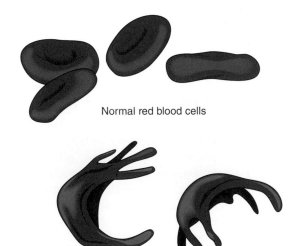

Normal red blood cells

Sickle cells

FIGURE 18.6 Normal red blood cells versus sickle cells.

sickling) may lead to death. Two clinic-pathological patterns have emerged: among (1) patients who developed exertional rhabdomyolysis and (2) patients who did not develop rhabdomyolysis.

Exertional Sickling

In a sickling event, the low oxygen levels and decreased pH lead to intravascular sickling within active vessels.[42] As sickling continues to decrease oxygen levels, the positive feedback loop triggers metabolic failure. This metabolic failure results in rhabdomyolysis and acute renal failure.

- *Symptoms:* muscle weakness, cramping, mild pain[43]
- *Signs:* collapse
- *Differential diagnosis:* heat stroke, heat exhaustion
- *Treatment:* For prevention, athletes should slowly build cardiorespiratory endurance and emphasize hydration. During an acute event, you should assess the athlete's vital signs, provide supplemental oxygen and hydration, cool the athlete, activate EMS, and notify health care professionals of rhabdomyolysis suspicion. If the athlete's core temperature is above 104°F (40°C), give her a cold-water immersion for 15 to 20 minutes before attempting transport to an advanced level of care.
- *Return to activity:* Athletes should receive physician's clearance before a gradual return to activity.

Rhabdomyolysis

Rhabdomyolysis is a breakdown of the skeletal muscular tissue due to trauma or extreme exertion which then releases enzymes and electrolytes that are difficult to metabolize in large quantities, potentially resulting in kidney failure. Rhabdomyolysis may also be a result of sickle cell anemia. As exertional sickling slows oxygen, patients may fall into rhabdomyolysis, leading to muscle breakdown, metabolic acidosis, lactic academia, myoglobinuria, renal failure, and disseminated intravascular coagulation.[42,43]

- *Symptoms:* cramping in abdominal area, back and extremities
- *Signs:* tenderness in abdominal area, back, extremities; rapid breathing conditions
- *Differential diagnosis:* Similar conditions include heat exhaustion, heat stroke, and cardiac conditions. Presentation differs from heat illness in that the athlete slumps to the ground and has normal appearance and air movement and a rectal temperature less than 103°F (39.5°C).

- *Treatment:* Immediate treatment requires activating EMS, cooling the athlete, monitoring vitals, and administering high flow oxygen (15 L/min).[43]
- *Return to activity:* Physician clearance is required before a gradual return to play.

Gastrointestinal System Conditions

The gastrointestinal system transports food and helps the body digest food and absorb. Progression of the following disorders may begin to inhibit some activities of daily living and physical activity. With accurate evaluation and appropriate management programs, patients may avoid progression of these disorders that would likely lead to surgical intervention.

Gastroesophageal Reflux Disease

Gastroesophageal reflux disease (GERD) is a condition of the retrograde flow of stomach contents into the esophagus.[44] GERD is classified as either nonerosive or erosive. Erosive GERD denotes esophageal mucosal histopathological changes.

- *Symptoms:* heartburn, regurgitation, dysphagia, nausea
- *Signs:* chest pain
- *Differential diagnosis:* peptic ulcer, tumor, cholelithiasis, angina
- *Treatment:* Initial treatment should begin with 8 weeks of **proton pump inhibitors (PPIs)**. If symptoms resolution was obtained, the treatment can be discontinued. The cornerstone of treatment is lifestyle modifications, including weight-loss counseling and avoidance of alcohol, tobacco, and foods that aggravate symptoms. Antacid and other antisecretory medications offer relief. Long-term treatment requires aggressive maintenance therapy using PPIs, surgery for patients with erosive GERD, and on-demand therapy or continuous maintenance therapy for those with mild erosive GERD.
- *Return to activity:* Athletes may continue to participate as tolerated.

Indigestion

Functional dyspepsia (indigestion) is a spectrum of symptoms localized to the epigastric region.[45] Dyspepsia may be acute or chronic. Functional dyspepsia is present whenever diagnostic workups do not identify any causal structural or biomechanical abnormalities. It is defined by the following:

- Persistent or recurring episodes (more than 3 episodes within the past 6 months)
- No organic cause on endoscopy
- Defecation does not ease symptoms
- Stool irregularities

- *Symptoms:* pain and burning, feeling bloated following a meal, early satiation, distention, nausea
- *Signs:* vomiting, coughing, hoarseness
- *Differential diagnosis:* GERD, irritable bowel syndrome, gastroenteritis
- *Treatment:* Treatment is supportive toward particular symptoms.
  - Proton pump inhibitors have favorable effects
  - Helicobacter pylori eradication treatment is an important option because of its curative potential.
  - *Phytotherapy:* Combinations of peppermint and caraway oil or a mixture of bitter candy-turf, wormwood, gentian, and angelica root are used, usually in combination with spasmolytic and sedative extracts, such as chamomile, peppermint, caraway, and lemon balm.
  - *Antidepressants and psychotherapy:* Amitriptyline reduces predominant symptoms of abdominal pain and mental comorbidity.
  - *Prokinetics:* none approved yet
- *Return to activity:* Athlete may continue to participate as tolerated.

Irritable Bowel Syndrome

Irritable bowel syndrome (IBS) is a chronic functional gastrointestinal disorder involving altered bowel habits with discomfort or pain but without detectable structural or biomechanical abnormalities.[46] Functional dyspepsia and IBS are functional somatic syndromes with chronic fatigue and fibromyalgia. IBS is considered multifactorial, with proposed mechanisms including gastrointestinal dysmotility, inflammation, visceral hypersensitivity, and altered microbiota.

- *Symptoms:* pain, bloating, constipation, fatigue
- *Signs:* changes in defecation, diarrhea
- *Differential diagnosis:* Similar conditions include celiac disease, lactose intolerance, gastroenteritis. IBS diagnostics are not recommended for patients except with weight loss, hematochezia, or iron deficiency.
- *Treatment:* Treatment should be multifaceted, involving exercise, diet modification, and pharmacotherapy. Traditional treatment has focused

on targeting individual symptoms. Newer medications focus on the molecular level, such as serotonin receptor agonists and antagonists and drugs that act locally on chloride channels (lubiprostone) and guanylate cyclase receptors (linaclotide) in the GI tract. Antidepressants are effective at reducing abdominal pain and global IBS symptoms. Eradication had statistically significant improvements in abdominal pain and diarrhea. Alternative therapies include aloe for constipation, peppermint oil, and probiotics.

- *Return to activity:* Increasing physical activity shows long-term benefits to patients with IBS. During flare-ups, patients should proceed with activity as tolerated.

Peptic Ulcer Disease

Peptic ulcer disease is most commonly caused by a *Helicobacter pylori* infection or use of nonsteroidal anti-inflammatory drugs (NSAIDs).[47] When a risk of gastric cancer is low and alarming symptoms are absent, the test-and-treat strategy is appropriate. Alarming symptoms include unexplained weight loss, progressive dysphagia, odynophagia, and gastrointestinal bleeding. Urea breath and stool antigen tests identify *H. pylori* infections.

- *Symptoms:* epigastric abdominal pain, bloating, abdominal fullness, nausea, vomiting
- *Signs:* weight loss, weight gain, hematemesis, melena
- *Differential diagnosis:* esophagitis, functional dyspepsia, gastroenteritis, GERD
- *Treatment:* Eradication of *H. pylori* is recommended for all patients. First-line therapy includes timing variations of PPIs, amoxicillin, clarithromycin, and tinidazole or metronidazole. Treatment length should be a minimum of 7 days. Sequential therapy is a 5-day course of PPIs and amoxicillin, followed by the addition of clarithromycin. Non-bismuth therapy or bismuth-based therapy may be added to either treatment approach.
- *Return to activity:* Athlete may participate as tolerated.

Gastroenteritis

Acute gastroenteritis is a diarrheal disease of rapid onset with or without additional symptoms and signs.[49] Both are caused by rotavirus, *E. coli*, or other microorganisms. Acute diarrhea is the passage of three or more loose or liquid stools per day for 3 to 14 days.[49]

- *Symptoms:* loose or liquid stool, nausea, abdominal pain
- *Signs:* fever
- *Differential diagnosis:* Similar conditions include food poisoning, appendicitis, diverticulitis, and cholecystitis. Stool samples are recommended only if there is an underlying chronic illness, symptoms last longer than 7 days, or in cases of a recent outbreak of gastroenteritis, bloody diarrhea, or travel to a high-risk area for gastroenteritis.
- *Treatment:* Treatment is centered on the prevention of dehydration with appropriate liquids, electrolytes, feeding, and the supplementation of zinc. Recently, the effectiveness of zinc supplementation has been debated.[49] Researchers have recommended the use of probiotics, racecadotril, and smectite.
- *Return to activity:* An athlete should be restricted until asymptomatic.

Crohn's Disease

Crohn's disease is a chronic inflammatory condition of the gastrointestinal (GI) tract.[48] Disrupted GI function results from genetics, immune susceptibility, environmental factors, and altered gut microbiota.

- *Symptoms:* abdominal pain, chronic diarrhea, weight loss, and fatigue
- *Signs:* abdominal pain in right lower quadrant, rectal bleeding, skin lesions
- *Differential diagnosis:* ulcerative colitis, infectious enterocolitis, NSAID-associated enteropathy
- *Treatment:* Rather than simply controlling symptoms, treatment aims for long-term remission and preventing surgery complications and disease progression. The most widely used medications are corticosteroids, immunosuppressants, biologicals, and antiadhesion molecules. Antibiotics should be issued only in cases complicated by fistulas or abscesses. Surgery is indicated for the patients with refractory medical disease and complications or obstructive symptoms and those or who are nonresponsive to therapy.
- *Return to activity:* For those patients with non-severe presentations, moderate exercise is safe and beneficial. During flare-ups, activity will be limited and potentially contraindicated.

Ulcerative Colitis

Similar to Crohn's disease, ulcerative colitis (UC) is a chronic inflammatory colon disease caused by an unknown immune response.[50] Risk factors are genetic, dietary, and environmental. Ulcerative colitis inflammation is limited to the colonic mucosa. It differs from Crohn's because patients with Crohn's disease have patches of normal mucosa.

- *Symptoms:* **hematochezia**, diarrhea, abdominal pain, **tenesmus**, malaise, weight loss
- *Signs:* fever
- *Differential diagnosis:* Crohn's disease, clostridium difficile infection, dysentery, colitis, gastroenteritis
- *Diagnostic confirmation:* by endoscopy
- *Treatment:* Treatment is based on the extent and severity of the inflamed tissue. It centers on inducing remission and preventing relapse.
  - For active disease, topical 5-aminosalicyclic acid (ASA), including suppository and enema, is recommended. Topical mesalamine enema formulations of 5-ASA also induce remission. Corticosteroids foams are effective to a lesser degree.
  - Taking oral 5-ASA and topical formulations together is superior to receiving either treatment alone. Oral treatment is effective for mildly to moderately active UC that extends proximal to the sigmoid colon. Surgery is indicated for patients who are not responding to conservative options and those with perforations, toxic megacolon, or uncontrollable bleeding.
- *Return to activity:* Approximately 50% of patients will have occasional interference in participation. Older patients and those with active inflammation and poorer quality of life are most likely to miss time. Athletes may participate as tolerated.

Genitourinary System Conditions

The genitourinary system consists of two kidneys, two ureters, one bladder, and one urethra. It also often includes the reproductive organs. The system has a number of functions, including excretion of waste; regulation of blood volume, pressure, and electrolyte levels; and the stimulation of red blood cell production. The female reproductive system produces eggs and transports them to the fallopian tubes and then to the uterus. If implantation does not occur, women menstruate. The male reproductive system transports, nourishes, and produces semen and sperm. Both the male and female reproductive systems are responsible for hormone production. Genitourinary conditions of either reproductive system may impede activities of daily living, limit physical activity, predispose people to other conditions, and potentially lead to infertility.

Endometriosis

Endometriosis is characterized by the growth of endometrium-like tissue within and outside of the pelvic cavity.[51,52] Fifty percent of adolescents with intractable dysmenorrhea or pelvic pain are diagnosed with the condition. Clinical presentation varies from no symptoms to severe symptoms. Diagnosis is delayed because of the lack of noninvasive methods for detection.

- *Symptoms:* Symptoms include chronic pain of pelvic, abdominal and low back regions; dysmenorrhea; dyspareunia; dyschezia; and subfertility. Symptoms are aggravated during menstruation.
- *Signs:* No visible signs exist.
- *Differential diagnosis:* ovarian cyst, neoplasms, pelvic inflammatory disease
- *Treatment:* A current stepwise pharmaceutical plan should start with oral contraceptives (OCs) or low-cost progestogen medications.[52] If OCs or low-cost progestogen medications are ineffective, higher-cost drugs may offer relief. Surgical ablation is also an option. OCs may be used for women whose chief compliant is dysmenorrhea and only when superficial peritoneal implants or ovarian endometriomas less than 5 cm large are present. Progestogens are preferred for women who have severe deep dyspareunia with infiltrating lesions.
- *Return to activity:* Athletes may participate as tolerated.

Dysmenorrhea

Dysmenorrhea, or painful uterine cramps with menstruation, is a common symptom to many gynecological conditions and may also be a primary disease.[52] Primary dysmenorrhea is pain without an organic disease. Secondary dysmenorrhea is associated with an underlying pelvic pathology, such as endometriosis and adenomyosis. Symptom presentation varies from mild to severe.

- *Symptoms:* lower abdominal cramping, lower abdominal and back pain, nausea, weakness, headaches

- *Signs:* vomiting, fainting
- *Differential diagnosis:* endometriosis and adenomyosis
- *Diagnostic confirmation:* requires history taking, physical exam, and ultrasound (to exclude the secondary causes of dysmenorrhea)
- *Treatment:* The goal of treatment is pain relief. Treatment involves NSAIDs as the first line of treatment, either alone or with oral contraceptives. Patients should try NSAIDs for at least three menstrual periods. Oral contraceptives suppress ovulation and endometrial proliferation. They relieve symptoms associated with heavy and painful periods and irregular bleeding. Progestins-only treatment reduces pain-causing endometrial atrophy and inhibits ovulation. Electrical stimulation and stretching reduce pain intensity and duration.
- *Return to activity:* Athletes may participate as tolerated.

Amenorrhea

Amenorrhea, or absence of a menstrual period, is classified as either primary or secondary.[53] Primary amenorrhea is the failure to reach menarche, either due to chromosomal irregularities or primary ovarian insufficiency. Secondary amenorrhea is the cessation of regular menses for 3 months or the presence of irregular menses for 6 months. Secondary amenorrhea is a warning sign of low bone accrual and mineral density.

- *Symptoms:* hair loss, acne
- *Signs:* dental erosion, **Russel's sign**
- *Differential diagnosis:* pregnancy, premature ovarian failure, various chronic illnesses
- *Treatment:* Treatment is based on the causes of secondary amenorrhea. A multidisciplinary health care team, including a dietitian and mental health professionals, among others, is needed for improved outcomes.
- *Return to activity:* There are no standardized guidelines for return to play. An athlete must be cleared psychologically and physically before beginning an individualized return-to-play protocol.

Polycystic Ovary Syndrome

Polycystic ovary syndrome (PCOS) is a metabolic, psychological, and reproductive disorder.[54] The diagnostic criteria are based on possessing two of three features: **hyperandrogenism**, ovulatory dysfunction, and polycystic ovaries.[54] PCOS affects 6% to 13% of women.

- *Symptoms:* increased growth of body or facial hair, amenorrhea or oligomenorrhea, infertility issues, weight gain, thinning or loss of scalp hair
- *Signs:* acne
- *Differential diagnosis:* thyroid dysfunction, adrenal hyperplasia, Cushing's syndrome, acromegaly
- *Treatment:* Sustained weight loss and other positive life changes improve menstrual function and reduce cardiometabolic risk factors. Hormonal (estrogen-progestin) OCs are first-line agents. Athletes should be screened for glucose intolerance and dyslipidemia.
- *Return to activity:* Athletes may participate as tolerated.

Functional Ovarian Cysts

Functional ovarian cysts are common and resolve within 2 months.[55] Rupture and hemorrhage may be a physiological event and a self-limited process.

- *Symptoms:* low blood pressure, fast heart rate, intense stomach pain, cramping, bloating, heaviness
- *Signs:* fever, vomiting
- *Differential diagnosis:* Similar conditions include appendicitis, ectopic pregnancy, endometriosis, and diverticulitis. Accurate diagnostics have allowed for conservative management.
- *Treatment:* Emergency department evaluation includes vital signs, hemoglobin level, ultrasound, and CT. Hospitalization is needed to monitor vitals and hematocrit levels and repeat imaging. Cysts may require surgical intervention.
- *Return to activity:* Activity may resume based on symptom resolution and as tolerated.

Urinary Tract Infections

Urinary tract infections (UTIs) account for 10% to 20% of all infections in primary care and 30% to 40% of patients treated in hospitals. The risk of contraction is 14 times higher for women than for men.[56] Risk factors include gender, prior UTIs, vaginal infection, sexual activity, use of spermicidal agents, trauma, diabetes, obesity, and anatomical abnormalities.[56,57]

- *Symptoms:* dysuria with changes in frequency, urgency, and **hesitation**
- *Signs:* The major sign is hematuria. Septic presentation includes fever, chills, nausea, vomiting, and back pain.
- *Differential diagnosis:* kidney infection, renal stones, vaginitis, pyelonephritis, pelvic inflammatory disease, herpes simplex

- *Treatment:* Treatment duration varies from 3 days to 6 weeks. Trimethoprim sulfamethoxazole, ciprofloxacin, and ampicillin are the most commonly prescribed therapeutic agents. For uncomplicated infections, 3 days of antibiotics are sufficient. For those with recurrent infections, nitrofurantoin is prescribed for 5 to 7 days even for asymptomatic patients. Cranberry, herbal preparations, and Canephron N all offer therapeutic benefits.
- *Return to activity:* Patients may not need to lose time. An uncomplicated UTI may resolve in 3 days. Patients with septic presentations may need to be withheld from activity until septic symptoms resolve.

Testicular Torsion

Testicular torsion is an acute injury resulting from the testicle spinning within the scrotum.[58] The motion cuts off the blood vessels. Time to intervention is essential. Without evaluation within the first 8 hours, the patient is likely to lose the testicle.

- *Symptoms:* Acute unilateral scrotum pain
- *Signs:* edema, tenderness, blue discoloration, elevated testis, absence of cremasteric reflex
- *Differential diagnosis:* epididymitis or orchitis, incarcerated hernia, varicocele, appendix testis torsion
- *Treatment:* An orchiectomy is performed with the potential for contralateral testicle injury.
- *Return to activity:* Return to activity is based on wound healing and resolution of symptoms and pain. Patients will not return to sporting activities for at least 2 weeks. Students should be able to return to school following a few days of rest.

Epididymo-orchitis

The epididymis part of the GI tract includes the testes, vas deferens, prostate, urethra, and bladder.[59] An infection that spreads to the testis is known as epididymo-orchitis. Infections are caused by sexually transmitted diseases (STDs), common pathogens, or retrograde flow of urine. In adolescents, trauma or repetitive activity may trigger the infection.

- *Symptoms:* scrotal pain; warm, erythematous skin
- *Signs:* swelling, unilateral tenderness, urethral discharge, tenderness on prostate palpation
- *Differential diagnosis:* testicular torsion, scrotal hernia, testicular cancer
- *Treatment:* Fluroquinolones, ceftriaxone, and doxycycline are all recommended as first-line option antibiotics. Empiric antibiotic treatment

is still recommended despite the push for diagnostic confirmation of STDs. Icing the area, drinking lots of fluid, and finishing the entire course of medication are all recommended for optimal resolution. Repetitive-activity infections are treated with rest, anti-inflammatories, and scrotal support.

- *Return to activity:* Athletes should return to activity following 48 to 72 hours of antibiotics.

Nervous System Conditions

The nervous system is divided into the central and peripheral nervous systems. The central nervous system contains the brain and spinal cord. The peripheral nervous system encompasses the nerves outside the spinal cord. The functions of the nervous system include receiving sensory information, generating responses, and coordinating actions. Depending on their severity, symptoms may be transient or potentially permanent. Quick evaluation and proper management help prevent lifelong complications.

Concussions

A concussion is a traumatic brain injury induced by biomechanical forces.[60] Direct blows to the head, face, or elsewhere send impulsive forces to the brain, resulting in a neurometabolic cascade. This cascade results in an ionic flux, leading to an energy crisis. The energy crisis alters axonal function and neurotransmission. These neuropathological changes indicate a functional disturbance and result in the presenting signs and symptoms. Concussions do not have to involve a loss of consciousness.

Signs and Symptoms

Concussion suspicion and diagnosis involves one or more clinical domains (table 18.4).

Differential Diagnosis

Concussions have a differential diagnosis with the following:

- Headache or migraine
- Anxiety
- Depression
- Post-traumatic stress disorder (PTSD)
- Attention-deficit/hyperactivity disorder (ADHD)
- Sleep dysfunction
- Subdural or epidural hematoma

Evaluation

To evaluate for a concussion, you should administer first aid, giving careful consideration to ruling out cervical spine injury. The presence of any of the following should raise the suspicions of a potential cervical-spine injury and may necessitate stabilization and immediate referral:

- Unconscious or altered level of consciousness
- Bilateral neurological complaints
- Spinous process pain
- Obvious spinal cord deformity[61]

An athlete demonstrating signs or symptoms of a concussion should be immediately removed from activity for further evaluation. If medical personnel or health care professionals are not immediately available, the athlete should be referred to an emergency medical facility for evaluation.

Assessment

Once first aid has been given, the concussion assessment must begin. Concussion assessment involves a combination of baseline or follow-up computerized neuropsychological testing and completion of the Sport Concussion Assessment Tool, version 5 (SCAT5), which

TABLE 18.4 Clinical Domains of Concussions

Physical	Behavioral	Cognitive	Sleep and waking disturbances
Headache Nausea Vomiting Blurred or double vision Seeing stars or lights Balance problems Dizziness Sensitivity to light or noise Tinnitus	Drowsiness Fatigue Irritability Depression Anxiety Irritability	Feeling slowed down Feeling in a fog Difficulty concentrating Difficulty remembering Slowed reaction time Retrograde amnesia Anterograde amnesia	Sleeping more than usual Difficulty falling asleep Difficulty staying asleep

includes the Glasgow coma scale, Maddocks questions, graded symptom checklist, cranial nerve testing, and balance assessments. It is important that no single tool is used for concussion evaluation. Following the initial evaluation, the patient should be continually revaluated until asymptomatic and scores return toward baseline.

Sport Concussion Assessment Tool, Version 5 (SCAT5)   The following red flags or observable signs denote removal from play and further evaluation:

- Neck pain or tenderness
- Double vision
- Weakness or tingling or burning in arms or legs
- Severe or increasing headache
- Seizure or convulsions
- Loss of consciousness
- Deteriorating conscious state
- Vomiting
- Increasingly restless, agitated, or combative
- Lying motionless
- Difficulties with balance, gait, or coordination
- Blank or vacant stare
- Facial injury after head trauma

The SCAT5 is available online.

Graded Symptom Checklist   Baseline symptoms should be obtained for comparison (table 18.5). If unable to record baseline measures, initial postconcussion symptoms should be tracked until the patient is asymptomatic.

Cranial Nerve Testing   A cranial nerve test should occur at regular intervals following a head injury until the clinician has determined the severity of the injury (table 18.6).

Romberg Test   The Romberg test assesses balance and coordination.

- Patient stands with feet shoulder-width apart.
- Examiner stands ready to support patient.

TABLE 18.5   Graded Symptom Checklist

	None	Mild		Moderate		Severe	
Headache	0	1	2	3	4	5	6
Sense of pressure in head	0	1	2	3	4	5	6
Neck pain	0	1	2	3	4	5	6
Nausea or vomiting	0	1	2	3	4	5	6
Dizziness	0	1	2	3	4	5	6
Blurred vision	0	1	2	3	4	5	6
Balance problems	0	1	2	3	4	5	6
Sensitivity to light	0	1	2	3	4	5	6
Sensitivity to noise	0	1	2	3	4	5	6
Feeling slowed down	0	1	2	3	4	5	6
Feeling in a fog	0	1	2	3	4	5	6
Difficulty concentrating	0	1	2	3	4	5	6
Difficulty remembering	0	1	2	3	4	5	6
Fatigue	0	1	2	3	4	5	6
Confusion	0	1	2	3	4	5	6
Drowsiness	0	1	2	3	4	5	6
Heightened emotion	0	1	2	3	4	5	6
Irritability	0	1	2	3	4	5	6
Sadness or depression	0	1	2	3	4	5	6
Nervous or anxious	0	1	2	3	4	5	6
Trouble falling asleep	0	1	2	3	4	5	6
Total number of symptoms				_____ of 22			
Symptom severity score				_____ of 132			

TABLE 18.6   Cranial Nerves and Their Functions

Number	Name	Function
1	Olfactory	Smell
2	Optic	Visual acuity
3	Oculomotor	Eye movements
4	Trochlear	Upward eye movements
5	Trigeminal	Facial sensation, chewing
6	Abducens	Lateral eye movements
7	Facial	Facial muscle movements
8	Vestibulocochlear	Hearing and balance
9	Glossopharyngeal	Pharyngeal muscles, taste
10	Vagus	Gag reflex, swallowing
11	Accessory	Shoulder shrug
12	Hypoglossal	Tongue movements

- Procedures
  - Patient closes eyes and abducts arms to 90 degrees with elbows straight.
  - Patient extends head and lifts one foot off the ground.
  - If patient achieves this position, the examiner instructs him to touch one finger to his nose.
- Positive test: Patient displays balance errors or general unsteadiness.

Balance Error Scoring System   The Balance Error Scoring System (BESS) is a battery of tests involving three different stances: double leg, single leg, and tandem stance. Each test is performed once on a firm surface and once on a foam surface (figure 18.7). For the tandem stance, the nondominant leg goes in back.

- Each test lasts 20 seconds. The maximum amount of errors for each trial is 10. During each test, the examiner counts errors made by the patient in performing the following:
  - Lifting the hands off the iliac crests
  - Opening the eyes
  - Stepping, stumbling
  - Moving the hip more than 30 degrees
  - Lifting the foot or heel up
  - Remaining out of the testing position for more than 5 seconds
  - If multiple errors occur at once, the examiner counts one error.
- Patients unable to hold the position for 5 seconds are assigned a maximum score of 10.

- A positive test indicates impaired cerebral function.

Rehabilitation

Rehabilitation involves controlled subsymptom threshold, submaximal exercise, controlled cognitive stress, pharmacological treatment, and school accommodations. Support exists for targeted therapy for vestibular dysfunction and cognitive therapy for persistent mood or behavioral issues. Once tests return toward baseline or the patient becomes asymptomatic, the patient may begin a return-to-activity protocol.

Return to Learn

The patient may struggle when returning to school. Some activities may increase symptoms. A graduated return-to-school strategy is as follows:

- *Stage 1.* The patient performs daily activities that do not produce symptoms. Start with 5 to 15 minutes at a time and build up.
- *Stage 2.* The patient performs school activities. School activities outside of the classroom include homework, reading, and other cognitive activities.
- *Stage 3.* The patient returns to school part time. She may need to start with a partial school day or take increased breaks during the day.
- *Stage 4.* The patient returns to school full time, gradually increasing school activities until a full day is tolerated.

Return to Play

The graduated return-to-sport strategy has to be completed before a full return to sporting activities occurs.

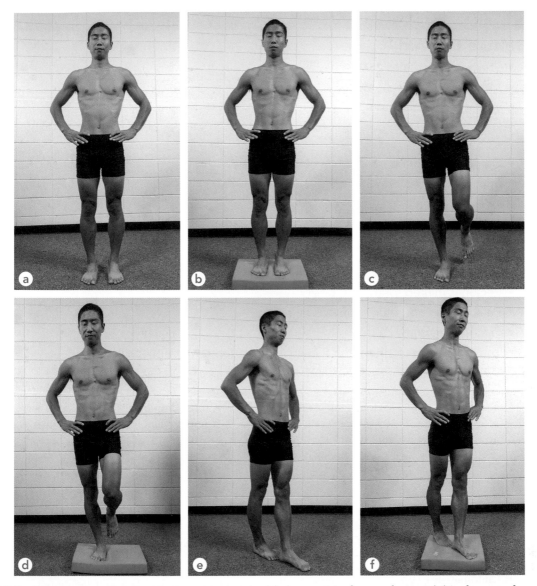

FIGURE 18.7   Balance Error Scoring System stances: double leg on *(a)* a firm surface and *(b)* a foam surface, single leg on *(c)* a firm surface and *(d)* a foam surface, and tandem stance on *(e)* a firm surface and *(f)* a foam surface.

The six-stage program is as follows:

- *Stage 1:* symptom-limited activity
- *Stage 2:* light aerobic exercise
- *Stage 3:* sport-specific activity
- *Stage 4:* noncontact training drills
- *Stage 5:* full contact practice
- *Stage 6:* return to sport

If symptoms are produced in a stage, the athlete should repeat the previous stage.

Epilepsy

Epilepsy is defined by a person's brain demonstrating a pathological tendency for recurrent seizures.[62,63] Epileptic seizures are produced by abnormal excessive or synchronous neural firing. While epilepsy is typically associated with grand mal seizures, there are four classifications of epileptic seizures: focal, generalized, unknown, and unclassified.

- Focal seizures are classified as aware or impaired awareness. The next step is denoting whether they are motor or nonmotor.
  - *Motor onset:* automatisms, clonic, atonic, spasms, hyperkinetic, myoclonic, and tonic
  - *Nonmotor:* autonomic, behavior arrest, cognitive, emotional or sensory
- Generalized seizures are either motor or nonmotor.

FOUNDATIONAL SKILL

Seizure First Aid

- Stay with the patient and time the seizure.
- Move away harmful objects.
- Turn the patient onto his side.
- Don't block airway; put something soft under the patient's head and loosen restrictive clothing.
- Do not restrain the patient.
- Stay with the patient until he is awake.[62]

Call 911 if any of the following occurs:

- Repeated seizures
- Difficult breathing
- Seizure occurs in water
- Person is injured, pregnant, or sick
- Person does not return to his usual state
- First-time seizure
- The seizure lasts longer than 5 minutes (for people with epilepsy)

- *Motor onset:* tonic-clonic, clonic, tonic, myoclonic, myoclonic-tonic-clonic, myoclonic-atonic, and atonic seizures, and epileptic spasms (either individually or in combinations)
- *Nonmotor (absence):* typical, atypical, myoclonic, and eyelid myoclonia

- *Symptoms:* nausea, hallucinations, déjà vu, transient numbness or weakness, migraines, visual symptoms[62,63]
- *Signs:* automatisms (lip smacking, picking at clothes, fumbling, unawareness of surroundings). Seizure presentations include the following:
  - Focal to bilateral tonic-clonic seizures (grand mal)
  - Absence: staring off into space
  - Atonic: limp loss of tone
  - Clonic: jerking alone
  - Tonic: tone
  - Myoclonic seizure: shocklike jerks
  - These may present individually or in combination with others signs.
- *Differential diagnosis:* syncope, hypoglycemia, transient ischemic attacks, multiple sclerosis
- *Treatment:* Anti-epileptic drugs are the first choice of treatment. Patients will usually require more than one medication. Depending on the type of epilepsy, there are several potential sur-

gical options, including vagus nerve stimulation implant and lobe or scar-tissue resection.
- *Return to activity:* Return to participation is at the neurologist's discretion. Resumption of activity may be based on the specific sport, with some clearances requiring a seizure-free period of 12 months.

Complex Regional Pain Syndrome

Complex regional pain syndrome is characterized by spontaneous and evoked pain, beginning in distal extremity, that is disproportionate in magnitude or duration to the typical course of pain.[64] Diagnosis often occurs in the pediatric population. Prominent autonomic and inflammatory changes occur. The patient must display one sign at the time of evaluation in two or more of the following categories: sensory, vasomotor, sudomotor or edema, and motor or trophic.

- *Symptoms:* hyperalgesia; altered patterns of hair, skin, and hair growth
- *Signs:* alterations in skin color, temperature, and swelling compared to the unaffected side; tremors; dystonia; edema; reduced strength; motor dysfunction; decreased range of motion
- *Differential diagnosis:* sensorimotor neuropathy, cellulitis, vasculitis, vascular insufficiency, lymphedema, deep vein thrombosis, Raynaud's phenomenon

- *Treatment:* Treatment requires a multidisciplinary approach involving medical, psychological, physical, and occupational components. During an acute inflammatory phase, oral corticosteroids are often used to decrease inflammation. Supplementary medications include anticonvulsants and analgesic antidepressants. If symptoms do not lessen with medication, ganglion blocks and spinal cord stimulation should be considered. Physical and occupational therapies should be implemented with the selected pharmaceutical program.

- *Return to activity:* Increasing aerobic activity is a therapeutic benchmark. Positive patient outcomes are associated with consistent exercise and physical therapy programs.

Eye Conditions

Each eye adjusts the amount of light received, focuses on images, and produces continuous images. Eyes detect light, leading to the conversion of the light into electrical impulses from the neurons to the brain. The cornea allows the transmission of light through the lens of the eye to the retina. The lens focuses the images on the retina. The retina transmits those light impulses via the optic nerve to the brain. With only the eyelid as the covering, the eye is easily accessible to trauma, debris, and outside infections. Also, the aging process leads to an inability to focus, reducing vision. Regardless of the cause, athletic trainers have to assess numerous changes to a patient's eyes to avoid a potential loss of vision.

Presbyopia

Presbyopia is a condition whereby a person loses the ability to focus on near objects due to a decrease in the elasticity of the lens. Presbyopia is commonly associated with age. Some diagnoses focus on pure vision loss rather than the visual loss requirements.[65] The normal age-related reduction in amplitude of accommodation reaches a point when clarity of vision cannot be sustained for long enough.

- *Symptoms:* headache, blurred vision, inability to focus, ocular discomfort, squinting, eye fatigue, drowsiness, diplopia
- *Signs:* loss of visual acuity
- *Differential diagnosis:* glaucoma, cataracts, macular degeneration
- *Treatment:* corrective lenses, Lasik surgery, pharmaceuticals, ciliary muscle electrostimulation
- *Return to activity:* correction and immediate return to activity.

Corneal Abrasions

Corneal abrasions are commonly encountered in sports.[66,67] They are defined as a defect in the epithelial surface of the cornea caused by mechanical trauma, foreign bodies, contact lens use, repetitive friction, or chemical or flash burns.

- *Symptoms:* **blepharospasm**, photophobia
- *Signs:* **epiphora**
- *Differential diagnosis:* penetrating injury, infective keratitis, corneal ulcers, conjunctivitis
- *Treatment:* Treatment includes topical NSAIDs and oral analgesics. Little evidence supports the use of antibiotic topicals, which are commonly prescribed to prevent resistant bacterial infection.
- *Return to activity:* Most patients heal in 24 to 48 hours.

Conjunctivitis

Infectious conjunctivitis is caused by either a bacterial or viral pathogen.[67] This common pediatric condition is characterized by dilation of the conjunctival blood vessels and corresponding inflammation. Conjunctivitis is most commonly caused by a virus, and adenovirus is the main contributor to the condition. In children, bacterial conjunctivitis is more common than viral.

- *Symptoms:* self-limiting pain, discomfort
- *Signs:* epiphora, hyperpurulent bacterial or serious eye discharge (figure 18.8)

FOUNDATIONAL SKILL

General Procedures for Removal of Foreign Bodies From the Eye

1. Inspect the eye to locate the foreign body.
2. Irrigate the eye with saline solution.
3. Use a moistened cotton tip applicator to gently sweep out the debris.
4. If unsuccessful, refer the patient to a physician.[67]

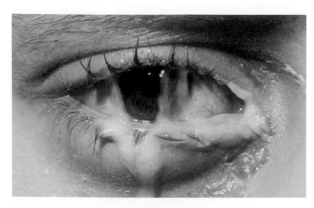

FIGURE 18.8 Conjunctivitis.

Ralph C. Eagle, Jr. / Science Source

- *Differential diagnosis:* infectious keratitis, endophthalmitis, glaucoma, cellulitis
- *Treatment:* For viral conjunctivitis, patients should start acyclovir ointment or ganciclovir gel. Topical steroids should be applied to exclude postviral keratitis. For bacterial conjunctivitis, either chloramphenicol eye drops 5% or framycetin sulfate drops 5% should be applied for 7 days. A warm compress can be applied to help with symptoms.
- *Return to activity:* The patient is contagious for 24 hours or until symptoms resolve.

Hyphema

Hyphema is the collection of blood in the anterior chamber of the eye.[69] This injury follows a blunt trauma that damages the iris or angle vessels. The typical mechanism is the result of a projective blow or punch that hits the exposed eye.

- *Symptoms:* blurred vision, dull ache, diplopia
- *Signs:* Red blood cells circulate in aqueous humor and set inferiorly (figure 18.9).

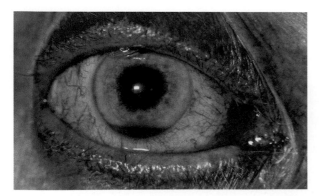

FIGURE 18.9 Hyphema.

SPL / Science Source

- *Differential diagnosis:* detached retina, eye contusion, traumatic iritis, traumatic microhyphema
- *Treatment:* grade 1 conservative treatment
  - Outpatient bed rest
  - Dilation
  - Re-evaluation every few days
  - Rise in intraocular pressure treated with topical or oral medication
  - Topical steroids
  - No NSAIDS
  - Report immediately if rebleed or decrease in vision occurs
- *Return to activity:* Patients should avoid vigorous exercise for several weeks and stop activity if symptoms reappear.

Glaucoma

After cataracts, glaucoma is the second leading cause of blindness globally.[70] Glaucoma patients demonstrate antibodies against retina and optic nerve proteins. Glaucoma involves progressive visual field loss due to the death of retinal ganglia and morphological changes in the retina.

- *Symptoms:* potential hearing loss
- *Signs:* gradual visual field loss, optic nerve changes
- *Differential diagnosis:* intracranial hypertension, ischemic optic neuropathy, optic atrophy, iritis, corneal ulcer, periorbital infections
- *Treatment:* Treatment involves eyes drops or systemic application of glaucoma medication, including carbonic anhydrase inhibitors, beta-blockers, and cholinergic agonists. Laser or surgical procedures should be a last option.
- *Return to activity:* The prognosis is best with timely diagnosis. Barring any safety concerns, there are no restrictions to activity.

Age-Related Macular Degeneration

Age-related macular degeneration is a preventable loss of central vision.[71] It is the most common cause of blindness. There are early and late stages based on morphological changes of the retina. Central vision is lost without changes in peripheral vision.

- *Symptoms:* vision loss, difficulties with dark adaptation, visual distortion, blurring, visual hallucination
- *Signs:* visual acuity loss

- *Differential diagnosis:* glaucoma, cataracts, polypoidal choroidal vasculopathy, macular telangiectasia
- *Treatment:* Antioxidant supplementation lowers the risk for the disease to develop and progress. Antioxidants to take include vitamins C and E, beta-carotene, zinc oxide, and 2 mg of cupric oxide. Inflammation should be targeted with tetracyclines, statins, and doxycycline.
- *Return to activity:* Consistent physical activity lowers the odds for development of macular degeneration.

Cataracts

A cataract is the **opacification** of either the lens of the eye or its membrane.[72] This clouding obfuscates the passage of light through the lens to the retina. Although this condition may occur across the life span, it predominately occurs in the geriatric population. Its severity varies with the potential for bilateral presentations. Earlier in its progression, the disease may not affect activities of daily living. The lens eventually becomes completely opaque.

- *Symptoms:* blurriness, decreased vision, diplopia, **polyopia**, seeing colored halos, photophobia, increased frequency of corrective lens changes
- *Signs:* decreased visual acuity
- *Differential diagnosis:* glaucoma, macular degeneration, refractive errors
- *Treatment:* Surgery is not indicated for patients with visual acuity of 6/24 or better; rather, pupillary dilatation or refractive glasses are the primary treatment options. If acuity is worse than 6/24 or the cataract is adversely affecting eye health, surgery is indicated as a last option.
- *Return to activity:* Initial treatment is correction with lenses or contacts. Because quality of life is hindered by the condition, surgery may be indicated for patients. Seventy to eighty percent of patients report excellent surgical outcomes.

Ear, Nose, Throat, and Mouth Conditions

Conditions of the ear, nose, throat, and mouth are often grouped together because of the organs' interconnectedness and several shared factors. Each area has a mucosal lining and contains special sensory organs. Conditions range from infectious processes and inflammation to acute trauma. Any of these conditions could negatively affect performance secondary to congestion, decreased visual acuity, decreased respiratory capacity, or swelling.

Allergic Rhinitis

Allergic rhinitis is an antibody-mediated inflammatory disease.[73] Episode patterns may be seasonal (pollens), perennial (mites), or episodic environmental (allergen exposures not normally encountered in patient's home or occupational environmental).

- *Symptoms:* nasal congestion, excessive mucus production, anterior or posterior rhinorrhea, itching
- *Signs:* sneezing paroxysm, allergic shiners, nasal and ocular pruritis
- *Differential diagnosis:* asthma, sarcoidosis, eosinophilia
- *Treatment:* Pharmacological therapy includes antihistamines (intranasal and oral), decongestants (intranasal and oral), corticosteroids (intranasal and oral), intranasal cromolyn, intranasal anticholinergics, and oral leukotriene receptor antagonists.
  - *For initial nasal symptoms:* Monotherapy with an intranasal corticosteroid is recommended rather than a combination of intranasal and oral antihistamine. An intranasal corticosteroid is recommended over a leukotriene receptor antagonist.
  - *For moderate to severe symptoms:* A combination of intranasal corticosteroid and an intranasal antihistamine is recommended.
  - For monotherapy, intranasal corticosteroids are more effective than oral leukotriene receptors. When a patient is already on intranasal corticosteroids, consider the addition of an antihistamine. The best additional therapy is an intranasal antihistamine, not an oral antihistamine.
- *Return to play:* The patient may participate as tolerated.

Acute Bronchitis

Acute bronchitis is a cough from an inflamed trachea and bronchi without evidence of pneumonia.[74] Viral infections are most likely responsible. The cough typically lasts 2 to 3 weeks.

- *Symptoms:* acute cough that may be accompanied by sputum production; signs of lower respiratory tract infections, including nasal congestion, headache, and fever
- *Sign:* wheezes or rhonchi on lung auscultation
- *Differential diagnosis:* Clinical diagnosis should rule out serious cases of asthma, chronic obstructive

pulmonary disorder (COPD), heart failure, or pneumonia. A temperature over 100°F (38°C) should prompt consideration of influenza or pneumonia.

- *Treatment:* No antibiotics are recommended for viral sinusitis, pharyngitis, or bronchitis. Over-the-counter medications are usually recommended for acute cough, including ibuprofen, acetaminophen, and steam inhalation. Expectorants, like guaifenesin, decrease cough frequency and intensity.

- *Return to activity:* As long as no fever is present, athletes should be allowed to participate as tolerated.

Pharyngitis

Pharyngitis is an inflammation of the pharynx.[75] The pharynx is the posterior aspect of the throat between the tonsils and larynx.

- *Symptoms:* Clinical diagnosis involves complaints of a sore throat and one of the signs in the following bullet point.

- *Signs:* redness of the posterior pharyngeal wall, pharyngeal or tonsillar exudate, swelling, cervical lymphadenopathy, or fever above 100°F (38°C; figure 18.10)

- *Differential diagnosis:* parainfluenza, rhinovirus, influenza, adenovirus

- *Diagnostic confirmation:* requires a rapid antigen test and a bacterial culture; a polymerase chain reaction offers a less sensitive test.

- *Treatment:* Due to the rise in resistant strains, antibiotics are recommended only for confirmed bacterial cases.

- *Return to activity:* For bacterial cases, infected athletes are considered contagious until they have completed 24 hours of antibiotics.

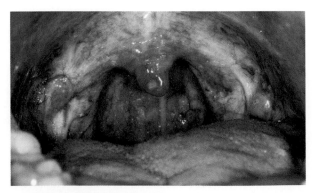

FIGURE 18.10 Pharyngitis.

Dr P. Marazzi / Science Source

Laryngitis

Laryngitis is an inflammation of the larynx. It accompanies many upper respiratory tract infections. Symptoms can last up to 3 weeks and may persist longer.[76]

- *Symptoms:* Clinical diagnosis involves complaints of hoarseness, sore throat, and difficulty swallowing.

- *Signs:* Bacterial laryngitis presents more frequently with purulent secretions.

- *Differential diagnosis:* dysphonia, epiglottitis, coryza

- *Treatment:* Treatment centers on supportive care. Both infection types benefit from vocal rest, analgesics, hydration, and humidification. Supportive OTC medications are mucolytics, decongestants, and glucocorticoid steroids. Bacterial infections benefit from antibiotic prescriptions.

- *Return to activity:* A patient may return to activity following cessation of the fever or 24 hours after the first dose of antibiotics.

Tonsillitis

Tonsillitis is an inflammation of the pharyngeal tonsils that may extend into the adenoid or lingual tonsils.[77] Most infections are polymicrobial, resulting from bacteria, viruses, yeasts, or parasites.

- *Symptoms:* Clinical diagnosis involves complaints of a sore throat and one of the following symptoms: fever, headache, malaise, difficulty swallowing, and snoring.

- *Signs:* Swollen tonsils (figure 18.11)

- *Differential diagnosis:* pharyngitis, epiglottitis, dental or peritonsillar abscesses

- *Diagnostic confirmation:* requires a throat swab, complete blood test, and rapid antigen test

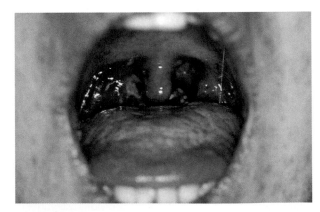

FIGURE 18.11 Tonsillitis.

Biophoto Associates / Science Source

- *Treatment:* Symptomatic control of viral infections focuses on pain, fever, and sore throat relief with analgesia, hydration, and NSAIDs. Bacterial infections require penicillin (amoxicillin) and fluoroquinolone (levofloxacin). If penicillin therapy fails, the patient may respond better to clindamycin or amoxicillin-clavulanate.
- *Return to activity:* Patients with bacterial infections are noncontagious following the first 24 hours of treatment.

Ruptured Tympanic Membrane

The tympanic membrane is a translucent membrane that separates the external and middle ears. Trauma may produce a rupture, tear, or perforation.[78] It is the most common type of trauma-induced otologic dysfunction.

- *Symptoms:* hearing loss, tinnitus, **otalgia**, vertigo
- *Signs:* **otorrhea**
- *Differential diagnosis:* chronic otitis media, otitis externa, cholesteatoma, myringosclerosis
- *Treatment:* Treatment ranges from observation to active treatments to surgical interventions. Surgery is indicated only for patients with perilymph fistula, facial paralysis, severe vertigo, or sensorineural hearing loss. Most patients heal spontaneously within 4 weeks. Treatments involve topical epidermal growth factors, enoxaparin, and ascorbic acid, which stimulate epithelization for closure and prevent formation of plaques. Infection prevention requires systemic antibiotics.
- *Return to activity:* Athletes may participate as tolerated.

Acute Otitis Externa

Acute otitis externa is a diffuse inflammation of the external ear canal, which may include either the pinna or the tympanic membrane.[79] Multifactorial infection mechanisms are regular cleaning, debris, trauma, sweating, allergy, and stress. Rapid onset of symptoms occurs within 48 hours of inflammation.

- *Symptoms:* otalgia, itching, feeling of fullness in the ear
- *Signs:* tenderness of tragus or pinna, diffuse ear canal edema or **erythema**, otorrhea, regional lymphadenitis, tympanic membrane erythema, cellulitis of pinna (figure 18.12)
- *Differential diagnosis:* ruptured tympanic membrane, eczema, seborrhea, dermatitis, herpes zoster oticus, TMJ syndrome, cholesteatoma

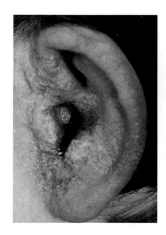

FIGURE 18.12 Otitis externa.
Biophoto Associates / Science Source

- *Treatment:* Topical antimicrobials and steroids should be administered for 7 days. Oral antibiotics have limited utility. Prevention includes limiting water accumulation and moisture retention in the external auditory meatus. Symptomatic control includes analgesics, acetaminophen or NSAIDS, potential oxycodone mix, sedation, and topical benzocaine for anesthesia.
- *Return to activity:* Athletes should respond within 72 hours of the initiation of treatment. Athletes should continue participation as tolerated.

Acute Otitis Media

Acute otitis media is the most common pathology in children requiring antibiotic prescription.[80] Both the direct and indirect costs annually total into the billions. Although antibiotic prescription is common in the United States for this condition, the growth of resistant pathogens call for more judicious use of antibiotics.

- *Symptoms:* otalgia, irritability, disturbed speech, vomiting, diarrhea
- *Signs:* middle-ear effusion, otorrhea, fever, cough, discharge (figure 18.13)
- *Differential diagnosis:* viral upper respiratory infection, acute otitis externa, bullous myringitis, spontaneous tympanic membrane perforation, mastoiditis
- *Treatment:* acetaminophen, ibuprofen, topical analgesics, narcotics with codeine or analogs, tympanostomy or myringotomy, amoxicillin, or azithromycin[69,70]
  - For patients 6 months to 2 years old, antibiotics should be issued for either certain or uncertain diagnoses.

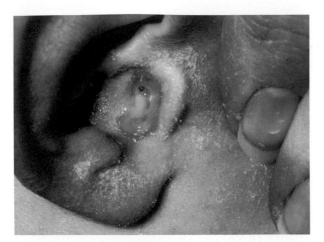

FIGURE 18.13 Otitis media.

Dr P. Marazzi / Science Source

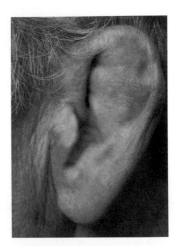

FIGURE 18.14 Cauliflower ear.

- For patients 2 years or older, antibiotics should be issued for severe confirmed presentation. For uncertain diagnoses or mild symptoms, the observation option should be used by the provider.
- If antibiotics are delayed, patients should have access with worsening symptoms.
- *Return to activity:* Once athletes are fever free, they may return to activity.

Cauliflower Ear

An acute auricular hematoma (cauliflower ear) is caused by a direct blow or repetitive friction to the ear. Hematomas form between the perichondrium and cartilage on the anterior ear. The hematoma disrupts blood supply to the cartilage. It results in necrosis, infection, and loss of cartilage. In the healing process, the subperichondrial hematoma results in chondrocytes and fibroblasts proliferating fibrocartilage. The fibrocartilage results in auricle distortion.

- *Symptoms:* otalgia, tinnitus
- *Signs:* edema, redness, warmth (figure 18.14)
- *Differential diagnosis:* acute auricular perichondritis, auricle pseudocyst, chondrodermatitis nodularis chronica helicis, relapsing polychondritis
- *Treatment:* Auricular hematomas require drainage followed by packing and padding. Correction of the cauliflower ear involves surgical intervention, but many either opt not to or delay the procedure to avoid time away from activity.
- *Return to activity:* Following drainage, athletes may return to activity with dressing and padding.

Systemic Disorders

Systemic disorders typically cause a functional glitch in a specific organ or organ system. However, their effects are widespread, affecting all body systems. You should know the medical history of your patients with regard to systemic disorders, since these conditions can cause complicating factors with regard to the way injuries present and heal.

Diabetes Mellitus

Diabetes mellitus is an endocrine disorder resulting in periods of hyperglycemia. Type 1 diabetes results in absolute insulin insufficiency.[83] Athletic trainers working in the traditional setting are more likely to encounter patients with type 1 diabetes. Type 2 diabetes develops over time, leading to cells becoming insulin resistant. Normal fasting levels are 60 to 100 mg/dL (3.3 to 5.5 mmol/L) and less than 140 mg/dL approximately 2 hours after a meal. For either type, maintaining near-normal glucose levels and blood pressure and demonstrating lipid control are tenets of treatment. Management is centered on maintaining appropriate glucose levels to avoid falling into hypoglycemia.

Hypoglycemia

Hypoglycemia is the most severe diabetic complication, and exercise is the most common exacerbating factor.[83] Exercise increases absorption of injected insulin and impairs release of glucose-counterregulatory hormones. Although exercise may cause bouts of hypoglycemia, consistent exercise and glucose management improves glucose sensitivity. If hypoglycemia is severe and prolonged, patients may suffer brain damage or death. Signs and symptoms occur at glucose levels less than 70 mg/dL (<3.9 mmol/L)

- *Symptoms:* tachycardia, palpitations, nervousness, headache, dizziness, blurred vision, fatigue, difficulty thinking
- *Signs:* sweating, trembling, loss of motor control, aggressive behavior, seizures, convulsions
- *Differential diagnosis:* anaphylaxis, seizures, stroke, head injury, cardiac pathology
- *Treatment:*
  - Mild hypoglycemia
    - Administer 10 to 15 g of a fast-acting carbohydrate.
    - Measure blood glucose.
    - Wait 15 minutes and remeasure.
    - If glucose level remains low, repeat the first step.
    - Wait 15 minutes and remeasure.
    - If blood glucose does not return to normal, activate EMS.
    - Once blood glucose level is within normal range, the athlete may consume a snack.
  - Severe hypoglycemia
    - Activate EMS.
    - Prepare a glucagon injection, following the directions on the kit. The kit is either a fluid-filled syringe and a vial of powder or an empty syringe requiring the powder and fluid.
    - Once the patient becomes conscious, provide food.
- *Return to activity:* For mild hypoglycemia, once the blood glucose level returns to normal and a snack is provided, the athlete may return to activity.

Hyperglycemia

Hyperglycemia occurs when the blood glucose levels exceed the renal glucose threshold level (>180 mg/dL).[83] After a hyperglycemic episode, athletes must avoid exercise. High-intensity exercise causes additional increases in blood glucose. Also, increases in catecholamines, free fatty acids, and ketones impair muscle glucose use and increase blood glucose levels. Lastly, psychological stress causes a rise in glucose levels. As ketones build up in the blood, the patient moves from mild hyperglycemia into ketoacidosis. Ketoacidosis leads to the more severe presentation of symptoms.

- *Symptoms:* nausea, dehydration, sleepiness, increased urination
- *Signs:* flushed warm skin, fruity or acidic breath, irregular breathing, disorientation, slowed reaction time
- *Differential diagnosis:* cardiac pathology, head injury, heat illness
- *Treatment:*
  - Mild hyperglycemia:
    - Assess urine for ketones.
    - Administer water or noncarbohydrate beverage; if ketones present, have athlete keep drinking and recheck urine in 15 minutes.
  - Severe hyperglycemia:
    - Call EMS.
    - Monitor vitals.
- *Return to activity:*
  - Fasting blood glucose level is greater than 250 mg/dL (13.9 mmol/L)
    - If ketones are present in blood or urine, exercise is contraindicated.
    - If ketones are not present, exercise is not contraindicated.
  - Blood glucose value is 300 mg/dL (16.7 mmol/L) and without ketones
    - Advise the athlete to exercise with caution and continue to monitor the condition.

Hypothyroidism and Hyperthyroidism

The thyroid gland produces hormones, resulting in a neuroendocrine cascade that triggers responses of the hypothalamus and anterior pituitary gland. Alterations in function affect energy expenditure, cardiac function, muscle physiology, protein synthesis, bone, and substrate.[84] Thyroid function works on a continuum, which may result in oversecretion (hyperthyroidism) or undersecretion (hypothyroidism), both of which present with nonspecific symptoms with varying severities.

Hypothyroidism

- *Symptoms:* nonspecific weight gain, fatigue, myalgia, depression, cold intolerance, constipation, menstrual irregularities, decreased exercise tolerance or performance
- *Signs:* dry skin, hair loss, proximal muscle weakness, bradycardia
- *Differential diagnosis:* iron-deficiency anemia, sleep **apnea**, depression, rheumatological diseases
- *Treatment:* lifelong thyroid hormone therapy
- *Return to activity:* There are no consensus guidelines for return to play. Athlete may be

allowed to participate as tolerated but will need monitoring by a physician to ensure adequate thyroid function.

Hyperthyroidism

- *Symptoms:* nonspecific weight loss, increased appetite, palpitations, heat intolerance, hyperdefecation
- *Signs:* diaphoresis, tremor, lid lag, proximal muscle weakness, tachycardia, **dysrhythmias**, hyperpyrexia
- *Differential diagnosis:* Graves' disease, subacute thyroiditis, toxic adenoma, hyperthyroxinemia, struma ovarii
- *Treatment:* Treatment centers on symptomatic control with the use of beta-adrenergic blockers and antithyroid medications. If medication management is unsuccessful or contraindicated, either radioactive thyroid ablation or thyroidectomy can be used.
- *Return to activity:* There are no consensus guidelines for return to play. Athletes will require physician clearance before returning to activity. Beta-blockers are not recommended for athletes. Athletes with hyperthyroidism are at increased risk for heat illness, **arrhythmias**, and fractures. Continued management is required to ensure a normally functioning thyroid and proper bone mineral density.

Pancreatitis

Acute pancreatitis is the most common gastrointestinal disorder necessitating hospitalization. It results in local and systemic inflammatory responses.[85] Twenty percent of cases develop into moderate to severe pancreatitis, with the potential for pancreatic necrosis.

- *Symptoms:* moderate to severe abdominal pain, nausea
- *Signs:* anorexia, fever, tachycardia, muscle guarding and rigidity, decreased bowel sounds
- *Differential diagnosis:* Similar conditions include peptic ulcer disease, cholecystitis, diabetic ketoacidosis, and myocardial infarction. Diagnosis requires two of the three following signs: (1) abdominal pain consistent with pancreatitis, (2) serum amylase or lipase of at least three times the normal limit, and (3) findings on imaging.
- *Treatment:* Primary management is fluid rehydration with lactated Ringer's (LR) solution. Pain control requires reassessment and adjustments to analgesia types and dosages. Endoscopic cholangiography or sphincterotomy are recommended

in cases of concomitant cholangitis. Cholecystectomy is performed for mild pancreatitis. Once pain begins to resolve, patients may start an oral diet. A soft, low-fat diet is recommended for patients with mild cases. Moderate to severe patients may require nasogastric feeding. Patients must receive nutrition education to know to avoid alcohol and high-fat food.

- *Return to activity:* Mild pancreatitis will resolve in a few days. If surgery is performed, return to activity may be delayed up to 2 months.

Sexually Transmitted Diseases

Despite making up a quarter of the sexually active population, 15- to 25-year-olds account for approximately half of the 20 million new cases of sexually transmitted diseases (STDs) that occur annually in the United States.[86,87] Patients often have asymptomatic infections until the occurrence of complications.[86,87] As the first point of contact for many patients, you must be familiar with signs and symptoms of common STDs to ensure proper referral to appropriate members of the health care team. Table 18.7 compares the most common STDs. You should educate clients with STDs about safe sex practices and the need for testing and treatment for themselves and any sexual partners to prevent the risk of reinfection.

Chlamydia

Chlamydia is the most frequently reported infectious disease in the United States.[87] It is most prevalent in people less than 24 years old. The most serious complications of chlamydia are pelvic inflammatory disease, ectopic pregnancy, and infertility. Some patients may already have subclinical upper reproductive tract infection. Asymptomatic infection is common in both sexes.

- *Symptoms:* pain, burning while peeing, pain with sex, lower belly pain
- *Signs:* yellowish, bleeding discharge; watery or milky discharge from penis; swollen testicles
- *Differential diagnosis:* Similar conditions include bacterial vaginosis, periurethral abscess, and prostatitis. Diagnosis occurs with first-catch urine or swab specimens.
- *Treatment:* Treatment options include azithromycin 1 g in a single dose or doxycycline 100 mg orally twice a day for 7 days, erythromycin 500 mg orally four times a day for 7 days, levofloxacin 500 mg once daily for 7 days, or ofloxacin 300 mg orally twice a day for 7 days.
- *Return to activity:* Athletes may participate as tolerated. Treatment is 95% effective, but reoccurrence is high.

TABLE 18.7 **Differential Diagnosis of the Most Common STDs**

Disease	Signs and symptoms	Differential diagnosis
Chlamydia	Both sexes: pain with sex, burning with urination, lower belly pain, yellowish bleeding discharge	Bacterial vaginosis Periurethral abscess Prostatitis
Gonorrhea	Both sexes: painful urination, increased discharge, pelvic pain Men: penis discharge, swelling of 1 testicle Women: vaginal bleeding, painful intercourse, abdominal pain	Chlamydia Bacterial vaginosis Genital herpes Candidiasis
Genital herpes	Both sexes: pain, dysuria, genital skin ulcers, swelling, lymphadenopathy, fever	Syphilis Candidiasis Herpes zoster Chancroid Hand, foot, and mouth disease Cervicitis or proctitis

Gonorrhea

Gonorrhea causes symptoms earlier in men than in women.[87] Women are asymptomatic until complications have occurred. If left untreated, an infected woman may suffer pelvic inflammatory disease, infertility, and ectopic pregnancy. Complications for men include epididymo-orchitis, reactive arthritis, and, rarely, infertility.

- *Symptoms:* Both sexes suffer from painful urination. Men may experience penis discharge (pus). Women may experience vaginal bleeding, painful intercourse, abdominal pain, and pelvic pain.
- *Signs:* penis discharge, increased vaginal discharge, swelling of one testicle in men
- *Differential diagnosis:* Similar conditions include chlamydia, bacterial vaginosis, genital herpes, and candidiasis. Genitourinary cultures are required for diagnosis, either with endocervical or urethral swabs.
- *Treatment:* A dual treatment with injection of ceftriaxone 250 mg and azithromycin 1 g taken orally is recommended.
- *Return to activity:* Athletes may participate as tolerated.

Trichomoniasis

Trichomoniasis is the most prevalent nonviral STD infection.[87] It is a parasitic infection that affects approximately 3.7 million people in the United States each year. The majority of infected people are asymptomatic or display mild symptoms.

- *Symptoms:* Most people have minimal or no symptoms, which may last for months to years. Men present with urethritis, epididymitis, or

prostatitis. Infected women present with urinary tract symptoms.
- *Signs:* penile discharge; diffuse malodorous, yellow-green vaginal discharge, with or without vulvar irritation
- *Differential diagnosis:* urethritis, chlamydia, gonorrhea, pelvic inflammatory disease, and bacterial or candida vaginosis
- *Diagnostic confirmation:* Vaginal, urethral, and urine testing are recommended; culture is the gold-standard diagnostic method.
- *Treatment:* Treatment is geared towards symptom reduction, which may reduce transmission risk. There is a high risk of reoccurrence, so patient education is necessary.
  - Metronidazole 2 g orally in a single dose or tinidazole 2 g orally in a single dose
  - Metronidazole 500 mg orally twice a day for 7 days
- *Return to activity:* Athletes will be able to participate as tolerated.

Syphilis

Syphilis is a systematic disease that is classified into stages based on clinical findings.[87] The stages of syphilis are primary, secondary, tertiary, and latent. Latent infections lack clinical presentation for an extended period of time. *Treponema pallidum* may also infect the central nervous system, resulting in neurosyphilis. Neurosyphilis may occur in any syphilis stage.

- *Symptoms:*
  - Tertiary syphilis involves aortitis, development of gummatous lesions, paresthesia, altered gait,

loss of coordination, muscle weakness, vision changes, and problems with bladder and sexual function.

- Early stages of neurosyphilis involve cranial nerve dysfunction, meningitis, altered mental status, and auditory or ophthalmic abnormalities.

- *Signs:*
  - Primary syphilis involves skin ulcers or chancre.
  - Secondary syphilis involves skin rash, mucocutaneous lesions, and lymphadenopathy.
  - Tertiary syphilis may involve a cardiovascular, neurological, or infiltration to any organ presentation.

- *Differential diagnosis:* genital herpes, chancroid, venereal warts, lymphoma, and pityriasis rosea

- *Diagnostic confirmation:* For primary, secondary, and tertiary syphilis, this is done with lesion exudate or tissues. Neurosyphilis may be diagnosed with a cerebral spinal fluid analysis.

- *Treatment:* Penicillin administered parenterally is the preferred drug. The solution used depends on the infectious stage and clinical manifestations of the disease. Benzathine penicillin G 2.4 million units IM in a single dose.

- *Return to activity:* An athlete must undergo treatment, remain asymptomatic, and have healed lesions before returning to activity.

Genital Herpes

Genital herpes is a lifelong viral infection caused by either herpes simplex virus 1 (HSV-1) or herpes simplex virus 2 (HSV-2).[87] HSV-2 accounts for most cases of recurrent genital herpes. HSV-1 infections are increasing in young women and account for a higher proportion of anogenital infections. Many infected patients have no or mild symptoms, but still intermittently shed the virus.

- *Symptoms:* pain, dysuria
- *Signs:* genital skin ulcers, swelling, lymphadenopathy, fever
- *Differential diagnosis:* syphilis; candidiasis; herpes zoster; chancroid; hand, foot, and mouth disease; cervicitis or proctitis.
- *Diagnostic confirmation:* requires specific virologic and type-specific cultures
- *Treatment:* Treatment should focus on the chronic nature of the illness rather than the acute episodes. Systemic antiviral drugs partially control symptoms and recurrent episodes or are used as a daily suppressive.

- Acyclovir 400 mg orally three times a day for 7 to 10 days or 200 mg orally five times a day for 7 to 10 days
- Valacyclovir 1 g can be taken orally twice a day for 7 to 10 days; extend treatment if healing is incomplete after 10 days.
- Suppressive therapy reduces the frequency of recurrences by 70% to 80%.
  - Acyclovir 400 mg orally twice a day
  - Valacyclovir 500 mg orally once a day or valacyclovir 1 g orally once a day

- *Return to activity:* On lesion presentation, an athlete must complete a minimum of 120 hours of systemic antivirals and have no new lesions for a period of 72 hours.

Vulvovaginal Candidiasis

Vulvovaginal candidiasis is often caused by *C. albicans*, other *Candida* species, or yeasts.[87] Approximately 75% of all women have one episode in their lifetimes, with 40% to 55% having more than one episode. Based on clinical presentation, diagnostic testing, and treatment response, vulvovaginal candidiasis is classified as either uncomplicated or complicated.

- *Symptoms:* pruritus, dyspareunia, external dysuria, pain
- *Signs:* abnormal discharge, redness, edema, fissures, excoriations, and curdy discharge
- *Differential diagnosis:* vulvar dermatitis, genital herpes, vulvar dermatoses
- *Diagnostic confirmation:* made with signs and symptoms plus (1) wet preparation of discharge demonstrating budding yeasts and (2) culture yielding positive yeast species
- *Treatment:* Uncomplicated infections are effectively treated with a short-course topical formulation. Longer doses are recommended for recurrent infections with the addition of an oral agent.
  - Over-the-counter treatment:
    - Clotrimazole: 1% cream 5 g for 7 to 14 days or 2% cream 5 g for 3 days
    - Miconazole: 2% cream 5 g daily for 7 days or 4% 5 g for 3 days
    - 100 to 200 mg suppository for 3 to 7 days
  - Prescription:
    - Butoconazole 2% cream or 5 g intravaginally in a single application
    - Terconazole: 0.4% cream 5 g intravaginally for 7 days, 0.8% 5 g intravaginally for 3 days, or 80 mg suppository for 3 days

- Oral agent: Fluconazole 150 mg orally in a single dose
- Recurrent infection requires cultures and responds well to short-duration azole therapies. Some specialists recommend a 7- to 14-day treatment with topical and oral cycles.
- *Return to activity:* An athlete may participate as tolerated.

Anogenital Warts

Anogenital warts are usually asymptomatic.[87] Human papillomavirus (HPV) 6 and 11 are the strains most commonly identified with the presentation of anogenital warts.[87,88] HPV 6 and 11 are also associated with conjunctival, nasal, oral, and laryngeal warts.

- *Symptoms:* pain, pruritic, redness
- *Signs:* appearance of one to several warts
- *Differential diagnosis:* condylomata lata, syphilis, verrucous carcinoma
- *Diagnostic confirmation:* by visual inspection and biopsy
- *Treatment:* Treatment is guided by wart size and number and the anatomic site of occurrence. Recommended regimens are imiquimod 3.75 or 5% cream, podofilox 0.5% solution, or sinecatechins 15%. Other options are provider-administered cryotherapy, surgical removal, or application of trichloroacetic acid or bichloroacetic acid.
- *Return to activity:* Athlete may participate as tolerated.

Human Papillomavirus

Human papillomavirus (HPV) enters the body through disruptions in the skin and mucosa.[88] The virus infects the basal stem cells. More than 180 subtypes of HPV exist. These variations trigger a variety of cutaneous and mucosal lesions and cancers. For prevention, a vaccine is available for adolescents. Two doses must be completed by age 13.

- *Symptoms:* pelvic or genital pain, pain or bleeding during intercourse, bleeding or spotting outside of menses
- *Signs:* cutaneous warts, anogenital warts, cervical dysplasia, palpable cervix lesions
- *Differential diagnosis:* corns, calluses, acrochordon, chancroid, herpes simplex
- *Treatment:* Treatment for cutaneous warts involves surgical or laser removal, cryotherapy, and irritant or immunomodulating medications.

Anogenital and oropharyngeal warts are treated similarly with cryotherapy, electrosurgical excision procedure, or cold knife excision. Malignancy requires resection and radiation.

- *Return to activity:* Symptomatic presentation of the virus will require specialist clearance.

Dermatological Conditions

Dermatological infections are transmitted through direct or indirect contact from a host to a susceptible person.[89] Outcomes are wide ranging from asymptomatic colonization to a lifelong systemic disease. Due to the nature of sports, athletes are at a higher risk for skin infections based on close physical contact with others and frequent degeneration of skin integrity. The three infection classifications are fungal, viral, and bacterial.

Fungal Infections

Fungal infections are caused by dermatophytes that survive on dead keratin cells in the stratum corneum of the epidermis.[89] Chronic perspirations, abrasive friction, and warm and moist areas lead to increased transmission risk. These infections present in many ways as denoted by the body area. Tinea capitis, tinea corporis, tinea cruris, and tinea pedis present on the head, body, groin, and feet, respectively.

Tinea Capitis

Tinea capitis appears on the head. Because of the presence of hair follicles, the condition is often difficult to promptly identify and treat.

- *Symptoms:* pruritus
- *Signs:* gray, scaly patches; mild hair loss (figure 18.15)
- *Differential diagnosis:* alopecia areata, seborrheic dermatitis

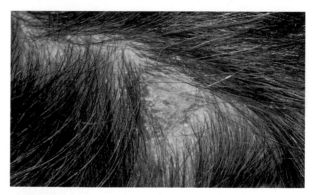

FIGURE 18.15 Tinea capitis.

Dr P. Marazzi / Science Source

- *Treatment:* The majority of cases require systemic antifungals, such as terbinafine, fluconazole, itraconazole, or ketoconazole.
- *Return to activity:* Infected patients require a minimum of 2 weeks of systemic antifungal treatment before return to activity.

Tinea Corporis

Tinea corporis, commonly called ringworm, is a dermatophyte infection on the body. Although lesions may occur in multiple locations, they do not frequently appear on the lower extremities.

- *Symptoms:* pruritus
- *Signs:* round, erythematous, scaly plaque with raised irregular borders and a central clearing (figure 18.16)
- *Differential diagnosis:* tinea versicolor, contact dermatitis, pityriasis
- *Treatment:* A topical antifungal should be applied 2 to 4 times a day. Topical agents include terbinafine, naftifine, ciclopirox, and oxiconazole.
- *Return to activity:* Athletes require at least 72 hours of treatment and a covered lesion before returning to sport.

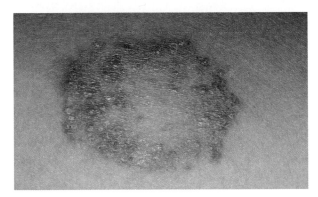

FIGURE 18.16 Tinea corporis.
Tom Myers / Science Source

Tinea Cruris

Tinea cruris, commonly called jock itch, breeds in the moist, macerating groin area. Patient education is essential to prevent occurrence and repeated infections.

- *Symptoms:* pruritus
- *Signs:* well-defined erythematous plaque in the groin and inguinal area (figure 18.17)
- *Differential diagnosis:* contact dermatitis, psoriasis, eczema

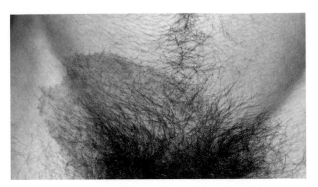

FIGURE 18.17 Tinea cruris.
Dr Harout Tanielian / Science Source

- *Treatment:* A topical antifungal should be applied 2 to 4 times daily.
- *Return to activity:* Athletes require at least 72 hours of treatment before returning to sport.

Tinea Pedis

Tinea pedis, commonly called athlete's foot, develops from macerated skin, which leads to marginated erythema and scaling.

- *Symptoms:* pruritis, burning
- *Signs:* erythema scaling, vesicle formation (figure 18.18)
- *Differential diagnosis:* psoriasis, candidiasis, erythemas, eczema
- *Treatment:* Tinea pedis often requires topical treatment throughout the athletic season. For larger lesions, oral antifungals (e.g., naftifine, oxiconazole, fluconazole, and itraconazole) help resolve active infections.
- *Return to activity:* Athletes require at least 72 hours of treatment before returning to sport.

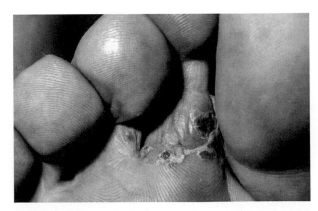

FIGURE 18.18 Tinea pedis.
Dr H.C. Robinson / Science Source

Viral Infections

The two most prevalent viral skin infections are herpes and molluscum contagiosum.[89] Both are often transmitted from skin-to-skin transmission with bodily secretions. Once infected, the patient will carry the virus for at least 2 years and potentially for a lifetime.

Herpes Infections

Herpes infections are transmitted through direct or indirect contact with a carrier.[89] The infections are caused by the herpes simplex virus. Due to their preexisting immunity, patients present with a wide variety of systemic signs and symptoms.

- *Symptoms:* malaise, prostration, polyarthralgia, polymyalgia
- *Signs:* fever, pharyngitis, conjunctivitis, widespread clustered vesicles on an erythematous base, lymphadenopathy, bacterial folliculitis (figure 18.19)
- *Differential diagnosis:* bacterial folliculitis, acute paronychia, herpes zoster, varicella
- *Diagnostic confirmation:* requires either a culture or Tzanck smear
- *Treatment:* Oral acyclovir, valacyclovir, and famciclovir are effective for acute infections.
- *Return to activity:* Patients have to complete a minimum of 120 hours of systemic antiviral medications and be free of systemic symptoms before returning to activity. There must be no new lesions for 72 hours and all lesions must have a firm adherent crust.

Molluscum Contagiosum

Molluscum contagiosum is a benign viral infection that is common in the pediatric population.[89] It is a self-limiting

viral infection that may spontaneously resolve after 2 to 4 years. Flare-ups of lesions result in papules anywhere on the body.

- *Symptoms:* potential redness, swelling
- *Signs:* several umbilicated flesh-colored to light-pink papules (figure 18.20)
- *Differential diagnosis:* basal cell carcinoma, cryptococcosis, verruca vulgaris
- *Diagnostic confirmation:* made by microscopic evaluation
- *Treatment:* sharp curette destruction
- *Return to activity:* An athlete may return following curette destruction and coverage with a gas-permeable membrane. Molluscum contagiosum flares usually resolve within 6 to 12 months.

Bacterial Infections

The majority of bacterial infections are caused by either *Streptococcus* or *Staphylococcus* strains.[89] Because asymptomatic people can be colonized with bacteria, it is

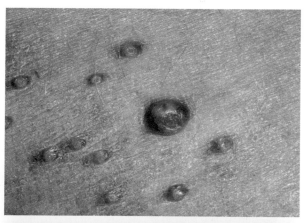

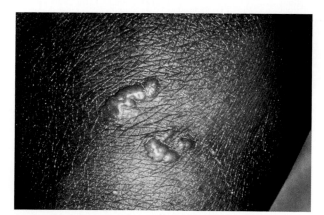

FIGURE 18.19   Herpes simplex virus.
Science Source

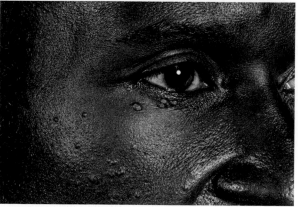

FIGURE 18.20   Molluscum contagiosum.
DR P. MARAZZI / Science Source; Dr M.A. Ansary / Science Source

essential to implement adherence to universal precautions and CDC recommendations.

Staphylococcus Aureus Infections

Approximately 30% of the population is colonized with *Staphylococcus aureus*, either in their anterior nares, axilla, or groin.[89] With skin trauma, these carriers may pass the bacteria into themselves or to others.

- *Symptoms:* pain
- *Signs:* Signs include redness, edema, and pus. Lesions are classified as follows:
  - Folliculitis involves perifollicular papules and pustules on hairy areas, especially ones that have been shaved, taped, or abraded (figure 18.21*a*).
  - Furuncles are perifollicular abscesses that may spontaneously rupture (figure 18.21*b*).
  - Carbuncles are multiple furuncles that combine into a purulent mass (figure 18.21*c*).
- *Differential diagnosis:* impetigo, drug-resistant skin infection, herpes
- *Diagnostic confirmation:* Suspicious lesions should be cultured for antimicrobial sensitivity.

- *Treatment:* Treatment should be dictated by culture and sensitivity testing. Simple folliculitis may respond to topical antibiotics. Furuncles and carbuncles will likely require incision and drainage. All infections will require an appropriate oral antibiotic prescription.
- *Return to activity:*
  - 72 hours of topical antibiotic therapy should be completed.
  - Athlete should be free of exudate from lesions and new lesions for at least 48 hours.
  - Active lesions may not be covered to allow participation.

Impetigo

Impetigo is a superficial bacterial infection that is caused by *Streptococcus aureus*.[89] Its presentation is either bullous or nonbullous lesions. Bullous lesions are superficial blisters surrounded by a scaly rim. Nonbullous lesions are thin-walled vesicles that rupture easily, resulting in yellow-golden crust.

- *Symptoms:* pruritus, pain

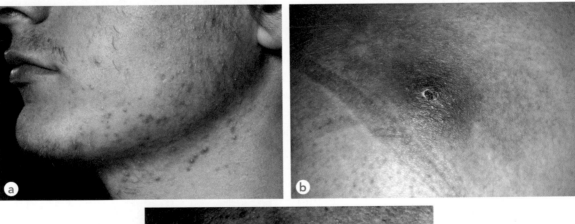

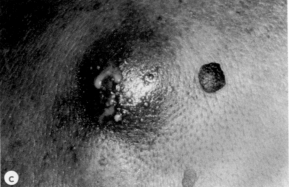

FIGURE 18.21 *(a)* Folliculitis, *(b)* furuncles, and *(c)* carbuncles.

(a) BSIP / Science Source; *(b)* Dr P. Marazzi / Science Source; *(c)* John Watney / Science Source

- *Signs:* bullous impetigo containing clear, yellow fluid that ruptures into a yellow, honey crust (figure 18.22)
- *Differential diagnosis:* cutaneous candidiasis, herpes simplex, scabies, dermatitis
- *Diagnostic confirmation:* Suspicious lesions should be cultured for antimicrobial sensitivity.

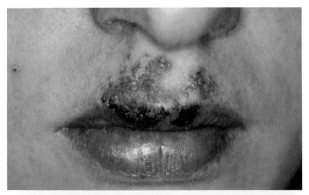

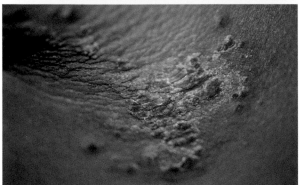

FIGURE 18.22 Impetigo.

Biophoto Associates / Science Source; DermPics / Science Source

- *Treatment:* Topical antibiotics, such as mupirocin, fusidic acid, and retapamulin, are effective against impetigo.
- *Return to activity:* Guidelines are the same as for *Staphylococcus aureus* infections.

Community-Associated Methicillin-Resistant Staphylococcus Aureus Infections

Community-associated methicillin-resistant *Staphylococcus aureus* infections (CA-MRSA) are the predominant skin infections presenting for evaluation at emergency departments.[89] As strains of the bacteria evolve, athletic trainers have to stay current with changes in standards of practice.

- *Symptoms:* pain, myalgia, nausea, chills
- *Signs:* CA-MRSA presents initially as folliculitis, furuncles, or carbuncles. The infection progresses from a small pustule or abscess, with increasing signs of systemic infection, such as rapid breathing, pulse, or a fever.
- *Differential diagnosis:* Similar conditions include *Staphylococcus aureus* infection, herpes, and impetigo. Any *Staphylococcus aureus* differential diagnosis must include MRSA.
- *Treatment:* Treatment should be dictated by culture, sensitivity testing, and local susceptibility profiles. Mild to moderate cases may still respond to beta-lactam agents. Since resistant profiles are evolving, fluroquinolones and macrolides or azalides are discouraged for CA-MRSA treatment.

EVIDENCE-BASED ATHLETIC TRAINING

CA-MRSA Transmission and Prevention

Examination of retrospective outbreaks has identified several contributing factors to transmission.[90] Infections are most likely directly spread between athletes who have direct skin-to-skin contact. An example would be that an infected offensive lineman would be more likely to transmit it to his defensive counterpart. Indirect transmission may occur through improper hygiene, cosmetic body shaving, and sharing of equipment and personal items. CA-MRSA isolates are prevalent in common-use athletic facilities. The CDC and NATA provide guidelines to reduce CA-MRSA and other skin infections.[89] Athletic trainers must have prevention and management plans that target organizational support, environmental cleaning, personal hygiene, wound management, education, and treatment. Despite the guidelines, research shows a wide variety of management responses, demonstrating the need for adherence to current best practices.

- *Return to activity:* Recognition and prompt referral are necessary to avoid systemic infections. As

with other bacterial infections, patients need to take at least 72 hours of oral antibiotic treatment.

CLINICAL BOTTOM LINE

- Athletic trainers must demonstrate competency in performing comprehensive evaluations for these or any general medical conditions. Comprehensive evaluations require ATs to perform a full physical examination, including observations, palpations, auscultations, and certain diagnostic tests.

- Athletic trainers must have proper disease knowledge and evaluation skills in order to communicate with all members of the patient's health care team.

- Athletic trainers have to view these illnesses and conditions from multiple angles. They should consider prevention, evaluation, referrals, standards of care, and safety for the client and others.

- When athletes have contagious conditions, they should be isolated from their teammates until the end of the contagious period.

- Because they treat patients across their life spans, athletic trainers should be familiar with common conditions for children, adults, and the elderly. By better understanding these conditions, athletic trainers may direct patients to the appropriate specialists and develop conditioning and athletic participation management plans.

- By understanding evolving best practices, athletic trainers are able to better advocate for their athletes with other health care professionals. Cases may be misdiagnosed or a patient may fail to respond to certain treatments.

- Disease and condition outcomes are largely dictated by timely recognition. Athletic trainers can largely affect outcomes with proper identification and evaluation and prompt referral.

- Athletic trainers must review the NATA position statements and other relevant materials regarding the mentioned conditions, illnesses, and infections.

 Go to HK*Propel* to complete the activities and case studies for this chapter.

CHAPTER 19

Psychosocial Interventions in Athletic Training Health Care

Paul Knackstedt, MS, Psy D, CMPC

CAATE STANDARDS

The following CAATE 2020 standards are covered in this chapter:

Standard 59

Standard 61

Standard 62

Standard 77

CHAPTER OBJECTIVES

After reading this chapter, you will be able to do the following:

- Summarize different psychosocial disorders common in physically active people

- Describe the psychosocial response to injury and how athletic trainers can help in the healing process

- Describe various mental training techniques commonly used in sports

- Discuss the athletic trainer's role in psychological first aid and the referral process

- Discuss how athletic trainers can work with patients with various mental disorders, help coordinate their care, and make referrals

- Discuss communication needed between the athletic trainer and the patient

- Review important communication skills for working with patients

- Explore the benefits of training and sport-performance interventions to increase emotional intelligence and improve skills

Historically, mental health disorders have been disregarded in this field due to expectations in athletic and military cultures that their members show strength, toughness, and endurance. Mental health conditions are the leading cause of disability in the United States,[82] and yet the populations served by athletic trainers face significant psychosocial barriers to using mental health services. A primary barrier is society's tendency to negatively view people with mental health conditions; this is a form of shaming known as **stigma**. Mental health stigma greatly contributes to decreased service use and often leads people to isolate themselves, feel guilty, and avoid reaching out for support.[82] As a result, athletes, members of the military, people in performing arts, and other physically active people may have difficulty expressing weakness or emotional vulnerability.

Athletic trainers are positioned perfectly to monitor patients during rehabilitation or at training and evaluate their progress on mental-health goals related to performance and their recovery from physical injury. For this reason, you need to be aware of the symptoms of mental health disorders, understand when to refer a patient, and know how to do so if needed. This chapter covers common mental health diagnoses and accompanying symptoms, which serve as a reference to help you best treat these populations.

Over the past several decades, research has consistently demonstrated a positive effect of **psychological skills training** on the rehabilitation process. Traditional psychological skills generally include goal setting, relaxation techniques, self-talk, and mental imagery. This chapter provides a basic level of understanding of psychological skills for athletic trainers. The information in this chapter should not give you the impression that you now have the skill level to apply these psychological skills on your own. Rather, when clients present with mental health issues, you should work with other members of the sports medicine team, specifically certified mental performance consultants (CMPC), psychiatrists, or licensed mental health care providers, including sport psychologists. This chapter will help you develop the awareness needed to identify areas of growth and assist in your clients' injury rehabilitation and general well-being by supplementing mental health skills that they may learn from a licensed professional.

Prevalence of Psychosocial Disorders

Mental health disorders do not enter our awareness relative to the kinds of obvious symptoms that often accompany a physical injury. Limping, swelling, bruising, and bleeding provide valuable information indicating that a physical injury has taken place; with mental health concerns, the symptoms are not as obvious. Athletes frequently respond to painful experiences and emotions by practicing the same coping skills that helped them reach a high level of success in sport—ignoring the pain, digging deep, and focusing on the task at hand. In an athletic culture where mental toughness and grit are emphasized, athletes often feel like they need to keep their pain in the dark and go through their struggles alone. Similar trends can be seen in military populations, where various forms of stigma reduce the likelihood that soldiers will seek support for mental health concerns.[1] As a result, athletic trainers and other members of the health care team need to be aware of the warning signs and symptoms of mental health issues that are common within the population they are working with.

Approximately 1 in 5 U.S. adults—48.3 million, or 18.5% of the U.S. population—experiences an issue related to mental health each year.[2] Injured patients are at an increased risk of suffering mental health concerns due to the stress and adjustment that accompany disability, including separation from sport or exercise, lack of freedom, decreased social support, and increased pain. In any given year, approximately 1 in 25 adults in the United States—9.8 million, or 4.0%—experience a serious mental illness that substantially interferes with or limits one or more major life activities.[2] In most cases,

---

EVIDENCE-BASED ATHLETIC TRAINING

NATA Consensus Statement: Mental Health Concerns at the Collegiate Level

The National Athletic Trainers' Association established a protocol for the recognition and referral of a student-athlete with a mental health concern.[87] Given the prevalence of mental health concerns nationwide, learning the signs and symptoms of mental health issues and how to refer patients are important foundational aspects of providing holistic care for athletic trainers.

The article discusses the effect of athletic injury on psychological stress and makes recommendations for follow-up with a mental health professional if difficulties emerge following an injury. The authors recommend that the athletic trainer work with a multidisciplinary team, including a physician, campus counseling service, community-based mental health provider, and psychiatrist. They recommend preparticipation physical examinations to screen for mental health concerns that may warrant follow-up care or evaluation.

The article lays out strategies for the athletic trainer to keep in mind when approaching a student-athlete with concerns about their mental well-being, including the importance of focusing on the athlete as a whole person, promptly referring them after they agree to attend counseling, and accompanying them to their first counseling session to ensure attendance. If a student is an imminent threat to harm themselves or others, it is important to make the appropriate mental health referral as soon as possible.

Confidentiality issues may arise in patient care systems where multidisciplinary care is emphasized as the gold standard. Patients should be informed that although mental health services are confidential, it may be helpful to notify another party of their attendance at appointments.

athletic trainers do not treat patients who are experiencing ongoing severe mental illness resulting in substantial limitations in major life activities, but because many mental illnesses manifest in patients during adolescence or their early 20s, athletic trainers may be the first health care provider to recognize the early symptoms of an emerging mental illness and start the referral process.

Student-Athletes

Research indicates mixed results regarding the prevalence rates of diagnosable mental health disorders in the athletic population compared to nonathletes. Sports medicine professionals have reconsidered the belief that athletes are protected from mental health disorders.[13] Although elite athletes receive the psychological benefits of exercise, social support, and mastery, the intense mental and physical demands of training and competition may make them susceptible to developing mental health issues.[14] The overwhelmingly stressful lifestyle of an athlete combined with the fact that their peak competitive years occur during adolescence and early adulthood, a significant time in human development, may create the perfect storm of risk factors that contribute to psychological distress.[15,16]

Athletes are exposed to a unique set of stressors[17-19] that the general population does not experience:

- Increased public attention through marketing efforts
- Mainstream and social media scrutiny
- Public photo shoots with fans
- Changes in support due to relocation
- Lack of financial opportunities due to athletic sacrifices
- Personal and team relationships
- Potential for injuries

The benefits of exercise on physical and mental health are well publicized;[20] however, a review found that intense physical activity performed at the elite athletic level might actually decrease mental well-being, increasing subsequent levels of depression and anxiety through subjective experiences of burnout, overtraining, and injury.[21,34] Based on a review, data indicate that rates of mental disorders such as anxiety and depression were seen at the same levels in elite athletes as the general population.[31] When the athlete population is divided into subgroups, athletes in the retirement phase of their careers[32] and those experiencing performance failure are at greater risk for elevated mental illness.[33]

Military Personnel

According to research, 1 in 4 active duty military personnel shows signs of a mental health condition.[76] Yet, approximately 40% to 60% of military personnel with a mental health concern do not seek treatment.[1] Common

EVIDENCE-BASED ATHLETIC TRAINING

NATA Consensus Statement: Mental Health Concerns at the Secondary School Level

The National Athletic Trainers' Association established a protocol for the recognition and referral of a secondary school student-athlete with a mental health concern[88] and developed a strategy for addressing mental health across institutions. Providers included a plan to address unique stressors, recognize behaviors to monitor, and cite special circumstances affecting psychological health.

Due to the high probability of secondary school students being affected by mental health concerns, athletic trainers should have a referral protocol in place. Secondary students experience similar stressors as collegiate student-athletes, including overtraining and burnout, injury, retirement from sport, performance challenges, dealing with success, and pressures to overspecialize. Be aware of the symptoms of common diagnoses and consider a referral if you see an increase in a student's presentation of a possible illness or condition. As always, the most important steps related to mental health are education, early recognition, and appropriate referral.

Bullying is defined as any unwanted aggressive behaviors toward a young person by another youth or group of youths (does not include siblings or current dating partner) that involves an observed or perceived power imbalance and is repeated multiple times or is highly likely to be repeated. Most people who are bullied are too embarrassed to tell anyone due to feelings of shame. In athletes, being bullied leads to loss of focus, tentative performance, anxiety, missed games or tournaments, and early retirement from sports. If you believe that a student-athlete is being bullied, consult with a mental health provider.

concerns for members of the military include depression, anxiety, post-traumatic stress disorder (PTSD), substance abuse, and traumatic brain injury (TBI). Substantial evidence suggests that military veterans face increased mental health concerns because readjustment to civilian life following wartime trauma is difficult. Coping with a physical injury is difficult for military personnel, who pride themselves on being fit and active and contributing to the organization. This increases the potential for patients to feel restless and struggle with some aspects of treatment compliance, since they may not be used to making changes to their activity level.

Barriers to Mental Health Services

Generally, in the United States, there are significant barriers to seeking, obtaining, and maintaining sufficient mental health care. Data reveal that among the 46.6 million adults aged 18 or older with any mental illness (AMI), 19.8 million (42.6%) received mental health services in the past year.[6] The National Survey on Drug Use and Health defines **mental health services** as inpatient or outpatient treatment or counseling or use of prescription medication for problems with emotions, nerves, or mental health.[6] Important demographic considerations from the survey include that more women with AMI (47.6%) received mental health services than men with AMI (34.8%).[6] Among people with AMI, fewer young adults received mental health services (38.4% of 18- to 25-year-olds) than older adults (43.3% of 26- to 49-year-olds and 44.2% of those aged 50 and older).[6]

Although more athletes are seeking professional support for issues related to performance and mental health than ever before, this has not always been the case. Historically, athletes have tended to deal with uncomfortable emotions in the same ways that they have been conditioned to treat discomfort and pain in the body: Ignore it, distract yourself, and tough it out. Athletes have found this to be an effective strategy for getting through adversity and quickly returning to play after injury. Barriers to athletes seeking help could be reinforced by cultural expectations of toughness, invulnerability, and the ability to battle through adversity.[62] Those who work closest with student-athletes, performing artists, and members of the military understand this culture and have responded by attempting to remove some of the barriers to mental health services and get these valuable services to those in need. In 2013, the NCAA's chief medical officer, Brian Hainline, started an initiative to address student-athlete mental health needs and begin to break down stigma and improve mental health services across the country. The initiative sparked a publication called Mind, Body, and Sport,[57] which included firsthand accounts from student-athletes, coaches, and mental health providers.

Patients often feel overwhelmed when attempting to find the motivation to add the task of daily rehabilitation to an already busy schedule. If they have endured a traumatic injury and are struggling with being separated from their social supports and feeling pressured to return to sport quickly, they may be receiving feedback like "You just need to be more mentally tough," "Stop being so dramatic," or "It's supposed to be hard." This feedback can be invalidating and deplete any remaining motivation they have, making it more difficult to build the confidence needed to overcome the daily hurdles involved in the

Mental Health Advocacy

Michael Phelps faced many challenges in his career on his way to becoming the most decorated Olympic athlete of all time and winning 28 medals, 23 of which are gold.[93] Despite being one of the world's most successful athletes, the American swimmer struggled with mental health and became very depressed in 2012 after the London Olympic Games.[91,92] Phelps said that after spending five days in his room and contemplating suicide, the decision to seek therapy saved his life.[92]

Phelps, along with a growing list of other high-profile athletes, are using their social recognition and influence to help raise awareness about the stigma and lack of access to mental health services that influence psychosocial outcomes. By disclosing his personal experience with depression and anxiety, Phelps strives to break down the barriers of seeking mental health treatment and normalize mental health concerns. He hopes his advocacy work can help society understand that depression can happen to anyone, even a 23-time Olympic gold medalist.

The most-decorated Olympian of all time has announced a new mental health advocacy partnership with an online therapy company that helps connect people to local mental health resources through the use of a mobile device. "For me, that's way bigger than ever winning gold medals . . . the chance to potentially save a life, to give that person an opportunity to grow and learn and help someone else, there's nothing better in life."[92]

process of long-term injury rehabilitation. As nice as it would be to have a one-size-fits-all model of treatment for injury, athletic trainers need to address the individual differences that make their patients unique, especially the psychosocial aspects that largely influence an athlete's rehabilitation progress.

Entirely denying the existence of mental health issues is a common barrier to seeking services.[63] Athletes are often concerned that admitting to any personal issues would lessen their chances of success by weakening a coach's confidence in their ability to perform, damaging teammates' perceptions of them, or lowering their self-efficacy.[64] This fear of stigma from an unsupportive coach or support staff member within the organization may prevent athletes from accepting that they need greater support or treatment for a mental health concern.[10]

Although research has shown that men and women experience similar rates of mental health concerns, the types of diagnoses may differ significantly. The gender gap in mental health service use has been connected to several factors, including men's attitudes about asking for help, structured social norms that are reconstructed during social interactions, and the reinforcement of masculinity norms in relationships with women.[80] Cross-cultural psychology has focused on differences in the ways people behave, express emotions, and cope with trauma across cultures.[98] Western views of mental health diagnosis and treatment may not be an exact fit across all cultures due to differences in the ways groups of people learn to express and cope with their emotions.

Common Mental Health Disorders

The DSM-5, the diagnostic tool published by the American Psychiatric Association, states that a mental disorder is a syndrome characterized by a clinically significant disturbance in a person's cognition, emotional regulation, or behavior that reflects a dysfunction in the psychological, biological, or developmental process underlying mental

functioning; this is usually associated with significant distress or disability in social, occupational, or other important activities.[71] The following sections discuss common mental health disorders that athletic trainers see when working with more traditional performing populations. By no means is this an exhaustive list, but conditions that occur in performers typically include more common types of mood disorders, anxiety disorders, attention-deficit/hyperactivity disorder (ADHD), substance use disorders, disordered eating, and impulse control problems. It is also important to consider that performers are impacted by subclinical levels of diagnosable disorders in ways that they may seek a referral to a mental health professional. This means that they experience less symptoms than the number required by the DSM-5 to qualify for diagnosis.

Mood Disorders

A **mood disorder**, also known as an affective disorder, is characterized by an elevation or lowering of a person's emotional state that severely affects function. The typical presentation of a mood disorder may include emotions that range from extreme lows to highs and irritability. The most common mood disorders are major depressive disorder and bipolar disorder (table 19.1). Other types of mood disorders not discussed in this chapter include mood disorder due to medical condition; mood disorder due to medications, drugs, or substance use; disruptive mood regulation disorder; seasonal affective disorder; persistent depressive disorder; and premenstrual dysphoric disorder. These other mood disorder diagnoses, although important to be aware of, are not as common as depression and bipolar disorder. Treatment for mood disorders includes a combination of counseling and psychopharmacological medication, depending on the severity of symptoms.

Depression

Depression is more than just feeling sad or wanting to cry. It can range from mild to severe depending on the number and severity of symptoms. Thoughts of suicide

Barriers to Seeking Mental Health Services

- Cultural stigma or societal perceptions about seeking treatment for mental health
- Socioeconomic barriers
- Lack of providers in their geographic area
- Poor understanding of mental illness
- Fear of having to take medication
- Poor self-awareness: unable to see the need for treatment
- Low perceived need: unsure if condition is severe enough for treatment
- Desire to handle problems on one's own

TABLE 19.1 **Comparison of Depression and Bipolar Disorder**

Mood disorder	Definition	Symptoms
Depression	Mood disorder resulting in low mood and loss of interest 5 of 9 symptoms present over 2-week period One symptom must include: • Depressed mood • Loss of interest or pleasure	Depressed mood or sadness Loss of interest Insomnia or hypersomnia Psychomotor agitation Fatigue Feelings of worthlessness or guilt Loss of appetite Increase or loss of weight Recurrent thoughts of death Difficulty concentrating Thoughts of suicide
Bipolar disorder	A category of mood disorder that causes extreme fluctuations in a person's mood, energy, and ability to function Includes bipolar I, bipolar II, and cyclothymic disorder Bipolar I: mania with or without an episode of depression Bipolar II: hypomania with an episode of depression Cyclothymic disorder: brief episodes of hypomania and depression	Mania symptoms: Abnormally elevated, expansive, or irritable mood and persistent activity or energy that is present nearly all day, every day, for at least a week Hypomania symptoms: Less intense than mania and lasts at least 4 days For mania or hypomania, accompanied by 3 of the following symptoms: • Inflated self-esteem or grandiosity • Decreased need for sleep • More talkative than usual • Flight of ideas or racing thoughts • Distractibility • Increase in goal-directed activity or psychomotor agitation • Excessive involvement in high-risk activities

are common during a depressive episode. If a patient discloses that they are having thoughts of suicide, make the appropriate referral to a trusted mental health professional for a thorough assessment. (Recommendations for referrals are presented later in this chapter.) Suicide is the 10th leading cause of death in the United States[2] and the 2nd leading cause of death for people aged 15 to 24.[4] If you notice several of these symptoms present in a patient over the same 2-week period, discuss what you are seeing with the patient or consult with a mental health professional.

In the United States, 6.9% of adults—16 million people—had at least one major depressive episode in 2015.[3] The rate of student-athletes developing depression have been found to be between 15.6% and 21%, with freshmen experiencing a higher rate of depression than other collegiate class years.[11, 12] Injured athletes have exhibited higher rates of depression symptoms than noninjured athletes, and may experience symptoms up to 2 months following injury.[38] A 2014 meta-analysis estimated the prevalence of major depression among U.S. military personnel by consolidating 25 epidemiological studies on the topic. Estimates of prevalence (standard error) were 12.0% (1.2) of participants currently deployed, 13.1% (1.8) of those previously deployed, and 5.7% (1.2) of those never deployed, signifying a slight increase in major depression prevalence following retirement from active duty.[83]

Patients with moderate to severe injuries often report emotional fluctuations, anxiety, anger, and frustration.[24] It is important to consider the wide array of possible responses to injury, especially those injuries that may require surgical procedures, separation from sport, and extended rehabilitation.[10] You should work to develop trust with your clients to help facilitate further conversations and increase the chances they will seek help for physical and psychological distress.

Confidence as an athlete is, in many ways, connected to participation and performance in sport. When athletes are setting goals, training, and competing within a sport context where they have important interpersonal relationships, they can maintain the proper balance of physical and mental endeavors. When an athletic injury occurs, a disruption in the balance of well-being can be expected for the majority of performers, especially in the early stages of athletic injury. An athlete's primary method of building their self-worth has been influenced by his ability to achieve reinforcement for their accomplishments and develop a sense of mastery. When they are separated from sport, patients need support to reframe the difficulties of the rehabilitation environment and embrace the challenge that lies ahead of them in recovering and returning to play.

Bipolar Disorder

Previously known as manic-depressive illness, bipolar disorder is a mental illness that causes a shift in a person's mood and energy. In any given year, an estimated 5.7 million American adults, or 2.6% of the population aged 18 or older, are diagnosed with bipolar disorder.[23]

Anxiety Disorders

Anxiety is a common psychosocial response to injury,[39] since uncertainty about the future occurs during every step of the injury and rehabilitation process (table 19.2). In the United States, 18.1% of adults experience an anxiety disorder, such as post-traumatic stress disorder, obsessive-compulsive disorder, and specific phobias.[2]

Anxiety is separated into the following:

- *Trait anxiety:* a stable characteristic; the level of unpleasant emotional or physical arousal across various situations

TABLE 19.2 Comparison of Various Anxiety Disorders

Anxiety disorders	Definition	Symptoms
Generalized anxiety	An anxiety disorder characterized by excessive worry, often accompanied by a combination of cognitive and physiological symptoms, including heart palpitations, shortness of breath, dizziness, sweating, and digestive issues	Excessive worry experienced more days than not for at least 6 months about a number of events The intensity of worry is out of proportion to the likelihood of the actual event. The patient finds it difficult to control the worry. The anxiety and worry are associated with at least 3 of the following: • Restlessness • Being easily fatigued • Difficulty concentrating or mind going blank • Irritability • Muscle tension • Sleep disturbance
Social anxiety disorder	Fear of being judged negatively, evaluated, or rejected in a social or performance situation	Marked fear or anxiety about a social situation with possible scrutiny by others The patient fears they will show anxiety symptoms that will be negatively evaluated. Social situations almost always provoke fear or anxiety. Social situations are avoided or endured with intense fear or anxiety. Fear or anxiety is out of proportion to the actual threat posed by the social situation. Fear, anxiety, or avoidance is persistent, lasting for 6 months or more.
Panic disorder	A condition in which debilitating anxiety and fear arise without reasonable cause	Recurrent, unexpected panic attacks during which 4 or more of the following are present: • Palpitations, pounding heart, or accelerated heart rate • Sweating • Trembling or shaking • Sensations of shortness of breath or smothering • Feelings of choking • Chest pain or discomfort • Nausea or abdominal distress • Feeling dizzy, unsteady, light-headed, or faint • Chills or heat sensations • Paresthesia (numbness/tingling sensations) • **Derealization** (unreality) or **depersonalization** (detachment) • Fear of losing control or going crazy • Fear of dying

- *State anxiety:* a transient characteristic; the level of unpleasant emotional or physical arousal in the current moment[41]

Patients who have high trait anxiety often respond to athletic injury with an increase in state anxiety post-injury.[42] State anxiety may fluctuate based on several factors, including injury severity and time lost from practice or competition.[25]

Injured athletes also experience anxiety as a result of the loss of regular interactions with teammates or coaches, who provide social support, or their perception that they are letting down family members, friends, coaches, and teammates.[43] Athletes are affected by anxiety disorders such as social anxiety (performance anxiety), panic disorder, and phobic anxiety, especially while recovering from an injury and returning to participation. Although it is less likely to occur in athletes, generalized anxiety and obsessive-compulsive disorder can also influence athlete mental health.[57] Anxiety disorders are treated with a combination of talk therapy and medication, with more severe symptoms requiring a greater level of care.

Social Anxiety Disorder and Performance Anxiety

Performance anxiety is related to anticipation of future events. People with extreme performance anxiety become physically and mentally overwhelmed during the execution of an action due to fear of evaluation and possible social rejection. Some performing artists are more likely to experience performance anxiety prior to their competition than others based on a variety of factors. A certain amount of performance anxiety is normal; many people can relate to the feeling of having butterflies before a big event. An amateur athlete is more likely to experience heightened anxiety that interferes with their ability to perform in competition due to their lack of experience managing arousal level in big competitions. Higher anxiety does not always translate to decreased performance if the competitor has learned ways to cope with anxiety through psychological skills. According to research on anxiety and mastery in music, under conditions of high state anxiety, performers with more years of training performed at a higher level than those with less training.[9] In a study examining anxiety and psychological skill use in amateur golfers, more physically skilled players used psychological skills to a greater degree than lesser-skilled players.[77]

Social anxiety disorder (SAD) produces fear in social and performance situations. One of the most common fears is public speaking, while other common triggers of anxiety include routine tasks like athletic, tactical, or musical performances. Sport and performance psychology services provide skills aimed at better preparing the mind of an athlete or performing artist for competition. Sport psychologists work with athletes and performing artists with social anxiety disorder at clinical and subclinical levels in order to find the best treatment options to improve their performance and help them find comfort.

Panic Disorder

The exact cause of panic disorder is unknown, but several theories are being researched to examine potential causes more deeply. Many experts agree that panic disorder is caused by a combination of factors, including biological and environmental influences. Research has supported theories that consider a person's genetic and contextual factors when considering a diagnosis of panic disorder.[81] Panic disorder includes unpredictable panic attacks. During a panic attack, a person experiences intense thoughts, feelings of being overwhelmed, and many physical symptoms, including racing heart, shortness of breath, shakiness, and sweating, that surface quickly and diminish within 20 minutes, which often leads to exhaustion.[57]

Attention-Deficit/Hyperactivity Disorder

An estimated 11% of school-aged children in the United States (6.4 million) are diagnosed with attention-deficit/hyperactivity disorder (ADHD) at some point in their lifetimes. The overall prevalence rate in adults is 4.4%, with men (5.4%) affected at a higher rate than women (3.2%).[84] ADHD is one of the most common disorders treated in athletes and presents with symptoms such as difficulty focusing, concentrating, learning, and sustaining attention.[57] Table 19.3 outlines the three types of ADHD.

Treatment for ADHD includes medication and counseling with academic coaching to improve time-management and organizational skills. Typical psychopharmacological treatments, including psychostimulants, are restricted by the NCAA. In order to participate in sports while using these types of medications, athletes require a thorough assessment by a psychologist as well as an annual physical exam.

Substance Use Disorder

Student-athletes most commonly use alcohol, marijuana, opiates, stimulants (e.g., caffeine, Adderall, Ritalin), nicotine, and performance-enhancing drugs. Males are more likely to use substances; overall, student-athletes are more likely to use substances during the off-season than during their competitive season.[57] Alcohol and drug use can commonly co-occur with other mental health disorders, such as mood disorders, anxiety disorders,

TABLE 19.3 **Types of ADHD**

Neurodevelopmental disorders	Definition	Symptoms
Attention-deficit/hyperactivity disorder: inattentive type	More common in females than in males Often looks like this person has trouble concentrating or paying attention to details	6 or more (5 or more for patients 17 years and older) of the following symptoms have persisted for the past 6 months: • Often fails to give close attention to details; makes careless mistakes • Often has difficulty sustaining attention in tasks or play activities • Often does not seem to listen when spoken to directly • Often does not follow through on instructions; fails to finish schoolwork, chores, other tasks • Often has difficulty organizing tasks and activities • Often avoids or dislikes tasks that require sustained mental effort • Often loses things necessary for tasks or activities • Is often easily distracted by extraneous stimuli (child) or by unrelated thoughts (adolescents and adults) • Is often forgetful in daily activities * Several symptoms were present prior to the age of 12 years
Attention-deficit hyperactivity disorder: hyperactive type	More common in males than in females Person fidgets and has trouble sitting still and managing impulses	6 or more (5 or more for patients 17 years and older) of the following symptoms have persisted for 6 months: • Often fidgets with hands, taps hands or feet, or squirms in seat • Often leaves seat in situations when remaining seated is expected • Often runs around or climbs in situations where it is inappropriate (child) or experiences feelings of restlessness (adults) • Often unable to play or engage in leisure activities quietly • Is often on the go, acting as if he is driven by a motor; appears unable to be comfortable • Often talks excessively • Often blurts out an answer before a question has been completed • Often has difficulty waiting his turn • Often interrupts or intrudes on others * Several symptoms were present prior to the age of 12
Attention-deficit hyperactivity disorder: combined type	Most common type of ADHD, although not necessarily the most severe (case-by-case basis) It includes symptoms of both inattentive and hyperactive types.	6 or more (5 or more for patients 17 years and older) of the inattentive symptoms present over the past 6 months 6 or more (5 or more for patients 17 years and older) of the hyperactive symptoms present over the past 6 months

and ADHD, reinforcing negative coping strategies and maintaining alcohol and drug use long after their competitive careers end. Among the 20.2 million adults in the United States who experienced a substance use disorder, 50.5% had a co-occurring mental illness.[2] Chronic drug use combined with certain biological risk factors and contextual stressors may trigger an adverse mental health event that can affect patient function. A diagnosis of substance-induced psychotic disorder (SIPD) can be made when psychotic symptoms include hallucinations or delusions and develop during or soon after drug use or withdrawal. If a patient appears to be experiencing significant perceptual issues, such as hallucinations or delusions, assess them for recent drug use and withdrawal and consider contacting emergency services for further assessment. Ensure the patient's safety before you allow them to leave the facility.

Impulse Control Problems

An impulse control disorder is a class of psychiatric disorder characterized by a failure to resist an urge. Impulse control problems often manifest in behavioral issues, erratic performance, and repeated instances of rule breaking, fighting, aggression towards others, interpersonal difficulties, and risky sexual behaviors.[57] Impulse control problems are often treated through a combination of talk therapy and medication management.

Disordered Eating

Disordered eating occurs in both genders, but is more common in females and in sports in which lower body weight and fat percentage improves performance—for example, gymnastics, diving, and ice skating (judged on aesthetics), wrestling, and distance running.[57] Treatment includes a combination of therapy, medical treatment, and nutrition education.

There are several different types of disordered eating, including anorexia nervosa, bulimia nervosa, body dysmorphic disorder, binge eating, avoidant/restrictive food intake disorder, pica, rumination disorder, other specified feeding or eating disorder, and unspecified feeding or eating disorder (table 19.4).

Anorexia Nervosa

Anorexia nervosa is a potentially life-threatening eating disorder where people do not consume enough calories, leading to significantly low body weight. People with anorexia usually have a fear of gaining weight. If that fear is not present, people with anorexia have persistent behaviors that interfere with their ability to add weight. A patient affected by anorexia may not be able to see the effect of her choices and notice how underweight they are currently.

There are two types of anorexia nervosa:

1. *Restricting type.* During the past 3 months, no recurrent episodes of binge eating or purging behavior (vomiting; misuse of laxatives, diuretics, or enemas) occurred. This subtype describes presentations in which weight loss is accomplished primarily through dieting, fasting, or excessive exercise.[71]
2. *Binge eating/purging type.* During the past 3 months, the patient has engaged in recurrent episodes of binge eating or purging behavior (i.e., self-induced vomiting or misuse of laxatives, diuretics, or enemas).[71]

Diagnosis of anorexia is multifaceted and typically requires a wealth of information collected over time to make an accurate assessment. Anorexia is often seen in conjunction with other mental health disorders, such as depression, anxiety, and obsessive-compulsive disorder. Multidisciplinary teams use a combination of physical exams, blood tests, mental health assessments, and standardized indexes like the body mass index (BMI) to diagnose anorexia nervosa. Adult BMI levels below 17.5% meet criteria for diagnosing anorexia. BMI alone is not enough to diagnose anorexia, but it can be used as one of many indicators for further care for a patient who may be struggling with disordered eating. There are also different levels of severity of anorexia based on BMI, ranging from mild (<17.5), moderate (16-16.99), and severe (15-15.99), to extreme (<15). A BMI below 13.5 can lead to organ failure, while a BMI below 12 can be life-threatening.

Bulimia Nervosa

Bulimia is a potentially fatal eating disorder that is defined by recurrent episodes of binge eating followed by intense feelings of guilt and shame and compensatory behaviors to accommodate for the binge. People with bulimia are very concerned about their body shape and weight. The etiology of bulimia nervosa is multifactorial, meaning that many causes can contribute to this disorder, including environmental stress, genetic factors, and neurochemical imbalances. Co-occurring psychological influences, such as anxiety disorders, depression, and low self-esteem, are also known triggers in patients reporting the presence of disordered eating behaviors.

Binge-Eating Disorder

Binge eating disorder (BED) is a severe, life-threatening, and treatable eating disorder characterized by recurrent episodes of eating large quantities of food, often very quickly and to the point of discomfort.

TABLE 19.4 Comparison of Disordered Eating

Type of disorder	Definition	Symptoms
Anorexia nervosa	Eating disorder where not enough calories are being consumed	• Restriction of energy intake relative to requirements, leading to significantly low weight • Intense fear of gaining weight or becoming fat, or behavior that interferes with weight gain • Disturbance in the way in which one's body weight or shape is perceived
Bulimia nervosa	Recurrent episodes of binge eating followed by intense feelings of guilt and shame	• Recurrent episodes of binge eating • Recurrent inappropriate compensatory behaviors in order to prevent weight gain, such as self-induced vomiting, overuse of laxatives or diuretics, fasting, excessive exercise • Eating more than most people would consider normal in a discrete time period (2 hr) • A sense of lack of control over eating during the episode (cannot stop eating) • Binge eating and compensatory behavior occur, on average at least once a week for 3 months • Self-evaluation is unduly influenced by body shape and weight
Binge-eating disorder	Recurrent episodes of eating large quantities of food, often very quickly and to the point of discomfort	• Recurrent episodes of binge eating • Eating more than most people would consider normal in a discrete time period (2 hr) • A sense of lack of control over eating during the episode (cannot stop eating) • The binge-eating episodes are associated with 3 or more of the following: • Eating much more rapidly than usual • Eating until feeling uncomfortably full • Eating large amounts of food when not feeling physically hungry • Eating alone because of embarrassment about how much one is eating • Feeling disgusted with oneself, depressed, or guilty after eating • Marked distress regarding binge eating is present • The binge eating occurs, on average, at least once per week for 3 months
Body dysmorphic disorder	Heightened distress caused by a preoccupation with a perceived defect in appearance	• Mental acts: social comparison • Repetitive behaviors: mirror checking, skin picking, excessive grooming, reassurance seeking

Body Dysmorphic Disorder

Body dysmorphic disorder (BDD) is heightened distress caused by a preoccupation with a perceived defect in appearance. This diagnosis has recently been recategorized in the DSM-5 and is now thought of as a type of obsessive compulsive and related disorder (OC-RD). OC-RD is more common in males than in females, especially in athletic populations in sports where muscularity and fitness are emphasized, such as wrestling, football, track and field, and swimming and diving, often resulting in unhealthy mirror checking, overexercising, and dieting. Generally, athletic trainers observe behaviors that demonstrate a patient's preoccupation with one or more perceived flaws or defects in appearance. Social comparison and overgrooming are typical in patients suffering from BDD. Patients with BDD are unable to be convinced that their concerns are imagined and not worthy of their constant attention. Another notable subtype of BDD is muscle dysmorphia, or the belief that one's body is too small and lacking sufficient muscle.

Behaviors to Monitor

Monitor for the following behaviors:[5, 56, 71]

- Overall lack of awareness of how stress affects them
- Acting out nonverbally to alert others something is wrong
- Changes in eating and sleeping habits
- Unexpected weight gain or loss
- Drug or alcohol use or abuse
- Withdrawing from social contact
- Talking about death or dying
- Problems focusing
- Becoming more irritable; anger management issues
- Negative self-talk
- Feeling out of control
- Mood swings, agitation, or irritability
- Overuse injuries or continually getting injured

Psychological Response to Injury

Sports medicine professionals tend to focus their attention on healing the physical damage from injury, but athletes may also have psychosocial wounds because of their injury that remain unhealed.[24] Athletic injury can contribute to an already stressful lifestyle, and injured athletes report feelings of tension, confusion, hostility, loneliness, fear, irritability, and anxiety.[25] Research has demonstrated a positive relationship between injury severity and negative mood in patients.[28] Several theoretical models have been proposed indicating that cognitive and affective elements may contribute to rehabilitation outcomes. Athletic trainers must understand how athletes respond to injury and the rehabilitation process, both physically and psychologically, in order to work with patients more effectively and help them deal with adversity in the future.[29]

The integrated model of psychological response to sport injury and the rehabilitation process (figure 19.1) is a conceptual model that explores the interrelated psychosocial process of cognition, affect, and behavior.[26] Based on this model, rehabilitation outcomes are affected by the initial injury and the subsequent changes in the patient's thoughts, feelings, and actions. Other contributions to the injury response are a variety of interacting personal and individual differences, such as gender, age, injury history, characteristics of personality, and athletic identity. Postinjury cognitive appraisals are at the center of the model and involve the patient's mental evaluation of aspects such as sense of loss, optimism, burnout, challenge, and self. **Cognitive appraisals** directly influence a

patient's affect-related psychosocial responses of emotion and behavior, as well as the patient's physical recovery. Emotional or affective responses to injury include mood disturbances such as depression, anxiety, low vigor, fatigue, grief, burnout, and fear of reinjury.[30]

Cognition and emotions directly affect the recovery process due to their influence on the injured athlete's behaviors—for example, attendance at rehabilitation sessions, adherence to prescribed exercises, substance abuse, exercise dependence, and suicidal behavior.[30] Treatment adherence is largely determined by an athlete's readiness and motivation to take on the rehabilitation of her injury.[35] Applying a behavior change model (typically used for increasing exercise behavior in sedentary people or eliminating substance use) for rehabilitation can help injured athletes increase self-efficacy, use pros of rehabilitation over the cons, and use behavioral processes instead of experiential processes.[37]

To rehabilitate their injuries responsibly, patients must accept the situation, adapt to new limitations, and create change with health-directed behaviors in multiple areas of life. The transtheoretical model [89] (TTM; figure 19.2) is helpful for improving outcomes as the patient works toward a goal. The TTM makes patients more aware of barriers and helps them identify how motivated they are to begin making the changes they need to make in order to see the outcomes they desire. Completing a brief initial assessment to identify ambivalence that may emerge throughout the process of therapy may be extremely helpful for finding ways to motivate the patient through various forms of adversity that they may face. The transtheoretical model has distinct stages: precontemplative, contemplative, preparation, action,

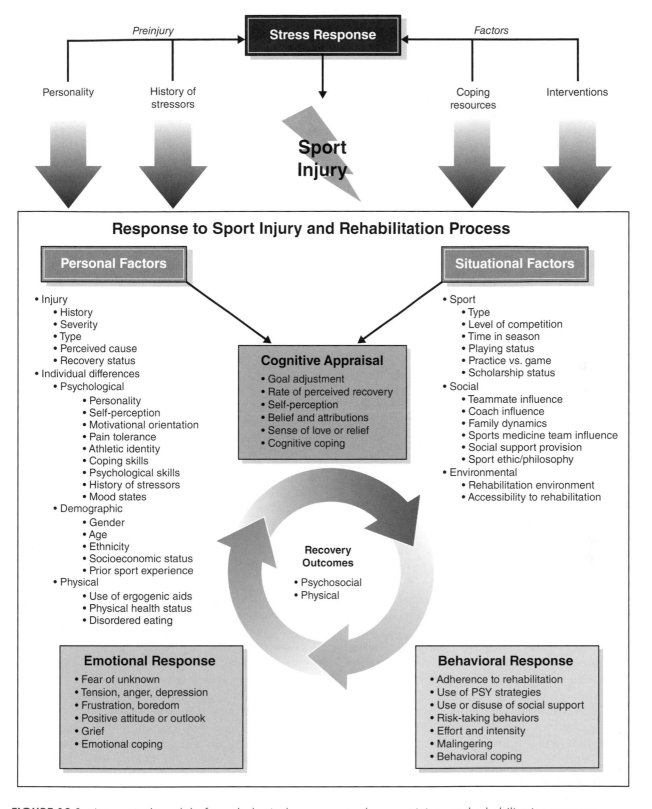

FIGURE 19.1   Integrated model of psychological response to the sport injury and rehabilitation process.

Reprinted by permission from D. Wiese-Bjornstal et al., "An Integrated Model of Response to Sport Injury: Psychological and Sociological Dynamics," *Journal of Applied Sport Psychology* 10, no. 1 (1998): 49.

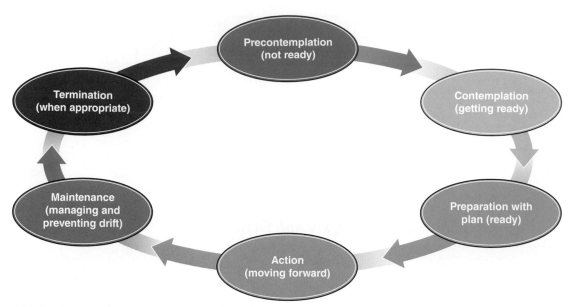

FIGURE 19.2 Stages of the transtheoretical model.

maintenance, and termination or eventual relapse of preexisting behavior (following several cycles through previous stages of change).[36] Motivation is vital to a successful rehabilitation, and athletic trainers need to find a way to help keep patients engaged and in the action stage of change throughout the rehabilitation process. When rehabilitation gets monotonous and motivation is lacking, some student-athletes ask their athletic trainer to adjust their rehabilitation exercises to keep things fresh, which helps them re-engage. Focusing on the present moment in the athletic training room through varied exercises and dynamic social relationships can help performers maintain motivation during their injury rehabilitation.

Due to the recurring nature of the behavior change processes, the TTM is conceptualized as a cycle rather than a linear process that has a distinct beginning and end. For example, many people have been directly or indirectly affected by family members struggling to make behavior change related to addiction, over-eating, or gambling. Some make progress with strategies to change their harmful behaviors and develop motivation to grow in a new direction while creating lasting change. Unfortunately, many people relapse and return back to the precontemplation stage. The cycle of arrows illustrates the frustration that many experience while working toward lasting behavior change.

Fear of Reinjury

Fear of reinjury may negatively influence the rehabilitation process. Patients may be concerned about returning to their preinjury level of performance.[48] Typically, a patient's fear of reinjury increases as they approach the scheduled date of return to activity or sport.[25,49,50] It makes sense that an athlete would be worried about performing all of the tasks of his job at the same level that they could previously while testing the injured body part at game-speed for the first time. You can help a patient address this fear of reinjury as their return-to-play date approaches by supporting open and honest communication about their worries. Confirm the physical healing that has taken place to help boost the patient's trust in his injured body part.

Fear of reinjury has been cited as contributing to lower sport confidence, difficulty giving maximal effort during rehabilitation or sport activity once the athlete has returned to play, or fear of being placed in an injury-provoking situation.[51] Fear of reinjury has also been noted as a common cause for retirement from athletic competition for athletes across all skill levels.[52,53,79] In a study by McCullough and colleagues, 50% of college athletes and 52% of high school athletes who had anterior cruciate ligament reconstructive surgery did not return to sport participation because of fear of reinjury.[79] If you can help a patient address their concerns by providing education about anatomical aspects of their specific injury, healing time, and structural integrity of the injured area, they may fear reinjury less when returning to play. Increasing the patient's awareness and acceptance that anxiety is a part of the process of returning from injury will help them move forward with the next steps.

Sociological Response to Injury for Athletes

Feelings of guilt and being ignored often accompany athletic injury because patients feel isolated and estranged from their team and sport during the rehabilitation process.[27] Some coaches limit injured athletes' access to team functions and decrease their level of social support following an injury. Depending on the patient's demographic and socioeconomic status variables, their coaching staff and teammates may represent their only source of support and may be even closer than family members. Remember to keep the whole patient as your primary focus, not just the affected body region. Injury is always about more than just the physical trauma that is endured; it is about what is lost and what could be at risk for the patient's future. People with strong social support networks often see positive influences in their health.

Athletes With Concussions

Several researchers have noted an increased incidence of depression associated with a history of concussion in retired boxers and professional football players.[44] Elevated levels of depression and mood disturbances have been documented in concussed patients.[45,46] Mainwaring and colleagues found that concussed patients reported total mood disturbances and depression three times greater than their baseline depression scores.[46] In addition, collegiate and high school patients diagnosed with concussion displayed depressive symptoms 14 days postinjury.

A person with post-concussion syndrome experiences objective declines in attention, concentration, learning, and memory. The patient also reports three or more subjective symptoms, which must have been present for at least three months. Common symptoms of post-concussion syndrome include the following:

- Become easily fatigued
- Disordered sleep
- Headache
- Vertigo
- Irritability or aggression on little or no provocation
- Anxiety, depression, or affective lability
- Changes in personality
- Apathy or lack of spontaneity

Because there is significant overlap between symptoms of post-concussion syndrome and common mental health disorders such as major depressive episodes and anxiety, it may be difficult to differentiate between the two at early stages following mild traumatic brain injury. If you have concerns about the potential for mental health symptoms like depression, anxiety, apathy, fatigue, irritability, trouble concentrating, insomnia, and personality changes, you should screen the patient and consider a referral to a mental health professional.

Psychosocial Interventions

The rehabilitation process can be a long and arduous journey for performers attempting to return from injury. Even the most determined can lose sight of their long-term goals, wane in motivation, and see a reduction in exercise adherence at certain phases of the return-to-play process. One way to address these issues is to apply psychosocial interventions in the rehabilitation setting, including effective communication, collaborative goal-setting exercises, relaxation training, mental imagery, and positive self-talk.[47]

Effective Communication

The involvement of multiple health care professionals in the typical rehabilitation setting, often-intense emotions, and urgency of treatment may cause challenges for coordinating patient care. Effective communication between patients, health care professionals, and athletic personnel is essential in order to facilitate patient-oriented collaborative care and keep everyone on the same page throughout the duration of recovery.

To improve communication skills in the athletic training setting, use the Bayer educational model's 4 Es:[54]

1. *Engage.* In order to open a line of communication and relate to the patient, you must first engage the patient in a way that they can easily understand. During the initial engaging step, do your best to see the patient as separate from their injury and work on building personal connections.

2. *Empathize.* Empathizing with the patient involves getting perspective and attempting to understand their views on the situation. Work to stay in the moment and show the patient that you are interested in their world. Do your best to be aware of your body language, including your eye contact and gestures of affirmation (head nodding or shaking). Learn about the cultural and social influences that may result in differences between your patients. Within an athletic culture, typical standards of communication include direct eye contact and confirmation that verbal messages have been received and understood.

3. *Educate.* The patient must understand a great deal of information concerning their injury in order to recover well. The education phase includes specific details of the injury, the anatomical region affected, the rehabilitation procedure, and the prognosis. If the patient is given the opportunity to ask questions, they will begin to invest in the rehabilitation process and take ownership of their role in recovery. One of your tasks is to make yourself available to provide

information and answer questions across multiple sessions.[58]

4. *Enlist.* Finally, you should enlist the patient and the team of health care professionals in making decisions and constructing an adherence strategy for rehabilitation. Instead of assigning roles, allow members of the team to express their thoughts on how they can contribute their skills to the injury plan of care; this will ultimately improve motivation for patients and providers.[58] Allowing patients to contribute to their rehabilitation plans, set goals, and give feedback about their treatment increases their sense of control over the injury process.

Collaborative Goal Setting

Setting goals is important following injury once rehabilitation is initiated. Although goal setting comes easily to many successful athletes, it is a skill that can be improved through training and collaboration. Patients and health care professionals have reported that goal setting enhances patient motivation.[59] A study of athletic trainers found that **goal setting** was one of the top two psychosocial strategies that injured athletes used to address stress, anxiety, anger, and treatment adherence issues.[60]

Consider these three main goals that directly apply to patient care in the rehabilitation setting:[61]

1. *Outcome goals.* **Outcome goals** are primarily focused on the result of the event, such as returning to play following an UCL rupture.[40]

2. *Performance goals.* **Performance goals** focus on short-term objectives that need to be achieved to reach the overall outcome goal.[40] In UCL rehabilitation following Tommy John surgery, a performance goal may be to increase elbow flexion range of motion by 15 degrees compared to the week before.

3. *Process goals.* **Process goals** pertain to individual skills that, if present, aid in completing goals and performing skills well.[40] In the UCL example, a process goal would be to bring present moment focus to the rehabilitation session in order to help the patient complete all repetitions in all sets assigned that day.

Communication and Referral Tips

If you want to model a culture where addressing personal vulnerability is seen as strong and valuable, you need to know how to identify and respond when mental health concerns inevitably arise. Here are 10 tips for addressing these concerns within your clients and institutional system.[56]

1. Be able to recognize symptoms of common mental health diagnoses, including anxiety, depression, and ADHD.

2. Build a referral network of competent providers in your local area and become familiar with the referral protocol for helping your patients use mental health services.

3. Speak with your local mental health providers to develop effective strategies on how to improve use of referrals for mental health services. Adapt your advice to the local culture.

4. Do your best to maintain patient privacy and approach treatment from a nonjudgmental stance.

5. Understand the boundaries of your role. Encourage the patient to seek help from a mental health professional while being genuine and compassionate.

6. Maintain communication with patients about their use of the mental health referrals and consider a release of information (ROI) to allow communication of confidential information between health care providers.

7. Help build a culture of openness and trust.

8. Adjust your feedback style to meet the communication needs of patients with mental health diagnoses.

9. Communicate with other health care providers in the patient's treatment team for treatment planning.

10. Continue to check in with patients who are separated from their competitive, recreational, or occupational activities as a result of injuries.

FOUNDATIONAL SKILL

Goal-Setting Principles

Keep in mind the following goal-setting principles:[58, 85, 86]

- Set specific goals.
- Set moderately difficult but realistic goals.
- Set short- and long-term goals.
- Set outcome, performance, and process goals.
- Write the goals down.
- Develop specific plans for achieving goals.
- Consider the patient's personality and motivation.
- Foster the patient's commitment to the goals.
- Provide goal support.
- Provide evaluation and feedback about the goals.

Relaxation Training

Patients who are unable to fully clear their minds, relax, and focus their attention on the tasks of rehabilitation may be distracted by physical, social, and performance stressors associated with their injury. Stressful situations result in a narrowing of attention, higher levels of distractibility, and increased muscular tension, all of which contribute negatively to recovery.[65] You can use the following **relaxation techniques** during return to play to help reduce distress and excess tension that may be complicating rehabilitation:

- *Diaphragmatic breathing.* **Diaphragmatic breathing** uses slow abdominal breaths to stimulate the vagus nerve and lower the stress response. The diaphragm is the large dome-shaped muscle at the base of the lungs. Slow belly breathing reduces the fight-or-flight response by decreasing activity of the sympathetic nervous system and improves heart rate variability (HRV), a measure of minute variations between beats of the heart.[72]
- *Progressive muscle relaxation.* **Progressive muscle relaxation** is an exercise that systematically tenses and relaxes individual muscle groups through directing conscious attention, active contraction, and relaxation. Jacobson provides a detailed script of progressive relaxation exercise that can be adapted for use in the athletic training room.[67]
- *Meditation.* **Meditation** is a skill that helps patients during rehabilitation because it provides relaxation training (e.g., diaphragmatic breathing and mental imagery) and emphasizes remaining in the present moment with an attitude of acceptance and nonjudgment.

Emotional Intelligence

Emotional intelligence is a term used to describe a conglomeration of social skills, including the ability to identify, understand, and manage emotions to manage stress, communicate effectively, empathize with others, overcome challenges, and work through conflict.[8] Emotional intelligence has received attention across various fields of psychology, including organizational and performance psychology. Emotional regulation is a related

FOUNDATIONAL SKILL

Areas of Emotional Intelligence

- Improved ability to manage thoughts and emotions
- Diverse skills for coping with stress
- Assertiveness and ability to express difficult emotions
- Being proactive instead of reactive in the face of adversity
- Maintaining goal-directed behavior following failure
- Expressing vulnerability and being open in intimate relationships[90]

concept and is defined as the ability to monitor one's own and others' feelings and emotions, to discriminate between them, and to use this information to guide one's thinking and actions to ultimately improve performance recovery.[94]

Meta-analytic studies have shown that measures of emotional intelligence are associated with enhanced performance,[95] well-being, and stress management.[7] Emotional intelligence has a more important role than general intelligence in various fields of study and attainment of competence.[97] Research is limited on the effectiveness of training programs that increase emotional intelligence, although this sort of training has been shown to be helpful in improving the efficiency of nursing care services and competence through decreased stress recovery.[89] Many emotional intelligence training programs have focused on sport-performance interventions, such as goal setting, self-talk, and mental imagery.[96] Developing effective and exciting ways to manage stress is vital to providing quality patient care and ensuring career longevity.

Mental Imagery

Imagery is a mental preparation technique used to create or recreate polysensory experiences within the mind to increase performance on subsequent efforts. It is also commonly known as visualization, mental rehearsal, simulation, and mental training.[40] People use **mental imagery** for a variety of reasons:[40]

- Building confidence
- Increasing motivation
- Managing arousal
- Improving concentration
- Controlling emotional responses
- Developing sport skills
- Practicing performance strategy
- Coping with pain
- Problem solving

As a health care provider, you should educate injured patients on the potential for mental imagery to influence their rehabilitation outcomes. Mental imagery is a skill that can be improved with training. The two most important aspects of mental imagery training are vividness and controllability.[40] By focusing on controlling the image, the patient can learn to create a story pertinent to his sport and challenges; for example, he has the ball in his hands as the clock winds down in the fourth quarter with the game on the line. By learning to control the imagery, the patient can make sure he envisions himself winning the game for his team instead of accidentally losing focus and making a mistake that results in loss of confidence.

Patients can increase the vividness, or the realism, of the imagery by integrating as many of their senses as possible.[40] The PETTLEP model of motor imagery by Holmes and Collins has a checklist of important aspects to include in a mental imagery script: physical, environment, task, timing, learning, emotion, and perspective.[69] Focusing on these elements during the execution of a skill will create a functional equivalence between imagery content and actual performance. For an expanded explanation, see Holmes and Collins.[69]

Self-Talk

Self-talk is anything that people say out loud or think about themselves.[68] There are three general forms of self-talk:

1. **Positive self-talk** is used in sport to help an athlete redirect attention toward a task, boost motivation and effort, and improve attitude (e.g., "Come on, you got this.").
2. **Negative self-talk** typically negatively influences performance, increases anxiety, and destroys confidence (e.g., "I can't believe you did that. You're worthless.").
3. **Instructional self-talk** does not have an influence on motivation and is meant to help improve focus on technical aspects of a movement (e.g., "Keep your knees shoulder-width apart, back straight, and head up.").

You must identify negative self-talk with your clients at an early stage and work to increase positive and instructional self-talk to help them break bad habits, initiate action, sustain effort, and acquire new skills.[40] It is easy for patients to get down on themselves during rehabilitation from an injury when they feel isolated from their teammates, friends, and family. Due to this increase in social isolation, you need to be aware of the likelihood that patients will exhibit negative self-talk and feelings of low self-worth. This may manifest itself with self-deprecating humor where they make jokes about themselves that may be funny at first. This may be the perfect opportunity to ask them about their ratio of positive to negative self-talk responses and what effect they think the joking has on them. It may also be a time to connect them with local mental health resources.

Working in a Multidisciplinary Team as an Athletic Trainer

In order to provide the most well-rounded patient care, you should use a multidisciplinary team approach. Working with a treatment team of professionals with various specializations will better address your clients'

Injury Rehabilitation and Psychosocial Skills Training

Research has demonstrated the effect of psychosocial skills training on injury rehabilitation, none more than the work of Ievleva and Orlick in 1991.[70] The authors used a survey to measure attitude, outlook, stress and stress control, social support, goal setting, self-talk, mental imagery, and healing beliefs and recommendations. Thirty-two former sports medicine clinic patients with knee or ankle injuries participated in the study. Nineteen percent of the participants had exceptionally fast recoveries, as evidenced by high scores on all psychosocial variables measured (positive attitude, outlook, stress and stress control, social support, goal setting, positive self-talk, and mental imagery). Participants who healed the slowest demonstrated low scores. Goal setting, self-talk, and imagery showed the greatest effect on recovery.[70]

Similarly, 60 white male athletes who suffered knee injury completed modules of stress inoculation training, including deep breathing, muscle relaxation, mental imagery, and positive self-talk aimed at reducing anxiety, decreasing pain, and minimizing days to return to play after injury. Results indicated that stress inoculation training led to significant differences in state anxiety and perceived pain levels in patients recovering from injury. The average number of days to recovery was also found to be significantly less in the intervention group compared to the control group.[66] This result shows that two very important variables in the injury recovery process are stress and anxiety and pain, which can be managed by practicing some stress inoculation skills.

physical and mental health concerns. Practicing psychology within sports medicine involves a number of interconnected factors, which can be seen in figure 19.3. Create a list of practicing health care professionals who provide patient services in your local area in case a patient is looking for a referral or you would like to add a consultant to your multidisciplinary team.[55]

The stigma for seeking support for a mental health disorder may be different for each person. Generally, within a population of athletes and active youths, physical injury and mental vulnerability are seen as weaknesses. Strength, endurance, and grit are emphasized daily, and athletes often get mixed messages about what it means to seek support for a mental health disorder. Athletes may also come from families that have specific beliefs about seeking treatment for mental health disorders; for example, a patient may benefit from a medication, but his family does not approve of the use of pharmacological medications.

Early intervention for mental illness is most effective, so do your best to get the client referred to a professional as soon as possible. Having a difficult conversation with a patient early in your relationship about your concerns related to his mental health may set you up to make greater progress in rehabilitation as your

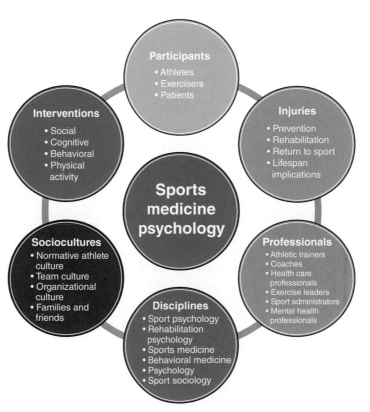

FIGURE 19.3 Various factors incorporated into a multidisciplinary approach involving psychological services in sports medicine.

relationship grows stronger. Discomfort when talking about mental health is normal. Have the facts, know the symptoms, and collect the relevant information from your patient. Your observations are the front line of defense and are extremely important to improving the wellness and performance of competitive artists. Listen and encourage conversation. Stop thinking about what to say next and try to be present with the patient. Lastly, be curious and do your best to avoid judgment.

Focus on the patient as a person, not just an athlete or an injury. This cannot be said enough. Do not refer to a patient as "my women's soccer ACL;" instead, refer to her by name. Get to know your patients, what makes them who they are, and what gets under their skin. You will need all of this information to help motivate them someday.

Confidentiality is extremely important when patients are seeking treatment with a mental health professional. If a patient receives a referral to a mental health professional from an athletic trainer, it is common professional practice to follow up with the client on referral. Do your best not to be intimidated by the possible discussion that could come from broaching this conversation.

At this point, it is up to the client whether they want to involve you in the exchange of confidential information shared with the mental health professional. A **release of information (ROI)** form signed by the patient and the mental health provider is required for you to receive information. Completion of this form indicates that the patient agrees to release confidential information, allowing the mental health professional to communicate any information that the patient permits with anyone listed on the ROI.

If a patient with mental health concerns signs an ROI, standard practice is to follow up with them about the referral. You should include continued assessment of symptoms and evaluation of function in your follow-up for mental health referrals. You can have a brief conversation with the patient to confirm that they have followed through on attendance, is developing a relationship with the therapist, and is noticing some symptom relief.

In making decisions about readiness to return from a mental health disorder, consult with the patient's mental health professional if possible. If you do not have a ROI, seek to develop a network of professionals across multiple disciplines whom you can consult in order to present hypothetical situations and receive a professional opinion.

CLINICAL BOTTOM LINE

- Athletic trainers are positioned to identify mental health concerns and facilitate referrals to mental health professionals.

- Psychosocial disorders that are common in a physically active population and as a reaction to injury include anxiety disorders, mood disorders, ADHD, disordered eating, and substance use disorder.

- Athletic trainers must first be aware of the local providers and institutional policies that dictate the provision of referrals for mental health services. Athletic trainers are strongly urged to check in with their employers to learn the protocol for referrals and obtain a list the network of mental health providers in the local area.

- A strong connection exists between high stress levels and injury incidence or poor rehabilitation outcomes. Athletic trainers can help patients improve injury outcomes by identifying skills they can use to decrease their stress levels.

- Mental skills training programs, including mental imagery, relaxation training, self-talk, and goal-setting techniques, are most influential for improving recovery time.

- The integrated model of psychological response to sport injury and rehabilitation is a conceptual model of injury response to an interrelated psychosocial process.

- Important personal contributions to the injury response include gender, age, injury history, characteristics of personality, athletic identity, and postinjury cognitive appraisals.

- Athletic trainers should speak with clients about confidentiality and recommend they complete a release of information. This can help coordinate rehabilitation care across multiple disciplines.

 Go to HK*Propel* to complete the activities and case studies for this chapter.

Go to HK*Propel* to download a foundational skill check sheet that covers the principles of goal setting.

CHAPTER 20

Special Populations

Monique Mokha, PhD, LAT, ATC, CSCS
Leamor Kahanov, EdD, ATC, LAT

CAATE STANDARDS

The following CAATE 2020 standards are covered in this chapter:

Standard 56

Standard 57

Standard 60

Standard 62

CHAPTER OBJECTIVES

After reading this chapter, you will be able to do the following:

- Recognize foundational concepts of sport health care for clients in special populations

- Identify the role of the preparticipation physical examination for athletes with different needs

- Identify the role of the athletic trainer in providing sport health care for clients in special populations

- Identify appropriate prevention and care for medical conditions specific to athletes with sensory, neurological, or intellectual disabilities

- Discuss laws pertaining to providing sport health care for clients in special populations

- Recognize the importance of communication skills in caring for clients in special populations

Active populations include people who may have disabilities or participate in physical job-related duties in addition to recreational and competitive athletics. A **disability** is an umbrella term for impairments, activity limitations, and participation restrictions. The definition of **special populations** is a bit more elusive depending on the professional discipline, but for the purposes of athletic training, it includes clients in a population subset based on job duties, age, gender identity, and disability. Athletic trainers must understand the physical and physiological characteristics of people with disabilities or from special populations to best address their health care needs.

This chapter is divided into two primary sections—special populations and disability—and provides a general overview of the special populations most commonly encountered in athletic training. The chapter addresses specific conditions associated with the identified special populations in addition to precautions, contraindications, modifications, and medications pertinent to working with people with specific challenges or needs. Athletic trainers engage many different special populations and may be specifically employed to provide health care to a special population group, such as military or factory personnel. Special populations also include groups identified by age, such as pediatric and masters populations. Clients from these populations may have additional physical or physiological differences that you must understand in order to provide optimal care. For a greater understanding of the athletic trainer's role in diagnosis, treatment, rehabilitation, and advocacy for people categorized in special populations, seek a more in-depth education.

Tactical Athletes

Athletic trainers are increasingly employed to assist **tactical athletes**, who are people in service professions (e.g., military, firefighters, law enforcement, and emergency responders). They typically have significant physical fitness and performance requirements associated with their work and face stressful, rigorous, and demanding challenges, often under life-threatening conditions. Additionally, tactical athletes carry heavy gear and equipment while doing their work.[51]

Tactical athletes experience musculoskeletal injuries more often than other employees who have work-related injuries. Reasons for increased risk of injury include external forces (e.g., other people), external equipment loads, the need to unexpectedly handle objects, and trips and falls.[4-7] Regardless of the tactical athlete's type of employment, the majority of musculoskeletal injuries occur during training due to the increased physical demands and unique specialized equipment.[8-13] The demands on tactical athletes (military, police, and firefighters) differ by activity type, cause and area of injury, and incidence (table 20.1). However, tactical athletes all experience common injuries, including strains, sprains, blisters, and fractures.[14-17]

Research suggests that conditioning conducted within the workplace may be more effective at returning personnel to work than clinically based work hardening.[52,53]

Interestingly, injured military veterans hold a significant spot on the United States' Paralympic roster. More than 50 military veterans competed in the Summer 2016

TABLE 20.1   Considerations for Tactical Athletes

Profession	Physical requirements	Most common injuries	Special considerations
Military	Carry heavy loads (e.g., body armor, equipment and supplies)	Physical training before assignment or deployment is the leading cause of injuries in military populations.[10-13,18-20] These musculoskeletal injuries often account for more injuries than those incurred in combat.[21] The lower extremity is the leading anatomical site of injuries (up to 80% of musculoskeletal injuries).[10-14,18,22,23] The lower back is the most common site of injury in combat.[18,21,25]	Psychological components (e.g., sense of confidence) of performing duties and returning to duty[18]
Urban and rural firefighters	Stair climbing Dragging and carrying (e.g., people and equipment)[25-30]	Carrying loads increases the risk of injury due to tripping.[25-27]	Firefighters may be required to manage a self-contained breathing apparatus. Firefighter gear and clothing may alter movements and mechanics, affecting skill performance and increasing risk of injury.[18]
Wilderness firefighters	Battle wilderness fires Battle firestorms[31]	Wilderness firefighters experience more musculoskeletal injuries than burns.[17,32]	
Police	Engage objects or a potential perpetrator Move in and out of vehicles Run through, over, and around obstacles Manage loads of equipment and body armor[8,10-13]	Musculoskeletal injuries often account for more injuries than actual combat.[21] The lower extremity is the leading anatomical site of injuries (up to 80% of musculoskeletal injuries).[14,22]	Physical assault from offenders

and Winter 2018 Games combined. The United States Olympic Committee launched the Paralympic Military Program in 2004. The program provides sport opportunities to support wounded, ill, or injured service members and veterans, including those with amputations, visual impairments, and traumatic brain injuries. It offers camps and clinics to connect this group to Paralympic sport.

Masters Athletes

Masters athletes (35 years of age and older) are a growing population. The athletic trainer and care team must take care to identify people from this group at risk of injury and disease in order to ensure their safe participation. Masters athletes tend to train at lower intensities than younger adult athletes, either due to age-related biological changes or injury. The three most frequently reported comorbidities are low back pain (25.3%), hypertension (22.9%), and knee osteoarthritis (15.3%). In a study of more than 2,500 masters athletes at the Senior Olympics, athletes with concurrent knee osteoarthritis were 3 times more likely to report a knee injury.[24]

Coronary artery disease (CAD) is the primary cause of sudden cardiac death in athletes over 35 years old, despite their high fitness level.[34] Therefore, thorough screening is of paramount importance. The Framingham Risk Score (FRS) is an algorithm that estimates the 10-year cardiovascular risk of a client and is used with masters athletes.[35] The preparticipation examination for masters athletes should include the FRS and an electrocardiogram. Exercise stress testing is indicated for people who are symptomatic or have a family history of premature CAD or an intermediate or high FRS.

Pediatric Athletes

Pediatric athletes (typically 6 to 18 years of age) sustain a variety of age-related traumatic and overuse injuries (table 20.2). Training errors, inadequate rest, muscle weakness and imbalances, early specialization, and improper technique are all potential causes of injuries in this special population.

Overuse injuries include growth-related disorders and those resulting from repeated microtrauma.[36] These injuries are preventable in young athletes with mindful monitoring of activity (e.g., pitch counts) and the use of a comprehensive, multidimensional approach. An example of a pediatric overuse injury is Little Leaguer's shoulder, a condition that results in **epiphysiolysis** of the proximal humerus. Little Leaguer's shoulder occurs in skeletally immature athletes who do a lot of overhead throwing. It is most commonly seen in baseball pitchers but may also occur in tennis players. Physeal (growth plate) fractures are classified according to the Salter-Harris scheme (see chapter 15).

Growth-related conditions include Osgood-Schlatter disease, Sever's disease, and other apophyseal injuries. Apophyseal injuries arise during growth spurts when bone growth exceeds the ability of the muscle–tendon unit to stretch sufficiently to maintain its previous level of extensibility. This causes increased tension where the tendon attaches to the bone. In the young athlete, training and competition increase distraction forces at the apophysis. These injuries are alleviated by rest and subside when the growth spurt is finished. Pain may be managed by reducing the volume of aggravating activities and applying ice.

Pregnant Athletes

Athletes can and do successfully compete while pregnant without experiencing adverse health effects. Most athletes with normal pregnancies can safely continue in team activities, although progressive modifications may need to be made after the 14th week.[54]

Age-Related Changes Affecting Athletic Performance

- Decreased production of anabolic hormones
- Decreased joint mobility
- Decreased muscle mass
- Decreased balance and coordination
- Increased intramuscular fat
- Increased recovery time
- Decreased muscle strength and power
- Decreased anaerobic and aerobic power
- Decreased reaction time
- Increased cardiovascular concerns

TABLE 20.2   **Common Injuries in the Pediatric Athlete**

Bone injury	Explanation	Signs and symptoms	Treatment
Osgood-Schlatter disease	Apophysitis at the tibial tuberosity	Gradual onset of pain, tenderness, and swelling at the tibial tuberosity that is worsened by running, jumping, and making quick changes in direction	Limited activity Knee strengthening and stretching Cross-training Knee strap or sleeve
Sinding-Larsen-Johansson syndrome	Apophysitis at the distal pole of patella (above the site of Osgood-Schlatter)	Gradual onset of pain, tenderness, and swelling at the distal pole of the patella that is worsened by running, jumping, and making quick changes in direction	Limited activity Knee strengthening and stretching Cross-training Knee strap or sleeve
Sever's disease	Apophysitis at the posterior calcaneus	Limpness Gradual onset of pain, tenderness, and swelling at the posterior calcaneus that is worsened by running, jumping, and making quick changes in direction	Limited activity Calf strengthening and stretching Cross-training Supportive shoes or orthotics
Little Leaguer's elbow	Apophysitis at the medial epicondyle of the humerus	Gradual onset of pain, tenderness, and swelling at the medial elbow that is worsened by throwing	Limited activity Wrist and shoulder strengthening Biomechanical evaluation of pitching (or serving) May require complete rest
Pelvic apophysitis	Occurs at a variety of hip muscle attachment sites (e.g., anterior superior iliac spine, ischial tuberosity) Tight hip and knee muscles, excessive foot pronation, and genu valgum may contribute to abnormal tension forces in the muscles and increase risk.	Limpness Gradual onset of pain, tenderness, and swelling at affected site on the pelvis that is worsened by running, jumping, and making quick changes of direction Could result in an avulsion fracture, which would present with acute pain and limited function	Limited activity Hip and knee strengthening and stretching Cross-training May require complete rest
Iselin's disease	Apophysitis at the 5th metatarsal	Limpness Gradual onset of pain, tenderness, and swelling at attachment of peroneus brevis on the 5th metatarsal that is worsened by running, jumping, and making quick changes in direction	Limited activity Ankle strengthening and stretching Cross-training May require immobilization (e.g., controlled ankle motion boot)
Slipped capital femoral epiphysis	Stress fracture to the growth plate of the proximal femur where the head shifts (slips) Condition can be stable or unstable (less common)	*Stable:* gradual onset of pain in the hip, groin, thigh, or knee that is worsened by running, jumping, and making quick changes in direction *Unstable:* acute onset of pain after a fall or injury; unable to bear weight	Surgery to prevent further slippage

Bone injury	Explanation	Signs and symptoms	Treatment
Greenstick fracture	Partial or incomplete fracture to any long bone	Acute pain, swelling, and loss of function consistent with closed fractures	Immobilization
Buckle (torus) fracture	Occurs at the distal radius when the radius compresses on itself	Acute pain, swelling, and loss of function consistent with closed fractures	Immobilization
Little Leaguer's shoulder	Stress fracture to proximal humerus at the growth plate	Gradual onset of pain in shoulder worsened by overhead throwing (late cocking and deceleration phases) Decreased performance	Total rest from throwing *Once cleared to throw by the physician:* Correct poor throwing mechanics Rotator cuff and scapula muscle strengthening Progressive throwing program
Legg-Calvé-Perthes disease	Blood supply is interrupted to the head of the femur, resulting in necrosis	Limpness Limited hip ROM Referred pain at hip, groin, thigh, or knee Must be recognized early to prevent permanent impairment	Limited activity Casting, bracing, hip strengthening, or surgery

Prevention Approach for Pediatric Overuse Injuries

- Alter sport for youth (e.g., volume, rules, equipment).
- Conduct thorough PPEs.
- Delay sport specialization (have athletes participate in activities with varied movement patterns).
- Identify risk factors for injury.
- Improve injury reporting and monitoring to understand epidemiology.
- Improve training and conditioning programs.
- Properly supervise and educate coaches on both coaching and medical aspects.

Athletes who are pregnant should be monitored for warning signs to terminate exercise:

- Abdominal pain, cramps, or contractions before the due date (preterm labor)
- Calf pain or swelling (need to rule out deep vein thrombosis)
- Chest pain
- Decreased movement of the baby
- Difficulty breathing (dyspnea) prior to exertion
- Dizziness
- Headache
- Muscle weakness
- Vaginal bleeding
- Vaginal leakage of clear fluid (amniotic fluid leakage)

There are also precautions to take after the 14th week of pregnancy. Athletes should avoid the following:[54]

- Training and competing in a supine position
- The Valsalva maneuver
- Activities with a high risk of falling

Certainly, injuries can occur to the pregnant athlete. At any stage during pregnancy, an extreme blow to (or fall onto) the abdomen can damage the placenta. Later in pregnancy, as the fetus moves higher in the womb and is unprotected by the pelvis, there is greater risk of damage to the fetus itself by direct impact during sport. Most medical experts agree that the kinds of falls and

Normal Physiological Changes During Pregnancy

The following physiological changes may affect an athlete's training and performance during pregnancy:

- Balance difficulties
- Breathing constraints (pressure of growing uterus on diaphragm)
- Increased caloric intake
- Increased cardiac output
- Joint hypermobility or laxity
- Weight gain

direct contact that typically occur during contact sports are unlikely to damage either the womb or the fetus. The choice to participate in contact sports ultimately belongs to the athlete but should be made in conjunction with her sports medicine team.

Other factors that should be considered are proper hydration and the athlete's prepregnancy health status. The latter refers to careful monitoring of preexisting medication use and health conditions, such as diabetes, asthma, and cardiac conditions. Further, the sports medicine team should recognize that pregnancy is an emotion-laden process for all women, especially for the female athlete. It is prudent to have psychological services available for the athlete as she manages the transitions into motherhood.

Introduction to Disability

Approximately 85.3 million people in the United States (27.2%) have a disability, and more than 3 million people with disability participate in physical activity and sport.[1] Physical activity and sport enhance overall health and quality of life for people with disabilities as well as provide a means for competition. Participants generally obtain the same health benefits from exercise and sport training as their able-bodied counterparts, such as increased cardiovascular conditioning, muscular strength, and self-confidence. Participation in physical activity and sport is not without inherent risks of injury and illness. Thus, the role of the athletic trainer to recognize, manage, and prevent injury and illness in these special populations is of paramount importance.

Athletic trainers may work with people with a variety of special needs that are present because of the client's work or sport demands or physical condition. For example, athletic trainers from the Warrior Research Center at Auburn University in Alabama provide injury identification, treatment, rehabilitation, and prevention services to members of the United States Army at Fort Benning, Georgia. In 2015, the Eastern College Athletic

Association became the first NCAA-sanctioned conference to adopt an inclusive strategy to provide new athletic opportunities for student-athletes with a variety of disabilities at the collegiate level. Other universities, such as the University of Alabama, the University of Texas at Arlington, and the University of Illinois, have staff athletic trainers who provide health care for wheelchair basketball teams. These diverse settings require the athletic trainer to be multiskilled.

International Classification of Functioning, Disability and Health

The International Classification of Functioning, Disability and Health (ICF) defines *disability* as an umbrella term for impairments, activity limitations, and participation restrictions. Disability is the interaction between people with a health condition and personal and environmental factors (figure 20.1).

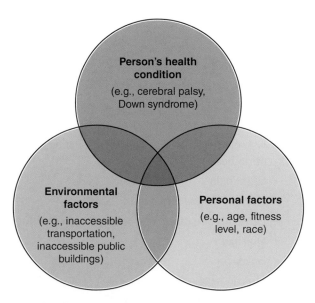

FIGURE 20.1 Disability intersection.

Disability is extremely diverse. Although some health conditions associated with disability result in poor health and extensive health care needs, others do not. However, people with disabilities have the same general health care needs as everyone else and therefore need access to mainstream health care services. Article 25 of the UN Convention on the Rights of Persons with Disabilities (CRPD) reinforces the right of people in this population to receive the highest standard of health care without discrimination.

In 2015, after recommendation by the Executive Committee for Education, the National Athletic Trainers' Association's board of directors approved the adoption of the World Health Organization's ICF with Children and Youth (ICF-CY) updates. In practice, this means athletic trainers consider not just the medical condition, anatomy, and physiology of the patient, but also his activities and personal and environmental elements. In short, a medical diagnosis is not enough to determine care. The ICF is a radical shift from emphasizing disability (cause) to focusing on level of health (impact).

Later sections of this chapter present health care information specific to groups of people with the same disability (e.g., visual impairment), but this is for ease of learning only. Remember that the client or athlete is a person who happens to have a disability. Thus, you should employ **person-first terminology**, which includes statements such as a person with a disability, person with cerebral palsy, athlete with a spinal cord injury, or athlete with an amputation.

Preparticipation Physical Examination

The purpose of the preparticipation physical examination (PPE) is to identify conditions that may place an athlete at increased risk and affect safe participation in organized sports.[2] (For a detailed discussion of PPEs, see chapter 8). Athletes must complete a thorough PPE so that baseline norms and risk of injury or illness can be established. The general approach of the PPE is similar for athletes with and without disabilities. However, athletic trainers working with people with disabilities may opt for a more focused exam, avoiding the mass or station approach, which is impractical for people with decreased mobility or who use wheelchairs.

When conducting the PPE, you may need a supplemental history form for athletes with special needs to assess conditions often associated with the special population. Take care to avoid **diagnostic overshadowing**, or attributing all symptoms to the primary condition or disability and overlooking other medical issues.[3] Although diagnostic overshadowing is a term typically applied to emotional, mental, intellectual, or learning disabilities,

---

FOUNDATIONAL SKILL

Conducting the PPE

Follow these additional recommendations when conducting the PPE for athletes with special needs:

- Position yourself at eye level with athletes in wheelchairs.
- Remember that it may be necessary to have a parent or guardian present to assist in obtaining an accurate history from an athlete with an intellectual disability.
- Ask an athlete with a spinal cord injury what movements are possible, which parts of the body have sensation, and if she has any current pain.
- Verbally explain exam components to an athlete with a visual impairment.
- Provide a guided tour of the facility.
- Obtain seizure history and document antiseizure medications, including type, dose frequency or use, and performance-related side effects.
- Allow an athlete with a visual impairment to place his hands on yours during a physical exam.
- Ensure proper fit and adequacy of prostheses, orthoses, sports wheelchairs, or other assistive devices.
- Use a team approach and seek further information from professionals with disability-specific expertise.
- Document residual limb care habits of athletes with amputations.
- Avoid diagnostic overshadowing.

athletic trainers should be aware of and avoid it when treating athletes with all disabilities.

Classification of Disability Sport Athletes

Sport opportunities for athletes with disabilities range from recreational to highly competitive to elite Paralympic sport. To ensure fair and equitable competition, athletes are classified, or grouped, into classes according to their activity limitation in a certain sport. This is similar, to a certain extent, to grouping athletes by age, sex, or weight. The system was designed to minimize the effect of impairments on sport performance and ensure that the success of an athlete is determined by skill, fitness, power, endurance, tactical ability, and mental focus. Some Paralympic sports are designed only for athletes with one eligible impairment type. For example, goalball is open only to athletes with visual impairment. Other sports, such as swimming and athletics, are open to athletes with any of the 10 eligible impairments outlined in the following sidebar. Athletes with the impairments listed are assessed by panels of 2 or 3 classifiers who have a medical background or are technical experts in their sport. Since some impairments change over time (e.g., visual acuity or **hypertonia**), an athlete may undergo evalua-

tion several times throughout her athletic career. Athlete classification is not without controversy.

Athletes With Visual Impairments and Blindness

Athletes with visual impairments (VI) have a range of visual acuity from legal blindness with partial sight to total blindness (table 20.3). Classification of VI is based on a Snellen chart measure of acuity (sharpness of vision) and assessment of field of vision (area seen with the eyes fixed straight ahead).

Causes of Visual Impairments and Blindness

Causes of VI may include tumors, albinism, injuries, and infectious diseases. In older people, common causes of blindness are diabetes, macular degeneration, glaucoma, and cataracts. Albinism is a lack of pigment in the iris and rest of the body, making the athlete sensitive to light and more susceptible to sunburn. Athletic trainers should advise the athlete to wear tinted glasses (indoors and outdoors), sunscreen, hats or visors, and long-sleeved shirts. Glaucoma is increased pressure

---

Eligible Impairments for Paralympic Competition

The following impairments are eligible for Paralympic competition:[60]

- *Ataxia:* uncoordinated muscle movements from a neurological condition, such as brain injury, cerebral palsy, or multiple sclerosis.

- *Athetosis:* unbalanced, uncontrolled movements and difficulty maintaining symmetrical posture due to brain injury, cerebral palsy, or multiple sclerosis.

- *Hypertonia:* inability of muscles to stretch properly and abnormal increased muscle tension, which can result from injury, illness, or a health condition such as cerebral palsy.

- *Impaired muscle power:* muscles or muscle groups cannot generate normal forces in one limb or the lower half of the body (e.g., caused by spinal cord injuries, spina bifida, or poliomyelitis).

- *Impaired passive range of motion:* movement is permanently reduced in one or more joints; acute conditions, joints that can move beyond average range of motion, and joint instability are not considered eligible impairments.

- *Intellectual impairment:* reduced intellectual abilities and adaptive behavior with an onset prior to age 18; expressed in conceptual, social, and practical adaptive skills.

- *Leg length difference:* bone shortening in one leg from birth or trauma.

- *Limb deficiency:* partial or complete loss of bones or joints; occurs from birth or because of trauma (e.g., car accident) or illness (e.g., bone cancer).

- *Short stature:* reduced standing height due to abnormal dimensions of bones or upper and lower limbs or trunk (e.g., due to **achondroplasia** or growth hormone dysfunction).

- *Visual impairment:* loss of vision due to eye structure impairment, optic nerve damage, or visual cortex damage.

TABLE 20.3   **Visual Impairments and Blindness Classifications**

Classification	Explanation
B1	Ranges from no light perception in either eye to light perception, but with inability to recognize the shape of a hand at any distance or in any direction
B2	Ranges from ability to recognize the shape of a hand to visual acuity of 20/600 or a visual field of less than 5° in the best eye with the best practical eye correction
B3	Ranges from visual acuity of more than 20/600 to visual acuity of 20/200 or a visual field of less than 20° and more than 5° in the best eye with the best practical eye correction
B4*	Ranges from visual acuity of more than 20/200 to visual acuity of 20/70 and a visual field larger than 20° in the best eye with the best practical eye correction

*B4 is a classification used only in events sponsored by the United States Association of Blind Athletes (USABA). B1 through B3 are used in events sponsored by both the USABA and the International Blind Sports Federation.

in the eye's globe caused by an inability of intraocular fluid to properly drain, which damages the optic nerve.

Understanding the cause of the VI is fundamental because some types of physical activity may worsen the impairment if adjustments to the training protocol or environment are not made. For example, contact sports such as goalball and judo are not recommended for those at risk for retinal detachment.

The cause of the athlete's VI should be noted during the PPE as well as the age at which he became visually impaired (congenital or later in life). This is also the time to determine the athlete's useful vision. About 80% of people who are blind have residual vision. Question the athlete about what he sees, in addition to conducting the visual acuity exam. Be sensitive to the fact that lighting in the athletic training facility may affect the athlete's ability to see.

FOUNDATIONAL SKILL

Communication With Athletes With VI

Here are some considerations for communication with athletes with VI:

- Always start an interaction by stating your name. For example, "Camilla, hi. It's Robert. I'm going to discuss your symptoms with you." Do not expect the athlete to recognize you by the sound of your voice.
- Ask the athlete if she needs assistance with mobility. Do not grab her arm; rather, offer your upper arm and allow the athlete to grasp it. Some athletes may prefer to grasp a shoulder.
- Provide the athlete with verbal cues that indicate changes in surface, location of the examining table, doors to be opened in or out, and steps up or down. Use tactile sense when performing an assessment; allow the athlete to follow your hands through the evaluation.
- Demonstrate a maneuver within the athlete's field of vision.
- Enhance visual cues: Conduct the assessment in a brightly lit area and use colored instruments or materials that contrast with the background (e.g., brightly colored stethoscopes and reflex hammers, colored tape around edges of furniture or doorways).
- Understand that athletes who have albinism and glaucoma can better distinguish solid-colored objects under nonglare lights and away from the glare from sunlight.
- Ask the athlete's preference when providing material that is usually in a written format, such as treatment instructions or medical staff contact information. Ask what works best (e.g., large print, Braille, audio clips, or computer software–based files).
- Keep the examination and treatment areas free of clutter and low-hanging objects.
- Face toward the athlete when asking questions or giving instructions.

Reprinted by permission from K. Walsh Flanagan and M. Cuppett, *Medical Conditions in the Athlete*, 3rd ed. (Champaign, IL: Human Kinetics, 2017), 462.

Medical Concerns for Athletes With Visual Impairments and Blindness

Generally, there are few special concerns in sports medicine regarding the athlete with visual impairment. First and foremost is the issue of communication. Work to enhance your communication with athletes with VI, since so much of the assessment is gained through the history. Remember that athletes with VI often cannot pick up nonverbal cues from the medical staff. Those whose onset of impairment was early in life may not have learned the socially accepted facial expression associated with each emotion or a nonverbal inference such as a head nod and a smile to denote comprehension of what practitioners are saying.

Athletes with VI sustained the second highest number of injuries (20% of all injured athletes) and fourth highest number of illnesses (12.8% of all ill athletes) at the 2016 Rio Paralympics.[38,39] Athletes with VI do not sustain disability-specific orthopedic injuries. However, proprioception in people who are blind tends to be worse than in those with partial sight, affecting the lower limbs and possibly resulting in abnormal gait and biomechanics.[40] Therefore, B1 athletes are more likely to sustain an injury than B3 athletes.[41] Common injuries include tendinopathies, sprains, and contusions. Sprains and contusions may be related to the VI, which makes the athletes more likely to bump into other players, barriers, or other objects in the training and competition areas. The areas most commonly affected are the thigh, knee, and shoulder.

The following general medical conditions may occur for athletes with VI:

- Athletes with glaucoma should avoid isometric activities, swimming under water, inverted body positions, use of antihistamines, excess fluid intake, and other practices that could increase eye pressure. Activities that elicit the Valsalva maneuver should be avoided. Further, take care with an athlete's use of acetazolamide and beta-blocker eye drops, often prescribed for glaucoma, both of which are prohibited by the World Anti-Doping Agency (WADA).[55]

- Precautions should be taken for athletes with diabetic retinopathy. For example, heavy weightlifting dramatically increases blood pressure and may cause retinal bleeding.

- Charles Bonnet syndrome affects 0.4% to 14% of people with an acquired VI. Reduced stimulus on the visual cortex triggers the syndrome, which can cause visual hallucinations, most commonly in the image of a person.[42] Refer an athlete who reports symptoms of Charles Bonnet syndrome to an ophthalmologist.

- Athletes with no light perception may experience a disruption in their circadian rhythms, which can result in reduced peak performance, sleep disorders, and reduced body temperature regulation throughout the day.[43]

- B1 and B2 athletes will have difficulty using urine color and volume as measures when self-monitoring hydration.

Some people who are blind exhibit **blindisms**, which are repetitive movements like hand waving, rocking, or finger flicking. There is no inherent harm in displaying blindisms other than the social stigma. Coaches, parents, and teachers commonly work with children who are blind to stop these movements in certain situations. Athletic trainers might encounter poor posture in people who are congenitally blind and have never seen others sit, stand, and move. Most adults develop proper posture through cueing and physical activity. Some novice athletes with visual impairments may have poor balance, fewer social skills, and low cardiovascular fitness. All of these aspects can improve with physical activity and sport.

Sports for Athletes With Visual Impairments and Blindness

Athletes with VI participate in a variety of sports with minimal to no adaptations. Paralympic sports for athletes with VI include cycling, alpine skiing, equestrian, paratriathlon, rowing, sailing, swimming, track and field, judo, goalball, and football 5-a-side. Goalball and football 5-a-side are only for athletes with VI. Beep baseball is also a sport played by athletes with VI. To provide appropriate health care, you should become familiar with the unique aspects of these sports, such as equipment, rules, playing surfaces, and movement requirements. For example, goalball is a quick-paced game played 3 against 3 on a gymnasium floor where the field of play is marked with tape overlaying string. Players wear eye patches and shades to equalize the VI. The offense throws or rolls a ball similar to a basketball with bells inside that is heard as it rolls on the floor. The defensive players dive laterally, using their bodies to block the ball from crossing their goal line. Players may wear knee, elbow, and hip padding. Spectators, coaches, and medical personnel must remain silent while the ball is in play. If a medical issue arises with a player, the referee will call a 45-second medical time-out, during which time the athletic trainer can assess the athlete.

Deaf Athletes and Athletes With Hearing Loss

In the United States, deaf people often do not consider themselves disabled, but rather members of a subculture of American society. As such, leaders of Deaf sport have chosen to dissociate from disability sport. Person-first terminology is typically not supported by these athletes. The preferred terminology is "Deaf," with an uppercase *D*.

- The term **Deaf** is associated with people who share the same social structures, cultural views, and history and use American Sign Language (ASL) as their primary mode of communication.[44]

- The term **hard of hearing** is used to identify people who have a milder form of hearing loss but can still communicate efficiently with the hearing community.

- **Hearing loss** is a general term that describes people who are hard of hearing or deaf. The term previously used for hardness of hearing was "hearing impaired," but this term is now considered an insult to the Deaf community because it emphasizes disability.

Deafness is a condition in which a person is unable to understand speech using the ears alone, with or without a hearing aid. An athlete who cannot detect the sound of a barking dog would have a severe to moderate hearing loss. Placing your fingers in your ears creates about a 25 decibels (dB) conductive loss. Hearing loss can range from mild to profound and is classified as one of three types.

- *Conductive:* hearing loss due to problems in the ear canal, eardrum, or middle ear (e.g., perforated eardrum, impacted earwax, foreign object, allergies, otitis media).

- *Sensorineural:* hearing loss due to problems in the inner ear, usually nerve related (e.g., head trauma, tumors, viral diseases such as measles or herpes simplex).

- *Mixed:* hearing loss caused by conductive damage in the outer or middle ear and sensorineural damage in the inner ear (e.g., head trauma, tumors, unintended side effects from medications).

To be eligible for participation in Deaf sports, athletes must have a hearing loss of 55 dB or greater.

Deaf athletes are not classified according to severity of hearing loss, and hearing aids are not permitted during competition.

Communication

People who are Deaf are at the greatest risk of miscommunication with people who are hearing. Therefore, communication is the primary factor related to the care of Deaf athletes and needs to be initially addressed during the PPE.[44]

In addition to the standard PPE history, ask the following additional questions during an examination with a Deaf athlete:

- Has the hearing loss progressed? Has it worsened, stayed the same, improved with aids?

- At what age did the loss occur?

- What method of communication does the athlete prefer (e.g., sign language, speech reading)?

- Does the athlete use hearing aids or have cochlear implants?

- Does the athlete use earplugs during swimming and water activities?

- Does the athlete have a history of ear infections?

- Is the hearing loss related to or accompanied by balance problems or vertigo?

General communication considerations for Deaf athletes are as follows:[37]

- Maintain eye contact and face the athlete in order to facilitate speech or lip reading; even the best speech readers will understand only about 30% of what is said.

- Orient the athlete to all aspects of the facility, paying special attention to exits and fire evacuation procedures.

- Speak normally if the athlete uses a hearing aid.

- Do not pretend to understand the athlete if her speech is unclear to you; instead, ask for repeats.

FOUNDATIONAL SKILLS

Hearing Test Points or Hearing Test Facts
- Intensity refers to the loudness or softness of sound; measured by decibels.
- Frequency refers to the perception of high and low pitch; measured in hertz (Hz).
- The audiogram includes only frequencies from 20 to 20,000 Hz.
- The frequencies (500, 1,000, 2,000 Hz) are emphasized in hearing tests.
- Persons who do not hear frequencies above 2,000 Hz have difficulty recognizing high-frequency sounds (the letters and sounds *s*, *sh*, *zh*, *th* as in think, *th* as in that, *ch* as in chair, *p*, *t*, *f*, *v*, and *h*).

- Use facial expressions, body language, gestures, and common signs such as thumbs up or down for "OK" and "not OK."
- Use instant texting, e-mail, or other similar electronic methods to communicate.
- Demonstrate any technique before performing it on an athlete.
- Use strobe fire alarms or other visual alerting devices in the facility so that the athlete has notification in the case of an emergency; point out these systems to the athlete.
- Use video, computer movie files, or other visual media as another form of demonstration.
- Loud or constant music or background noise, even at low levels, reduces hearing aid effectiveness and may even cause the athlete to develop headaches.
- Use visual and tactile cues.
- Avoid visual noise, such as extra physical or visual movements behind a person who is speaking.
- Learn basic American Sign Language.

Medical Concerns for the Deaf Athletes

A variety of hearing aids exist for the Deaf. Hearing aids do not clarify or make speech sound clearer; they simply amplify sound. The four basic types of hearing aids worn are as follows:

1. On the chest or body
2. Behind the ear
3. In the ear
4. On the eyeglasses

The practitioner is responsible for determining alternative techniques for communication. Athletic trainers working with Deaf athletes should know the American Sign Language alphabet and a few common signs. The alphabet and common signs, as well as many videos, are available on the Internet to help you sign accurately.

Cochlear implants are recommended for those people for whom a hearing aid is not helpful. The implants are surgically placed in the inner ear and are activated by an external speech processor worn on a belt or in a pocket. A microphone is worn externally behind the ear as a headpiece (figure 20.2). Sound is translated by the speech processor into distinctive electrical signals that travel up a thin cable to the headpiece and are transmitted across the skin via radio waves to the implanted electrodes in the cochlea. The auditory nerve is stimulated and information is transmitted to the brain, where it is interpreted. Newer models do not have external wires. Although cochlear

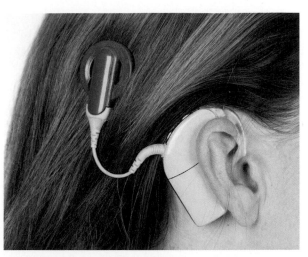

FIGURE 20.2 Cochlear implant.
ELizabethHoffmann/Getty Images

implants are not promoted by the National Association for the Deaf, they are increasingly implanted in children with sensorineural loss. The external apparatus should be removed during exercise to reduce the chance of electrostatic discharge. Athletes with cochlear implants must also stay away from plastic or rubber mats, balls, and equipment to prevent electrostatic discharge that can damage the electrodes.

Once communication barriers, type and care of hearing aids or implants, and any related conditions (e.g., balance problems, ear infections) have been addressed, sport health care will not be any different than for an athlete who is not deaf or hard of hearing.

Athletes With Amputations

For people with amputations, physical activity provides psychological and physical benefits, such as improvements in coping, mood, self-esteem, muscular strength, balance, and cardiovascular endurance.[45] The ability to continue to participate in sports and recreation is a major concern for people with amputation immediately following the surgery.[44] A decline in activity level after an amputation can lead to conditions such as low self-esteem, contractures, obesity, and diabetes.[45] Fortunately, opportunities are increasing for people with amputations to participate in all levels of recreational and competitive sports.

Amputations are categorized by location:

- AE: above the elbow (transhumeral)
- BE: below the elbow (transradial)
- AK: above the knee (transfemoral)
- BK: below the knee (transtibial)]

A number is used for identification in sport classifications:

- A1: AK double
- A2: AK single
- A3: BK double
- A4: BK single
- A5: AE double
- A6: AE single
- A7: BE double
- A8: BE single
- A9: Combined lower and upper limbs

The most popular sports for athletes with amputations are track and field and swimming. In track and field, the rules for individual events are the same as for able-bodied competition. The athletes may use prostheses, but no other assistive device is allowed. Prosthesis use is optional in most events but is not permitted in the high jump. Athletes with double amputations most often compete in wheelchair tennis or basketball events.

Sports governing bodies have rules regarding participation with prosthetic devices. At present in the United States, the National Federation of State High School Associations does not prohibit wearing these devices and leaves the decision to each state association. The National Collegiate Athletic Association has guidelines and standards regulating the use of artificial limbs in its sports medicine handbook. Factors considered in their use include the type of amputation and prosthesis, the potential harm to other players, and the question of an unfair advantage for the athlete because of the prosthetic device.

Causes of Amputations

Limb deficiency may be congenital or acquired from trauma or disease. Common indications for amputation include a necrotic extremity associated with peripheral vascular diseases or diabetes; life-threatening emergency conditions related to cancer, war injuries, or infection; and congenital deformity or injuries to the brachial plexus. Athletic trainers must consider the underlying general medical issue (e.g., diabetes, cancer) in the athlete that led to the amputation as well.

Medical Conditions for Athletes With Amputations

The primary medical problems in athletes who have had amputations are skin breakdown and phantom pain (table 20.4). However, the intact limbs are at risk for injuries such as Achilles tendinopathy, stress fractures, plantar fasciitis, and upper limb overuse injuries.[46] People with amputations have an increased prevalence of osteoarthritis than those without amputations.

TABLE 20.4 Common Medical Conditions for Athletes With Amputations

Condition	Description	Treatment
Skin breakdown	Abrasions, blisters, rashes, contact dermatitis, cysts, folliculitis, verrucous hyperplasia (warts), fungal infections due to skin irritation between the prosthetic's socket and residual limb surface or poor hygiene	Use fragrance-free soap or antiseptic cleaner, talcum powder, or silicone-based skin lotions Dry thoroughly Ensure proper prosthetic fit Rest from prosthetic (if severe) Refer to physician
Choke syndrome (stump edema syndrome)	Venous and lymphatic congestion that produces edema and hemorrhage in the distal stump, usually from an incorrectly fitting prosthetic that is "choking" the area	Ensure proper prosthetic fit Use shrinkers
Phantom sensation and phantom pain	Sensations of size, position, movement, itchiness, heat, cold, and touch in the amputated part; when pain is present, this is termed "phantom pain."	Refer to physician. Treatment varies from mirror-limb exercises to pharmacological agents.
Contractures or muscle tightness	Shortening of the muscles, tendons, and other tissues	Use a combination of heat, soft tissue massage, and mobility exercises. Ensure proper prosthetic fit.
Low back pain	Discomfort of the muscles and other tissues of the low back, typically due to altered biomechanics in activities of daily living or sport	Use a combination of pain-relieving interventions (e.g., heat, cold, TENS), soft tissue massage, mobility and strength exercises, and balance and coordination training. Ensure proper prosthetic size, type, and fit.

CLINICAL SKILL

Wrapping and Bandaging Amputations

Typically, the athlete or athletic trainer will use two 4-in. (10-cm) elastic bandages and wrap them diagonally to prevent occluding blood supply, making sure that there are at least 2 layers of bandage but that no layer directly overlaps the other. Also, they will keep the bandage free of wrinkles and creases and ensure that there is no bulging or puckering of the skin. The limb may be rewrapped every 4 to 6 hours or when the bandages loosen.

1. Apply the bandage with the limb extended to prevent contractures.

2. All turns of the bandage should be diagonal (i.e., figure-eight pattern), versus circular, to promote circulation (figure 20.3).

3. Wrap the bandage less firmly in the distal to proximal direction on the stump. No skin should be showing except for the joint itself, which usually is not bandaged at all.

4. Wrap right up to the crease of the buttocks and around the waist (like the common hip spica wrapping technique) of an athlete with an above-the-knee amputation.

5. No pain should be associated with the wrapping.

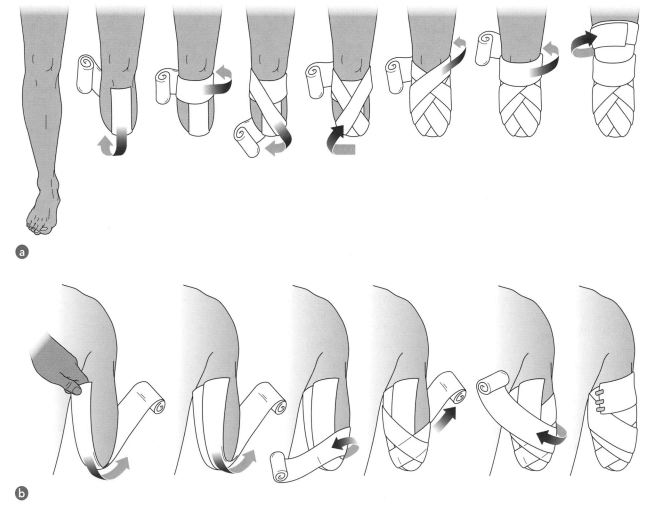

FIGURE 20.3   (a) Lower extremity wrapping and (b) upper extremity wrapping.

Although athletes should adopt good hygiene habits, washing the residual limb more than one time a day makes the skin moist and predisposes it to breakdown. Younger athletes with amputations have special needs because their appliances are small and require frequent adjustments to accommodate for growth. However, skin breakdown is less frequent at younger ages. It is outside the scope of this chapter to discuss the advances in sport prosthetic devices. Thus, athletic trainers should work with a prosthetist who is well versed in sport prosthetic technology. Sometimes a carefully designed prosthesis can serve for both activities of daily living and sports participation. Other times, protheses are highly specific for different sports; if used incorrectly, they can result in injury.

You may need to assist in or perform wrapping of the residual limb. Although athletes and athletic trainers may have subtle differences in the way they wrap, the basic technique for providing edema control and support without restricting circulation is the same.

Encourage athletes to wash their bandages by hand and squeeze them rather than wring out the water. They should spread them out on a flat surface to dry. Bandages should never be put in a dryer. Some athletes may use **shrinkers**, which are elastic compression socks that are pulled over the residual limb. Shrinkers are not as effective as wraps in controlling edema, but they are easier to use. Shrinkers and bandages should fit tightly, but not be painful or restrict blood flow. Avoid allowing athletes to roll or fold down the top of the shrinker, which compromises its effectiveness.

Athletes With Spinal Cord Injury

Spinal cord injury (SCI) results in complete or partial loss of motor and sensory function below the lesion accompanied by short-term and long-term effects on bowel, bladder, and sexual function. It also potentially results in altered body composition, neuropathic pain, spasticity, autonomic dysfunction, and secondary health conditions such as osteoporosis, type 2 diabetes, and cardiovascular disease. Thus, participation in sport and physical activity is beneficial beyond competition value. Sports are also associated with a high rate of employment, demonstrating their value from personal and societal perspectives for people with SCI. Athletes with SCI have been at the forefront of the Paralympic movement, having participated in the very first Paralympic Games in 1960. Many of the 22 Paralympic sports were originally created for people with SCI. Sports like tennis, fencing, and athletics are performed in a wheelchair and generally use the same rules as for able-bodied sports. Sports like alpine skiing and cross-country skiing are performed with specific equipment tailored for athletes

with SCI. Wheelchair rugby, wheelchair basketball, and sledge hockey are sports that engage athletes with SCI as well as other physical disabilities (e.g., amputations, orthopedic impairments).

SCI results from some form of injury or disease to the vertebrae or the nerves of the spinal column (figure 20.4). Other causes of SCI include the following:

- **Spina bifida** is a congenital SCI in which the neural tube does not close completely during the first 4 to 6 weeks of fetal development, leaving an opening in the spinal column. Spina bifida occurs most often in the low back and is more prevalent in females than males. People with spina bifida have muscle weakness or paralysis below the affected area. Spina bifida has three categories:

  1. *Occulta.* This is the least severe and most common type; has no visible symptoms.
  2. *Meningocele:* Meninges protrude through the opening at the spine, forming a cystlike swelling.
  3. *Meningomyelocele.* This type is the most severe; spinal cord and meninges protrude through the opening at the spine, forming a cystlike swelling.

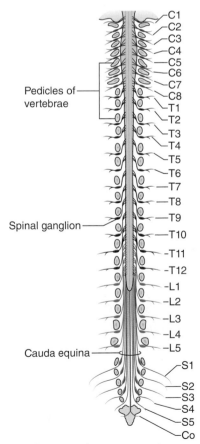

FIGURE 20.4 Spinal nerves with corresponding cervical levels.

- **Poliomyelitis**, or **polio**, is caused by a viral infection that affects motor cells of the spinal cord. Sensation and bowel and bladder control are not affected in the athlete with polio. The severity and degree of paralysis depends on the number and location of the motor cells destroyed by the virus.

SCI is usually accompanied by some degree of paralysis. The degree of paralysis is based on the level and type of lesion:

- *Incomplete SCI.* Some sensation or movement may occur below the level of lesion.

- *Complete SCI.* No sensation or movement occurs below the level of lesion.

- *Tetraplegia (i.e., quadriplegia).* The lesion occurs above T1, involves the cervical spine, and affects all four limbs. A person with tetraplegia has no trunk control or sitting balance and usually uses a high-backed sports wheelchair.

- *Paraplegia.* The lesion occurs below T1, affecting the lower extremities. A person with paraplegia has full use of the upper extremities and may or may not have trunk control and sitting balance.

In general, the lower the level of the lesion on the spinal cord, the greater the functional ability of the athlete. The lower the level of lesion in the spine, the lower the seat back height of the athlete's wheelchair. This is because lower lesions indicate greater trunk control and balance. The opposite is true with higher level lesions.

The extent of a SCI is generally described by means of a 5-point grading system. The American Spinal Injury Association (ASIA) advocates an impairment scale for classifying an athlete (table 20.5).

Medical Concerns for Athletes With SCI

Athletes with SCI present with a variety of general medical and musculoskeletal concerns for the athletic trainer to consider (table 20.6). Some are familiar (e.g., carpal tunnel syndrome, shoulder impingement) and some are unique to or at higher risk in this population (e.g., autonomic dysreflexia, latex allergy).

Athletes with SCI have higher resting heart rates and lower blood pressures than able-bodied athletes. An athlete with tetraplegia may be as low as 90/60 mmHg. Peak heart rates for people with tetraplegia typically do not exceed 130 beats per minute. As part of the PPE, blood pressure should be obtained in two of three positions, as applicable: supine, sitting, and standing.[47] A change of less than 10 mmHg between positions is acceptable.

Autonomic Dysreflexia

Autonomic dysreflexia (AD) is a condition unique to people with SCI with lesions above T6, although attacks are possible in athletes with lesions to T10. AD causes the athlete's blood pressure rises to dangerous levels (systolic blood pressure can reach 300 mmHg);[56] if untreated, it can lead to stroke or death. In a clinical context, it is defined as a sudden rise in systolic blood pressure of >20 mmHg above baseline.[57] It is caused by a painful, irritating, or strong stimulus below the level of SCI lesion, such as an insect bite, bone fracture, or distended bowel or bladder. Other physiological causes of AD include a urinary tract infection, bowel impaction, epididymitis or scrotal compression, menstruation, gastritis or gastric ulcers, or appendicitis. External causes of AD include constricted clothing, uniform, shoes, or equipment; contact with sharp objects; blisters; sunburn; or ingrown toenails.

Pressure ulcers are areas of skin breakdown that occur when the underlying tissue has been damaged due to loss of blood flow. In athletes with SCI, they are common in the buttocks and sacral regions. Athletic trainers should assist the athlete with routine skin inspections to prevent pressure sores. There are several stages of pressure sore staging classified by the National Pressure Ulcer Advisory Panel:[59]

- *Suspected deep tissue injury.* This is a localized area of discolored (purple or maroon), intact skin or a blood-filled blister that occurs due to damage of the underlying soft tissue from pressure or shear. The area may be preceded by tissue that is painful, firm, mushy, boggy, and warmer or cooler than the adjacent tissue.

TABLE 20.5 **ASIA Impairment Scale for Spinal Cord Injury**

Grade	Impairment	Description
A	Complete	No sensory or motor function is preserved in segments S4-S5.
B	Incomplete	Sensory function present, but no motor function is preserved below the neurologic level of injury; includes the S4-S5 segments.
C	Incomplete	Motor function is preserved below the neurologic level and >50% of the key muscles below neurological level have muscle grade < III.
D	Incomplete	Motor function is preserved below the neurologic level and >50% of the key muscles below the neurologic level have a muscle grade ≥ III.
E	Normal	Motor and sensory functions are normal.

TABLE 20.6   **Common Medical Conditions in the Athlete With SCI**

Condition	Explanation	Signs and symptoms	Treatment
Autonomic dysreflexia	Sympathetic condition only occurring in athletes with lesions T6 or above. Noxious stimulus triggers severe, life-threatening hypertension	Headache Flushed skin Chills Sweating Anxiety Hypertension	Locate and mitigate the cause. Place athlete in as upright a position as possible. Loosen clothing and equipment. Administer oral nifedipine or GTN spray.* Call emergency medical transport.
Thermoregulation	Impaired ability to control body temperature. Sweating and shivering do not occur below the level of lesion	Same as for able-bodied athletes but less specific since sweating and shivering are impaired	Same as for able-bodied athletes
Urinary tract infection	Bacterial infection, usually due to distended bladder or catheter issues (kinks in tubing)	Nonspecific, but may include general feeling of unease, low-grade fever	Administer antibiotics and address the cause of the infection, including encouraging more frequent monitoring of catheter
Fractures	Increased risk of bone fractures and delay of healing in paretic (paralyzed) areas due to loss of bone mineral density	Signs and symptoms of autonomic dysreflexia. Possible deformity. Remember that patients cannot experience pain in paretic areas.	Same as for able-bodied patients, with the addition of treating autonomic dysreflexia, if present
Latex allergy	Athletes with spina bifida have increased prevalence of latex allergies.	Hives Itchy skin Stuffy or runny nose Difficulty swallowing Wheezing Anaphylaxis, if severe	Administer calamine lotion or hydrocortisone cream, antihistamine, or epinephrine. Call emergency medical transport.
Pressure sores	Breakdown of skin and underlying tissues from prolonged pressure. Usually occur on buttocks or sacral areas	See the following section on stages for more information.	Refer athlete ASAP to primary care physician or dermatologist. Encourage daily inspection of skin to prevent or monitor sores.
Overuse upper extremity injuries	Nerve entrapments, tendonitis, tendinopathy, and strains due to repetitive movements of daily living (e.g., pushing chair, reaching up, transferring) or sport (e.g., serving, shooting, pushing)	Same as for able-bodied patients	Same as for able-bodied patients, with special emphasis on evaluating technique, protective gear (e.g., gloves), and equipment (e.g., sport chair fit)
Shunt issues	Shunts used by athletes with spina bifida may become infected or fail, causing seizures or other changes.	Swelling or redness along shunt tract. Pain at site of surgical repair. Headache. Changes in personality, vision, or performance	Refer the athlete to his primary physician or neurologist

*Glyceryl trinitrate (GTN) spray is contraindicated in athletes who use it already for erectile dysfunction.

EVIDENCE-BASED ATHLETIC TRAINING

Boosting

Some athletes intentionally invoke AD immediately before competition in an attempt to gain a physiological advantage; this is known as **boosting**. Therefore, precompetition clinical and blood pressure checks are randomly performed. Of respondents surveyed at the 2008 Paralympic Games, 66% had experienced AD and 16.7% had intentionally boosted. Boosting is banned by the World Anti-Doping Agency.

- *Stage I.* This is intact skin with nonblanchable redness of a localized area, usually over a bony prominence. Darkly pigmented skin may not have visible blanching; its color may differ from that of the surrounding area.

- *Stage II.* In this stage, partial thickness loss of dermis presents as a shallow, open ulcer with a red or pink wound bed, without slough. It may also present as a serum-filled blister that is either intact or ruptured.

- *Stage III.* This stage involves full-thickness tissue loss. Subcutaneous fat may be visible, but bone, tendon, and muscle are not exposed. Slough may be present, but it does not obscure the depth of the tissue loss. May include undermining and tunneling.

- *Stage IV.* This is full-thickness tissue loss with exposed bone, tendon, or muscle. Slough or eschar may be present on some parts of the wound bed. Often includes undermining and tunneling.

- *Unstageable.* This stage is defined as full-thickness tissue loss in which the base of the ulcer is covered by slough (yellow, tan, gray, green, or brown) or eschar (tan, brown, or black) in the wound bed.

Athletes With Cerebral Palsy

Cerebral palsy (CP) is a chronic neurological disorder caused by a lesion in the brain that affects movement and posture. CP occurs before, at, or soon after birth and is not hereditary or progressive. It affects the ability to move and maintain balance and posture because of the damage to those areas of the brain that control muscle tone and spinal reflexes. The disorder varies from mild, evidenced by general clumsiness and a slight limp, to severe, in which the affected person is dominated by reflexes, unable to ambulate without a motorized chair, and nonverbal. There are three types of CP (table 20.7).

The Cerebral Palsy International Sport and Recreation Association uses a classification system based on an individual athlete's functional ability. There are 8 classes (CP1 through CP8); CP1 to CP4 are athletes who use wheelchairs and CP5 to CP8 are athletes who are ambulatory.[48] This system also includes athletes with other conditions characterized by nonprogressive brain lesions, such as stroke and traumatic brain injury.

TABLE 20.7 Types of Cerebral Palsy

Type of cerebral palsy	Description
Spastic CP	• Most common • Characterized by hypertonic muscle tone during voluntary movement • Flexor muscles stronger than the extensor muscles • Exaggerated myotatic reflex • Scissors gait
Athetoid CP	• Second most common type • Characterized by constant, purposeless, and unpredictable movement that is caused by fluctuating muscle tone • Patient may have lack of head control (i.e., rolling from side to side) and trouble with speaking, eating, and writing. • Most patients are tetraplegic; some use wheelchairs and others walk with an unsteady gait. • Signs and symptoms increase with stress and fatigue.
Ataxic CP	• Results from disorders to the spinal cord and brain • Varies from mild to severe • Diagnosed only in people who can walk unaided • Balance and coordination disturbances

Athletes with CP may be further grouped according to how many limbs are affected and what functions they have.

Athletes with CP have a high incidence of exhibiting **pathological reflexes**. In infants, the involuntary, predictable muscle and postural tone shifts that occur are normal and considered important for development. However, reflexes that are not integrated at the developmentally appropriate times become pathological and affect the smoothness and coordination of movement. During an examination, the athletic trainer should be aware of what reflexes the athlete has not integrated so that he can be positioned in such a manner as not to elicit reflexes that may interfere with the examination. A comprehensive discussion of the more than 25 primitive reflexes that might be present in this population is beyond the scope of this chapter. However, one example is the asymmetrical tonic neck reflex (ATNR). The ATNR is also known as the fencing reflex because, when activated, the upper extremities assume the "en garde" position of fencers. Rotation or lateral flexion of the neck causes extension of the arm on the face side and simultaneous flexion on the nonface side. When addressing the athlete, the athletic trainer should position herself in front of the athlete to avoid head turning that elicits the reflex.

Athletic trainers should remember that these reflexes are involuntary motions or postures; although they are not painful, they can compromise certain body positions. Communication with the athlete can be enhanced by understanding the reflexes and working around the stimuli that elicit them.

Medical Concerns for Athletes With CP

Some people with CP may have associated medical conditions, such as the following:

- Deafness
- Vision disturbances
- Impaired hand–eye coordination
- Intellectual disabilities
- Seizures

Seizure conditions are common in athletes with disabilities. Athletic trainers should know that exercise decreases the incidence of seizures; thus, athletes with CP should not be discouraged from participation based on seizure history. Seizures and seizure medications should be identified at the PPE and then carefully monitored.

- Seizure medications are chosen for a patient based on the type of seizure.
- Athletic trainers should familiarize themselves with the side effects of the medications, which can include impaired attention span, ataxia, nystagmus, strabismus, and cognitive impairment. Carbamazepine is often recommended for this athletic population, but should be used with caution because it has been known to cause hyponatremia.[49]
- Compliance with seizure medication is extremely important, and athletic trainers may need to prompt athletes to take medications at correct times, especially when routine is disrupted (e.g., travel for competition).

Although seizures during aerobic activity are rare, athletic trainers should still be on alert to provide appropriate intervention.

Athletes With Intellectual Disabilities

The American Association for Intellectual and Developmental Disabilities defines intellectual disability as "significant limitations in both intellectual functioning (reasoning, learning, problem solving) and in adaptive behavior, which covers a variety of everyday social and practical skills."[50] This disability originates before the age of 18 and has a lasting effect on development. The intelligent quotient (IQ) test is a major tool in measuring intellectual functioning, which is the mental capacity for learning, reasoning, and problem solving. A test score below or around 70 indicates a limitation in intellectual functioning. Athletic trainers may work with athletes at all levels of function; however, 85% of people with intellectual disabilities are categorized as mildly impaired. Causes of intellectual disabilities range from fetal alcohol syndrome to chromosomal abnormalities, and some causes are unknown. The cause, if known, should be noted during the PPE and monitored in some cases, such as seizure disorders.

Down syndrome is the most common chromosomal abnormality that causes intellectual disability. It is an autosomal chromosomal condition that results in a host of medical concerns in addition to those seen in athletes with other intellectual disabilities. Medical conditions associated with Down syndrome include atlantoaxial instability balance deficits, obesity, poor hand–eye coordination, postural or orthopedic posture problems (e.g., kyphosis, clubfoot, lordosis), joint laxity, vision concerns (e.g., strabismus, nystagmus, cataracts), and cardiac issues (e.g., ventricular septal defect, atrioventricular canal defect, mitral valve prolapse).

Communication

Terminology and directions used in the assessment of athletes with intellectual disabilities need to be clear and concise. Here are some tips for good communication practices with athletes with intellectual disabilities:

- Always speak to and interact with the athlete in an age-appropriate way. For example, avoid giving instructions in a singsong voice to a teenaged or adult athlete. If you need to guide an athlete to an area, avoid taking her by the hand (unless she is a child), since this is not age appropriate.

- Demonstrate the task first and then give the athlete simple, one-step instructions, repeating or rephrasing as necessary while the athlete moves through the task.

- Ask the athlete to repeat the instructions to ensure that she understands.

Medical Concerns for Athletes With Intellectual Disabilities

People with intellectual disabilities vary widely in their abilities and the medical issues they experience, making generalizations difficult. Assessment during the PPE is the best method of determining normative values for each athlete. Some of the more common medical concerns are as follows:

- Atlantoaxial instability (occurs in Down syndrome only)
- Cardiac issues (e.g., atrial septal defects, ventricular septal defects)
- Hypothyroidism (common in people with Down syndrome)
- Joint laxity
- Obesity
- Pain insensitivity
- Posture or orthopedic concerns (e.g., kyphosis, clubfoot, lordosis)
- Seizures
- Vision concerns (e.g., strabismus, nystagmus, cataracts)

Let's look at a few of these more closely.

- Cardiac issues. Echocardiograms may be indicated to screen for cardiac defects, such as atrioventricular septal defects, ventricular septal defects, and atrial septal defects. Maximal heart rates of people with intellectual disabilities are 8% to 20% lower (10 to 15 bpm) than expected, and people with Down syndrome have even lower maximal heart rates.

- Atlantoaxial instability (AAI) is a condition present in approximately 17% of people with Down syndrome. AAI is characterized by instability between the atlas (C1) and axis (C2) that results from either a bony or ligamentous abnormality. Neurological symptoms can occur when the

spinal cord or adjacent nerve roots are involved. Therefore, people with Down syndrome must be screened for AAI prior to participation. This is done with an X-ray. If present, restrictions such as no soccer heading, butterfly swim stroke, and inverted diving are made.

- Seizures occur in approximately 20% of people with mild intellectual disabilities. The PPE should include inquiries about seizure control methods and medications.

- Approximately 25% of people with intellectual disabilities show signs of pain insensitivity or indifference that places them at increased medical risk. People with intellectual disabilities have died from appendicitis and bowel obstruction that went undiagnosed because they did not indicate being in pain. Further, people with intellectual disabilities may not be able to verbally communicate their symptoms clearly.[58] Athletic trainers should carefully check for signs of trauma and not rely exclusively on what the athlete reports.

- Anticonvulsive, hypnotic, neuroleptic, and antidepressant medications are commonly used in this population. Hypothyroidism is common in people with Down syndrome, and many of these athletes may be receiving thyroxine replacement therapy. Side effects of some of these hypothyroidism medications can cause angina until a stable dose has been determined.

- Vision problems are common in people with intellectual disabilities, necessitating a careful visual examination during the PPE.

Athletes With Les Autres

Les autres is a French term meaning "the others." It is used to describe athletes with a range of conditions that result in locomotive disorders—such as dwarfism, muscular dystrophy, osteogenesis imperfecta, and juvenile rheumatoid arthritis—that don't fit into the traditional classification systems of the established disability groups previously presented. There are two general categories: short stature and impaired passive range of motion. Within each category, there are specific conditions.

Short Stature

Athletes in the short stature category are considered to have reduced standing height due to dwarfism (table 20.8). Dwarfism can be caused by any of more than 200 conditions. Causes of proportionate (trunk and limbs are in proportion to one another) dwarfism include metabolic and hormonal disorders such as growth hormone deficiency.

TABLE 20.8 **Types of Dwarfism**

Type of dwarfism	Definition	Concerns
Achondroplasia	Most common type; congenital condition where the athlete has a relatively long trunk and shortened upper parts of the arms and legs[33]	Lumbar lordosis and swayback, genu varum, pes planus, and increased joint mobility
Spondyloepiphyseal dysplasias	Group of conditions characterized by a shortened trunk, which may not become apparent until a child is between the ages of 5 and 10	Club feet, cleft palate, hip osteoarthritis, weakness of the hands and feet, and a barrel-chested appearance
Diastrophic dysplasia	Rare, congenital condition where the athlete has shortened forearms and lower legs, known as mesomelic shortening	Limited range of motion, cleft palate, and ears with a cauliflower appearance (not to be confused with hematoma auris).

The most common types of dwarfism, known as skeletal dysplasias, are genetic. Skeletal dysplasias are conditions of abnormal bone growth that cause disproportionate dwarfism. Disproportionate dwarfism means the trunk is of typical size, while the limbs are shorter.

Impaired Passive Range of Movement

This subgroup of les autres athletes includes athletes with reduced range of movement in one or more joints that is caused by an illness such as juvenile arthritis or a congenital deficiency such as arthrogryposis (joint contracture). However, joint instability (e.g., dislocation) and acute conditions of reduced range of movement (e.g., arthritis) are typically excluded.

Common Medical Concerns for Athletes With Les Autres

Research is severely lacking on rates of sports injury and illness among athletes in the les autres category. The following conditions are suggestions for the athletic trainer to consider:[33]

- Reduced muscle tone, resulting in decreased strength and endurance
- Breathing limitations due to smaller thoracic cavity
- Scoliosis or low back pain
- Genu varum that may affect gait and sport biomechanics
- Ear infections are common in athletes with dwarfism.
- Spinal stenosis is common in athletes with dwarfism.

Sports for Athletes With Les Autres

Equestrian, powerlifting, swimming, table tennis, and track and field are Paralympic sports for people with short stature. Paralympic sports for people with reduced passive range of motion include archery, boccia, cycling, equestrian, paracanoe, paratriathlon, powerlifting, rowing, sailing, shooting, swimming, table tennis, track and field, wheelchair basketball, wheelchair fencing, and wheelchair tennis. Outside of the Paralympics, athletes may participate in a variety of additional sport and recreational activities.

CLINICAL BOTTOM LINE

- Athletic trainers must understand the foundational concepts of working with athletes with disabilities to ensure that they provide the appropriate prevention, assessments, and accommodations for the specific disability or special population.
- The use of augmented physical examination forms to identify common comorbidities associated with specific special populations is essential to help athletic trainers prepare their response to medical issues that may arise as a component of physical activity, competition, or disability.
- The role of the athletic trainer in working with special populations is to provide medical care for varying medical conditions, anatomy, and physiology of people with disabilities or special populations in order to help the client participate in physical activity or life situations. Specifically, the athletic trainer needs

to understand personal, environmental, and equipment specifics for people with special needs to manage prevention, care, and rehabilitation.

- Differing special populations require specificity in care:
  - For athletes with amputations, athletic trainers may need to adjust or augment taping and wrapping to accommodate for an amputated limb.
  - Tactical athletes may need additional modifications and rehabilitation specific to carrying a large load of equipment, working in excessive heat or environmental conditions, or gait and postural issues associated with extensive standing or walking.
  - Athletes who are blind need focused, consistent communication from the athletic trainer. Enhanced visual cues are necessary, both in the field and in the athletic training room, to enhance performance and decrease secondary injury.
  - Athletes with hearing loss may also need more focused communication to assist with facial expressions and speech reading. Augmenting prevention treatment and rehabilitation with videos and pictures is helpful when describing processes and desired outcomes.
  - Due to the wide variety of intellectual disabilities athletes may have, general modifications are difficult to create. Thus, athletic trainers should give specific attention to each athlete and his needs and ability to communicate and understand. Potential caregiver access or support is essential to ensuring proper medical care.
- The right of people in special populations to receive the highest standard of health care without discrimination has been ratified by the UN convention. Likewise, the NATA approved the adoption of the World Health Organization's ICF, whereby an athletic trainer considers not only the medical condition or anatomy and physiology of a patient, but also his activities and life situation.
- Athletic trainers should employ person-first terminology to emphasize the client, not the disability.
- Athletic trainers may need to modify their communication strategies when working with clients in special populations. For example, communication with an athlete who is blind is very different from communication with one who has Down syndrome. The common components of communication include making the patient feel comfortable by stating your name, identifying why you are assessing the athlete, maintaining direct eye contact, and speaking directly to the athlete.

 Go to HK*Propel* to complete the activities and case studies for this chapter.

Therapeutic and Medical Interventions

Part V provides information regarding therapeutic and medical interventions, with each chapter in the section focusing on one particular aspect. In order to provide patient-centered, holistic care, athletic trainers will need to simultaneously apply concepts and practices from each of these chapters. Therapeutic interventions are a principle component of an athletic trainer's practice. Key information on therapeutic modalities, therapeutic exercise, and pharmacological interventions is introduced in chapters 21, 22, and 23, respectively. A comprehensive overview of medical interventions for athletic trainers also includes casting, which is presented in chapter 24. Unique to this textbook is discussion on emerging therapeutic interventions and key concepts that are currently used in athletic training practice. Athletic trainers must be able to integrate therapeutic options and broadly apply these concepts to work with a diverse range of patients. The information provided in part V serves as a foundation for professional practice.

CHAPTER 21

Therapeutic Modalities and Interventions

Leamor Kahanov, EdD, ATC, LAT

CAATE STANDARDS

The following CAATE 2020 standard is covered in this chapter:

Standard 73

CHAPTER OBJECTIVES

After reading this chapter, you will be able to do the following:

- Understand legal concerns
- Identify classifications of therapeutic modalities
- Understand therapeutic modality safety
- Discern evidence-based data regarding use of therapeutic modalities
- Describe maintenance and purchasing parameters

Many settings require athletic trainers to use therapeutic modalities for rehabilitation and treatment. Therapeutic modalities are highly regulated based on state practice acts; thus, practitioners must understand the legal liabilities. Depending on the state's regulations, the athletic trainer may be designated to coordinate and monitor the use of therapeutic modalities. Athletic trainers must determine the optimal implementation of modalities to achieve desired patient outcomes and maintain patient safety. To ensure continuity of care, they should work with other health care providers, such as physical therapists, occupational therapists, and physicians, on the implementation and continued use of therapeutic modalities.

A **therapeutic modality** is the application of an implement or device that causes physiological changes that improve or facilitate normal function. They are routinely used by athletic trainers in the treatment and rehabilitation of injuries. This chapter provides a foundational overview of the therapeutic modalities most commonly applied for active populations. Additional education is required to gain proficiency in clinical application and the critical decision-making skills needed to appropriately and effectively incorporate therapeutic modalities into the treatment and rehabilitation of active people.

Therapeutic modalities are placed into five classifications based on different forms of energy:

1. Thermal
2. Electrical
3. Electromagnetic
4. Sound
5. Mechanical

Legal Considerations of Therapeutic Modality Application

Knowledge of therapeutic modalities and their indications and contraindications is of paramount importance for using them appropriately and ensuring patient safety. Laws governing the use of therapeutic modalities vary by state and medical practice acts. Due to this variance, knowledge of therapeutic modality application is superseded by each state's medical practice act.[1] Athletic trainers must adhere to state law when considering therapeutic modalities and thoughtfully apply them based on the best available evidence.

Each energy form is transmitted differently when in contact with human tissue (table 21.1). In general, energy is reflected, refracted, absorbed, and transmitted; however, in human tissues, energy must be absorbed in order to produce any therapeutic physiological effect.[2]

Thermal Modalities

Thermal energies include both heat and cold therapies. The transfer of thermal energy occurs through conduction, convection, radiation, and conversion (see table

TABLE 21.1 **Overview of Therapeutic Modalities**

Modality classification	Types	General physiological effects and indications	General contraindications

Thermotherapy: heat	Moist heat pack
	Electrical heat
	Warm whirlpool
	Paraffin
	Fluidotherapy
		Decrease
		  Muscle spasm
		  Pain perception
		  Joint stiffness
		Increase
		  Blood flow
		  Metabolic rate
		  Collagen elasticity
		  Capillary permeability
		  Edema
			• Thrombophlebitis
			• Sensory deficits
			• Acute injury or infection
			• Malignant tissue
			• Should not be used over the eyes, carotid sinus, anterior neck, or r eproductive organs

Thermotherapy: cold (cryotherapy)	Ice massage
	Cold-water or ice immersion
	Ice or cold pack
	Cryokinetics
		Decrease
		  Muscle spasm
		  Pain perception
		  Blood flow
		  Metabolic rate
		  Collagen elasticity
		Increase
		  Joint stiffness
		  Capillary permeability
		Debated
		  Edema reduction
			• History of vascular impairment, such as frostbite or arteriosclerosis
			• Cold allergy
			• Hypertension
			• Raynaud's disease
			• Rheumatoid arthritis
			• Limb ischemia

Electrical	Interferential
	low-intensity stimulation (microcurrent/MENS)
	Iontophoresis
	High-voltage galvanic stimulation (HVGS)
	Transcutaneous electrical neuromuscular stimulation (TENS)
		Decrease
		  Muscle spasm
		  Pain perception
		  Joint stiffness
		  Muscle atrophy
		Increase
		  Blood flow
		  Metabolic rate
		  Collagen elasticity
		  Capillary permeability
		  Edema
			• Altered tissue sensation
			• Presence of an implanted electrical device (i.e., pacemaker)
			• Malignant tissue
			• Epilepsy
			• Thrombosis
			• Skin conditions
			• Open wounds
			• Should not be used over the eyes, carotid sinus, anterior neck, or reproductive organs

Modality classification	Types	General physiological effects and indications	General contraindications
Electromagnetic	Diathermies	*Decrease* 　Muscle spasm 　Pain perception 　Joint stiffness *Increase* 　Blood flow 　Metabolic rate 　Collagen elasticity 　Capillary permeability 　Edema	• Altered tissue sensation • Presence of an implanted electrical device (i.e., pacemaker) • Malignant tissue • Epilepsy • Thrombosis • Skin conditions • Open wounds • Should not be used over the eyes, carotid sinus, anterior neck, or reproductive organs
Mechanical	Traction Intermittent compression Massage	*Decrease* 　Muscle spasm 　Pain perception 　Joint stiffness *Increase* 　Blood flow 　Metabolic rate 　Collagen elasticity 　Capillary permeability 　Edema	
Sound	Ultrasound	*Decrease* 　Muscle spasm 　Pain perception 　Joint stiffness *Increase* 　Blood flow 　Metabolic rate 　Collagen elasticity 　Capillary permeability 　Edema	
Infrared modalities	Low-level laser LED (light-emitting diodes)	*Decrease* 　Muscle spasm 　Pain perception 　Joint stiffness *Increase* 　Blood flow 　Metabolic rate 　Collagen elasticity 　Capillary permeability 　Edema	

21.2). When using all forms of energy therapy, athletic trainers must screen their patients for contraindications and carefully monitor the application process to avoid tissue damage.

Thermotherapy

Thermotherapy is the application of heat for the prevention, treatment, or rehabilitation of injuries and diseases. Heat is typically applied in order to increase collagen

tissue extensibility, relieve muscle spasms, decrease pain or muscle spasm, reduce inflammation postacutely, and increase blood flow.[2] Table 21.3 lists thermotherapy modalities.

Cryotherapy

Cryotherapy, the application of cold, is a generally accepted practice in sports medicine for trauma and pain control following acute injury. Cold is intermittently

TABLE 21.2 **Thermal Energy Transmission**

Transmission	Definition	Example of modality
Conduction	Transfer of heat from a warmer object to a cooler object	Moist heat packs Electrical heating pads Cold and ice packs Ice massage Paraffin bath
Convection	Transfer of heat through the movement of fluids (either gas or liquid)	Whirlpool Fluidotherapy
Radiation	Transfer of heat from one object to another through the air	Lasers Diathermy
Conversion	Transfer of energy from one form to another that produces heat	Ultrasound Electrical stimulation Lasers Chemical agents (counterirritants)

TABLE 21.3 **Thermotherapy Modalities**

Modality	Definition	Indications	Application	Contraindications and considerations
Hydrocollator packs or moist heat packs 	Cotton packs containing silica gel are immersed in a controlled hot water bath at a temperature of 160°F to 170°F (71°C to 77°C) and then placed on the body.	Reduction of pain-spasm cycle Heat pack is limited by the size of the surface area and adipose tissue (acts as a thermal insulator).	Remove the moist heat pack from the hot water bath, drain it, and cover it with a towel (may be commercial). Apply to the affected area of the body for 15-20 min. Select a heat pack approximately the same size of the affected surface area on the body.	Watch for heat sensitivity or burns from a moist heat pack when hot.
Warm whirlpool 	Immersion in water 102°F to 108°F (39°C to 42°C) that is agitated	Reduce postacute inflammation Decrease pain Decrease spasm Increase tissue extensibility	Place patient in a comfortable position. Submerge the body part in the water 8-10 in. (20-25 cm) away from the jet so that the jet stream swirls around the appendage. Do not place the jet stream directly on the body part. Maximum length of treatment is 20 min.	Contraindicated for acute inflammation. Full-body immersion should not occur in water 104°F (40°C) or hotter. Whirlpool must be cleaned and maintained daily to ensure safety and disinfection.

Modality	Definition	Indications	Application	Contraindications and considerations
Paraffin bath	Paraffin and mineral oil mixture maintained in a commercial heater at 126°F to 130°F (52°C to 54°C)	Used for small extremities (e.g., fingers, toes)	For both methods, the appendage should be thoroughly cleaned prior to treatment. *Method 1* Dip the body part 8-10 times, allowing each layer to dry before redipping. Wrap the body part in a plastic bag and place it in a towel. Rest the body part for 30 min or until heat is no longer generated. *Method 2* Soak the body part in the paraffin unit for 20-30 min, being careful not to touch it to the hot sides or bottom of the unit. Remove the body part from the paraffin unit and allow the wax to dry in order to remove easily.	Contraindicated for acute inflammation. Monitor for heat sensitivity and discomfort.
Fluidotherapy	Dry heat at 100°F to 113°F (38°C to 45°C) housed in a unit that contains dry cellulose particles that allow air to circulate.	Decrease pain Increase tissue extensibility Decrease spasm Decrease postacute swelling	Place the patient's appendage in the fluidotherapy unit. Adjust the air turbulence for patient comfort. Treatment time is 15-20 min.	

applied to minimize the inflammatory process and control pain from day 1 to 2 weeks postinjury. For optimal effects, cold is applied in conjunction with rest, ice, compression, and elevation.[2-13]

The application of cryotherapy and the concomitant effects depend on the type of cold used, length of time, and the size of the area.[14-18] In general, the longer the exposure to cryotherapy or cold, the deeper the cooling. The athletic trainer must explain to her patients what sensations to expect on cold application:[12]

- 0-3 min: Patients will feel cold.
- 2-7 min: Patients will feel mild to moderate burning and aching.
- 5-12 min: Patients will feel numbness.

Table 21.4 lists cryotherapy modalities.[2,19-22]

Electrical Modalities

Electrotherapy is a passive form of treatment where many different forms of electrical stimulation are applied,

TABLE 21.4 **Cryotherapy Modalities**

Modality	Indications	Application	Contraindications and considerations

Ice massage or ice cup	Use over small body areas:
	  Tendons
	  Muscle
	  Bursae
	  Myofascial trigger points
	  Skin (for numbing)
		Hold the ice cup so the exposed ice touches the designated area.
		Rub the ice cup over the skin in overlapping concentric circles or an area of 4-6 in. (10-15 cm) for 5-10 min or until the patient feels numbness in the affected area.
			People who have adverse reactions to cold should avoid this treatment.

Ice or cold water immersion	Immersion is preferred when circumferential cooling is required or desired.
	Use for the following body parts:
	  Fingers
	  Hands
	  Arms
	  Toes
	  Feet
	  Legs
	  Lower extremity
		Size of whirlpool depends on body size.
		Water temperature should be between 50°F and 60°F (10°C to 15°C).
		Immerse for 10-15 min or until area is numb or the pain spasm cycle is disrupted.
			Return to activity should be assessed based on proprioceptive ability of the athlete and extensibility of tissue needed for activity. Overcooling may lead to frostbite and time parameters should be adhered to.

Ice pack or ice bags (wet)	Provides the best cooling opportunities.	Place crushed ice in a damp towel or bag and place on the desired body area. Plastic wrap or Flexi-Wrap may be placed around the ice bag or pack to secure it in place. Treatment time is 15-20 min.	
Ice pack or ice bags (dry)	Use when wet ice packs or bags, which are optimal, are contraindicated due to compromised skin conditions or inappropriate due to treatment location.	If using an ice bag: Place crushed ice or ice cubes in a plastic bag with the air removed. If using a chemical gel pack: Break the inner seal (follow pack directions) to create cold. Plastic wrap or Flexi-Wrap may be placed around the ice bag or pack to secure it in place. Treatment time is 15-20 min.	Chemical gel packs may leak or cool excessively, leading to burns. To mitigate burning with patients sensitive to cold, wrap the pack in a single layer of towel.
Cryokinetics	Combination technique where exercise is conducted with a cold application. The intent is to numb the body area (analgesia) to progress movement.	Numb the body area with any cryotherapy modality; patient communicates when area becomes numb (typically occurs in 12-20 min). Numbness will last 3-5 min where exercise is performed. Reapply cold therapy for 3-5 min until numbness returns. Repeat 5 times.	Closely monitor progression, intensity, and activity level so as not to induce additional injury.

Primary Electrical Modalities for Pain Modulation Theories

The way we experience pain is complex, and many pain control theories exist. The two main theories governing use of electrical modalities are as follows:[26-30]

Gate Control Theory
- *Definition:* Pain is experienced at the origination of the stimulus. This input then travels to the brain. Painful input can be prevented from travelling through the nervous system if something blocks it or closes the gate. Creating an alternate stimulus to the gate is theorized to block the pain stimulus from travelling.
- *Modality application:* Typically, TENS (high-frequency) or IFC at 80 to 150 pps.

Endogenous Opiate System (EOS) Stimulation
- *Definition:* The experience of pain initiates the endogenous opioid system, which functions to relieve pain sensation. Enacting the EOS system allows the body to produce three opioids that mask the pain experience: beta-endorphins, met-enkephalins and leu-enkephalins, and dynorphins. The ability to initiate an EOS may reduce the patient's pain.
- *Modality application:* TENS at 1 to 5 pps (brief intense).

primarily to reduce pain and spasming but also to increase tissue healing. Examples include active participation to enhance muscle contraction and strength, such as neuromuscular electrical stimulation (NMES) and Russian stimulation. Electrical stimulation is used for several purposes, depending on the type of electrical modality, intensity, and selected parameters:

- Pain control
- Muscle contraction
- Muscle pumping
- Muscle strengthening
- Minimizing atrophy
- Muscle reeducation

Electrical stimulation is never the only component of treatment or rehabilitation; it is used to augment intended outcomes. Advanced training and skill development are needed to appropriately identify, apply, and actuate a treatment or rehabilitation plan that includes electrical modalities (table 21.5). Athletic trainers should check the medical practice acts in their state to determine appropriateness of use in practice. Electrical modalities are listed in table 21.6.

Biofeedback measures muscular contractions through visual and auditory signals to assist patients in strengthening and muscular and postural control. The athletic trainer uses a biofeedback device that identifies the patient's muscular contractions and then guides the patient through neuromuscular relaxation or muscle reeducation.[31]

TABLE 21.5 **Types of Electrical Currents**

Current	Definition	Indications	Types of modalities
Monophasic: direct current (DC)	Current that flows in one direction	Pain modulation Decrease muscle spasms Muscle reeducation Increase range of motion (ROM) Wound healing Increase blood flow	NMES General electrical stimulation Iontophoresis
Biphasic: alternating current (AC)	Current that alternates	Pain modulation Stimulate muscle contractions	TENS Interferential NMES
Pulsatile	Three or more pulses (bursts) followed by periods of rest that repeat in regular intervals		Russian stimulation Interferential/premodulated

TABLE 21.6   **Electrical Modalities**

Modality	Indications	Application	Contraindications and considerations
TENS (transcutaneous electrical neuromuscular stimulation)[23-27]	Manage acute and chronic pain	High frequency (>50 Hz) with an intensity below motor contraction (sensory intensity) or low frequency (<10 Hz) with an intensity that produces motor contraction	Cancer Damaged skin Pregnancy Epilepsy Infection Thrombosis Should not be used near the eyes, genitals, oral cavity, or carotid sinus
Iontophoresis	Electrical stimulation that is used to help administer medication for: Analgesia Decreased inflammation Wound healing Edema	10-20 min treatment Active electrode (commercial or reusable) applied with medication with a dispersive pad Current flow and density are determined by medication and area size.*	Chemical burns are the most common consideration and should be monitored. People with known skin sensitivities may wish to avoid iontophoresis.
Low-intensity stimulation (LIS) or microcurrent electrical nerve stimulator (MENS)	Analgesia Restored cellular balance Tissue healing Facture healing	Extremely small microcurrent (less than 1 mA) of electrical impulses transmitted to nerves	LIS/MENS is currently applied based on theory. Evidence is lacking. Theory is that current intensities are too small to excite the peripheral nerves.
Neuromuscular electrical stimulation (NMES)	Creates muscle contraction to do the following: Decrease muscular spasm Retard muscle atrophy Strengthen muscles Promote blood flow to enhance tissue healing	Typically 75 pps (pulses per sec): 12 sec on, 50 sec off for 15-20 min	Consideration: Primarily used for muscle reeducation but less noxious than Russian stimulation Contraindications: Cancer Damaged skin Pregnancy Epilepsy Infection Thrombosis Should not be used near the eyes, genitals, oral cavity, or carotid sinus

Modality	Indications	Application	Contraindications and considerations
Russian stimulation	Produces same outcomes as NMES but may be more tolerable	2,500 Hz, AC current bursts modulated every 10 msec	Cancer Damaged skin Pregnancy Epilepsy Infection Thrombosis Should not be used near the eyes, genitals, oral cavity, or carotid sinus
Interferential current (IFC)	Decrease pain Decrease muscular spasm Improve localized blood flow	Place electrodes around the affected area so that the target tissue is centered. Apply currents for 10-20 min: 20-25 pps for muscle contraction and 50-120 pps for pain management	Consideration: The effect is similar to other electrical stimulation currents but may create a larger area of stimulation. Contraindications: Cancer Damaged skin Pregnancy Epilepsy Infection Thrombosis Should not be used near the eyes, genitals, oral cavity, or carotid sinus
High-voltage galvanic stimulation (HVGS) or high-volt pulsed stimulation (HVPS)	Relieve pain Improve blood flow Relieve muscle spasm Improve joint mobility Heal ulcers	Pulse rate: 80 pps Treatment duration: 20-30 min	Safer and more comfortable than Russian stimulation Penetrates deeper than low-voltage currents Effective for direct stimulation of deep nerves and muscles Does not produce contraction in the denervated muscle Partially innervated or totally innervated muscle responds well

*Practitioners should seek additional training and knowledge and research their state's legal parameters prior to any implementation of electrical modalities.

Electromagnetic Modalities

Electromagnetic energy modalities typically involve a high-energy source that is transmitted by the movement of photons.[2,32-35] Diathermy and infrared modalities are the most common forms of electromagnetic modalities used by athletic trainers to enhance tissue healing by increasing cellular activity.

Diathermy

Diathermy therapies are used when a heating effect in the tissues is desired without motor or sensory stimulation.[36-40]

Diathermy therapies are high-frequency modalities that use radiation with more than 1 million cycles per second. The high radiation cycles increase tissue temperature, generating heat that is absorbed by body cells, and produce regenerative tissue healing effects.[37-40] Table 21.7 lists diathermy modalities.

Light Therapy

Literature regarding light therapy has focused on low-level laser therapy (LLLT) for tissue healing properties;[41,42] more recently, light-emitting diodes (LEDs) have

indicated promise in therapeutic treatments with the same effects.[42-46] Light amplification by stimulated emission of radiation (LASER) produces both visible and infrared light. High-powered lasers are used medically in surgeries for cauterization and incisions. LLLT, also known as cold lasers, emits little to no thermal effects but enables tissue healing. Parameters for LLLT and LED vary based on the type of gas and light used and the intended tissues; thus, to ensure patient safety, athletic trainers should do further study before applying light therapy. Infrared modalities are listed in table 21.8.

TABLE 21.7 Diathermy Modalities

Modality	Indications	Application	Contraindications and considerations

Shortwave diathermy[18-21]	Tissue heating
	Tissue extensibility
	Postacute tissue healing
		Continuous or pulsed:
		  heating up to 3 cm
		Treatment times:
		  20-30 min
			More effective than ultrasound for larger areas
			Use if pressure from transducer is contraindicated
			Contraindications for heat apply

TABLE 21.8 Infrared Modalities

Modality	Indications	Application	Contraindications and considerations
Low-level LASER[41,42, 46-53] (light amplification by stimulated emission or radiation)	Wound healing Analgesia Anti-inflammatory	Make gentle contact with the skin perpendicular to the target tissues. Base dosage on pulse frequency and treatment time and review it based on laser type and gas prior to implementation. Further information is necessary to conduct laser therapy.	May be performed on open lesions, burns, and ulcers. No deleterious effects currently reported. Do not use near the eyes. Contraindications: Pregnancy Cancerous tissue Growing cartilage (in youth) Skin disease Epilepsy Cardiac problems Deep vein thrombosis
LED[41,43-53] (light emitting diodes)	Wound healing Analgesia Muscle fatigue	Parameters are similar to laser and should be followed accordingly.	Comparison of laser and LED is inconclusive as to differences or similarities in outcomes.[22] LED is a less expensive modality.

EVIDENCE-BASED ATHLETIC TRAINING

Infrared Laser Wavelength and Tissue Depth of Penetration

Therapeutic infrared laser wavelengths are in the optical spectrum, which ranges from the red spectrum to near infrared (NIR) wavelengths (600-1,070 nm). Depending on the amount of energy or power delivered, expressed in joules (J), the tissue depth of penetration varies from 0.5 to 3 mm.[55-57]

- Orange spectrum light has a wavelength of 600 nm and penetrates 0.5 to 1 mm.
- Red spectrum light has a wavelength of 600 to 650 nm and penetrates 0.1 to 2 mm.
- Deep red spectrum light has a wavelength of 650 to 950 nm and penetrates 2 to 3 mm.
- NIR light has a wavelength of 950 to 1,000 nm and penetrates 1 mm.

Sound Modalities

Ultrasound is a deep-heating modality that is inaudible to the human ear. Ultrasound functions by creating a mechanical vibration through sound waves that pass into tissue and create thermal physiological effects. Frequency of ultrasound wave productions is between 700,000 and 1 million cycles per second. Waves can penetrate up to 5 cm deep. Ultrasound travels well though homogenous tissue and can therefore reach deeper depths than electromagnetic radiation or superficial heat, where the transfer of energy has a greater absorption.

Both nonthermal and thermal effects of ultrasounds are used for tissue healing. Heating tissue theories vacillate between the need for a raised tissue temperature between 40°C and 45°C for at least 5 minutes and the quantity of tissue increases in baseline temperature, yet the evidence is vague. Regardless, literature indicates that ultrasound tissue temperature increases depend on the tissue type, presence of adipose tissue, MHz, and time application. Heating occurs with both pulsed and continuous ultrasound. Unlike other heating modalities, ultrasound also has nonthermal effects. Little evidence exists that identifies the effect of ultrasound intensity on final tissue temperature; thus, clinicians should be cautious. However, it is generally accepted that the lower the intensity (W/cm^3), the shorter the treatment duration; the lower the frequency (MHz), the greater the depth of penetration. In order to transmit the acoustic energy, a coupling medium is required. These include water, oils, topical analgesics, gel packs, gel pads, and varying types of gel. The evidence indicates that all coupling mediums have similar transmission outcomes.[58-64]

Ultrasound may also be used with other modalities, such as hot packs, electrical stimulation, and exercise. Advanced inquiry and physiological understanding are needed to appropriately apply these skills and concepts with patients.

An ultrasound machine is shown in figure 21.1 and various ultrasound techniques are shown in figure 21.2. Ultrasound modalities are listed in table 21.9.

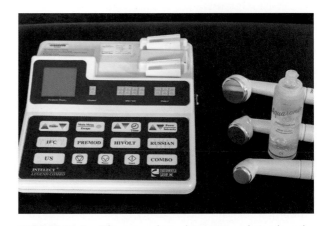

FIGURE 21.1 Ultrasound machine, transducer heads, and gel.

EVIDENCE-BASED ATHLETIC TRAINING

Depth of Ultrasound Penetration

Ultrasound penetration is based on intensity and frequency. The following are general guidelines for frequency depth:

1 MHz: depth of 2 to 5 cm

3 MHz: depth of 0.5 to 1.5 cm

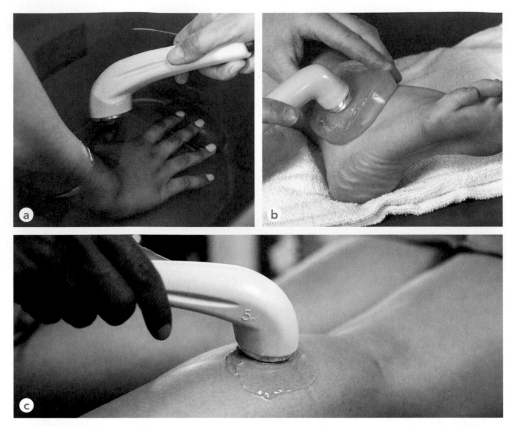

FIGURE 21.2   Ultrasound techniques: *(a)* water technique, *(b)* bladder technique, and *(c)* traditional technique.

TABLE 21.9   **Ultrasound Modalities**

Modality	Indications	Application	Contraindications and considerations
Nonthermal ultrasound (sometimes called pulsed)	Soft-tissue repair Bone healing	Continuous: 0.1-0.2 W/cm^3 Duty cycle 20%: 1 W/cm^3 (also aids fracture healing)[65] 1 or 2 times a day for 6-8 days; if acute, every other day[66-70]	Areas of bone growth/epiphyseal plates Pacemakers Fracture healing Vascular disease Ischemic tissue Neurologically compromised/decreased sensation Pregnancy Cancer Should not be used over the eyes, genitals, or oral cavity
Thermal ultrasound (sometimes called continuous)	Increase tissue extensibility Decrease joint stiffness Reduce muscle space Modulate pain Increase blood flow	Treatment time: 5-10 min at 1-3 MHz, depending on depth desired Continuous ultrasound intensity	
Phonophoresis[72-74]	Delivery of medication into tissues (typically anti-inflammatory medications) Benefit: no damage to tissue and noninvasive	Both thermal and nonthermal parameters (previously mentioned) may be used.	
Low-intensity pulsed ultrasound (LIPUS)[74-77]	Nonunion fractures	1.5 MHz, pulsed at 30 mW/cm^3	Contraindication: same as for ultrasound. Evidence is lacking for use in prevention Useful for nonunion fractures

Ultrasound Treatment Protocols

Appropriate application of ultrasound requires attention to patient preparation, equipment safety, correct parameters, and patient safety in sequence.[76-83]

- Select thermal or nonthermal technique based on the patient's needs.
- Verify the unit is on 0 prior to turning it on.
- Apply a coupling agent no bigger than 16 square in. (40 cm^2) in diameter to the treatment area.
- Monitor time based on the identified treatment duration.
- Maintain continuous contact between the soundhead and the treatment area, moving the soundhead in a circular overlapping manner. A speed of 3 to 4 cm/sec is ideal.
- Maintain continuous conversation with the patient. Turn off the unit if the patient experiences pain or extreme heat.
- Clean the patient's body to remove all coupling agents after the treatment is complete.

Mechanical Modalities

Mechanical modalities use an object to provide motion that creates a therapeutic effect. In the context of athletic training, this object can be the clinician's hands or implements that provide a force to soft-tissue structures. Common mechanical modalities in athletic training include traction, massage (including instrument-assisted soft-tissue mobilization, or IASTM) and intermittent compression (table 21.10).

Soft-Tissue Mobilization

Soft-tissue mobilization (STM) is a form of manual therapy that addresses soft-tissue injury. STM uses both specially designed instruments and hands-on techniques to enhance healing, reduce pain, and increase range of motion. STM may be implemented using specific techniques that are applied during appropriate tissue healing times.

TABLE 21.10 Mechanical Modalities

Modality	Definition	Indications	Application	Contraindications and considerations
Mechanical traction: Manual traction:	Creation of tension that is applied to a body segment. Traction may be manual or mechanical.	Most commonly used for the spine. Also used for the following: Nerve root impingement Vertebral disc herniation Spondylolisthesis Decrease muscle spasm Ligament sprain Pain reduction	Traction application varies depending on device or manual technique used	Unstable spine Ligament instability Arthritis Osteoporosis Severe anxiety Cauda equina syndrome Osteomyelitis Artery insufficiency

> continued

Table 21.10   *>continued*

Modality	Definition	Indications	Application	Contraindications and considerations
Intermittent compression[2,71]	Unit that provides external pressure to reduce edema.	Edema Lymphatic dysfunction Improve circulation	Application and setting vary depending on appendage. The sleeve should be applied prior to inflation. The patient should be in a comfortable position, which may include elevation when indicated. Inflation to an appropriate setting is then indicated. Continued observation is necessary to ensure compression is not constricting blood flow or creating a neural response.	Deep vein thrombosis Compartment syndromes Vascular insufficiencies Fracture Pulmonary edema Congestive heart failure Combine with elevation for the best results. Pressure should not exceed the patient's diastolic blood pressure. Current evidence is thin regarding treatment protocols.

Instrument-Assisted Soft-Tissue Mobilization

Instrument-assisted soft-tissue mobilization (IASTM) is a manual therapy that uses instruments to facilitate the healing process by assisting in the formation of new extracellular protein matrices (i.e., collagen).[84-87] IASTM originated in China as the ancient technique of Gua Sha, in which the skin was scraped with instruments such as smooth bone, stones, and spoons; today, the technique uses manufactured set of tools (figure 21.3).[88-91] IASTM is used for soft-tissue mobilization (e.g., scar tissue, myofascial adhesion) to decrease pain and improve ROM and function. The use of an instrument over the skin is thought to reduce the stress imposed on the practitioner's hands and body and provide a mechanical advantage in soft-tissue mobilization. Some experimental studies and case reports suggest that IASTM can significantly improve soft tissue function and ROM following sports injury and reduce pain, potentially decreasing the duration of rehabilitation and the time needed to return to activity.[92-96] However, case reports account for the majority of literature and the totality of the experimental research on IASTM is inconclusive. IASTM research and outcome reliability are still evolving.

Massage

Massage for medical purposes is defined as the manipulation of the body's soft tissues through techniques

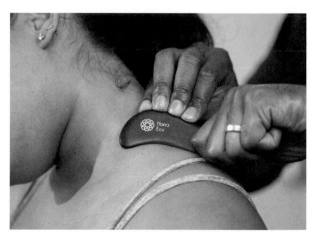

FIGURE 21.3   IASTM tools.

that bring about specific responses, including stroking, rubbing, kneading, compressing, and applying percussion and vibration.[97] In general, the evidence for the use of massage for physiological and psychological purposes is variable, but provides a framework for use.[98,99] Responses to massage are mechanical, physiological, and psychological (table 21.11).

The fundamentals of massage are distilled into five categories, each with a specific indication and desired physical response (table 21.12). General contraindications for massage include acute injury, surgery or illness, deep vein thrombosis, frostbite, contagious skin conditions, open wounds, and burns.

TABLE 21.11   **Responses to Massage**

Response	Effect	Example
Mechanical[98-101]	Venous and lymphatic drainage Mild stretching	A patient post surgery who is immobilized for 3 weeks may receive massage (post incision healing) to maintain elasticity of the scar, skin, and connective tissue.
Physiological[98-101]	Increase circulation Assist in tissue healing process (postacute) Increase nerve conductivity Decrease inflammation (postacute) Relaxation (**effleurage**) Stimulation (vibration and **tapotement**)	Postacute quadriceps strain (14 days) in a geriatric tennis player with a residual hematoma, decreased ROM, and pain with contraction. Massage is indicated to increase extensibility and decrease the hematoma.
Psychological[100,102-104]	Confidence between provider and patient Decrease anxiety Increase perception of recovery	A high school swimmer has anxiety prior to each race based on past experience with a back injury that has not reoccurred for 3 months. Sport massage prior to competition has reduced the anxiety level of the athlete and helped him maintain performance.

TABLE 21.12   **Massage Techniques**

Technique	Indications	Application	
Effleurage (stroking)	Relaxation Sedation	Hands move in unison to stroke the designated tissues. Light and deep methods exist.	
Petrissage (kneading)	Increase tissue extensibility in muscular tissue	Pick up muscle and skin between thumb and forefinger, rolling and twisting in opposite directions. Alternate hands.	
Friction	Increase circulation to joints, scars, adhesions, and fascia Decrease muscle spasms	Using the heel of the hand or fingers, apply pressure in a small circular motion. The purpose is to stretch the underlying tissue through friction.	

> continued

Table 21.12 >*continued*

Technique	Indications	Application
Tapotement (percussion)	Stimulate tissue to increase blood flow and tissue extensibility.	Techniques include cupping, pinching, and hacking.
Vibration	Relaxation and soothing Stimulation of tissue (sport massage)	Rapid movement creates a quivering or trembling effect on the tissue.

Specialty massage exists to increase tissue extensibility (deep transverse friction massage) and relax hyperactive muscle spaces (acupressure massage). These techniques are used with increasing frequency in sport massage, a treatment modality specifically for the active population that enhances physiological and psychological responses to benefit performance.[97] Sports massage is performed on a designated body area rather than the whole body, since full-body massage may relax the patient to the extent that she is not able to be responsive in activity.[98-105]

Evolving and Emerging Therapeutic Modalities

Evolving and emerging therapeutic modalities are ever evolving. As such, you should consistently review current and new evidence to determine the best practices for patient care. Additional approaches not specifically addressed in this chapter include the following:

- *Whole-body vibration.* This is a mechanical intervention that creates body vibrations by standing on a vibration platform, holding vibration apparatus (i.e., dumbbells or pulley systems), or directly applying a vibration unit to a specific muscle belly or tendon. The literature suggests promising outcomes in increasing leg strength,[106-109] proprioception, balance, and spinal reflex neuropathways.[110-118]

- *Therapeutic magnets.* This alternative medical practice uses static magnets for the purpose of alleviating pain. The magnets may be in the form of bracelets, necklaces, or individual magnets that are placed on body areas with a compression-type wrap. Current literature indicates a lack of efficacy.[119-122]

- *Cupping.* This alternative medicine practice uses suction cups of various forms for the purpose of pain reduction, tissue healing, and tissue extensibility. Variations include flash cupping, moving cupping, and wet cupping. The ancient form of cupping involves heating a glass cup and placing it on the skin to create a vacuum. More recent interventions use a cup with suction to create a vacuum. The literature on cupping efficacy is variable and indicates some benefits depending on the technique and purpose.[123-131]

- *Infrared heat lamps.* Also known as heat lamps, infrared heat lamps are used to treat pain,[128,132,133] muscle strains, skin lesions (i.e., acne, rashes and infections),[134] and nose, ear, and sinus infections.[133,135] The infrared bulb may penetrate 3 to 9 in. (8-23 cm). Infrared is the light waveband longer than 760 nm and up to 1 mm.[136] Although a therapy used for decades, a resurgence in recent years has occurred with limited evidence of efficacy.[128-135]

- *Vapocoolant spray.* Vapocoolants, or cold sprays, are used for topical pain relief, often associated with trigger points, or to anesthetize skin prior to injections. Current literature indicates a lack of efficacy for trigger-point or pain management.[137-141]

- *Platelet-rich plasma (PRP) therapy.* PRP therapy is purported to accelerate the healing of injured tendons, ligaments, muscles, and joints through injecting a concentration of a patient's own platelets. PRP injections theoretically use a patient's own platelets to heal musculoskeletal injury. PRP treatment appears promising for some musculoskeletal diseases, but evidence of efficacy is variable depending on the injury and specific indication.[142]

- *Pneumatic compression device (PCD).* PCD is a mechanical, inflatable device with compression garments including sleeves, gloves, or boots to achieve therapeutic improvement of venous circulation. PCD is typically employed for patients with edema or those who are at risk of deep vein thrombosis or pulmonary embolism. Advantages from daily treatments using a PCD are likely to be even greater. PCD is purported to improve exercise performance and speed muscle recovery, but the literature provides little support for the articulated benefits.[143-145]

- *Blood flow restriction therapy.* Blood flow restriction is a therapeutic technique that applies external cuff pressure to a limb to occlude venous outflow while at the same time maintaining partial arterial inflow. The efficacy of blood flow restriction therapy in the literature is variable with a lack of strong study design but may prove promising for elderly populations.[146-148]

These modalities lack robust evidence and outcomes to suggest that current uses are effective, yet continuous investigation and outcome studies may alter practices in the future. Athletic trainers should review the evidence routinely.

Purchasing and Maintaining Equipment

Therapeutic modality equipment requires routine maintenance, calibration, and electrical checks to ensure that it is safe and delivers accurate treatment

---

FOUNDATIONAL SKILL

Effective Therapeutic Massage

Athletic trainers must understand how to provide effective therapeutic massage. Ensure that the patient is comfortable and in a proper position on the table.

- Place padding where needed below the patient.
- Ensure that the table as at an adequate height for your comfort during the massage.
- Respect the patient's privacy by draping a sheet over any body parts not being massaged.
- Ensure that the room is a comfortable temperature.

  Use a confident yet gentle touch to maintain the patient's physical and psychological comfort. Massage lubricants may be needed to easily slide your hands over the identified body area.

- Rubbing or friction of a dry body area may irritate the skin.
- Petroleum-based lubricants and oil liniments are best used for therapeutic massage.

parameters. A plan for routine upgrades and purchase of new equipment is necessary to ensure the safety of patients and use of contemporary, viable equipment.

Equipment should be evaluated annually to assess damage and remaining life and safety. As much as possible, equipment should meet evidence-based guidelines. Therapeutic modality assessment includes a visual check for broken or frayed electrical cords, calibration and electrical checks from a licensed technician, and an assessment of evidence-based use. In addition, a facility designee should review research on new and upcoming rehabilitation devices or modifications and advise the facility on the need for potential purchases that should be added to the annual budget and long-term replacement budget.

CLINICAL BOTTOM LINE

- Patient safety is of the utmost importance when using therapeutic modalities. To ensure patient safety, athletic trainers should know and routinely check current state laws to determine legality of use and reassess the best available evidence on appropriately applying treatment.

- Thermal therapies, such as hot packs (moist heat packs) and warm whirlpool, are typically applied to increase collagen tissue extensibility, relieve muscle spasms, decrease pain or muscle spasm, reduce inflammation postacutely, and increase blood flow.

- Cold therapies, such as ice packs and cold whirlpool, are primarily used after acute injury to mitigate the inflammatory process. For optimal effects, they should be used in conjunction with rest, ice, compression, and elevation. Cold modalities are also used to modulate pain for subacute and chronic injuries.

- Electrical energy modalities have diverse treatment modes and units, but they all generally produce beneficial effects that assist with pain control, muscle contractions, muscle strengthening, minimizing atrophy, muscle reeducation and tissue extensibility. Careful selection of electrical modality and a healthy understanding of the evidence are necessary to appropriately apply these concepts to enhance patient care.

- Diathermy and infrared modalities are the most common forms of electromagnetic modalities used by athletic trainers. They enhance tissue healing by increasing cellular activity. Diathermy heats tissue with vibration to modulate pain and increase tissue extensibility and healing, whereas infrared modalities lack the thermal component to augment tissue healing.

- Ultrasound is a sound energy modality that is inaudible to the human ear. It provides deep heating and its thermal effects increase tissue extensibility, decrease joint stiffness, reduce muscle spasm, increase blood flow, and assist with pain modulation. It is also used to heal tissue without the thermal components of sound energy.

- Mechanical energy modalities use an object such as the clinician's hands (massage or traction) or an implement (traction, intermittent compression) to provide a force to soft-tissue structures, creating a therapeutic effect. The use of mechanical energy modalities may assist in the tissue healing process (postacute), increase nerve conductivity, decrease inflammation (postacute), decrease anxiety, or produce relaxation.

- Evolving, emerging, and alternative modalities, such as magnets and whole-body vibration, lack evidence of effective outcomes; therefore, they should not be unilaterally implemented into therapeutic rehabilitation regimens. More investigation on interventions is required.

 Go to HKPropel to complete the activities and case studies for this chapter.

Go to HKPropel to view videos of ultrasound applications and various therapeutic interventions.

CHAPTER 22

Therapeutic Exercise in Rehabilitation

Mitchell Wasik, MS, ATC, LAT

Leamor Kahanov, EdD, ATC, LAT

CAATE STANDARDS

The following CAATE 2020 standard is covered in this chapter:

Standard 73

CHAPTER OBJECTIVES

After reading this chapter, you will be able to do the following:

- Define therapeutic exercise

- Differentiate between therapeutic exercise and exercise for conditioning

- List various components of therapeutic exercise

- Identify different approaches to rehabilitation programs

- Describe how to purchase and maintain therapeutic equipment

Therapeutic exercise is integral in injury rehabilitation and maintenance. Athletic training practice in all settings requires an understanding of therapeutic exercise. Athletic trainers may need to educate patients regarding home programs, implement therapeutic exercise programs, or facilitate therapeutic exercise on site. To ensure continuity of therapeutic care, athletic trainers may also need to work with other health care providers, such as physical therapists, strength and conditioning professionals, occupational therapists, and physicians. Athletic trainers are often in the role of coordinating and monitoring care, which often includes therapeutic exercise intervention.

Athletic trainers are obligated to provide optimal care for patients, which includes assessing patient needs to determine the therapeutic exercise interventions essential for achieving desired clinical and patient outcomes. This chapter provides a foundational understanding of therapeutic exercise in evidence-based practice in athletic training, focusing on research modes and models. For more information on advanced therapeutic exercise regimens and concepts, investigate the sources cited in each section further.

Therapeutic Exercise Overview

Therapeutic exercise is a component of rehabilitation that addresses the return of injured patients to pain-free function or activity. The purpose of therapeutic exercise is to restore normal function to an injured anatomical area or chronic physical dysfunction by incorporating a wide range of physical activities that focus on restoring and maintaining strength, endurance, flexibility, stability, and balance. Therapeutic exercise differs from general fitness exercise or training and conditioning, which affect overall health and reduces the likelihood and influence of injury.[1-6] However, components of general fitness and conditioning are included in therapeutic exercises for the purposes of rehabilitation of injury and return to the patient's normal function. Fitness and wellness are discussed in chapter 9. People who lack cardiovascular fitness, optimal strength, and range of motion have a greater incidence of injury and may incur a longer recovery.[1-6]

To ensure that a patient is ready to return to activities of daily living or exercise and sport, therapeutic exercise addresses the following aspects of rehabilitation:

- Inflammation
- Pain
- Range of motion
- Strength
- Endurance
- Power
- Neuromuscular control
- Balance
- Cardiorespiratory fitness

Athletic trainers address these aspects of rehabilitation through a planned process that includes multiple techniques to facilitate return to participation in activity or sport. Therapeutic exercise may be distilled into specific components, each of which manages a specific aspect of physical function:

- Balance and postural control
- Neuromuscular control
- Physical inactivity and immobilization
- Range of motion and tissue extensibility
- Therapeutic strengthening, endurance, and power exercises
- Tissue healing

This chapter identifies the most common therapeutic exercises and facilitated techniques. Further study is necessary to ensure patient safety and accurately implement patient-centered rehabilitation programs.

Physical Inactivity and Immobilization

Initially, you should address your patients' physical inactivity and immobilization to minimize loss of strength and flexibility while decreasing pain and inflammation. Incurred injury affects two aspects of the human condi-

tion: general fitness and specific loss, which may include function, strength, and range of motion to the injured area. The human body is intended to maintain dynamic movement for proper functioning of muscles, ligaments, joints, the cardiorespiratory system, and neural integration with the aforementioned systems.[7] The effects of immobilization on anatomical and orthopedic function result in the loss of muscle mass, strength, coordination, and endurance. Appropriate implementation of therapeutic exercise can mitigate the effects of immobilization or disuse of an anatomical area.

General conditioning is also affected when activity is ceased. Continued exercise—both general and specific to the injured area—without aggravation of the injury is optimal for maintaining function; facilitating this sort of exercise is part of your role as an athletic trainer. A decrease in function occurs for all body systems with immobilization. Muscle **atrophy** (reduction of muscle mass) occurs within 24 hours of immobilization or disuse. Joints need the compression that occurs from motion to lubricate the articular cartilage and provide nutrition to the surfaces. Without nutrition, joints degenerate, neuromuscular fibers decrease recruitment, and strength and power diminish, reducing function (table 22.1). Within the limits of the injury, general fitness and motion should be maintained.

Rehabilitation Program Essentials

Rehabilitation begins with a well-conditioned person before injury or illness. The better conditioned the patient is in terms of cardiovascular fitness, strength, and range of motion, the better her rehabilitation outcomes will be. Regardless of a patient's overall fitness level, after acute injury or a surgical intervention, an initial acute first aid and injury management process that includes pain and inflammation control is crucial to early successes in rehabilitation.[18] In addition, to ensure a safe return to physical activity, you should work with patients to reestablish neuromuscular control, address range of motion, and restore muscular strength and endurance. During therapeutic rehabilitation, you should also assess balance and postural control, core strength, and cardiorespiratory endurance as appropriate for the patient. Lastly, promote a return to physical activity after the patient has successfully passed functional testing (see table 22.2).

Rehabilitation Phases Based on Tissue Healing

Therapeutic rehabilitation is generally planned based on tissue healing phases (see figure 22.1). Rehabilita-

TABLE 22.1   **Effects of Physical Inactivity and Immobilization**

Anatomical area	Effect	Rehabilitation or intervention
Muscle (general)[7-11]	Atrophy (loss of muscle mass) occurs. Protein synthesis is reduced without movement.	Immobilization in an elongated position leads to less atrophy than in a shortened position.
Type I muscle fibers	Type I (slow-twitch) fibers develop fast-twitch characteristics.[7] The number of fibers is reduced.	Isometric contractions and some types of electrical stimulation may reduce atrophy.
Neuromuscular	Stimulation of muscle fibers are decreased due to a reduction of motor nerve recruitment and stimulation.[12,13]	Movement reactivates motor neurons within 1 week.[8]
Joints	Lubrication is reduced, resulting in degeneration of articular cartilage.	A continuous passive motion machine, hinged braces, and some electrical stimulation can reduce the loss of articular cartilage.[9]
Ligaments and bone	Strength decreases.[10-13]	After immobilization, high-frequency, short-duration exercise increases the hypertrophy of collagen fibers, with full remodeling achieved in 1 to 2 years.[12-15]
Cardiorespiratory	Decreases occur in stroke volume, maximum oxygen uptake, and vital capacity with immobilization. Resting heart rate increases by 1 half-beat per minute each day of immobilization.[16,17]	Addressing movement and general fitness within the limits of the immobilization will minimize negative outcomes.

TABLE 22.2   **Rehabilitation Components**

	Rehabilitation components	Effect from injury	Outcome
Acute injury: postoperatively and throughout rehabilitation	Control and minimize inflammation	Swelling, secondary cellular or tissue death	Decreased pain
	Control and minimize pain	Altered use of body part, disuse, malcoordination	Restoration of normal function
	Address neuromuscular control	Joint mechanoreceptors, muscle mechanoreceptors	Restoration of control and normal function
Address after pain and inflammation are under control	Range of motion (ROM)	Decreased ROM due to pain, tissue damage, protective reflex	Restoration of normal, pain-free ROM
	Muscular strength	Decreased strength due to tissue damage or pain	Restoration of normal, pain-free strength
	Muscular endurance	Decreased endurance due to pain or decreased strength	Increased duration of pain-free strength
Evaluate and address as appropriate	Balance and postural control	Decreased proprioception, decreased neuromuscular control	Increased pain-free balance and muscle coordination
	Cardiovascular endurance	Decreased due to protective disuse	Minimize and maintain throughout healing.
	Core strength	Reflexive malcoordination due to pain	Maintain basic core function through base-level exercises.

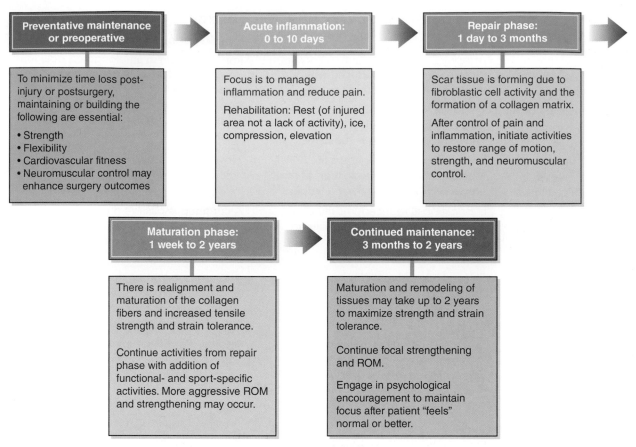

FIGURE 22.1   Rehabilitation phases based on tissue healing time.

tion phases can include 4 to 6 components, depending on the author of the plan, yet all plans are based on the known tissue healing parameters identified in chapter 15.

Different tissues have slight variances in healing times, which are also influenced by the health and age of the patient. Additional advanced knowledge of these parameters and how they contribute to healing is required for disseminating any rehabilitation regimen. Tissue healing times depend on severity of injury, the patient's overall health, initial injury care, and additional health care issues or disability (see chapter 15).

FOUNDATIONAL SKILL

Rehabilitation Plan Process

1. Determine the level of pain using a pain scale. Use the pain level to determine an appropriate therapeutic rehabilitation for reducing pain.

2. Assess the joint's range of motion (ROM). Determine what may be limiting the joint's ROM. Based on your findings, create a treatment plan by selecting appropriate therapeutic interventions to return to full ROM.

3. Determine the strength of all the muscles that surround the injury or site of chronic dysfunction. Based on the strength findings or imbalances, select appropriate strengthening exercises.

4. Before implementing ROM and strengthening exercises, determine what therapeutic rehabilitation interventions may achieve both outcomes. For example, squats can increase ROM in the knee and strength in the thigh.

5. Continually reevaluate pain, ROM, and strength with the rehabilitation plan to maximize rehabilitation efficacy and reduce time needed to return to activity.

Rehabilitation plans should be individualized for each patient. Rehabilitation planning can involve a complex decision-making process that encompasses patient goals, patient evaluation and reevaluation, and appropriate exercise and therapy selection. Further study beyond the foundational information provided in this chapter is necessary for implementing rehabilitation planning. After diagnosis, acute injury, or surgery, the athletic trainer will use the patient assessment to create a rehabilitation plan that includes a time line and outlines the types of therapy necessary for return to activity. A rehabilitation plan includes the following, in order of assessment:

1. Pain level
2. Range of motion
3. Strength
4. Dysfunctional movement patterns (typically chronic issues)

Therapeutic Strengthening, Endurance, and Power Exercises

Components of therapeutic exercise include muscular strengthening, endurance, and power exercises, which may also address ROM or tissue extensibility and neuromuscular activity.[23-25] Strengthening concepts can be used across the phases of rehabilitation if appropriately applied based on tissue healing, patient feedback, and safety. This concept is called **progressive strengthening** or **progressive resistance exercises**. Athletic trainers should consider tissue healing and strength when developing rehabilitative strengthening exercises. The degree of tissue healing and strength has implications for the type of strengthening protocol so as to limit aggravating the healing process.

The basic concepts of strengthening and conditioning for fitness also apply to rehabilitation. **Isotonic, isometric**, and **isokinetic** strengthening are primary techniques used for both rehabilitation and conditioning.

Isotonic

- Muscle contraction that occurs with constant tension as the muscle changes length
- Contractions can be **concentric** (muscle shortening) or **eccentric** (muscle lengthening)

Isometric

- Strengthening where joint angle and muscular length do not change
- Activities include free weights and resistance bands with manual resistance

Isokinetic

- Contraction similar to isotonic (concentric and eccentric), but done at a constant speed
- Typically used during the remodeling and maturation phase
- Activities include isokinetic machines

The following strengthening techniques can be used both concentrically and eccentrically, based on tissue strength and phase of rehabilitation:

Concentric Muscular Contraction

- Shortening of a muscle that is contracting; critical for power
- Activities include free weights, resistance bands, isotonic exercise machines, and manual resistance

Eccentric Muscular Contraction

- Elongation of muscle while contracting to an opposing force (deceleration)
- Activities include free weights, resistance bands, isotonic exercise machines, and manual resistance.

For a review of fitness and wellness concepts, see chapter 9.

Neuromuscular Control

Neuromuscular control is an umbrella term identifying the body's ability to efficiently create and reduce force through movement control using a combination of **proprioception**, kinesthetic awareness, and dynamic stability. It is an essential component of therapy and reconditioning that is applied in all phases of rehabilitation. Understanding a body's position in space or the joint angle is imperative to establishing normal functional movement and timing after injury. The components for establishing neuromuscular control are as follows:[8]

Criteria for Return to Full Activity	
No pain	Full range of motion
No inflammation	Neuromuscular control
Full strength	Ability to meet all activity-specific demands

- *Proprioception:* stationary awareness or knowledge of where a body part is in space (e.g., knowing that your arm is at 90 degrees of abduction when the arm is stationary).
- *Kinesthetic awareness:* the body's ability to sense position in space through and during movement (e.g., the ability to move your arm to 90 degrees of abduction).
- *Dynamic stability:* the ability to maintain proper joint position throughout motion (e.g., moving your arm to 90 degrees of abduction while maintaining the body in an anatomically correct

position so as not to create undue joint stresses that might result in shoulder impingement).

- *Agility:* muscle preparation and reaction to sensory movements that are appropriate in scope and strength.

Neuromuscular control exercises involve a range of activities that include balance and functional movements[26-28] (figure 22.2). These activities include proprioceptive exercises, which are a component of neuromuscular control. Proprioceptive exercises require either repetition of activities in order to reestablish a pattern of movement or a step-by-step progression from

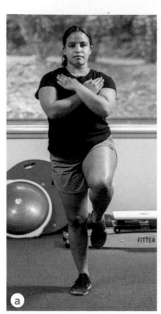
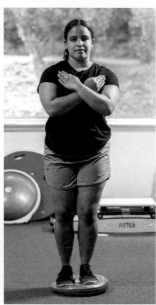
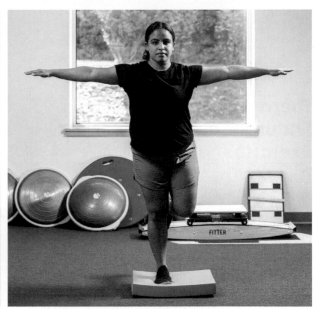
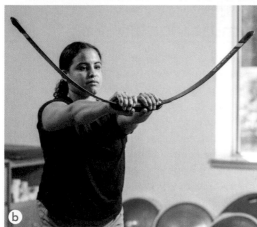
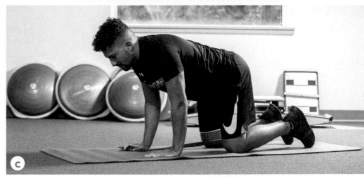
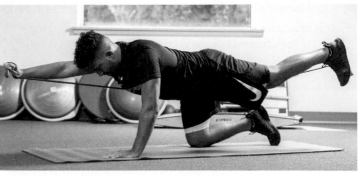

FIGURE 22.2 Neuromuscular control exercises: *(a)* balance progression, *(b)* upper extremity and core, and *(c)* lower extremity and core.

simple to complex movements associated with the need for increased strength (table 22.3). Note that kinesthetic awareness and dynamic stability are developed through proprioceptive exercises with movement. The connection from the central nervous system to the activity action is critical for controlled movement of sensory patterns.

Practitioner-Assisted Therapeutic Exercise

Beyond strengthening, therapeutic exercise includes multiple modes of activities and techniques that are often practitioner initiated and assisted. Athletic trainers choose the appropriate activities based on the injury or physical dysfunction in order to enhance healing and return to activity and minimize additional injury. Which practitioner-assisted therapeutic exercises are used depend on the tissue healing parameters. Table 22.4 identifies specific genres of practitioner-assisted therapeutic exercises.

Open and Closed Kinetic Chain Exercises

Open and closed kinetic chain exercises are needed to fully rehabilitate a person back to activity.

- Exercises are considered **open kinetic chain (OKC) exercises** when an extremity is free to move in space and not fixed to an object. An example of an OKC is an isotonic exercise machine where the lower leg swings freely (figure 22.3a). One advantage of OKCs is that strengthening can be isolated to specific areas or muscles.

- Exercises are considered **closed kinetic chain (CKC) exercises** when an extremity is fixed to an object like the floor or a wall. Lunges and push-ups are good examples of closed kinetic chain activities (figure 22.3b). Advantages of CKCs include kinesthetic awareness, balance, the use of functionally specific exercises, and increased joint stability during the exercise.

TABLE 22.3 Proprioception Repetition Versus Progressions

Proprioceptive repetition	Proprioceptive progression
Example 1. Lower extremity Stand on 1 leg with eyes open for 30 sec Repeat 4 times	Example 1. Lower extremity 1. Stand on 1 leg 2. Stand on 1 leg with eyes closed 3. Stand on 1 leg while bending over to pick up an object
Example 2. Upper extremity Hold a Bodyblade with palm facing down and shoulder flexed to 90 degrees for 30 sec Repeat 4 times	Example 2. Upper extremity 1. Hold a Bodyblade with palm facing down and shoulder flexed to 90 degrees 2. Hold a Bodyblade with shoulder flexed, palm facing down and shoulder flexed to 90 degrees, then supinate hand 90 degrees 3. Repeat process, horizontally abducting arm 4. Repeat process, pronating hand so palm is facing down 5. Advanced: Slowly go through a throwing motion with the Bodyblade

EVIDENCE-BASED ATHLETIC TRAINING

Neuromuscular Control Efficacy on Performance and Strength

Neuromuscular control is integral in rehabilitation and contributes to various components of the process in the facilitation of return to activity.[26,29,30]

- Evidence supports the benefits of neuromuscular training for enhancing performance in agility, jumping, and balance training.
- Evidence is inconsistent on the benefits of neuromuscular control training compared to plyometric or strength training on the effects of strength and power.
- Evidence supports that neuromuscular training after injury may prevent recurrent ankle and knee injuries.

TABLE 22.4 **Types of Rehabilitation Exercises**

Rehabilitative exercise	Benefits	Contraindications	Example of use
Open and closed kinetic chain (OKC; CKC) exercises	Muscle strengthening, cocontractive movement control	Restrictions in ROM, acute pain, poor neuromuscular control	17-year-old high school athlete with ankle sprain OKC: strengthening lower leg CKC: improving balance
Aquatic exercise	Reduced weight-bearing, reduced impact, low risk of injury	Open wounds, fear of water, current illness	63-year-old with a total knee replacement in need of progressive weight-bearing exercise, cardiovascular exercise, and strengthening of hip and leg
Proprioceptive neuro-muscular facilitation techniques	Increase neuromuscular coordination, increase ROM	Acute inflammation, acute pain, excessive joint laxity, infection	30-year-old postsurgical ACLR with loss of coordinative hip and leg muscle contraction
Joint mobilization	Decrease joint pain, increase joint ROM	Acute joint injury, acute inflammatory situation	30-year-old male with ACLR needs knee extension joint mobilization to ensure full extension
Traction	Decompress joint, decrease neuromuscular tension	Acute injury, excessive pain	56-year-old woman with L4-L5 degenerative disc disease
Myofascial release	Promote relaxation, decrease pain, increase ROM	Acute injury, inflammation, open wound, fracture healing, arthritis	19-year-old swimmer with myofascial restriction in L rotator cuff
Strain/counterstrain	Promote very gentle tension release, reduce neuromuscular pain	Pain	45-year-old woman with trapezius spasm
Instrument-assisted soft-tissue mobilization	Decrease scar tissue, increase fibroblast activation	Active infection/inflammation, DVT, active implant	63-year-old with total knee replacement to reduce scar tissue so skin doesn't limit ROM
Positional release	Decrease muscle spasm, decrease fascial tension, decrease pain	Healing wounds, fractures, infections, hypersensitive skin	17-year-old with fractured humerus removed from sling has pain in upper trapezius
Soft-tissue mobilization	Reduce scar formation, increase soft tissue motion and extensibility	Acute injury, hypersensitive skin, pregnancy, osteomyelitis, pain	17-year-old with fractured humerus removed from 6 weeks of immobilization

Placement of OKCs or CKCs within the rehabilitation phases is critical to patient safety and depends on the type of injury or surgery experienced and the type of activity the patient wants to return to. Advanced knowledge in rehabilitation is necessary for deciding where and when to incorporate OKCs and CKCs into the rehabilitation plan.

Aquatic Exercise

Aquatic exercises (figure 22.4) are appropriate for all phases of rehabilitation because the buoyancy and hydrostatic pressure are easily varied depending on the patient's needs. Aquatic therapy benefits patients by reducing weight for functional activities, promoting strengthening,

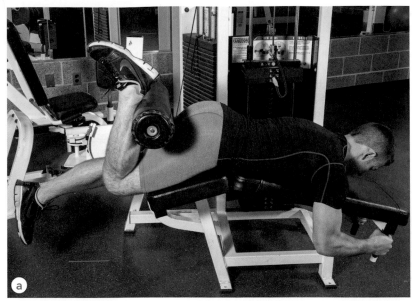
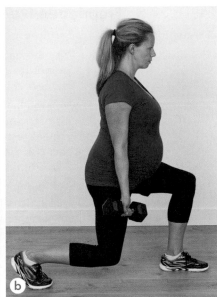

FIGURE 22.3 *(a)* Open and *(b)* closed kinetic chain exercises.

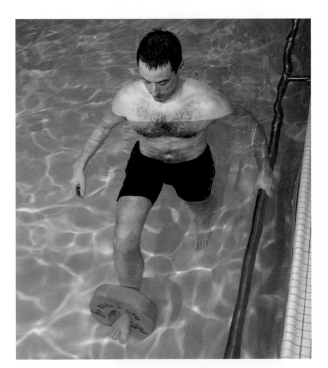

FIGURE 22.4 Example of an aquatic exercise.

and increasing range of motion, neuromuscular control, endurance, and cardiovascular fitness.[16,31-33]

Proprioceptive Neuromuscular Facilitation

Proprioceptive neuromuscular facilitation (PNF) is a rehabilitation technique that is primarily used to increase both active and passive range of motion through neuromuscular engagement by relying on reflexive stretching. Multiple PNF techniques exist and are selected by the practitioner based on the needs of the patient, injury, and contraindications. Table 22.5 provides an example for the hamstring. This technique requires manual interaction with the practitioner to elicit the initial stretch and contraction through a designated movement pattern[34-39] (figure 22.5). Selection of the movement pattern is typically based on the type of movement outcomes desired; for example, rehabilitation to return to an overhead throw may be best achieved using a D1 pattern. In order to benefit the patient, athletic trainers must have advanced knowledge of and familiarity with the prescribed PNF movement patterns, pattern selection, and activation.

EVIDENCE-BASED ATHLETIC TRAINING

PNF Efficacy

- Evidence indicates benefits of PNF for stroke patients in movement, specifically walking.[40,41] PNF is enhanced by virtual reality.[40]
- PNF may lead to improvements in behavior, mood, depression, and anxiety.[42]
- The evidence for PNF as a stretching technique indicates no difference from other stretching techniques.[42]

TABLE 22.5 **Proprioceptive Neuromuscular Stretching Techniques**

Stretching technique	Example
Hold-relax	With the hamstring on stretch, asks the patient to push against you, creating an isometric contraction, for ~10 sec. Instruct the patient to relax, and then gently increase the hamstring stretch. Repeat 2 or 3 times.
Hold-relax-contract	With the hamstring on stretch, ask the patient to push against you, creating an isometric contraction, for ~10 sec. Next, instruct the patient to relax. After the patient relaxes the isometric contraction, have him contract the quadricep for ~5 sec. Ask the patient to relax while you gently increase the hamstring stretch. Repeat 2 or 3 times.
Hold-relax-swing	With the hamstring on stretch, ask the patient to push against you, creating an isometric contraction, for ~10 sec. Instruct the patient to relax. After the patient relaxes the isometric contraction, have him contract the quadriceps while you gently increase the hamstring stretch. Repeat 2 or 3 times.
Indications	To aid in the release of neuromuscular tension to allow a greater gain in ROM
Contraindications	Joint instability, acute injury, inflammation, disease to tissue being stretched, infection

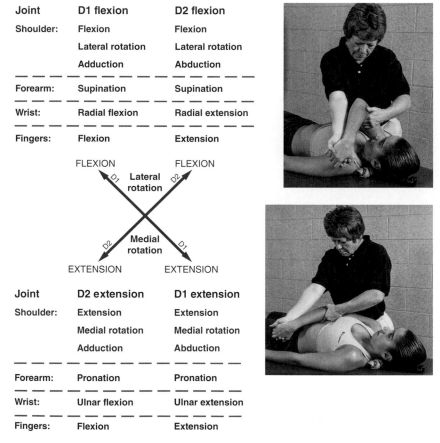

FIGURE 22.5 Upper-extremity PNF movement patterns.

Joint Mobilization

Joint mobilization is a type of manual therapy that stretches or mobilizes muscle and joint tissue to increase range of motion (figure 22.6). Joint mobilization is a passively applied technique. Many theories exist as to which joint mobilization techniques increase range of motion and enhance function. There are several gentle joint mobilization techniques:

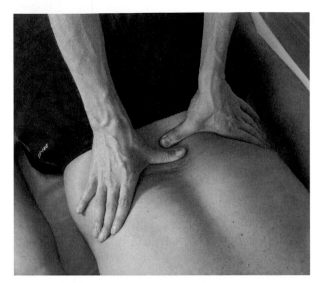

FIGURE 22.6   Example of joint mobilization.

- *Kaltenborn:* passive treatment of joint mobilization that uses sustained stretching; may include some painful motions.[43-45]
- *McKenzie:* uses joint mobilization movement and static positioning to encourage appropriate joint motion in the lumbar spine.
- *Maitland:* passive treatment of joint mobilization that uses oscillations.[46]
- *Mulligan:* passive treatment of joint mobilization that uses sustained stretching with the intent to not illicit pain.[43-45]

In joint mobilization techniques, the practitioner applies a gentle force, moving the physiological component of a joint's range of motion. Athletic trainers should understand the differences between the theories and select a technique based on the anatomical area and patient's need (e.g., pain versus restriction).

To appropriately apply joint mobilization, further study is needed beyond the foundational information. In addition to joint mobilization theory, practitioners must understand both joint mechanoreceptors and accessory motions to apply the therapy appropriately. Regardless of the theory, properly selecting the type of joint mobilization per joint mechanoreceptor is a key factor in pain modulation and should be part of advanced practitioner education.[46-49] A deeper understanding of accessory motions that include the concave–convex rule is concomitantly necessary to appropriately apply joint mobilizations during the rehabilitation phases.

Traction

Traction is a therapeutic modality used to reduce tension on a body segment through distraction. Clinically, traction may be performed both manually and mechanically.

Manual traction is performed by a clinician with appropriate education and training on the appropriate positioning and distraction techniques for extremities and the spine. Mechanical traction employs machines that may include pulleys, ropes, or tables (see table 21.10).

Myofascial Release

Myofascial tissue is a matrix of connective tissues that surrounds all muscles, organs, and glands. Myofascial tissues has high concentrations of collagen that is extensible; thus, injury may inhibit the extensibility of muscles and tendons.[50-53] Myofascial release is used to relax the myofascial tissues and may also relieve soft-tissue adhesions and scar tissue. It may be performed by a practitioner, through self-release (e.g., foam roller or tennis ball), or reciprocal inhibition and stretching (figure 22.7).[51,54,55] Other techniques to enhance the extensibility of the myofascial system include strain/counterstrain, positional release, and soft-tissue mobilization.

- *Strain/counterstrain.* This positional technique is used to alleviate neurogenic muscular pain. It

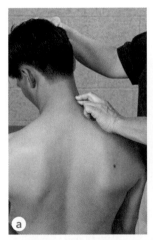 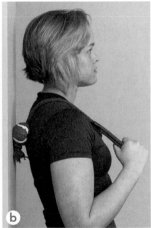

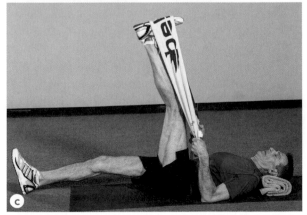

FIGURE 22.7   Examples of myofascial release: *(a)* practitioner, *(b)* self-release, and *(c)* reciprocal inhibition and stretching of the gastrocnemius.

FOUNDATIONAL SKILL

Budget Plan for Equipment Replacement, Accrual, and Maintenance

Annually identify the following based on inspection of facility and the evidence:

- Highly expendable items replaced yearly (resistance tubing or putty)
- Items that need to be replaced every 2 or 3 years (exercise balls, rubber-coated weights)
- Items that need to be replaced every 5 to 10 years (isotonic weight machines, traction device, treatment tables)
- Items that need routine maintenance

---

uses a position that shortens the affected muscle for 90 seconds to 3 minutes.

- *Positional release.* This technique uses a position of patient comfort. It targets the somatic dysfunction that may be the source of myofascial pain.
- *Soft-tissue mobilization (STM/IASTM).* This hands-on technique is used to decrease pain and increase healing and function in soft tissues (i.e., muscles, tendons, fascia, and ligaments).

Purchasing and Maintaining Therapeutic Exercise Equipment

Rehabilitation equipment can range from expendable items such as resistance tubing to high-priced computer-driven isokinetic or proprioceptive devices. Regardless of the state of the rehabilitation facility, a plan for routine upgrades and new equipment is necessary to ensure the safety of patients and eliminate equipment that is no longer viable according to the latest evidence-based research.

Each year, a designee should be assigned to review all of the facility's equipment to assess damage and determine its remaining life span and safety. This process will help the team identify potential purchase needs to incorporate into the annual budget and long-term replacement budget. In addition, the designee should review the research on new and upcoming rehabilitation devices or modifications that could be added to the facility.

Lastly, as part of the inspection process, the designee should identify all items that need maintenance and make a list of routine maintenance activities on the relevant equipment.

CLINICAL BOTTOM LINE

- Therapeutic exercise is a planned rehabilitation process that includes multiple techniques to facilitate return to participation in physical activities or sport.
- Therapeutic exercise is implemented to restore normal function to an injured anatomical area for both athletes and the general population. It differs from conditioning and training, which are intended to maintain or achieve overall general positive health and reduce the likelihood and effect of injury and illness.
- Therapeutic rehabilitation is generally planned based on the tissue's healing phases, with specific phases that include 4 to 6 components, depending on variations in the phase delineation. Regardless of the phase, the components of therapeutic rehabilitation address the following:
  - Physical inactivity and immobilization
  - Inflammation
  - Pain
  - Range of motion
  - Strength
  - Neuromuscular control
  - Balance
  - Cardiorespiratory fitness

- As a means to facilitate a rehabilitation program, therapeutic exercise has many approaches that require an advanced practitioner to apply critical decision making to discern appropriate use of varied clinical applications. Practitioners need to make decisions based on tissue healing parameters, strengthening, tissue elasticity, and functional activity needs.

- Based on the aforementioned parameters, therapeutic exercise selection may include any of the following clinical applications:
  - Rehabilitative exercise
  - Proprioceptive neuromuscular facilitation techniques
  - Aquatic exercise
  - Open and closed kinetic chain exercises
  - Joint mobilization
  - Traction
  - Myofascial release
  - Strain/counterstrain
  - Instrument-assisted soft-tissue mobilization
  - Positional release
  - Soft-tissue mobilization

- Maintenance of therapeutic equipment is of paramount importance for patient safety, appropriate budgeting, and the use of current evidence-based rehabilitation techniques. For each facility, an appropriate designee should annually review equipment to identify replacement needs.

 Go to HK*Propel* to complete the activities and case studies for this chapter.

CHAPTER 23

Pharmacological Interventions

Leamor Kahanov, EdD, ATC, LAT

CAATE STANDARDS

The following CAATE 2020 standards are covered in this chapter:

Standard 74

Standard 75

CHAPTER OBJECTIVES

After reading this chapter, you will be able to do the following:

- Define the term *drug*
- Identify methods for drug administration and dispensation
- Explain the difference between administration and dispensation
- Identify legal concerns for administering medications to active populations
- Categorize drugs for different therapeutic uses
- Describe ergogenic aids for improving performance
- Describe the athletic trainer's role in drug-testing policies
- Describe the athletic trainer's role in drug management

Pharmacology, which is the science of drug action, effect, and uses, requires interprofessional collaboration to ensure that the patient receives the correct medications in the correct dosages according to current legal parameters. A **drug** is a chemical that causes a physiological effect when introduced into the body. Drugs may be used in the prevention, treatment, or diagnosis of an injury, illness, or disease. Many medications originated from natural sources, such as bark, roots, leaves, and plants, yet current drugs are often synthetically produced. Use or application of drugs for therapeutic interventions must be managed and administered with adequate knowledge of the legal parameters. Athletic trainers must understand and adhere to state and federal regulations to provide the best health care to patients in a legal and safe manner. This chapter provides a foundational understanding of pharmacology in athletic training. For more details on evidence-based practice and research principles, investigate the sources in each section further.

Pharmacokinetics and Pharmacodynamics

Clinical decisions regarding the type, dose, route of administration, and length of time are complex and based on the pharmacokinetics and pharmacodynamics of a drug. Administering and dispensing practitioners should have a robust understanding of a drug's mechanics and effects on the body to provide the appropriate drug or advice for patients.

Common Drug Preparations in Athletic Training Environments

Capsule: a gelatin-based, oblong-shaped container that holds drugs

Elixir: a sweet alcohol liquid solution used to deliver drugs

Extract: drug made from vegetable or animal matter

Gel: a clear or transparent semisolid that liquefies when applied to skin

Liniment: drug mixed with alcohol, oil, or soapy emollient for skin application

Lotion: a liquid solution containing medication that is applied to skin

Lozenge: a round or oval disc containing a combination of drugs that dissolve in the mouth

Ointment: a semisolid that delivers drugs or medication to the skin or mucous membranes

Pill: an oval or round disc containing a combination of drugs intended for ingestion

Powder: finely ground drugs that may be used both internally or externally

Suppository: drugs mixed with gelatin and shaped for insertion into the body (typically the rectum) that dissolves at body temperature

Syrup: liquid solution of sugar used to deliver drugs or medication

Tablet: a powdered drug compressed into a small disc

Tincture: a water and alcohol solution used to deliver drugs made from plants

Pharmacokinetics is how the body processes a drug. Drugs follow a routine process through the body (figure 23.1):

1. They are introduced in the body through a process called administration.

2. They move through the body through a process called distribution.

3. They are absorbed in the body through metabolism.

4. They are removed from the body system through elimination.

Many factors affect administration, distribution, metabolism, and elimination, including age, weight, underlying comorbidities (other illnesses), genetic response to drugs, and drug chemical composition.

A drug delivery system is a combination approach between dose and route of administration to determine the best approach, formula, or technology for transporting the drug for the intended therapeutic effect.[1-6] A drug route of administration refers to the way in which drugs are introduced into the body:

- *Buccal:* between the gum and cheek
- *Inhalation:* breathed into the lungs by mouth or nose
- *Intravenous:* inserted into a vein through IV or injection
- *Intramuscular:* injection into a muscle
- *Intrathecal:* injected between the vertebrae
- *Nasal:* through the nose, typically a spray
- *Oral:* by mouth
- *Rectal:* through the rectum
- *Sublingual:* under the tongue

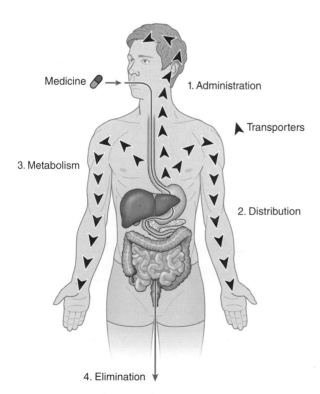

FIGURE 23.1 Pharmacokinetics.

- *Transdermal:* through the skin, often with a patch or cream
- *Vaginal:* through the vagina

Typically, an athletic trainer who is legally able to administer a medication will do so in one-dose applications through oral and dermal routes.[7-10]

Drug distribution is the movement of a drug to and from the bloodstream and other tissues in the body. Drugs penetrate and leave different body tissues at varying rates and are often designed to target tissues based on the chemical construction of the tissue. **Drug absorption** is the movement of a drug or medication through the body systems from the point of introduction (site of administration) to the bloodstream.[1-6] Absorption is a consideration of the drug introduction and delivery system and is based on the site and route of introduction into the body and the dosage of the medication. Intravenous drug introductions require no absorption; oral, dermal, and rectal introductions must be absorbed through the body systems.[1-6] As an athletic trainer, your role is to administer medications specifically as directed on an **over-the-counter (OTC)** one-dose package.[7,8]

Drug metabolism is the chemical changes that occur in the body after the drug's introduction. Most drugs are metabolized through the liver, creating inactive compounds that are then excreted. Drug excretion primarily occurs through the kidneys as urine. However, some drugs are excreted through saliva, sweat, and feces. The rate at which a drug is metabolized or excreted is called the half-life. The half-life is the basis for how often to administer a drug so that it remains at therapeutic levels, called a steady state.[1-6]

Pharmacodynamics is the study of how a drug affects the body; it also looks at the relationship between drug concentration and therapeutic action, which includes time, intensity, and adverse effects.[1-6] **Bioavailability** is the amount and rate at which a drug dose reaches the action site unchanged or, in other words, is completely absorbed in the body. A medication that reaches the action site unchanged has a bioavailability of 100%. Drugs administered intravenously have a bioavailability of 100% as opposed to those administered by other routes such as oral, rectal, or transdermal. The bioavailability

of a medication route is essential in calculating dosages for administration.[1-6] Athletic trainers who are legally allowed to administer medications must use the dosage amounts identified for the OTC medications.[7-10]

Legal Issues and Regulations

Athletic trainers are often in the position of managing both OTC and prescription drugs and medications, whether working in a health care facility, travelling with an athletic team, or supervising patients. Laws and regulations governing drugs are multifaceted, and you should know and understand the federal, state, and international parameters of drug dispensation, administration, storage, record keeping, disposal, and maintenance. In addition, each health care facility may have additional regulations, and competitive sport bodies (i.e., NCAA, International Olympic Committee [IOC]) also have discrete regulations. This chapter does not detail specific laws from states and sport authority regulating bodies, which are extensive. Athletic trainers working or volunteering in venues that require drug management must understand all the laws and regulations of that state, governing body, and facility.

Administration and dispensation of drugs represent distinctly different delivery functions controlled by federal and state laws. Administering a drug is providing a patient with a single dose of medication for immediate use.[7-13] For example, you might provide a single dose of OTC acetaminophen (Tylenol). Providing more than a single dose of OTC medication to a patient is considered dispensing under the federal definition, which is illegal for an athletic trainer in all 50 states.[7-13] Dispensing medication is federally defined as providing both prescription and OTC medication to a person beyond a single dose. Only licensed practitioners identified under state and federal regulations may dispense drugs. Failure to adhere to federal and state law is a violation and may lead to legal issues for the licensed dispensing practitioner, athletic trainer, clinic, school, or health care entity.[7-13]

Federal and state laws are enacted for patient safety. You must understand the foundational laws that protect patients in order to ensure patient safety. Here are the federal regulations governing pharmaceutical care:

FOUNDATIONAL SKILL

Dispensation of Medication

It is illegal for athletic trainers to dispense medication. According to federal law, only pharmacists and physicians can dispense medication unless another person is designated by each individual state; some states allow nurse practitioners and physician assistants to do so.[7-10] Under no circumstances can a physician instruct an athletic trainer to dispense medication.

- *Federal Food, Drug, and Cosmetic Act (FDCA) of 1938:*[14] regulates the quantity, strength, bioequivalence, and labeling of prescription and nonprescription drugs
- *Durham-Humphrey Amendment of 1951:*[15] separates prescription from nonprescription drugs
- *Federal Anti-Tampering Act of 1983:*[16] created 7-point label requirements and tamper-resistant packaging on all nonprescription medications
- *Omnibus Reconciliation Act (OBRA) of 1990:*[17] mandates drug review, patient medication records, and verbal patient education as part of dispensing of prescription medications

Managing a Formulary

Typically, athletic training settings are formularies in the management of drugs. A **formulary** is an entity that maintains a list of drugs that are available (provided or sold), while a **pharmacy** is an entity that sells, dispenses, and prepares medications (**compounding**).[1,3-6,11,66,67] Management of drugs in an athletic training setting requires that each facility have a policy and procedure manual that is aligned with federal and state laws and guidelines and also creates explicit guidelines for employees. The policy and procedure manual should include guidelines for drug ordering, receiving, storage, securing, dispensing, administration, transportation, disposal, record keeping, inventory, and audits. It should be approved by the employment agency and reviewed annually by a minimum of a physician, pharmacist, and lead or head athletic trainer.[7-10,12]

A component of managing a formulary is ensuring that nonprescription drugs administered or dispensed have the required appropriate labeling:[7-10,12]

1. The name of the product
2. The name and address of the manufacturer, packer, or distributor

3. The net contents of the package
4. The established name of all active ingredients and the quantity of certain other ingredients, whether active or not
5. The name of any habit-forming drug contained in the preparation
6. Cautions and warnings needed to protect the consumer
7. Adequate directions for safe and effective use

Ordering

Ordering OTC medications may be accomplished through medical supply companies. You should confer with the team physician or clinical administrator to determine the medications identified as part of the health care center's formulary. Any prescription drugs must be ordered by the designated physician or practitioner and locked in a storage location; only the designee should have a key.[8]

Receiving

The process for receiving and reconciling medication should be outlined in the facility's established guidelines. Incoming medications should be verified for quantity, drug name, dosage, and lot number and rectified with the existing accurate list of all possible medications in the facility to ensure that all the medications are accounted for.

Storage

Storage of medications is regulated by federal and state laws in addition to best practices and guidelines. Medication storage is specific to the facility, but medication generally should be stored in a locked cabinet away from patient access. Ensuring medication potency and efficacy requires that the storage area remain temperate (i.e., it should not get too hot or cold), dry, and dark. Some medications may need refrigeration; the same safety

International Regulations

The World Health Organization (WHO) originally set standards to use Latin nomenclature and dosages identified with the metric system in order to standardize drug dosage identification in mostly European nations. Each nation has a governing body that identifies and regulates the drugs for the country.[18,65]

- British drug standards for drug administration and dispensation are managed by the British Pharmacopoeia Commission under the direction of the General Medical Council. This governmental body sets the standards for drugs in the United Kingdom.[19]
- The Canadian Formulary (CF), published by the Canadian Pharmacists Association and recognized by the Canadian Food and Drugs Act, identifies the drugs and standards for Canada.[20]

guidelines for patient access apply to refrigerators where medication is stored.

Securing, Dispensing, and Administering Medication

When securing, dispensing, and administering medication, you must follow both federal and state guidelines in addition to facility protocols. The steps to ensuring secure dispensation and administration are as follows:

- Verify the prescription or directions from the medical provider.
- Check and double check that the medication is accurate per prescription or directions.
- Check to make sure that the correct dosage, directions, lot number, and federally required packet information appear on the medication.
- Check and double check that the accurate information is in the patient's chart.
- Validate that medication removal process was followed for medication reconciliation processes.

Transportation

Transportation of medication is state regulated; thus, transferring medication across state lines may violate laws. Review federal and state laws on transporting medications for the purpose of athletic competition.

Disposal

Disposal of medication should be outlined in the facility's established guidelines. Guidelines for disposal of OTC and prescription drugs should include recommendations from the dispensing pharmacist. You should maintain an authorized collection receptacle for drug disposal and return unused and expired medications to a designated pharmacy.[21-23] Avoid flushing medications down the toilet or throwing them away in common garbage bins, which can contaminate the water supply.[21-23]

Record Keeping

Per federal law, the health care facility must keep records available for all prescription drugs for a minimum of three years. Drug records should include the administration and dispensation of all medications, inventory received and disposed of, and a current balance of medications. The policy and procedure manual should outline the timeline for audit and reconciliation of the drugs.

Patient records for administration and dispensation of drugs must list information both on a log sheet for drugs and in the patient's file and should include the following:[7-10,12]

- Patient's name
- Date
- Injury or illness
- Drug administered or dispensed
- Dose
- Quantity
- Lot number

Inventory

A formulary managed by an athletic trainer must maintain accurate records of inventory separate from individual patient charts. Prescription medications should be maintained by the designated physician or practitioner. The quantity of drugs remaining available for administration must match the number on the tally sheet for each

---

FOUNDATIONAL SKILL

Medication Administration

Follow these guidelines when administering medications:[7-10,12,14,16,17,24,25]

- Take a thorough history from the patient.
- Refer patients with any potentially significant medical issues to a physician.
- Consult a physician prior to providing any OTC medication for clients taking additional medications.
- When working with athlete clients, consult the banned substance statutes for any relevant athletic governing body (i.e., state high school associations, NCAA, IOC).
- Provide OTC medications in single-dose packages with appropriate labeling.
- Provide verbal directions per the written directions on the single-dose packet.
- Ensure that the patient understands the dose schedule.
- Keep appropriate medical records for each administration.

medication if audited by accreditation teams or state or federal authorities. Although a hard copy approach is acceptable, many computer programs are available that automatically calculate inventory. Inventory accountability should include the following:[7,8]

- A running tally of the quantity available for each medication
- The date and quantity of each dispensation
- Name of drug and lot number
- Expiration dates for each medication (Expired medications must be removed from stock.)

Audit

An audit of a pharmacy is a formal review from an outside regulatory body or entity to ensure compliance with federal, state, and institutional regulations. Audits can include a review of processes, reconciliation of drug accounting, agreements, insurance claims, and overall document verification. Medications and drugs that are maintained in an athletic training setting may also be subject to external audits.

Drug Testing

Drug testing in athletic training settings may be delineated by the institution or an athletic association, such as the National Collegiate Athletic Association (NCAA)[25,26] or the United States Olympic Committee (USOC), or run by the United States Anti-Doping Agency (USADA).[25] Drug testing may be done to detect recreational, performance-enhancing, OTC, or prescription drugs. Delineation of the type of drug is based on the institution and level of athlete. Banned drug lists associated with specific levels of athletes, such as the NCAA or USADA, are updated regularly and should be referenced to ensure the safety of the athlete.[25,27] Since the specific parameters of drug testing vary greatly, the institution should publish policies in a policy and procedure manual that is available to both employees and athletes.[7-9,11,12,26,28,29]

The following guidelines are for athletic trainers involved in drug testing:[30-32]

- The institution should determine if the athletic trainer or athletic training room is the responsible party for drug testing based on neutrality. Responsible parties for drug testing are decided by each institution based on state laws and regulations and institutional counsel advice.
- The athletic trainer, if involved, should follow the guidelines outlined in the institution or medical facility's policy and procedures document.

Common Medications in Athletic Training

The availability of OTC medications and prescription drugs through a licensed provider is widespread in active populations. Your role in the context of prescription medication, given that dispensing is illegal, is reviewing patient history, monitoring treatment and outcomes, and referring the patient if negative side effects arise. New drugs are continually being developed and approved by the Food and Drug Administration (FDA), so you should monitor the list of banned or illegal drugs for inclusion of new drugs, changes to dosages, and elimination of drugs available for patient use. The following sections provide information on the most commonly used drugs in athletic training. You must have a general understanding of drug classifications and definitions in order to effectively communicate with health care providers and maintain accurate records.

Prescription Medications

Prescription drugs must be prescribed by a state licensed practitioner. The medication is dispensed through a licensed pharmacist or by a physician during an office or hospital visit.[7-9] You will often need to communicate with a licensed provider regarding prescriptions. You must understand drug classifications and common abbreviations (table 23.1) to ensure accurate communication and minimize mistakes.

Prescription medications are sorted into five classifications (schedule I to V), which were created by the federal government and dictated by the Controlled Substance Act (CSA), to delineate a drug's medical use and abuse or dependency potential.[2,3,5,11,34] The determining factor for scheduling a drug is based on the abuse or dependency rate.[3,5,6]

- Schedule I drugs have a high potential for abuse and dependency but no accepted medical use. Examples include heroin, LSD, and ecstasy.
- Schedule II drugs have a high potential for abuse and dependency and are considered dangerous but have an accepted medical use. Examples include OxyContin, fentanyl, Vicodin, Adderall, and Ritalin.
- Schedule III drugs have a low to moderate potential for abuse and dependency. Examples include Tylenol with codeine, testosterone, and ketamine.
- Schedule IV drugs have a low potential for abuse and dependency. Examples include tramadol, Ambien, Valium, Ativan, Darvocet, and Xanax.
- Schedule V drugs have a lower potential for abuse and dependency but still contain limited amounts

TABLE 23.1 **Common Drug Abbreviations**

Abbreviation	Denotation	Abbreviation	Denotation
Aa	Of each	Pc	After meals
Ac	Before meals	Po	By mouth
Ad lib	As much as desired	Prn	As needed
ASA	Aspirin	Q	Every
Bid	Twice a day	Qd	Every day
BW	Body weight	Qh	Every hour
C	With	Q2h	Every 2 hours
Cc	Cubic centimeter	Q3h	Every 3 hours
Caps	A capsule	Qid	4 times a day
Cr	Controlled release	Qod	Every other day
D	Days	Rect	Rectally
D/C	Discontinue	Rx	Take
Elix	Elixir	s	Without
Et	And	Ss	One half
Fldxt	Fluid extract	SC	Subcutaneous
Gm	Gram	Sig	Label
Gt	A drop	SL	Sublingual
Gtt	Drops	Stat	Immediately
Hr	Hour	Syr	Syrup
Hs	At bedtime	Tab	Tablet
IM	Intramuscularly	Tib	2 times a day
IV	Intravenously	Tid	3 times a day
L	Liter	Top	Topical
Od	Once daily	Wk	Week
OTC	Over the counter	U	Unit

of narcotics. Examples include Robitussin AC, Lomotil, and Lyrica.

Over-the-Counter Drugs

Drugs that are considered safe for self-administration without a prescription or medical guidance are called over-the counter (OTC) drugs. OTCs are available to consumers primarily at drug, grocery, and convenience stores or online. You may store OTC medications on site

as part of the medical or clinical environment and provide guidance to patients. If you manage OTC drugs in your work environment, you must adhere to federal and state safety and administration laws.[9]

Anti-Inflammatories

Nonsteroidal anti-inflammatory drugs (NSAIDs) and analgesic drugs are often used in an athletic training setting to decrease pain and inflammation. NSAIDs are

Generic and Brand-Name Drugs

Both prescription and OTC drugs can be generic or brand name. Generic drugs contain the same active ingredients in strength, administration route, and quality as brand-name drugs but do not have the trade name. Brand-name drugs are protected by a patent and have a trade name. Once a brand-name drug's patent expires, generic drugs can be sold using a nontrade name.[1,3,5,6,11]

used primarily to treat acute injuries but can also be used to treat chronic pain.[3,5,6,11,68] Typically, NSAIDs are used short term to address pain and inflammation associated with sprains, strains, and muscle injury. NSAIDs can also be used to assist with dysfunction and pain associated with tendinitis and tendinosis.[3,5,6,11] Prolonged use of anti-inflammatories may have long-term negative effects that include bacterial resistance and offsets the balance of microorganisms that regulate the gastrointestinal tract, potentially leading to chronic illnesses. Table 23.2 lists common NSAIDs and precautions.

Muscle Relaxants

Muscle relaxants are used to reduce muscle spasms in order to reduce pain.[3-5,11,38] Although muscle relax-

ants are not NSAIDs and have no anti-inflammatory, antipyretic, or analgesic effects, their use may be to ultimately reduce pain associated with spasticity.[6] Common muscle relaxants are listed in table 23.3.

Respiratory Drugs

Athletic trainers are responsible for understanding the effect of drugs on the respiratory system in order to monitor usage and effect on individual activity. You should know about OTC respiratory drugs to best assist patients in selecting appropriate medication. Identifying signs and symptoms of side effects for patients using prescription respiratory drugs is an essential duty for athletic trainers.[3,5,11,29]

TABLE 23.2 Common NSAIDs and Analgesics

Classification	Use or action	Drug generic (brand name)	Side effects
Acetaminophen	Analgesic Antipyretic	Tylenol	Prolonged use can cause liver damage Do not use with alcohol
Salicylates	Analgesic Antipyretic Anti-inflammatory	Acetylsalicylic acid (aspirin) Magnesium salicylate (Doan's pills) Choline salicylate (Arthropan)	GI distress or disease Nausea Tinnitus Prolonged bleeding Reye's syndrome
Nonsalicylate nonsteroidal anti-inflammatory*	COX-1 and COX-2 inhibitor Anti-inflammatory Analgesic Antipyretic (antifever)	Ibuprofen (Advil/Motrin) Flurbiprofen (Ansaid) Celecoxib (Celebrex) Oxaprozin (Daypro) Piroxicam (Feldene) Indomethacin (Indocin) Etodolac (Lodine) Naproxen (Naprosyn/Aleve/Anaprox) Nabumetone (Relafen) Ketorolac (Toradol) Diclofenac (Voltaren/Cataflam)	May have hypersensitivity from cross-sensitivity to aspirin or other NSAIDs Skin rash Itching Visual disturbances Weight gain Edema Black stool Dark urine Headache
Opioid analgesics*	Acute pain typical after an accident or surgery	Morphine Hydromorphone (Dilaudid) Oxycodone (OxyContin) Oxycodone/acetaminophen (Percocet) Codeine (Codeine) Propoxyphene (Darvon) Acetaminophen/propoxyphene (Darvocet)	Addictive (schedule V drugs; switch to nonopioid pain relievers as soon as possible) Nausea Visual disturbance Drowsiness Mental cloudiness Vomiting Constipation Respiratory distress Depression

*NSAIDs and analgesics may be both OTC and prescription, depending on strength.

Based on Asperheim (2011); Mangus and Miller (2005); Coombs et al. (2015); Holgado et al. (2018); Jankowski et al. (2015); Ziltener, Leal, and Fournier (2010).

TABLE 23.3   **Common Muscle Relaxants**

Condition, illness, or disease	Use or action	Drug generic (brand name)	Side effects
Skeletal muscle relaxants[39]	Decrease spasticity or pain from muscle spasms	Methocarbamol (Robaxin) Diazepam (Valium) Cyclobenzaprine (Flexeril) Carisoprodol (Soma)	Drowsiness Allergic reactions such as swelling in the throat or extremities Trouble breathing Hives Chest tightness Light headedness or fainting Liver damage

Respiratory drugs act on and affect three areas of the body:

1. The respiratory center in the brain to depress breathing, often caused by opioids and barbiturates

2. The mucous membrane lining of the respiratory tract to suppress coughing or to liquefy mucus for expulsion

3. The lungs to increase bronchiole size and assist with breathing

You will most commonly encounter medications for bronchiole size due to asthma or a reaction to allergens or mucous membranes (because of coughs and colds).[29,40-42] Respiratory drugs that affect the brain are primarily depressants from the opium (morphine, codeine) and barbiturate (phenobarbital) groups and are not provided for therapeutic interventions in the active populations.[6] Table 23.4 identifies appropriate drugs for asthma-related respiratory therapy. Portable handheld inhalers are common in an active population to address exercise-induced bronchospasm. Metered-dose inhalers (MDIs) and dry powder inhalers (DPIs) are the two most common inhalers used by active clients. MDIs and PDIs provide a single dose of medication.

Allergy Drugs

Allergies generally exist due to the body's sensitivity to a foreign substance (antigen) that produces an antibody to specifically target that substance. The body's

FOUNDATIONAL SKILL

Using a Meter-Dosed Inhaler

1. Inspect the inhaler for any damage to the casing or mouthpiece.
2. Shake the inhaler.
3. Exhale all air from the lungs.
4. Place spacer mouthpiece or the inhaler in the mouth.
5. Begin inhaling slowly through the mouth and then press down on the inhaler (figure 23.2). Do not breathe in through the nose. If using a spacer, wait 5 seconds to breathe in after compressing the inhaler.
6. Breathe in slowly and deeply for 3 to 5 seconds.
7. Take the inhaler out of your mouth. Hold your breath for a count of 10 or as long as possible.
8. If a second puff is prescribed, wait for 30 seconds before taking it.
9. If using a corticosteroid inhaler, rinse out your mouth with water.[29, 40-42]

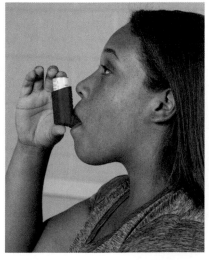

FIGURE 23.2   Using an inhaler.

TABLE 23.4   **Common Asthma Respiratory Inhalants**

Condition, illness, or disease	Use or action	Drug generic (brand name)	Side effects
Asthma: short-acting beta-agonists	Acute symptoms	Albuterol inhalation powder (ProAir RespiClick) Albuterol inhalation solution (AccuNeb) Albuterol inhaler: Proair HFA (Proair HFA) Albuterol inhaler: Proventil (Proventil) albuterol inhaler: Ventolin (Ventolin) Levalbuterol (Xopenex) Cromolyn inhalation arformoterol (Brovana)	Scheduled use is not recommended. Long-acting beta-2 agonists should not be used for acute treatment. Use of more than one canister a month may indicate overuse; patient should be referred to a licensed practitioner.
Asthma: long-acting beta-agonists	Acute symptoms	Formoterol inhalation powder (Brovana) Formoterol inhalation solution (Foradil) Indacaterol (Perforomist) Olodaterol (Arcapta) Salmeterol (Striverdi) Arformoterol (Serevent)	Minor side effects: • Throat irritation and hoarseness (caused by inhaled corticosteroids in combination medicines) • Rapid heartbeat or palpitations • Headache and dizziness • Nausea, vomiting, and diarrhea • Anxiety • Nervousness or tremor (such as unsteady, shaky hands) Side effects that need immediate attention: • Fast, pounding, or irregular heartbeat • Muscle cramps • Increased thirst or urination
Asthma: corticosteroids (maintenance)	Maintenance medication Considered most effective treatment for symptoms of persistent asthma and first line of controller medications (WHO, NHLBI)	Beclomethasone MDI, non-breath actuated (Qvar) Budesonide inhalation powder (Pulmicort) Budesonide inhalation suspension (Pulmicort) Ciclesonide (Alvesco) Flunisolide inhalation aerosol (Aerospan) Fluticasone furoate inhalation powder (Arnuity) Fluticasone propionate inhalation aerosol, powder (Flovent) Fluticasone propionate inhalation powder: ArmonAir (ArmonAir) Mometasone 110 mcg inhalation powder (Asmanex Twisthaler)	May increase severity of asthma and risk of asthma-related deaths. Oral candidiasis can be reduced by using a spacer and rinsing the mouth with water after inhalation.
Asthma: corticosteroids (acute attack)	Acute attack management	Hydrocortisone (Solu-Cortef): IV for immediate use Prednisone: prolonged effect (oral)	Both are RX. May be oral or IV. Anti-inflammatory effect may take up to 6 hr.

Condition, illness, or disease	Use or action	Drug generic (brand name)	Side effects
Asthma: combination products	Long-term and acute management	Albuterol/ipratropium inhalation spray (Combivent) Budesonide/formoterol (Symbicort) Fluticasone/salmeterol inhalation aerosol, powder (Advair) Fluticasone/salmeterol inhalation powder (AirDuo) Fluticasone/vilanterol (Breo) Fluticasone furoate/umeclidinium/vilanterol (Trelegy) Glycopyrrolate/formoterol (Bevespi) Indacaterol/glycopyrrolate (Utibron) Mometasone/formoterol (Dulera) Tiotropium/olodaterol (Stiolto) Umeclidinium/vilanterol (Anoro) Albuterol/ipratropium inhalation spray (Combivent)	Minor side effects: • Throat irritation and hoarseness (caused by inhaled corticosteroids in combination medicines) • Rapid heartbeat or palpitations • Headache and dizziness • Nausea, vomiting, and diarrhea • Anxiety • Nervousness or tremor (such as unsteady, shaky hands) Side effects that need immediate attention: • White patches on tongue or in mouth • Signs of infection (such as fever, persistent sore throat) • Mental/mood changes (such as nervousness) • Trouble sleeping • Vision problems (such as blurred vision)

Based on Prentice (2017); Starkey (2013); Asperheim (2011); Houglum (2000); McFadden and Gilbert (1994); Ari et al. (2009); Fanta et al. (2009); Fanta, Bochner, and Hollingsworth (2014); Morton and Fitch (1992).

reactions to the antigen also produce histamines, which cause the common symptoms of allergies: red, watery eyes; sneezing; rash; and asthma.[28,47] A severe allergic reaction—including a drop in blood pressure, cardiac issues, swelling, and respiratory constriction—is called anaphylaxis and requires immediate emergency care. Antihistamines, corticosteroids, and mast cell stabilizers are the primary drugs used for allergies (see table 23.5).[3,5,6,13,28,33,47] Prescription medications for allergies depend on the diagnosis and treatment regime. OTC medications are also available and may be found on site in the athletic training room.[42]

Athletic trainers may administer OTC for allergies only in the following situations:[9,10]

- The patient indicates she has not taken any other medications in the past 4 to 24 hours (time spacing depends on type of medication).
- The patient indicates no allergies to medications.
- The patient does not have liver or kidney disease.
- The patient does not have a cough or cold.

Gastrointestinal Drugs

Gastrointestinal issues are often complicated and may identify more significant underlying disease processes. Gastrointestinal disorders are often associated with stomach hyperacidity, poor eating habits, or food incompatibility.[3,6,11,51-53] You must be able to identify the appropriateness of OTC medications and when a referral is required. Most antiemetics are prescription drugs. Laxatives should be used under physician supervision, since consistent constipation may be a sign of an underlying disorder. Systemic antidiarrhea medications often contain opiate derivatives or anticholinergic agents and should be ordered by a physician. Table 23.6 identifies common gastrointestinal medications.

Athletic trainers may administer OTCs for gastrointestinal issues only if patients *do not* have the following:[3,5,6,11,51-53]

- Diarrhea lasting more than 24 hours
- Nausea associated with abdominal or chest pain
- Projectile, prolonged, or severe vomiting
- Prolonged or severe abdominal pain or tenderness

Patients who have any of the following medical conditions should consult with a physician immediately:[3,5,6,11,51-53]

- Peptic ulcer disease
- Reflux disease
- Diarrhea

TABLE 23.5 **Common Drugs for Allergies and Colds**

Classification	Common conditions in athletic training	Drug generic (brand name)	Side effects
Antihistamines: pills and liquids	Allergies: runny nose, itchy and watery eyes, swelling, rashes	Diphenhydramine Chlorpheniramine Cetirizine (Zyrtec Allergy) Desloratadine (Clarinex) Fexofenadine (Allegra Allergy) Levocetirizine (Xyzal) Loratadine (Alavert, Claritin)	Drowsiness
Antihistamines: nasal sprays		Azelastine (Astelin, Astepro) Olopatadine (Patanase)	Drowsiness fatigue Bitter taste
Antihistamines: eye drops		Azelastine (Optivar) Emedastine (Emadine) Ketotifen (Alaway) Olopatadine (Pataday, Patanol, Pazeo) Pheniramine (Visine-A, Opcon-A, others)	Headache Dry eyes Burning
Decongestants and antihistamines: pills and liquids		Cetirizine and pseudoephedrine (Zyrtec-D) Desloratadine and pseudoephedrine (Clarinex-D) Fexofenadine and pseudoephedrine (Allegra-D) Loratadine and pseudoephedrine (Claritin-D)	Not recommended for people with the following conditions: Pregnancy High blood pressure Cardiovascular disease Glaucoma hyperthyroidism
Decongestants: nasal sprays	Runny nose and watery eyes	Oxymetazoline (Afrin, Dristan, others) Tetrahydrozoline (Tyzine)	Repeated use can result in worsening congestion
Corticosteroids: nasal sprays	Allergy-related inflammation	Budesonide (Rhinocort) Fluticasone furoate (Flonase Sensimist, Veramyst) Fluticasone propionate (Flonase Allergy Relief) Mometasone (Nasonex) Triamcinolone (Nasacort Allergy 24 Hour)	Bitter smell or taste Nasal irritation Nosebleeds
Corticosteroids: inhalers	Allergy-induced asthma	Beclomethasone (Qvar) Budesonide (Pulmicort Flexhaler) Ciclesonide (Alvesco, Zetonna) Fluticasone (Advair Diskus, Flovent Diskus, others) Mometasone (Asmanex Twisthaler)	Mouth and throat irritation Oral yeast infections
Corticosteroids: eye drops	For itchy, watery, red eyes when other options are ineffective	Fluorometholone (Flarex, FML) Loteprednol (Alrex, Lotemax) Prednisolone (Omnipred, Pred Forte, others)	Physician monitored: Cataracts Glaucoma Infections
Corticosteroids: pills and liquids	Severe allergy symptoms	Prednisolone (Prelone) Prednisone (Prednisone Intensol, Rayos) Methylprednisolone (Medrol)	Cataracts Osteoporosis Muscle weakness Stomach ulcers Increased blood sugar Delay growth in children Exacerbates hypertension

Classification	Common conditions in athletic training	Drug generic (brand name)	Side effects
Mast cell stabilizers: nasal sprays and eye drops	Allergies: runny nose, itchy and watery eyes; used when antihistamines are ineffective	Cromolyn (Crolom: nasal spray) Lodoxamide (Alomide) Pemirolast (Alamast) Nedocromil (Alocril)	Generally safe but require several days to reach full effect

Most drugs are available in both prescription and OTC formats.
Based on Prentice (2017); Starkey (2013); Asperheim (2011); Price et al. (1995); Wadler and Hainline (1989).

TABLE 23.6 **Common Gastrointestinal Medications**

Classification	Common conditions in athletic training	Drug generic (brand name)	Side effects
Antacid	Stomach hyperacidity	Aluminum hydroxide (Alternagel) Magnesium hydroxide (Phillips' Milk of Magnesia) Calcium carbonate (Caltrate, TUMS)	Constipation Laxative effect (Milk of Magnesia)
Antiemetics	Nausea	Dimenhydrinate (Dramamine) Meclizine hydrochloride (Antivert) Prochlorperazine maleate (Compazine) Trimethobenzamide hydrochloride (Tigan) Ondansetron hydrochloride (Zofran) Granisetron hydrochloride (Kytril)	Drowsiness Dry mouth Ringing in the ears Muscle restlessness Heartburn Dark-colored tongue
Cathartics (laxatives)	Constipation	Magnesia magma (milk of magnesia) OTC Magnesium citrate solution (citrate of magnesia) OTC Castor oil OTC Senna (Senokot) RX Dulcolax RX/OTC	Inappropriate use may lead to electrolyte imbalances.
Antidiarrheal	Diarrhea	Loperamide (Imodium A-D, Diamode) Bismuth subsalicylate (Pepto-Bismol, Kaopectate, Maalox) Lactobacillus acidophilus (Acidophilus)	Nausea Drowsiness Dry mouth Constipation
Emetics	Used to empty stomach contents quickly; often used for poisoning.	Ipecac syrup	Vomiting Diarrhea
Histamine-2 blockers	Stomach acidity, ulcers	Cimetidine (Tagamet) Ranitidine (Zantac) Famotidine (Pepcid)	Headache Dizziness Diarrhea
Proton pump inhibitors	Gastroesophageal reflux disease (GERD)	Omeprazole (Prilosec)	Headache Dizziness Diarrhea

Based on Prentice (2017); Asperheim (2011); Mangus and Miller (2005); Koon, Atay, and Lapsia (2017); Swoboda (2003); Waterman and Kapur (2012).

- Constipation
- Intestinal gas

Antibiotics

Penicillin, the first antibiotic, was discovered by Sir Alexander Fleming in 1928 when working with the mold *Penicillum*.[6] The discovery that mold has many disease-producing microorganisms has led to the development of antibiotics, which are derived from living cells that inhibit the proliferation of microorganisms that cause infections or diseases. The majority of antibiotics are developed from molds, bacteria, and yeasts, yet synthetic antibiotics are also available. [3-6,11,30,48-50]

Antibiotics are characterized into two general categories: [3-6,11,33,54-56]

1. Wide-spectrum antibiotics, which are effective against many organisms
2. Narrow-spectrum antibiotics, which are effective on only select organisms

The resistance of microorganisms to antibiotics is a growing concern. Primary theories for this phenomenon are over-prescription and inaccurate use of antibiotics, which allows microorganisms to mutate to resist the drugs. [3-6,11,33,54-56] Inaccurate use can result from patient failure to adhere to the length of the prescription, typically 10 days, or from physician prophylactic use. [5,11,33,54-61] As

an athletic trainer, your role is to refer patients you suspect have a bacterial infection to a licensed practitioner and monitor potential signs and symptoms of adverse reactions. Patients should be under the care of a physician or licensed practitioner for any life-threatening infections. Antibiotics should be used to treat infections for serious illnesses like pneumonia or sepsis. Antibiotics are not necessary for rashes, dizziness, nausea, diarrhea, or yeast infections. Table 23.7 identifies common antibiotics. [57]

Oral antibiotics are not approved in the United States for OTC sale. [61] Topical antibiotics used for skin abrasions, burns, or minor cuts are available OTC and may be found on site in the athletic training room. [7,8,12] Common OTC topical antibiotics include the following: [3,5,6]

TABLE 23.7 Common Antibiotics and General Uses

Classification	Use or action	Drug generic (brand name)	Side effects
Penicillin*	Bacterial infections: streptococcal, pneumococcal Other respiratory infections Gonorrhea Syphilis Meningitis Urinary tract infections Ear infections	Amoxicillin (Amoxil) Amoxicillin (Augmentin) Ampicillin Azithromycin (Zithromax)	Cardiovascular abnormalities Tendon ruptures Photosensitivity Diarrhea Nausea Vomiting Anaphylaxis
Tetracyclines	Prevent bacteria from reproducing (bacteriostatic)	Doxycycline Tetracycline Minocycline	Nausea Vomiting Diarrhea Itching of the rectum or vagina Swollen tongue Black or hairy tongue Sore or irritated throat Headache Hives Skin rash Chest pain
Cephalosporins	Kills bacteria Strep throat Ear infections Urinary tract infections Skin infections MRSA	All cephalosporins start with cef-, ceph-, or kef- Ceftibuten (Cedax) Ceftriaxone (Rocephin) Ceftazidime (Ceptaz) Cefotaxime (Claforan) Cefpodoxime (Vantin) Cefdinir (Omnicef) Cefixime (Suprax) Cefdinir (Omnicef Mini-Pac) Cefditoren (Spectracef) Ceftizoxime (Cefizox) Cefoperazone (Cefobid) Ceftazidime (Fortaz) Ceftazidime (Tazicef)	Stomach discomfort Nausea or vomiting Diarrhea Yeast infection or other fungal infection Blood abnormalities Rash or itching

Classification	Use or action	Drug generic (brand name)	Side effects
Quinolones (not recommended for patients under age of 18)	Inhibit synthesis of bacterial proteins Sinusitis Urinary tract infections	Ciprofloxacin (Cipro) Levofloxacin (Levaquin) Moxifloxacin (Avelox)	Tendon, muscle, and joint damage
Lincomycins	Effective against bacteria that can live without oxygen Pelvic inflammatory disease Bone and joint infections Respiratory tract infections Malaria	Clindamycin (Cleocin) Lincomycin (Lincocin)	Diarrhea Nausea or vomiting Rectal itching Skin rash Tinnitus Dizziness
Macrolides (new generation of antibiotics developed to overcome bacteria resistance)	Community-acquired pneumonia Pertussis (whooping cough) Uncomplicated skin infections	Azithromycin (Zithromax) Clarithromycin (Biaxin) Erythromycin (Erythrocin, Ery-Tab, E.E.S. 400) Fidaxomicin (Dificid)	GI distress Diarrhea Nausea or vomiting
Sulfamides (resistance is currently widespread)	Targets bacteria that can live without oxygen Urinary tract infections Prevention of pneumocystis pneumonia Ear infections	Sulfamethoxazole-trimethoprim Sulfasalazine Sulfisoxazole	Diarrhea Nausea or vomiting Rectal itching Skin rash Headache Dizziness Pale skin Tiredness
Glycopeptide	Treat methicillin-resistant *Staphylococcus aureus* (MRSA) Complicated skin infections	Dalbavancin (Dalvance) Oritavancin (Orbactiv) Telavancin (Vibativ) Vancomycin (Vancocin)	Diarrhea Nausea Headache Taste disturbance Foamy urine
Aminoglycosides	Inhibits bacterial synthesis	Gentamicin (Garamycin) Tobramycin (Tobi) Amikacin (Amikin) Paromomycin (Humatin)	Hearing loss Ringing in the ears Increased thirst Skin rash Unusual drowsiness, Dizziness or weakness
Carbapenems	Kills bacteria Pneumonia Kidney infections Multi-drug resistance – hospital acquired	Imipenem (Primaxin IM) Meropenem (Merrem) Doripenem (Doribax) Ertapenem (Invanz)	Diarrhea Nausea Vomiting Skin rash

*Note: Certain penicillin are more effective on certain bacteria or infections, and a licensed practitioner or pharmacist should be consulted. Hypersensitivity and allergies to penicillin should be queried during history taking and noted on any patient chart and by the licensed practitioner.

Based on Prentice (2017); Rowland and Tozer (2010); Starkey (2013); Asperheim (2011); Mangus and Miller (2005); Wadler and Hainline (1989); Burstein et al. (1993); Fayock et al. (2014); McGrew (2007).

- Neosporin
- Bacitracin
- Polysporin
- Triple antibiotic (generic)

Viral and Fungal Drugs

Fungal infections in athletic training are primarily skin related (dermal) and infect the foot (tinea pedis), nails (onychomycosis), and other exposed skin surfaces.[3,5,6,12] Antifungal topical creams, sprays, and powders can be used to treat infection and mitigate its spread. Oral antifungal medication is available OTC and by prescription (table 23.8).[3,5,6,12] You should refer patients to a physician or licensed practitioner when an infection becomes chronic or red, painful, and irritated, which may signify a concomitant bacterial infection.[62]

TABLE 23.8 **Common Antiviral and Antifungal Medications**

Classification	Common conditions in athletic training	Drug generic (brand name)	OTC/RX
Antifungal	Tinea capitis	Terbinafine (Lamisil) Ketoconazole (Nizoral) Itraconazole (Sporanox) Fluconazole (Diflucan)	RX
	Tinea corporis and tinea cruris	Terbinafine 1% (Lamisil) Ketoconazole 2% (Nizoral) Clotrimazole 1% (Lotrimin) Naftifine 1% (Naftin) Oxiconazole 1% (Oxistat) Ciclopirox .77% (Loprox) Fluconazole (Diflucan) Terbinafine (Lamisil)	OTC OTC OTC RX RX RX RX RX
	Tinea pedis	Ketoconazole 2% (Nizoral) Clotrimazole 1% (Lotrimin)	OTC OTC
Antiviral	Herpes simplex	Abreva Acyclovir Allantoin (Camphor) Blistex Docosanol Zovirax	OTC RX OTC OTC OTC RX

Based on Prentice (2017); Starkey (2013); Asperheim (2011); Huff (1998); Zinder et al. (2010).

Commonly Abused Drugs and Supplements

The use and abuse of performance-enhancing and recreational drugs are your responsibility to monitor, specifically if you have clients who are athletes.[9,24,25] The legal use of drugs in quantities outside of regulation guidelines and the abuse of drugs have a profound effect athletes' ability to compete as well as health considerations. Regardless of your work setting, if you suspect drug abuse, refer the client to a physician, preferably one with expertise in drug abuse management.

You need to understand the use of legal and illegal drugs to enhance performance in addition to recognizing recreational drug abuse that mitigates a person's overall health. Many of the commonly abused drugs or supplements are found in OTC medications or are readily available in drug or health-food stores (table 23.9). Refer to banned drug lists (i.e., NCAA, USOC) to determine in what quantity a drug or supplement becomes banned or detrimental to a patient's health.[9,24,25]

Special Considerations

Athletic trainers are often employed in settings that are unique in health care such as high schools, colleges or universities, and professional and international sport environments. These special populations require varied considerations for athletic trainers.

Blood Doping

Blood doping is a method of increasing blood volume by removing an athlete's blood, storing it, and then reinfusing into his body 6 weeks later. Blood doping is not a drug but an ergogenic aid to increase hemoglobin concentration and improve endurance performance. The risks of the process include infection due to transfusion, kidney damage, liver dysfunction, hepatitis or other blood infections, and circulatory or metabolic shock due to blood overload. Risks increase further when blood from a donor is used rather than the recipient's own blood. Athletic organizations such as the NCAA or USOC have strict guidelines and testing to minimize the use of blood doping. For more information, refer to their recommendations.[24,25]

TABLE 23.9   **Commonly Abused Drugs and Supplements**

Drug or supplement	Common drugs	Athlete use	Action	Signs and symptoms of overuse
Stimulants	Ephedra Caffeine Methamphet- amine Cocaine	Reduce fatigue Increase competi- tiveness	Stimulate central nervous system Increase blood flow	Loss of judgment Headaches High blood pressure Irregular heartbeat Anxiety Tremors

Amphetamines	ADHD medica-
	tions (i.e., Ritalin)
	Narcolepsy
	medications (i.e.,
	Adderall)
		Quickness
		Reduces fatigue
		Excitement
		Attentiveness
			Stimulate central
			nervous system
				Dry mouth
				Euphoria
				Insomnia
				Anorexia
				Reduced mental activity
				Impaired motor skills
				Increasingly irrational
				  behavior
				Repetitive behaviors
				Long-term use may create
				  hallucinations or paranoia.

Caffeine	Coffee Tea Sports drinks Cocoa	Increased energy Delayed fatigue Improved athletic performance	Stimulates central nervous system Diuretic Stimulates gastric secretion	Potential for dehydration Heart palpitations Headache Nausea Tremors

Creatine	Creatine
	supplement
		Increases athletic
		performance
		from muscle
		development
			Muscle building
			Heightened
			muscle
			contraction
				Weight gain
				Dehydration
				Increased risk of heat-
				  related illness
				Long-term use may create
				  kidney dysfunction.

Anabolic steroids	Tetrahydrogestri-
	none (THG)
	Androstenedione
		Increase muscle
		mass
			Derivative of
			testosterone
			Promotes growth
			and development
			of reproductive
			tissues
			Increases protein
			synthesis, muscle
			mass, and bone
			maturation
				Hair loss
				Liver dysfunction
				Kidney dysfunction or
				  disease
				Heart disease
				Changes in mood
				Increases irritability
				Severe acne
				Aggression, depression or
				  suicidal tendencies

Human growth hormone (HGH)	HGH	Increases muscle
		mass
			Increases muscle
			mass, skin thick-
			ness, connective
			tissue mass, and
			organ weight
			Decreases body
			fat
				Premature completion of
				  bone growth
				Enlargement of bone
				  thickness
				Enlargement of the bones
				  of the face
				Diabetes
				Heart disease
				Goiter
				Menstrual disorders
				Impotence
				Decreases life span by up
				  to 20 years

Based on Houglum (2000); Miller et al. (2005); Fanta et al. (2009); Fanta, Bochner, and Hollingsworth (2016); Brady, McCauley, and Back (2016); Dolovich et al. (2005).

Signs and Symptoms of Substance Abuse

Signs and symptoms of substance abuse include the following:[29,42,44,45,63,64]

- Sudden personality changes
- Changes in peer group
- Change in social or leisure activities
- Mood swings
- Increasing isolation from friends and family
- Defensiveness when discussing medications
- Negative attitude
- Missing appointments with increasing frequency
- Decreasing grades
- Sudden weight changes
- Alcohol routinely smelled on breath or body
- Decreasing personal hygiene

Minors

Minors should not receive OTC medications without parental consent.[9] Prescription medication dispensation is subject to state laws for minors.[9] You should have an understanding of state laws regarding minors before administering or dispensing any drugs.

EpiPens and Short-Acting Beta-Agonist Inhalers

EpiPens and inhalers are dispensed by licensed practitioners directly to the patients.[8,9] You may assist in educating the patient on their use after a pharmacist or licensed practitioner has provided the initial education.[9] Protocols for use as an emergency medication are based on facility-established protocols under the direct supervision of a physician. To maintain on-site facility protocols, a DEA certificate that identifies practitioner oversight and responsibility is recommended.[9] Established protocols may allow you to administer emergency medication under delineated circumstances.

Phoresis Treatments

You may be asked to administer topical applications known as phoresis treatments under the direction of a physician.[9] Each facility must have an established protocol for administration of phoresis treatments.[9] State laws and statutes should be consulted prior to administration. As with EpiPens and prescription inhalers, a DEA certificate should be kept on file in the facility.[8,9]

Team Travel

Athletic trainers who travel and manage OTC or prescription medication should carry a formulary signed by a supervising physician.[9] The formulary should identify the communication plan between the athletic trainer and physician during both domestic and international travel.[9]

CLINICAL BOTTOM LINE

- Drugs are a chemical substance that, when introduced into the body, produce a physiological effect. Drugs in the United States may be administered or dispensed depending on the strength and nature of the chemical substance and the effects produced on the body.
- The athletic trainer is legally allowed to perform drug administration only, which is defined as providing over-the-counter medications in one-dose packets. Dispensing medication entails providing patients with more than one dose of either over-the counter or prescription medication or any amount of prescription medications.
- Only a licensed practitioner identified by the state or federal definition may dispense drugs.
- Nonsteroidal anti-inflammatory drugs (NSAIDs) and analgesic drugs are often administered by an athletic trainer in one-dose OTC packets in order to decrease pain or create analgesia. NSAIDs may be

used for both acute and chronic injuries in the short term; however, monitoring the symptoms of possible side effects is essential for maintaining the health of the patient. Typically, NSAIDs are administered to decrease dysfunction and pain associated with tendinitis and tendinosis.

- Ergogenic aids are often used by the athletic population to enhance performance. These aids may cause concomitant health care issues that are significant in addition to the regulatory and legal implications. Some ergogenic aids are illegal; other are banned by athletic associations (i.e., NCAA, USOC). The athletic trainer should monitor clients for signs and symptoms of abuse, which generally include behavioral changes, weight changes, and increasing isolation or aggression.

- Drug-testing policies and procedures should be outlined in a manual approved by the institution. Athletic trainers should adhere to any additional requirements from athletic associations, such as the NCAA and USOC.

- People working in the athletic training setting must adhere to federal and state laws regarding drug storage, packet labeling, and disposal. Patient records must include the patient's name, date, injury or illness, drug administration or dispensation, and the drug's dose and lot number. All information must be listed on a log sheet and transferred to the patient's file.

 Go to HK*Propel* to complete the activities and case studies for this chapter.

Go to HK*Propel* to download foundational skill check sheets about administring medications and using a meter-dosed inhaler.

CHAPTER 24

Clinical Casting

Bryce B. Gaines, LAT, ATC

CAATE STANDARDS

The following CAATE 2020 standard is covered in this chapter:

Standard 78

CHAPTER OBJECTIVES

After reading this chapter, you will be able to do the following:

- Understand basic pathologic fracture alignment

- Identify the stages of bone tissue healing and articulate how they relate to immobilization duration

- Discuss the general clinical objectives of casting as a therapeutic treatment

- Identify appropriate materials for successful application and removal of casts and splints

- Recognize basic casting techniques for the upper and lower body and the common injuries treated by these applications

- Discuss benefits, risks, and contraindications of cast application

- Identify solutions for common problems encountered with casting

- Recognize cultural, social, and economic nuances of the patient-centered model of care that may affect implementation of casting as a treatment strategy

The climate of health care in the United States is changing at an ever-increasing rate. Care is shifting from professionally mandated treatment plans to a more patient-centered approach based on collaborative treatment methodology and accessibility. As a part of that change, athletic trainers are gaining respect among the allied health professions for their knowledge of musculoskeletal evaluation, injury assessment and rehabilitation, and protective intervention. This combination of abilities has moved the profession out of the world of sports and into clinical practices as athletic trainers are called to be experts on musculoskeletal evaluation, durable medical equipment, orthotic devices, and other treatment strategies that were once afforded only to the athletic population. Casting is a practice that lends itself closely to preventive and protective taping skills already well established in the athletic training profession. It is a common treatment strategy used in orthopedic practices nationwide. Their understanding of casting gives athletic trainers an appreciation for the nuances of fracture care and management as well as the ability to provide a clinical service that ultimately improves the patient's experience and the orthopedic practice's throughput. Finally, casting further establishes the athletic trainer as a knowledgeable and capable member of an interdisciplinary health care team.

Casting is a commonly used method for immobilizing a joint or multiple joints to achieve the following:[2,3,11]

- Immobilize a tissue injury or pathology to promote appropriate healing

- Prevent the tissue from incurring additional injury or stress

The most common application for casting is to provide immobilization and stabilization for fractured bones. However, casting can be used to encourage changes to soft tissue structures and provide a mechanism for sustained, low-load, long duration stretching through position-specific splinting. Due to the rigid properties of casting materials, it is also ideal for providing external stability to displaced fracture patterns following reduction. Casting allows the reduction to be maintained to achieve the most functional positioning of the affected tissues while natural remodeling takes place.[3,8]

For fracture care, casting is most effective in the subacute phase of injury. In the initial acute phase, the body's inflammatory response is a contraindication for casting (explained further later in this chapter). Once the initial inflammatory response has subsided, or is at least well controlled, the body part can be immobilized more predictably and, therefore, safely.[1,11]

Basic Principles

Before applying any cast, or when planning how to effectively immobilize any body part, you must observe certain principles in order to measure how productive cast application will be. Ask yourself the following questions.

Is the fracture displaced or nondisplaced?

Displaced fractures occur as the result of high-velocity injuries and result in misaligned segments of the injured bone. Displacement can be partial or complete and can present as translational (sagittal plane motion), angulation, rotation, or shortening.[4] Fractures that maintain anatomical alignment are considered to be nondisplaced. Correction, or realignment, of displaced segments is called **fracture reduction**. This is not to be confused with reduction of a joint dislocation. In joint dislocations, there is a disruption of complementary surfaces of two separate articulating bones. Reduction in the context of joints

---

EVIDENCE-BASED ATHLETIC TRAINING

Tissue Healing Time Line

Tissue healing occurs along a continuum, with no set start or end time between phases.[10] Understanding the general stage of a patient's healing based on time measured from onset of injury provides valuable information as to which interventions will have a significant effect on your desired outcome as the treating health care practitioner.

- The inflammatory response phase begins at the time of injury, when the tissue experiences disruption of blood vessels,[17] and lasts 3 or 4 days.[10,17] Once platelets activate outside of the blood vessel by binding to exposed collagen fibers, chemoattractants are released, recruiting platelets, erythrocytes, and fibrin to form a clot and initiate the inflammatory phase.[17] The cellular makeup of the clot established during the inflammatory phase will serve as the foundation for the next phase of healing.[10,17]

- The fibroblastic repair phase, which begins as early as 4 days postinjury and extends to 6 weeks afterwards,[10] is responsible for increased cell proliferation, capillary budding and revascularization, and the synthesis of the extracellular matrix that fills in the damaged tissue lost during the inflammatory phase.[17] This process is essential for providing the scaffolding necessary for new bone growth and formation during remodeling. It is during this portion of the healing process that structural integrity is regained.[17] When motion at the fracture site is prevented and fractured bone ends are held in place following injury, primary mineralized tissue repair can occur, which affects the structural stability of callus formation.[17]

- In the maturation or remodeling phase, beginning around 4 to 6 weeks postinjury,[4,10] the callus formed during the repair phase continues to condition and harden through osteoclastic destruction of necrotic tissue and osteoblast proliferation of lamellar bone tissue.[17] Wolff's law states that bone will adapt to imposed stress.[10] As such, the end of remodeling is ultimately based on the size of the callus formed during the repair phase; a small callus translates to relatively quicker remodeling. Full remodeling can take 6 months to 2 years or longer depending on the age, health, and activity level of the patient.[10,17]

involves reestablishing the relationship between those complementary surfaces. With fracture reduction, the aim is to reestablish anatomical alignment between two (or more) bone segments that had previously composed one bone. This delineation is important in choosing the appropriate casting materials and technique.

Will I be able to immobilize the necessary anatomy above and below the injury?

A fractured bone can no longer be expected to behave as a uniform segment. Because the body has mass, and therefore weight, any motion of the segment will create load distal to the injury site, which could result in disruption of the articulating surfaces of the fracture. In order to control or prevent motion of an injured bone, you must immobilize either *(a)* the joints proximal and distal to extra-articular fractures or *(b)* the bones proximal and distal to intra-articular fractures.[11] Proximal humeral fractures are an example of a fracture site that is difficult to immobilize by cast application. Advanced techniques for doing so exist but describing them is beyond the scope of this text.

What are the other load-producing forces (deforming forces) acting on the bone?

Bones are the struts on which our muscle forces act to create leverage and generate motion. Once a bone is fractured, any muscle force applied through it has the ability to displace the fracture. Your casting technique should attempt to account for these deforming forces

---

EVIDENCE-BASED ATHLETIC TRAINING

General Follow-Up and Immobilization Duration by Region

Hand
- *Non- or minimally displaced proximal phalangeal shaft fractures of middle fingers.* Follow up 2 weeks later for cast check and X-rays. Continue immobilization for 4 weeks.
- *Fractures of the thumb.* Follow up 1 to 2 weeks later for cast check and X-rays. Continue immobilization for 4 weeks (scaphoid fractures casted until the union is visualized after 6 to 24 weeks[3]).
- *Fractures of fingers.* This is typically managed with buddy taping or splints[1,3,4,9,10,11]

Wrist
- *Stable fractures of carpal bones (except scaphoid and lunate) and distal one-third radius and ulnar.* Follow up 2 weeks later for cast check and repeat X-rays. Continue immobilization for 3 to 4 weeks in pediatric patients and 4 to 6 weeks in adults until healing is visualized.

Forearm and Elbow
- *Stable fractures of distal humerus and proximal/midshaft radius and ulna.* Follow up 5 to 7 days later for cast or splint check and repeat X-rays. Continue immobilization for at least 2 weeks.

Ankle and Foot
- *Isolated stable malleolar fractures, tarsal fractures, and metatarsals.* Follow up 2 to 4 weeks later for cast check and repeat X-rays. Continue immobilization with partial weight-bearing for 4 weeks (non-weight-bearing for tibial fractures).

Knee and Lower Leg
- *Stable fractures of the tibia, fibula, or patella.* Follow up 5 to 7 days later for repeat X-rays and transition patient to removable splint or hinged brace with non-weight-bearing or toe-touch weight-bearing for 4 weeks (progression to partial weight-bearing for 8 to 12 weeks for tibial plateau fractures).

Unstable fracture patterns of the upper and lower extremities are typically managed surgically, except if the patient is elderly, has significant comorbidities, or elects to accept the risks of conservative management. In such cases, serial follow-up at weekly intervals is recommended to ensure optimal cast fit and fracture reduction. Total time of immobilization can be 4 to 6 weeks, possibly longer if callus formation is not appreciated on X-ray.

and mitigate them as much as possible. Limiting motion at the joints is insufficient. Common examples of this phenomenon are as follows:

- Palmar displacement of the distal fragment in metacarpal fractures due to the pull of the interossei muscles[3,7]
- Dorsoradial displacement or collapse of distal one-third radius fractures because of tension from the brachioradialis[3,8]

Will I limit motion at other nonaffected joints?

Immobilization of a joint leads to stiffening of the muscles, tendons, ligaments, and the joint capsule surrounding them, resulting in decreased functionality. This cost is acceptable when the result is achieving a necessary environment for bone healing. However, immobilizing unaffected, uninjured joints will increase the overall functional deficit of the body part and increase the patient's need for rehabilitation after immobilization[11] (i.e., decreased function in one finger is not as inhibiting as having decreased function in three fingers of the same hand; rehabbing one finger is easier and less painful than rehabbing three or more fingers of the same hand). Cast only what you need to and promote motion in the surrounding unaffected joints.

Are there any comorbidities to account for with this patient?

If there are other circumstances involved that need to be monitored and casting will prevent appropriate monitoring of these conditions, consider a different immobilization technique. Common contraindications include the following:

- Allergic reactions
- Distal neuropathy
- Eczema
- Open sores or wounds
- Paralysis
- Skin sensitivities (Raynaud's syndrome or heat sensitivity)

Materials for Application

Once you have determined the need for casting and the effectiveness of cast application, the next step is ensuring you have all the necessary supplies:

- Stockinette
- Fiberglass casting tape
- Webril padding
- Plaster casting tape
- Medical shears or bandage scissors
- Gloves (nitrile or latex)
- Water
- Foot stand (for lower extremity casting)

Understanding the benefits and limitations of differing available materials (figure 24.1) will aid your decision making and ultimately lead to the most appropriate combination of materials to achieve your desired goal and provide the most comfortable experience for your patient.

Stockinette and Webril products come in cotton and synthetic forms. Different suppliers will promote varying benefits for one as opposed to the other, but the main differences are expandability and breathability of the materials. Since it is a natural material, cotton is more breathable and expands more readily than does its synthetic counterpart, making it the more appropriate choice if pressure reduction is needed in the cast.[8] These qualities also cause cotton to break down more quickly, so it may not be the best choice for a long-term application. In warm climates or summer months, patients may request waterproof padding material so they can participate in water-based activities. Waterproof padding should be used only in situations where the prospect of additional swelling is minimal[16] and in water activities involving clean water (i.e., bathing, showering, pool use), not in natural waters.

When deciding which material or technique to use, consider the following factors:[1,5]

- Type of injury
- Goal of immobilization
- Stage of healing
- Availability of materials
- Patient access to follow-up care

In addition to types of padding material, various rigid casting materials present different opportunities for application depending on your desired outcome (table 24.1). Fiberglass cast material is lightweight and significantly stronger than plaster;[8,11] unfortunately, it does not mold as easily as plaster. Fiberglass is also water-resistant. When paired with a waterproof liner and padding, it can allow for water-based recreation to some degree. Plaster, although not as strong as fiberglass, is a substantial immobilizer. It can be more readily molded to varying contours and positions, making it preferable to fiberglass when a custom mold for fracture reduction needs to be achieved.[11] Unlike fiberglass, plaster breaks down in water, even after fully cured; therefore, it must be kept dry.

In more acute injuries where swelling will likely develop, when significant swelling is already present, or there will be a short time (1 week or less) from time

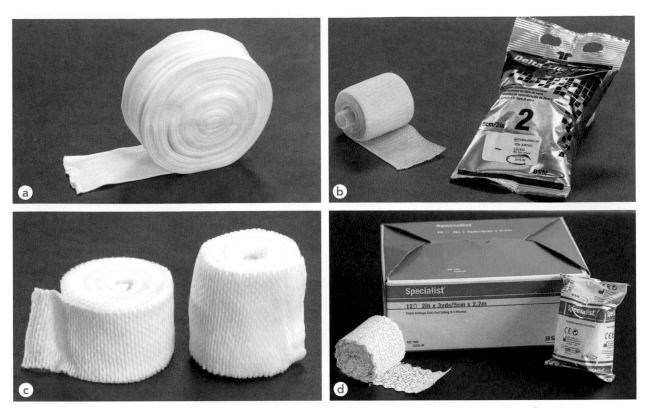

FIGURE 24.1 *(a)* Stockinette, *(b)* fiberglass casting tape, *(c)* cast padding, and *(d)* plaster casting tape.

TABLE 24.1   **Benefits and Drawbacks of Common Rigid Materials**

Material	Pros	Cons
Fiberglass	• Excellent stabilizer • More breathable • Water-resistant • Less messy • Easily transportable • Will cure without water	• Not as forgiving to substantial angles • Can inspire noncompliance • Expires more quickly • Expensive
Plaster	• Great stabilizer • Easily customizable • Long shelf life • Easily transportable • Less expensive	• Very messy • Needs water to set up • Not breathable (uncomfortable) • Heavy in weight • Poor resistance to moisture
Prefabricated fiberglass splint	• Available in precut lengths • Easy set up • Ideal for temporary immobilization in acute setting • Less constrictive	• Poor stabilizer compared to circumferential casting • Limited fine contouring • Bulky to transport • Expensive

of application to follow-up, you can choose an Ortho-Glass application or another noncircumferential splint. This technique will allow for increasing and decreasing amounts of swelling, which is common for the initial inflammatory phase. It will also allow for easy access to the affected body part to address wounds, apply modalities, or monitor any other comorbidity that may exist.[1,11]

If swelling is well controlled and any existing contra-indications mentioned previously have been accounted for, you may move forward with cast application as an immobilization technique. To find out more about splinting applications, refer to *Athletic Taping, Bracing, and Casting*, 4th ed.,[9] or *Ortho-Glass: Splinting Course Manual*.[13]

Being Prepared

When applying a cast, first make sure you have all necessary materials ready at hand. Remember, your patient is injured. Holding any position, even for a short time, will probably be mildly to moderately uncomfortable. Measure, cut, and prepare any aspects of application that you can in advance while the patient is comfortable.

The properties of different materials and how they can best be implemented to achieve optimal care of your patient are key concepts in mastering the skills of casting and splinting. That said, you may find that, in your particular setting, you have access to only one type of casting material, stockinette, or padding. Limited access to resources can occur for any number of reasons, but your ability to provide quality care and treatment should not be completely subject to this obstacle. Whatever materials are available, make sure you take the time to examine them and familiarize yourself with their capabilities. With creativity and ingenuity, you may find that you can easily achieve a technically solid cast by deconstructing a length of preformed fiberglass splinting and separating the layers of cast tape to perform a full, circumferential short-arm cast.

General Application Tips

Every body part and fracture pattern has a specific technique that provides the most ideal healing environment for the affected tissues. Although every application is unique, the mechanics of casting are similar throughout: proper material selection based on body part and patient dimensions, appropriate wrapping technique for cast padding and cast material, the basics of cast molding, and the basics of cast removal.

Choosing Your Materials

Casting materials such as stockinette, plaster rolls, fiberglass rolls, and padding are available in varying widths to accommodate different sizes of body parts.

- 1-in. (2.5-cm) stockinette can be used to cover fingers or toes.
- 2-in. (5-cm) stockinette and padding are generally used for the hands and wrists and people who have smaller ankles.
- 3- in. (8-cm) stockinette and padding are to be used for larger arms and most ankle injuries.
- Stockinette and padding 4 in. (10 cm) and wider are mostly reserved for people with very large arms and applications of the lower extremity.

Selecting the appropriate materials is very important for ensuring patient comfort and avoiding an adverse patient experience. For example, materials that are too bulky may create folds and creases, which become points of friction within the cast. These could cause collections of sweat and skin irritation and result in painful blistering.

Wrapping Techniques

When wrapping cast padding or cast material, avoid unnecessary folding or overlapping. This could result in an undesired number of layers, bulkiness, points of friction, and overall discomfort. There should be a minimum of 4 layers of padding between the skin and the cast material.[15] Use more layers over bony prominences or if the cast will be worn for a long period of time. Remember that the padding material will settle and thin as it is compressed between the cast's hard shell and the skin and as it absorbs sweat and then dries out. Creating a thick, fluffy layer of padding initially may lead to a loose-fitting cast when the padding settles, causing poor immobilization. However, too little padding will result in skin irritation and may lead to abrasions, blistering, and a need for cast replacement. Four layers of soft roll are generally agreed on in the literature as being substantial enough to provide adequate padding and skin protection from the saw blade at time of removal and result in the least amount of fit distortion once settling has occured.[15]

When applying padding or cast material, pay close attention to your tension on the material. Wrapping too tightly could cause neurovascular compromise; wrapping too loosely could result in an ill-fitting cast and poor fracture stabilization. To achieve the most comfortable tension, place the material roll against the surface with the roll opening away from the patient's body (figure 24.2) and roll the material (padding or casting) along the surface, allowing it to unravel.

Apply the padding and casting material using the cover-by-half method, which creates the sturdiest material configuration and the most uniform compression across the span of the casted field. It is achieved by layering the material such that the upper edge of the current layer falls at 50%, or half, the width of the previous layer. The desired result is a kind of barber pole effect of the padding

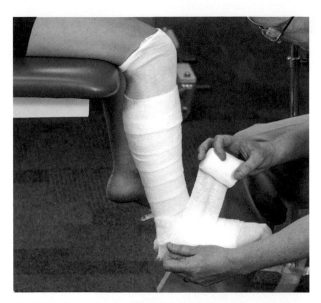

FIGURE 24.2 Proper material application technique with minimal tension and the roll facing away from the patient's body.

or casting material laid flat on the body's surface. Once you have wrapped one full length of the extremity using this pattern, you will have applied two layers of padding or casting material. Repeat for the desired number of padding or casting layers.

Molding

Once you have applied casting material, you must mold the cast quickly to appropriately fit and secure the anatomy. Although using the roll-on technique with the casting material will create the general shape of the cast, molding the material will tailor it to the affected body part and fracture site to establish necessary fixation and stabilization.[8] Mold the cast with the palms of your hands whenever possible. Molding with your fingers will produce a rippling in the cast material from the gaps between the fingers, which may result in inconsistent pressure across the casted surface. Also, a cast that is more cylindrical, as opposed to one closely resembling the natural anatomic structure, will be less effective at restricting rotational motion within the cast, which will

allow for deforming forces to be placed across the fracture site and possibly result in displacement. In the upper extremity, for example, the **cast index** is the ratio of the sagittal width to the coronal width on the inside edges of the cast at the fracture site.[6,8] Although adipose tissue proliferation and muscle hypertrophy may alter forearm shape, the forearm skeletal structure and musculature generally have a narrower width in the sagittal plane than in the coronal plane; therefore, the molded cast should reflect this shape. A cast with an index less than or equal to 0.81 was found to have a 20.42% lower displacement rate than those with an index greater than 0.81.[6] A cast index of 1 would be a perfectly cylindrical cast. Regardless of the appearance and shape of the body part, you must understand the fracture location and orientation as well as the overlying anatomy when applying and forming a cast in order to account for and minimize the effects of all of the factors previously reviewed in the casting basic principles.

To achieve proper fixation of a displaced fracture when molding a cast, you will need to create three static points of contact within the cast surrounding the fracture (figure 24.3). The first and second points of contact will need to be

- proximal and distal to the fracture site,
- applied on the surface opposing the apex of the fracture, and
- applied in the same direction as the apex of the fracture.

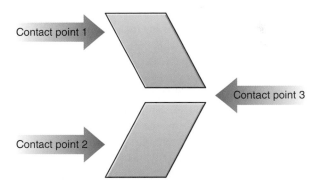

FIGURE 24.3 Three-point fracture reduction.

FOUNDATIONAL SKILL

Molding Versus Reducing

Although properly molding a cast to ensure stabilization of a reduced fracture is essential for optimizing healing, the action of reducing a fracture does not fall within the scope of practice for athletic trainers. Please do not confuse molding with reducing. Fracture reduction is a manipulation that should be performed by a health care practitioner whose scope of practice covers such procedures. Once the reduction has been achieved, the cast can be molded to maintain the reduction.

FOUNDATIONAL SKILL

Wet Versus Dry Materials

Fiberglass casting material cures more quickly when it is wet, but it is also able to cure without water application. If you are applying a cast that you are unfamiliar with or one where the positioning or angles are difficult to achieve, consider applying the cast without wetting the material first. This will allow you maximum time to manipulate the material as desired. You can apply water later using your hands or a spray bottle and perform your mold.

These two points will provide counterpressure to the third contact force. The third point of contact will be applied at the apex of the fracture in the direction of reduction. This will reestablish anatomical alignment and ensure that the fracture holds reduction within the cast.

Cast Removal Procedures

Perhaps as significant to the patient experience as having a cast applied is the process of having it removed. After cast removal, patients expect healing and a return to normalcy on both the physical and psychological levels. For this reason, avoid regarding this step as a mere formality; instead, make an effort to appreciate and empathize with your patient's experience.

Remember that most patients have never had a cast removed before. This may be the first time someone has put sharp or powered tools near their skin, and they may therefore feel apprehensive about having the cast taken off. They may be frightened that the saw blade or scissors will cut them. Take the time to explain in detail that you are going to remove the cast, how you are going to do it, and what tools you will be using to do so (figure 24.4). Set an honest expectation of what the patient will experience. Although the saw is capable of causing friction burns, or even lacerations, if enough pressure is applied, explaining how the tools will feel on their skin, the safety measures built into the tools you are using (e.g., the blunted points of tape or bandage scissors, the oscillating motion of the saw blade), and the techniques you will use to ensure their safety will go a long way toward putting the patient at ease. Encourage your patient to relax as much as possible. For small children, restraint may be necessary. Discuss this with the child's parent or guardian before recruiting their assistance; parents and children find it off-putting to walk into the room with a team of people they are unfamiliar with.

The general removal technique is to make longitudinal cuts on opposing sides of the cast, creating two full-length pieces (anterior and posterior or medial and lateral; figure 24.5a). Then, use the cast spreader (figure 24.5b) to part the fiberglass pieces. Next, use medical shears to cut

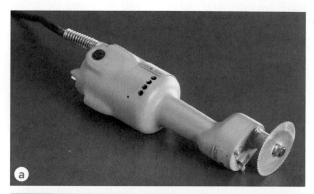
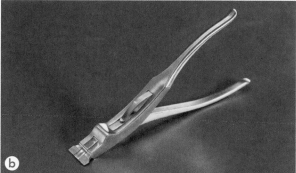
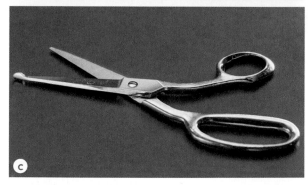

FIGURE 24.4 *(a)* Cast saw, *(b)* cast spreader, and *(c)* bandage scissors.

the underlying padding material (figure 24.5c). Cut the cast and padding completely so that the patient does not have to use any force to remove the extremity from the material. The particulars of how to remove each type of cast are outlined in their respective sections.

Cast-Cutting Techniques

Basic Cutting Technique
- Begin proximally.
- Hold the saw so the blade is at a right angle to the surface you are cutting.
- Apply downward pressure such that the saw sinks through the material but does not deform the cast surface.
- Once a full-thickness cut is made, lift the blade out, move distally one cutting length of the blade, and repeat.

Advanced Technique: The Roll
- Begin proximally.
- Hold the saw with a flexed wrist and the blade at a right angle to the cast surface.
- Apply downward pressure such that the saw sinks through the material but does not deform the cast surface.
- Once the downward cut is made, using your finger as the saw guide, extend your wrist or roll the saw blade distally.
- Once the full-thickness cut is made, lift the blade out, reposition your wrist, and begin the next cut at the distal end of the previous cut, repeating the same motion.

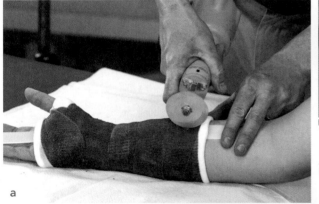
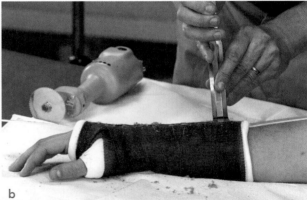
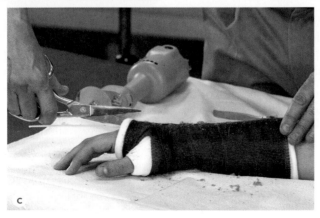

FIGURE 24.5 General cast removal technique.

Pro Tip

Once you have made a complete cast cut, use your thumb to press firmly along the edge of your cut. If the edge of the cast you are pressing on flexes independently of the opposing edge, you have achieved a full-thickness cut. If it does not flex, you have not achieved a complete cut. Press along the full length of your cut to ensure it is complete before performing your next cut or attempting to spread the cast.

Upper Extremity Casts

Upper extremity injuries are very common in sports as well as in the general population. A 2009 study found that each year 1.1 in 100 people in the United States presents to the local emergency department for an upper extremity injury, 29.2% of which are fractures.[14] As such, casting and splinting of the upper extremity is a common practice in the clinical setting.

Short Arm Cast

The short arm cast is the most basic upper extremity application covered in this chapter. It serves as the cornerstone construct that is adapted to create each additional upper extremity casting technique covered in the following sections. This cast is used to restrict motion at the carpal, radiocarpal, and distal radial or ulnar levels for fractures affecting the applicable skeletal anatomy.

Common Injuries
- Carpal fractures
- Distal radius and ulna fractures
- Distal radius fracture
- Radial styloid fractures

Supplies
- 2 or 3 rolls of 2″ casting material
- Forearm length of 2″ to 3″ stockinette
- 2 or 3 rolls of Webril padding
- Basin of water
- Scissors
- Gloves

Positioning

Unless specifically instructed otherwise, any nondisplaced fracture with an acceptable degree of angulation should be cast in the **position of function**, which is 30 degrees of wrist extension and with the thumb opposed to midway between maximal radial and maximal palmar abduction.[1,3,11] It is sometimes referred to as the full-can position. This position allows for some degree of usefulness of the affected

FOUNDATIONAL SKILL

Upper Extremity Relaxation

When applying a cast to the upper extremity, remember to have the patient relax the extremity in order to achieve appropriate molding and stabilization. A patient supporting the weight of her own extremity is tensioning the surrounding muscle, which can result in patient discomfort and fatigue and increased muscle bulk, making for improper fit. At least 3 points of support are ideal: The first two are your own hands and the third is a fixed surface supporting the elbow.

Pro Tip

Fractures that are dorsally angulated or radially angulated or need to be reset due to dorsal or radial displacement often tend to settle in those directions as they heal. For this reason, avoid casting them in extension because this may lead to displacement in the cast and poor positioning for healing. Cast this injury in slight flexion and ulnar deviation;[8] the resultant tension of the radiocarpal ligamentous structures (known as ligamentotaxis) will help to prevent adverse settling of these fracture patterns.

hand once the cast has been applied, which is important for encouraging use of the fingers in that hand. If the patient feels absolutely incapacitated with that hand, he will be less apt to engage it, leading to further atrophy and the development of stiffness in unaffected joints. This position is easily achieved by handing an item to the patient that is roughly the size of a soda can and asking him to hold it as if he were going to drink it.

Application

1. Have patient sit with his elbow on a counter (arm-wrestling position), or lie supine with his elbow securely and comfortably situated on the table surface. Position his wrist and hand in the position of function, as described previously.

2. Cut a length of stockinette 2 or 3 in. wide (depending on the patient's arm size) that will cover from just proximal to the middle finger PIP joint to the antecubital crease.

   - Once you have applied the stockinette, cut a small slit at the thumb MCP to allow the thumb to stick out (figure 24.6*a*).

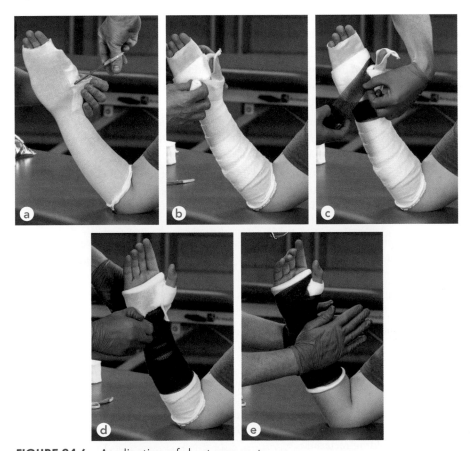

FIGURE 24.6   Application of short arm cast.

- Optional: For patient comfort, you can use a finger length of 1-in. stockinette to cover the thumb. This will be rolled down later as a buffer between the cast material and the skin.

3. Apply cast padding using a circling pattern:
   - Using the roll-on technique, begin distally and circle the hand with the far edge covering just distal to the metacarpal heads; apply 3 layers.
   - Begin wrapping proximally, using the cover-by-half technique.
   - Tear, cut, or fold the padding to pass through the web space of the thumb (figure 24.6b), making sure to maintain the aforementioned layering technique and creating another barrier for comfort when you lay the cast material through the web space.
   - Continue to wrap proximally until the proximal edge of the Webril is 1 finger-width distal to the antecubital crease.
   - Repeat this until you have created at least 4 layers of padding material. Be sure to apply additional padding over bony prominences such as the radial styloid, ulnar styloid, and along the dorsal aspect of the thumb metacarpal, which are common locations of irritation.

4. Put on gloves and apply cast material using the same roll-on and cover-by-half techniques used for the cast padding (figure 24.6c).
   - The distal edge of the cast material should lie just proximal to the metacarpal heads posteriorly and fall right at the palmar crease anteriorly. This will prevent swelling from collecting in the knuckles and allow for MCP flexion of the fingers, keeping the hand semifunctional and preventing undue stiffness.
   - Be sure that the edges of the casting material fall within the borders of the padding material so that the fiberglass does not come into contact with the skin.
   - When maneuvering through the thumb and index web space, you can use either a cutting or folding technique to decrease the width of the material. Ideally, the cast material should fall proximal to both the thumb (1st) and index finger (2nd) metacarpal heads to allow for motion at these joints.
     - Cut the material from the proximal edge such that the open end falls around the anterior and posterior aspect of the base of the thumb. This tends to generate less bulk but is sometimes difficult to do and takes more time.
     - Fold the cast material to decrease the material width as it passes through the space, then allow it to fan open again across the palm (or the dorsum of the hand depending on your wrapping preference) as you lay the material down ulnarly.
   - Apply 2 initial rounds, then continue wrapping proximally, observing the overlap-by-half technique. End the application when you are 3 finger-widths distal to the antecubital crease, using your scissors to cut the remaining material left on the roll. At this point, you will have applied 2 layers of casting material.

5. Using the flats of your hands, apply gentle, consistent anterior and posterior pressure at the fracture site such that the fracture is roughly in the center of your palms. This creates even pressure just proximal to, at the level of, and just distal to the fracture.
   - Hold this position until the casting material is stiff enough to maintain the desired shape once you remove your hands.
   - Remember that the portion of material that came off the roll first has been exposed to air the longest, so it will cure the earliest. Apply your mold to this portion of the cast first since you will have the least amount of time to manipulate it, then move on to less mature portions of the cast for molding.

6. Once the cast maintains the desired shape without pressure from your hands, you can pull the stockinette at either end of the cast toward the middle of the cast. The padding material that extends beyond the edges of the casting material will roll up (or down) and form a padded edge to the cast so as not to irritate the skin (figure 24.6d). This is why you should always make sure your cast material lies within the borders of the padding material.

7. Next, open a new roll of casting material and apply it, using the same roll-on and cover-by-half techniques used for the previous layers of padding and casting material.

   • Make sure that the edges of the casting material do not approach the edges of the padding too closely. (Pro tip: Mind your lines.)

   • Make sure that the open edges of the retracted stockinette are secured under the layers of cast material so that the padding does not unravel or become undone. (Pro tip: Lock down your edges.)

   • This final layer is for added strength and support of the cast as well as the overall look of the finished product.

8. Mold the final layer as in step 5 (figure 24.6*e*), then allow 5 to 8 minutes for the cast to stiffen.

   • Instruct the patient not to move or use the arm during the early curing process, since the cast will still be malleable.

   • The cast will take at least 12 hours to fully harden, but it will stiffen to a point that the average person cannot manipulate it within 40 minutes.

Removal

1. Have your patient sit comfortably or lie supine. Make sure that you can comfortably hold the casted arm in your nondominant hand and easily alter the arm position while maintaining patient comfort.

2. Visualize the path of your cuts. You will need to make them on opposing sides of the arm—either volarly and dorsally or radially and ulnarly—to create two separable pieces of the cast.

3. If your patient is very apprehensive about having the blade contact his skin, you can insert a cast strip guard underneath the cast along the desired path of your cut.

4. Hold the casted appendage firmly. Using a cast saw, cut proximal to distal using the in-out or roll technique described earlier in this chapter.

5. Once you have completed opposing cuts, use the cast spreader to widen the cuts.

6. Use your tape or bandage scissors (always holding the blunted side against the patient's skin) to cut the underlying stockinette and Webril padding along both seams. Do not cut only one seam and hinge the cast open.

7. Remove the cast by pulling the two resultant pieces apart with a symmetrical, predictable motion. This is important because some patients move as soon as they feel the space to do so, which may result in unintentional injury exacerbation if they move in a way that they think would avoid hitting you or the cast.

Thumb Spica

The thumb spica application is very closely related to the short arm cast, with one modification: It includes partial or complete immobilization of the thumb.

Common Injuries
• Scaphoid fractures
• Intra-articular and nonarticular fractures of the proximal or distal thumb phalanges
• Thumb MCP UCL injuries

Supplies
• 2 or 3 rolls of 2″ casting material
• Forearm length of 2″ or 3″ stockinette
• 2 or 3 rolls Webril padding
• 1″ stockinette sleeve approximately 1.5 times the patient's thumb length
• Basin of water
• Scissors
• Gloves

Positioning

Patient can either sit with her elbow fixed firmly against a table or firm surface (arm-wrestling position) or lie supine with her shoulder abducted and elbow bent to 90 degrees so that the forearm is perpendicular to the table surface and pointed directly toward the ceiling. Unless otherwise instructed by the overseeing provider, you should place the wrist and hand in the position of function, which is the wrist slightly extended and the thumb opposed.

Application

1. Have the patient sit with the affected arm in arm-wrestling position or lie supine with the arm positioned as described previously. Her hand and fingers should be in the position of function.

2. Cut and apply the protective stockinette layer.

   • Apply 1 in. stockinette to the affected thumb. Cut the proximal edge of the thumb sleeve vertically to allow the sleeve to drape anteriorly and posteriorly over the thenar web space (figure 24.7*a*).

   • Cut and apply 2 or 3 in. of stockinette sleeve so that it extends from just proximal to the middle finger PIP joint to the antecubital crease. Cut a hole adjacent to the thumb MCP joint to allow the thumb to poke through (figure 24.7*b*).

3. Apply 2 in. Webril starting at the distal end of the affected thumb.

   • The distal edge of the Webril should extend just beyond the tip of the thumb or just distal to the IP joint (depending on what joints are to be immobilized) but not beyond the length of the stockinette sleeve.

   • Wrap 3 layers around the thumb to start, then work proximally using the overlap-by-half technique. Cut, tear, or fold the Webril at the proximal edge to accommodate the thenar web space.

   • As you reach the hand, the distal edge of the Webril should lie just distal to the metacarpal heads.

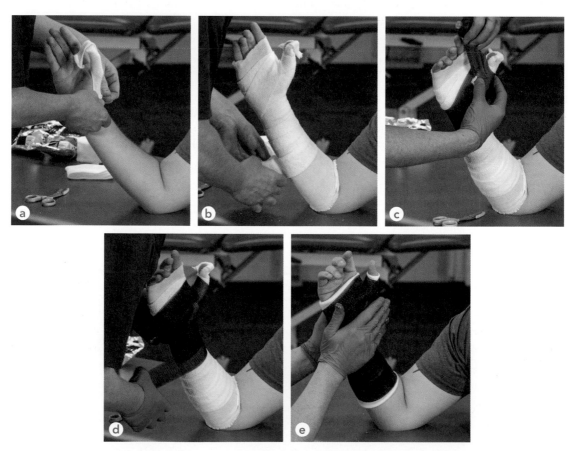

FIGURE 24.7 Application of short arm thumb spica cast.

- Continue to wrap proximally, using the roll-on and cover-by-half methods, until you reach the antecubital crease. Wrap 3 or 4 layers.
4. Put on gloves, prewet cast material if desired and apply casting material beginning at the thumb.
   - The distal edge of casting material should lie at the level of desired immobilization, either just distal to the tip of the thumb or just proximal to the IP joint (figure 24.7c).
   - Apply 2 rounds, then wrap proximally using the overlap-by-half technique.
   - Cut or fold the proximal edge of the cast tape to accommodate the thenar web space. Make sure that the edges of the cast material do not extend beyond the borders of the padding material.
   - Continue to observe the cover-by-half technique as you apply the hand portion of the cast. Dorsally, the cast should lie just proximal to the metacarpal heads and fall right at the palmar crease anteriorly so as to allow for MCP motion at the other 4 fingers (figure 24.7d).
   - Roll on the casting material until you are 3 finger-widths distal to the antecubital crease.
5. Using a hand grip similar to that of arm wrestling, hold the patient's hand and encourage her to mirror your hand positioning without applying significant force. Using the flat surface of your free hand, form a posterior mold at the level of the fracture.
   - When the material has stiffened enough to maintain its mold, use both hands to form the appropriate forearm mold.
6. Once the cast maintains the desired shape without pressure from your hands, you can pull the stockinette at either end of the cast toward the middle of the cast: down over the thumb, down over the palm, and up over the forearm. The padding material that extends beyond the edges of the casting material will roll up (or down) and form a padded edge to the cast so as to not irritate the skin. This is why you should always make sure your cast material lies within the borders of the padding material.
7. Next, open a new roll of casting material and apply it with the same roll-on and cover-by-half techniques, you used for the previous layers of padding and casting material.
   - Make sure that the edges of the casting material do not approach the edges of the padding too closely (i.e., mind your lines).
   - Make sure the open edges of the retracted stockinette are secured under the layers of cast material so that the padding does not unravel or become undone (i.e., lock down your edges).
   - This final layer is for added strength and support of the cast as well as overall look of the finished product.
8. Mold the final layer as in step 5 (figure 24.7e), then allow 5 to 8 minutes for the cast to stiffen.
   - Instruct the patient not to move or use her arm during the early curing process, since the cast is still malleable.
   - The cast will take at least 12 hours to fully harden, but it will stiffen to a point that the average person cannot manipulate it within 40 minutes.

Removal

An anterior-to-posterior cut pattern should be sufficient for removal. If a cut needs to extend to the thumb, extend your longitudinal cut through the proximal and distal ends, then choose a point along that cut in the palm of the hand where you can make a straight line from the current cut through the end of the thumb extension. Do the same for the posterior aspect of the cast. Do not attempt to cut along the web space, since the size of the blade does not allow for easy or comfortable positioning with an average-sized adult hand. Attempting to do so may injure your patient.

Long Arm Cast

The long arm cast extends from the wrist or hand above the elbow to the level of the deltoid insertion (if possible), but at least proximal to the level of the bulk of the biceps brachii. With this cast, the goal is to prevent wrist flexion, extension, pronation, and supination, as well as elbow flexion and extension.

Common Injuries
- Middle one-third or proximal one-third radial shaft fractures
- Combined middle or proximal radial and ulnar shaft fractures
- Capitellar fractures
- Condylar or supracondylar fractures

Supplies
- 2″ to 4 stockinette
- 1″ stockinette (optional)
- 2″ and 3″ Webril padding
- Tape
- Scissors
- At least four 2″ cast rolls
- Two 3″ cast rolls
- Spray bottle of water
- Gloves

Positioning
Have the patient lie supine with the shoulder comfortably abducted to tolerance, as much as 90 degrees, and the elbow flexed to 90 degrees or a desirable range as instructed by supervising physician, depending on the fracture pattern. Forearm positioning is based on physician instructions and the following guidelines for forearm fractures:

- *Proximal one-third:* Immobilize in slight supination.
- *Middle one-third:* Immobilize in neutral.
- *Distal one-third:* Immobilize in pronation.

The goal is to decrease or negate the pull of pronator (distal) or supinator (proximal) forces, which will act as deforming forces during healing. Have the patient passively maintain this position with hanging traction, using finger distraction devices applied to the index and middle fingers. Alternatively, an assisting provider can hold the patient's hand by the same two fingers.

Application
1. Position patient comfortably, lying supine with the arm suspended as previously described.
2. Cut and apply a length of 2- or 3-in. stockinette that will extend the full length of the upper extremity, from the axilla to the PIP joints of the fingers. Cut a hole at the thumb MCP joint to allow for opposition (figure 24.8a).
   - Use 2-in. stockinette for small children, 3 in. for most adults, and 4 in. for people with large upper arms. You may also apply combinations of widths in an overlapping manner for people with small forearms and large upper arms, such as length of 2-in. stockinette for the forearm and length of 3-in. stockinette for the upper arm.
   - If the cast is to include the thumb or if you wish to create a padded border for the thumb, you can place 1-in. stockinette over the thumb now.
   - Use scissors to make a transverse cut across the antecubital crease, such that the stockinette does not form a fold. Place the material so it lies flat.
3. Begin distally, using 2-in. Webril padding. Apply padding using the roll-on and cover-by-half techniques.
   - The distal edge of the padding material should lie just proximal to the PIP joints of the fingers. Apply 3 layers, then work proximally. Cut, tear, or fold material to account for the thenar web space.
   - Roll the padding until you are within 2 finger-widths of the antecubital crease. Place the patient's elbow in 90 degrees of flexion and then, using the remainder of the first roll, wrap the elbow with a

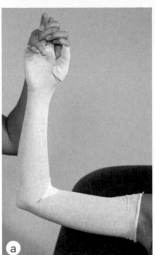 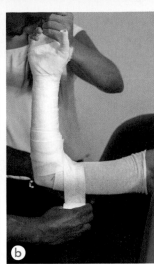 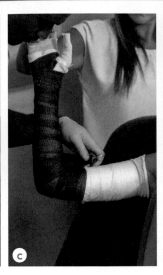 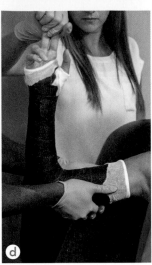

FIGURE 24.8 Application of long arm cast.

figure-eight pattern. The crossing of the figure eights should fall over the antecubital crease so that the padding material does not fold (figure 24.8b).

- Switch to 3-in. padding and perform 1 figure eight to cover all exposed parts. Pad proximally as high as possible to just superior to the level of the deltoid insertion.
- Repeat this process to achieve at least 4 total layers of padding. Add extra padding at the ulnar styloid, radial styloid, olecranon process, and medial and lateral epicondyles by tearing off small squares of padding material.
- Finish by adding 1 or 2 padding layers at what will be the proximal border of the cast.

4. Wearing gloves, open 1 roll of 2-in. cast material. Reposition the patient as necessary so as to limit the need for movement once the cast material has been applied. Begin distally, using the roll-on and cover-by-half methods. Do not wet the fiberglass cast material prior to application.

- The distal edge of the casting material should lie at the palmar crease anteriorly and just proximal to the metacarpal heads posteriorly. Apply 2 layers and then work proximally.
- Cut or fold the cast material to accommodate the thenar web space.
- Continue to wrap proximally until the roll is finished.
  - If the forearm is short, you may reach the elbow before the roll is complete. Wrap using the cover-by-half technique to within 2 finger-widths distal to the antecubital crease, then begin using a figure-eight pattern to include the elbow.
- If the patient's forearm is large, switch to 3-in. cast material once the previous roll is complete. Begin the next roll by continuing in the same fashion until you are 2 finger-widths distal to the antecubital crease. Then begin using a figure-eight pattern to cover the elbow (figure 24.8c).
- Apply 2 layers to cover the elbow, then wrap proximally, with the final layer ending at the level of the deltoid insertion if possible.

5. Since you did not wet the cast material when you began, the curing time is increased. Using the spray bottle, wet the cast at the level of the fracture and apply uniform pressure, using the palms of your hands.

- Once the facture level has been appropriately molded, apply water to the forearm and wrist (if you have not already done so) and mold to create the appropriate cast index and wrist positioning.
- Spray the proximal portion of the cast and mold it to mimic the anatomical structure of the brachial region: tapered at the top, narrower in the frontal plane, and wider in the sagittal plane.
- Apply your supracondylar mold.

- For a supracondylar fracture, you will apply this mold first.
- Place your palms on the medial and lateral aspects of the elbow, such that the hypothenar eminences are immediately proximal to the medial and lateral epicondyles (figure 24.8*d*).
- This mold is of particular importance because it prevents inferior translation of the cast, making sure it maintains its position on the upper extremity.

6. Once the brachial mold, the supracondylar mold, and the forearm mold (not necessarily in that order) are set to the point that they can hold their shape without the pressure from your hands, fold the stockinette over the proximal and distal edges of the cast to create padded proximal and distal edges.

7. Open a new 2-in. casting roll and apply the 3rd and 4th layers of casting material, using the methods described in step 4 and the molding techniques described in step 5.
   - A 2-in. roll is easier to work with in the smaller angles of the hand and wrist, while the 3-in. width covers more effectively in the larger anatomy of the elbow and upper arm.
   - Be sure to mind your lines and lock down your edges, both proximally and distally.
   - Once you have applied the full layer, distal to proximal, wet the cast with the spray bottle and mold it to allow for uniform curing.

8. Allow the material to set for 8 to 10 minutes so that the cast, though not fully cured, has reached a point that it cannot be deformed by patient effort.

Removal

This application is most easily removed with medial and lateral longitudinal cuts down the length of the cast. Do not attempt to cut in a curved path, since you may risk bending the blade. Begin proximally and cut distally beyond the intersection of the humerus and elbow, then cut from the elbow to the forearm so that both cuts are straight.

Ulnar and Radial Gutter

These are specialized applications for immobilization of the wrist, metacarpals, and index through small fingers. Immobilization of the thumb or 1st metacarpal would be achieved using the thumb spica application.

Common Injuries
Fractures of the 2nd to 5th metacarpal base, shaft, or neck

Supplies
- 1″ stockinette
- 2″ stockinette
- 2″ Webril padding
- Two or three 2″ casting rolls
- Tape or bandage scissors
- Water

Positioning
Have the patient sit with the elbow fixed on a firm surface in the arm-wrestling position or lie supine with the arm abducted to 90 degrees and the elbow flexed to 90 degrees. Place the patient's wrist in a position between 15 and 25 degrees of extension and the involved fingers in the **intrinsic plus position** (MCP joints flexed to as close to 70 to 90 degrees as is comfortably achievable). This involves the index and long fingers for a radial gutter and the ring and small fingers for an ulnar gutter. For the purposes of this technique, the following description details the ulnar gutter cast application.

Application
1. Have the patient sit with the affected arm on a table in arm-wrestling position or lie supine with the hand, wrist, and fingers placed as described previously.

2. Cut a length of 2-in. stockinette that will extend from beyond the tips of the fingers to the antecubital crease. Cut a hole at the thumb MCP joint to allow the thumb to poke through. Cut another hole at the index finger MCP joint to allow the index and ring fingers to poke through.

   • Because the joint proximal to the fracture site is the CMC joint, this cast can be made in gauntlet form, which means it does not have to extend as far proximally on the forearm as the short arm application.

   • Apply 1 finger length of 1-in. stockinette to cover the thumb and the index and long fingers as a pair.

   • Pair the ring and small fingers and wrap them in the remaining length of the 2-in. stockinette (figure 24.9a).

3. Apply Webril padding, beginning at the fingers and working proximally.

   • Begin by laying 2 strips of 2-in. cast padding, one on top of the other, longitudinally from the tip of the ring finger to the base of the wrist posteriorly. Next, layer 2 strips palmarly, extending from the tip of the ring finger to the wrist.

   • Wrap 2 layers of padding around the distal end of the ring and small fingers so that the distal edge of the padding extends just beyond the tip of the ring finger. Then work proximally, using the cover-by-half technique (figure 24.9b).

   • Cut or tear the padding to accommodate the web space so that you can maintain the cover-by-half pattern.

   • At the level of the palm, extend the padding across the palm and thenar web space. Cut or tear the padding to accommodate the thenar web space.

   • Continue to work proximally until you reach the mid forearm (for a gauntlet cast) or 1 or 2 finger-widths distal to the antecubital crease (for a short arm cast).

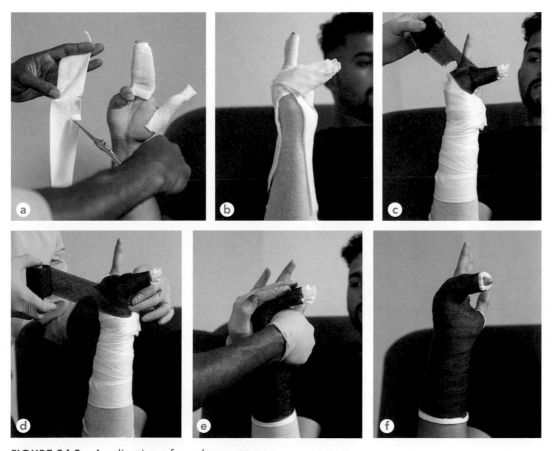

FIGURE 24.9 Application of an ulnar gutter.

- The fingers are already covered by 4 layers at this point: 2 longitudinal layers volarly and dorsally, then cover-by-half layers down the length of the fingers. Beginning at the hand, repeat your padding application to achieve 4 total layers.

4. Put on gloves and begin applying cast material, following the same roll-on technique and sequence as you used for the padding material.

- Begin at the fingers, wrap 2 layers such that the distal edge of the casting material extends just beyond the tip of the ring finger.
- Continue to wrap proximally, overlapping by half. Cut or fold the cast material to accommodate the interphalangeal web space (figure 24.9*c*).
- Be sure that as you approach the flexion angle of MCP joints, you ensure that the casting material lies in a gradual curve volarly, with no folds, creases, or buckles (figure 24.9*d*).
- Extend your wrap across the palm or posterior of the hand when the distal edge of the cast material lies at the palmar crease. Cut or fold the cast material to accommodate the thenar web space.
- Continue to wrap proximally, using the roll-on and cover-by-half methods until you are within 2 finger-widths of the edge of the Webril padding border.

5. Use your hands or a spray bottle to wet the applied layer of casting roll and form the intrinsic plus mold (figure 24.9*e*).

- Place the thenar eminence of your hand at the 4th and 5th metatarsal heads anteriorly.
- Place the palm of your remaining hand against the posterior of the cast such that you can mimic the desired angle of the fingers in the cast by overlaying them with your own fingers.
- Pronate or supinate your anterior molding hand and flex or extend your posterior molding hand to achieve the desired wrist angle.
- Hold this position until the cast is set enough that it can hold the mold without pressure from your hands.

6. Pull the excess stockinette at the ends of the cast back over the cast edges to form a padded edge at the ring and small fingertips, the base of the index and middle fingers, the thumb, and the proximal aspect of the cast.

7. Use a new roll of cast material and repeat the previous casting application as described in step 3.

- Be sure to keep the cast roll's edges within the defined border (i.e., mind your lines) so that the completed cast does not irritate the patient's skin. Make sure the open edges of the retracted stockinette are secured under the layers of cast material so that the padding does not unravel or become undone (i.e., lock down your edges).
- Once you have applied the final layers, distal to proximal, wet the cast material, smooth the edges and surface, and reapply molds (figure 24.9*f*).

8. Allow the material to set for 8 to 10 minutes so that the cast, though not fully cured, has reached a point that it cannot be deformed by patient effort.

King and colleagues describes a less restrictive technique in the management of **boxer fractures**, which involve fractures of the 5th metacarpal neck with apex dorsal angulation.[7] The casting technique is closer to that of the short arm application, but includes applying hanging traction to the injured finger for 5 to 10 minutes to achieve reduction, then extending the distal border of the ulnar aspect of the cast to cover the proximal one-third of the proximal phalanx of the small finger. With the small finger still in traction, a 3-point mold is performed to maintain the reduction.[7]

Removal

This application can be removed using an ulnar and radial cutting approach. When cutting into the palmar aspect of the cast, pick locations that can easily accommodate the full cutting length of the blade and where you can connect two established openings with a straight cut (i.e., between the thumb and index finger openings, or down the radial aspect of the finger extension to the opening at the base of the fingers).

Lower extremity injuries are significantly cumbersome and limiting to manage for the average person because, in many cases, the patient will be limited, if not completely restricted, from weight-bearing on the affected extremity, or they will be allowed to weight-bear in an application that does not allow for normal kinematics of the foot, ankle, or knee. Protection of fractures of the lower leg, ankle, and foot differ from the upper extremity because it is far easier to impact these injuries with a thoughtless gesture. Putting a foot down to balance is an instinctual and less conscious action than would be lifting an object of weight with a casted hand. Additionally, as the full-weight-bearing structures of the body, the amount of force absorbed by, and exerted across, these structures are many times greater than that of the upper extremity. For these reasons, casting of the lower extremity will involve more robust amounts of materials as well as careful instruction on adherence to limitations and activity modifications.

Short Leg Cast

Similar to the short arm cast in the upper extremity, the short leg cast is the most basic and most common application of the lower extremity; therefore, it serves as the building block for the lower extremity applications that will be covered in this text. This application is used to restrict motion of the talocrural, subtalar, tarsal, metatarsal, and even the MTP joints.

Common Injuries
- Distal fibular fracture
- Nondisplaced and stable, medial, lateral, or bimalleolar fracture
- Syndesmotic sprains
- Lisfranc sprain

Supplies
- 3″ or 4″ stockinette
- 2″ and 3″ Webril padding
- 2″ and 3″ cast rolls
- Scissors
- Foot stand
- Gloves
- Bucket of water
- Rigid, flat surface
- Cast saw

Positioning

The patient should be casted with the ankle in a talar and subtalar neutral position or as close to this position as is tolerable. The patient will likely be resistant to maintaining this position, so you should explain to him why this position is important to help enlist his cooperation.

Application
1. Have the patient sit with his legs over the edge of a plinth table, positioned far enough forward on the table so that you can easily pass your hands between the posterior aspect of his lower leg and the edge of the table (figure 24.10a).
2. Cut and apply a length of 3- or 4-in. stockinette, as determined by the size of body part. The stockinette length should extend from the popliteal fold proximally to 3 or 4 finger-widths beyond the toes distally. Cut a slit in the stockinette across the anterior ankle to eliminate the fold (figure 24.10b).
3. Set the cast stand (if available) under the patient's affected extremity and position him for padding and cast application.

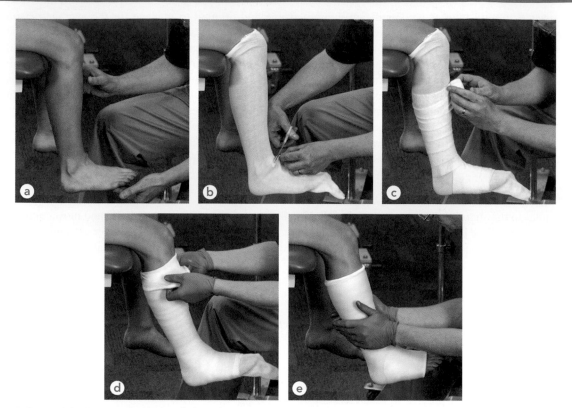

FIGURE 24.10 Application of short leg cast.

- Slide the foot plate of the stand under the stockinette. This will prevent the casting material from drying to the equipment. Elevate the stand so that the patient's foot rests on the foot plate and his knee is flexed to 90 degrees. The foot plate should be aligned to the plantar surface of the 1st and 2nd ray.

- The ankle should be aligned in neutral and should be in line with the tibial tubercle.

4. Using 2-in. Webril padding, begin wrapping distally. Apply 2 or 3 layers such that the distal edge of the padding falls just proximal to the great toe's IP joint.

   - Angle the direction of the roll so that the applied layers reflect the natural alignment of the toes.

   - Wrap across the top of the foot to start, then move around the lateral aspect and underneath the foot toward the medial arch. Wrapping in this direction accentuates the natural arch of the foot.

   - For toe-plate construction, begin your initial layers of padding 2 finger-widths distal to the toes. Angle your padding to follow the natural anatomy of the toes.

5. Work proximally, using the roll-on and cover-by-half methods, until you reach the anterior ankle.

   - Use a figure-eight pattern to pad the ankle, with the crossing aspect of the pattern falling at the anterior ankle.

   - To avoid bulkiness, use C-strips to apply any further necessary padding, wrapping posteriorly over the heel. Apply an additional 1 or 2 strips over the medial and lateral malleoli, since these bony prominences may become sensitive.

6. Using a 3-in. Webril roll, continue to wrap the ankle and tibial shaft, working distally to proximally and using the roll-on and cover-by-half methods (figure 24.10c).

   - Continue to wrap proximally until the proximal edge of the padding borders the soft tissue of the hamstrings posteriorly or reaches the tibial tubercle anteriorly. Apply 2 layers.

7. Repeat steps 4 to 6, using Webril to achieve a minimum of 4 layers of padding material.

8. Wearing gloves, open and wet a 2- or 3-in. roll of casting material (depending on the patient's foot size and preference). Reposition the patient, if necessary, and then begin applying the material distally at the toes.

- For a regular application, begin the roll at the metatarsal heads.
- For toe-plate construction, begin the roll 1 or 2 finger-widths beyond the end of the tips of the toes, but within the edge of the previously laid padding.

9. Use the roll-on and cover-by-half methods to enclose the foot and ankle, working in the same pattern you used to apply the padding.
   - At 2 finger-widths before the ankle, use a figure-eight pattern, laying the crossing of the figure eight across the front of the ankle.
   - Cover all padding material, taking care to make sure the cast roll is laid flat on the padding surface.
   - Use additional rolls as needed. Continue wrapping until you have uniformly applied 2 layers of casting material. End the cast layer 2 or 3 finger-widths distal to the tibial tubercle.

10. Lift the patient's leg slightly to remove the foot stand from under the padding and casting material.
    - Place the patient's foot on a flat, rigid surface to mold the cast to the plantar aspect of the foot, making sure to keep the ankle and subtalar joints in neutral.
    - Use the palms of your hands to form the malleolar molds.
    - This will ensure that the cast will not have uneven displacement across the weight-bearing surface.

11. Fold the stockinette over the edges of the casting material proximally and distally to create a padded edge to the cast (figure 24.10*d*).
    - For toe-plate applications, make sure that the folded stockinette covers a fair amount proximal to the MTP joints.

12. Apply the 3rd and 4th layers of casting material using the roll-on and cover-by-half methods, being sure to mind your lines. For a toe-plate application, do not wet the cast material prior to application.
    - You can replace the stool for your or the patient's comfort if necessary, but your initial layers should hold your molds at this point, so it isn't necessary.
    - Smooth the cast and redefine your molds for the outermost layer (figure 24.10e).

13. For a toe-plate application, once you have applied the last layer of casting material, cut the portion of the cast covering the toes. Leave a protective plate under the plantar aspect of the toes but expose the toes superiorly. The resulting cut looks a lot like a CAM walking boot.
    - Cut along the lateral edge of the small toe to the 5th MTP joint. To perform the cut, use scissors if the cast has not cured and a cast saw if it has.
    - Starting at the base of the initial cut, cut across the top of the MTP joints, trying to roughly mirror the natural angle to the 1st MTP.
    - Make a horizontal cut along the medial aspect of the great toe to meet with your transverse cut. Remove the excised piece.
    - If you choose, you can pull back the stockinette further to reveal the toes and lock down the edge of the stockinette by covering it with a layer of casting material.

14. Allow the material to set for 8 to 10 minutes so that the cast, though not fully cured, has reached a point that it cannot be deformed by patient effort.

FOUNDATIONAL SKILL

Success Is About the Angles

When wrapping a conical-shaped body part, as is the case when transitioning from the ankle to the bulk of the calf, angle your roll so that the material lies flat. Attempting to apply a straight, transverse layer will result in padding or casting material that hangs loosely and bunches under subsequent layering leading to inconsistent, nonuniform pressure in the cast. Holding your roll so that it unravels downward to start will create a loop that is narrower inferiorly and wider superiorly, allowing for a flat, clean layer.

Removal

The short leg cast can be removed using medial and lateral cuts.

1. Start proximally and cut longitudinally along the medial aspect of the cast, positioning your cut such that your path will fall immediately anterior to the medial malleolus. End your longitudinal cut 1 or 2 finger-widths inferior to the medial malleolus.

2. Perform a transverse cut along the medial arch of the foot so that the path of this cut intersects your previous cut at a point inferior and anterior to the medial malleolus.

3. Begin proximally again and cut longitudinally along the lateral aspect of the cast, positioning your cut such that your path will fall posterior to the lateral malleolus. End your longitudinal cut 2 or 3 finger-widths inferior to the lateral malleolus.

4. Perform a transverse cut along the lateral aspect of the foot so that the path of the cut intersects with your previous cut at a point generously inferior and posterior to the lateral malleolus.

5. Part the cast at the medial and lateral seams using the cast spreader and cut the underlying padding and stockinette using tape scissors.

6. Completely separate the anterior and posterior portions to remove the cast.

Short-Leg Weight-Bearing Application

This application is nearly identical to the short-leg application; the only difference is the fabrication of a posterior slab as the initial layer of cast that, when dried, provides extra support in weight displacement and force translation through the cast. This application is most commonly used for stable, nondisplaced distal fibular fractures, syndesmotic sprains, or significant ankle sprains. It is sometimes used when a CAM boot is either unavailable or not covered by insurance or if patient compliance is a concern.

Supplies
- 3″ or 4″ stockinette
- 2″ and 3″ Webril padding
- 2″ and 3″ cast rolls
- Scissors
- Foot stand
- Gloves
- Bucket of water
- Rigid, flat surface
- Cast saw

Positioning

The patient should be casted with the ankle in talar and subtalar neutral position or as close to this position as is tolerable. The patient will likely be resistant to keeping this position, so you should explain to her why this position is important to help enlist her cooperation.

Application

1. Have the patient position her affected extremity on the foot stand and apply stockinette and cast padding as described for the short-leg application.

2. Using 3-in. cast material, apply 2 rounds at the proximal end of the cast: 1 that will form the upper border and 1 inferior round using the cover-by-half method.

3. Apply another 2 rounds at the distal end of the cast over the toes in the same fashion, working proximally.

4. Using the same roll, create your posterior slab for support:
   - Unroll a length of cast material that will extend from the spot 1 to 2 finger-widths inferior to the upper border of the cast down to the plantar surface of the metatarsal heads.
   - Once this length is established, fold the roll back on itself to create a length that is 4 to 6 layers thick.

- Apply this slab along the posterior of the lower leg so that it lies along the length as measured.
- Secure it by applying another 2 rounds at the proximal and distal ends of the cast.
- Apply the cast material as described previously for the short-leg application.

Removal

Cast removal process is exactly the same as for the short-leg application.

Long Leg Cast

This cast application invariably requires the assistance of at least 1 practitioner to hold the limb in position while materials are being applied. These casts can be considerably uncomfortable to apply for the patient due to the location of the injury, the weight of the lower extremity, and the available purchases for hand placement and positioning while the cast is being applied. You must account for all these considerations before starting the application. A patient needing this cast will also need training in using crutches, which is covered in chapter 12.

Common Injuries
- Midshaft tibia fracture
- Proximal tibia fracture
- Tib/fib fractures (in children)
- Tibial plateau fracture
- Patellar fracture

Supplies
- 3″, 4″, and 6″ stockinette
- 3″ and 4″ Webril padding
- 2″, 4″, and 6″ cast rolls
- Water
- Tape scissors
- Gloves
- Cast stand

Positioning
- If the patient can tolerate sitting with his knee in flexed position and the fracture pattern allows for this position, begin with the patient seated with his foot positioned on a foot stand. Once you have applied the lower leg portion of the cast and achieved the desired mold, you will then have the patient quickly transition to a supine lying position, where an assisting practitioner can hold the leg in position while you apply the more proximal portion of the cast. The patient's knee should be flexed between 20 and 30 degrees and the ankle and subtalar joints should be in neutral. Because of the necessary change in position, be sure that both of these positions can be easily, swiftly, and comfortably achieved in the location you've selected.
- If the patient cannot tolerate a seated position, then you will have to fully apply the cast with him in a supine lying position. You will have to perform the ankle and knee positioning and molds with the patient free standing and must establish them as the casting material is applied. Position changes after the casting material is applied will result in defects in the cast.

Application
1. Position the patient as described previously based on his comfort and fracture pattern.
   - If using a cast stand, make sure the ankle is positioned in both talocrural and subtalar neutral.
   - If the patient is supine, have your assistant hold the leg up with the knee slightly flexed, supporting weight on the ball of the foot and the posterior thigh, just above the popliteal fossa.

2. Apply a length of stockinette that will extend from the proximal one-third of the thigh (ideally, only 4 or 5 finger-widths distal to the greater trochanter or as proximal as you can go) to 3 finger-widths beyond the toes distally.

   • Make a transverse cut across the front of the ankle to prevent bunching.

   • Make another transverse cut across the back of the knee to prevent bunching.

3. Select your Webril width based on the size of the patient's anatomy and apply your first 2 layers of padding. You will wrap only to the tibial tuberosity.

   • Begin padding distally, with 2 or 3 layers covering the toes. Work proximally using the roll-on and cover-by-half techniques.

   • When you reach the angle of the ankle, use a figure-eight pattern to cover the heel (as explained for the short-leg application).

   • Continue to apply the padding, working proximally and making sure the padding material lies flat on the skin.

   • Repeat this padding technique to apply layers 3 and 4 to the lower leg, stopping at the tibial tuberosity.

4. Apply casting material as though you were doing a short leg cast. Do not wet the material to start (figure 24.11*a*).

   • Begin such that the distal edge of your cast roll falls at the metatarsal heads.

   • Work proximally using the roll-on and cover-by-half techniques.

   • Use a figure-eight wrapping pattern to cover the heel.

   • Wrap the material, working distal to proximal, until you are 2 or 3 finger-widths inferior to the edge of your padding border.

5. Using the palms of your hands, mold the cast to reflect the patient's natural anatomical profile.

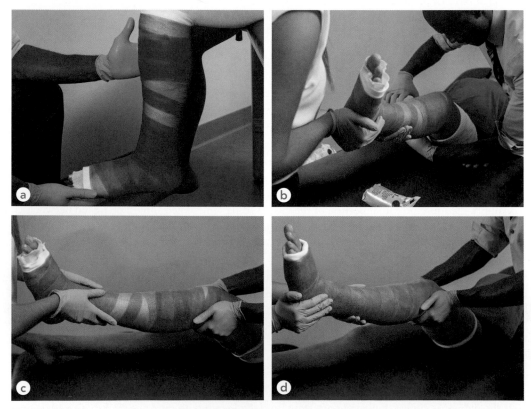

FIGURE 24.11 Application of a long leg cast.

6. Remove the cast stand (if using one) and flatten the plantar aspect of the cast.

7. Once this portion of the cast can hold the mold, have the patient recline to a supine position and begin applying the proximal portion of the cast (figure 24.11*b*).
   - Have your assistant hold the patient's lower leg and maintain the desired degree of flexion in the knee; this position must be held steadily.
   - Using the appropriate width of Webril, begin your padding by wrapping 2 layers that cover the top border of the previously casted portion of the leg by 1 full width.
   - Work proximally, using the roll-on and cover-by-half methods.
   - Repeat this process to apply the desired number of padding layers (at least 4).
   - Wrap an additional 1 or 2 layers at the proximal edge.

8. Select your larger-width casting roll as appropriate based on the patient's limb size and apply it to form the proximal portion of the cast.
   - Wet the cast material and begin this layer 1 full roll-width distal to the added cast padding layer from the previous step.
   - Wrap proximally, using the roll-on and cover-by-half methods. Ensure that the appropriate knee position is well maintained and held steadily.
   - Apply layers 2 or 3 finger-widths distal to the edge of the padding material.
   - Repeat to achieve the 3rd and 4th layers of casting material to the proximal leg.
   - Fold the excess stockinette at the toes proximally over the distal end of the cast and fold the excess at the thigh distally over the cast to create padded edges.
   - Select a large width of cast roll, wet it, and lock down the edge of the stockinette distally, and then quickly wrap the leg distal to proximal. *Do not* use a cover-by-half technique. Lay the material just so the edges cover each other and attempt to cover as much of the leg as quickly as possible (figure 24.11*c*).

9. Use the palms of your hands to form a supracondylar mold and smooth the cast profile (figure 24.11*d*).
   - Using the thenar eminences, mold the cast above the patient's knee to approximate the flare of the medial and lateral femoral condyles.
   - Mold the cast to the middle and distal thigh so that it is not perfectly cylindrical.

10. Hold the position to allow the material to set for 8 to 10 minutes so that the cast, though not fully cured, has reached a point where it cannot be deformed by patient effort.

Removal
This cast can be removed using medial and lateral cuts along the length of the cast. Because of the angle created at the knee, it may be difficult to cut in a curved path. Also, due to the length of the cast and the thickness with which the cast was layered, the blade is very likely to heat up during the removal process. You may need to take brief breaks from cutting to allow the blade to cool. If the blade heats up excessively, it may create discomfort for the patient or even break, which could result in injury to yourself or the patient.

Pro Tip
The transition to applying the proximal portion of the cast has to take place very swiftly. Once the lower cast cures to a certain point, the adherence of the proximal portion to the distal portion will not be uniform, and the resultant application will be unstable at the junction of the upper and lower segment. Not wetting the cast initially affords you some time to make this union.

Postcasting Care Considerations

When placing the patient in a cast, it is vitally important that you clearly convey to her the considerations and limitations that she must observe in order for the cast treatment to be effective. Your ability to make these considerations relatable is integral to patient compliance and treatment success. Casting is an unfamiliar experience for the vast majority of people, and your patient will not be aware of just how much her daily life and activities will be affected by wearing a cast. Providing insight and solutions to common problems in advance will help your patient feel comfortable in dealing with limitations and inconveniences when they arise.

Crutch Training

When a lower extremity cast is applied, weight-bearing restrictions are typical. Crutch fitting and training are necessary to instruct the patient on appropriate crutch use and have her demonstrate the ability to safely maneuver prior to ending the encounter. Neglecting to do so could result in the patient putting an undue amount of pressure on the injured extremity and displacing the fracture within the cast or could cause some other form of injury. The foundations of crutch fitting are addressed in chapter 12.

Driving

Due to the immobility of the foot, ankle, or knee when in a short or long leg cast, a person's ability to effectively operate a vehicle is significantly compromised. You must discuss these limitations with the patient. In some states, having a cast applied to *any* extremity, upper or lower, will deem the driver compromised, since he will not be able to react as an able-bodied driver would. This could result in injury to the patient or someone else. In the event of a law enforcement stop or an accident, the patient will be subject to laws within the local jurisdiction regarding operating a motor vehicle while impaired. Suggest that your patient make arrangements for transport with a friend or family member or familiarize himself with available rideshare services.

Compartment Syndrome

The most important and potentially the most negative issue that may arise as a result of casting is a condition known as **compartment syndrome**. This occurs when an injury is casted, usually in the acute to subacute phase of healing, and swelling is either present at the time of cast application or reoccurs after the cast has already been applied.[3] Because cast material is circumferential and rigid, this method of immobilization does not allow for significant tissue expansion. This means that in the event of swelling of the affected area, the cast will create an unmovable counterforce against the body's natural process. This constriction causes increased pressure in the soft tissues of the affected body part and can cause blood flow restriction and compromise of neurological structures that can lead to hypoxia in the muscle, soft tissue, and neurological tissue.[3,4] If the pressure is not relieved in an efficient manner, damage incurred by these tissues could become irreversible, leading to debilitating functional deficits. You should educate your patient on the signs of compartment syndrome and what to do in the event that he is experiencing said symptoms:[2,3,4,10,11,12]

- *Pain.* The fracture has been immobilized and is protected by the cast. Therefore, the patient should experience little to no pain over the affected site. Inform him that there may be some soreness due to prolonged immobilization, which is common for muscles that are not being used.
- *Pallor (skin coloration).* This is when skin distal to the cast experiences a change in color compared to an uninvolved contralateral extremity. Coloration could be white or lighter in appearance, reddened, or blue or purple, all of which denote circulatory interruption, either by blood being held in the tissues or blood not being able to reach the tissues.
- *Paresthesia (numbness and tingling).* This sensation is akin to the extremity going to sleep and is most commonly felt by people hitting the funny bone or lying with the extremity in a compressed position for a long period of time.
- *Pulse (pulselessness).* Is there a pulse present proximal and distal to the cast?
- *Paralysis.* The extremity is not responding to your patient's desire to move it.
- *Swelling.* Swelling distal to or proximal to the borders of the cast indicates that the body tissues around the affected area are attempting to swell.

If your patient experiences any of these signs of compartment syndrome, he should do the following:

Elevate the Affected Body Part Above the Level of the Heart

- *Upper extremity.* Place the hand on top of the head, hang the hand on the opposite shoulder, hold the arm above shoulder height, or sit with the arm across the back of the chair or couch.
- *Lower extremity.* Lie down on a bed with the foot elevated on pillows, lie down on a couch with the foot elevated on the arm or back of the couch, or lie on the floor with the foot against a wall or held in the air.

Observe Symptoms for 10 Minutes

- If symptoms improve:
  - Maintain elevated position until symptoms completely resolve.
  - Avoid gravity-dependent positions.
  - Contact the physician's office to inform her of this occurrence.
- If symptoms do not improve:
  - Contact the physician's office to inform her of this occurrence and ask for instruction.
  - If the office is closed, go to the nearest urgent care or emergency department for cast removal and examination.

Casting Acute Injuries

When casting swollen body parts, the following two approaches are often used:

1. The cast can be applied with little to no tightness. This will allow for only minimal additional swelling at best. If the patient's swelling surpasses the extra room afforded by applying the cast loosely, the now-tightened cast may pose a threat for the development of acute compartment syndrome, and the cast will have to be removed.
2. Monovalve, bivalve, or triple-cut techniques can be used to give the cast[12] the ability to expand in size or open completely and to be adjusted for swelling.

The monovalve (also called univalve) technique consists of applying a cast and then performing a longitudinal cut along one side using a cast saw. This technique is best used for low- to medium-energy injuries because swelling tends to be less substantial, and can account for a decrease in pressure of approximately 30%.[3,4,8] A bivalve technique involves making 2 longitudinal cuts on opposing sides of the cast, as if to remove it but leaving the underlying padding and stockinette intact. This can result in a pressure decrease of approximately 60% to 70%.[3,8,9] Lastly, a triple-cut technique would achieve maximum pressure reduction by performing the bivalve technique and cutting the underlying padding (figure 24.12).[8,9,12]

For bivalved, triple-cut casts, use Webril to pad the roughened edges and place each piece in a length of stockinette, forming two splints, if you will. Reassemble the cast over the affected body part and wrap it with elastic bandages to hold it on. Bivalving is an option only for stable fracture patterns.

When casting a swollen extremity, educate the patient that once the initial inflammation phase has passed and the swelling begins to subside, the cast will loosen. This is to be expected. However, if the cast loosens to a point where the body part is mobile within the cast, then the cast is no longer suitable for the intended purpose and must be replaced. A poorly fitting cast creates an opportunity for the fracture to displace within the cast[8] and progressively heal in a poor position if it is not attended to in a timely fashion.

Other Care Considerations

- Keep the cast dry. Many pharmacies and online shopping outlets offer products for protecting casts in water for both the upper and lower extremity. Although some of them are very good, patients should be cautious of any water-related activity. The fiberglass shell is water-resistant on its own, but the underlying padding is not. Since the deeper portions of the cast are not exposed to air, any moisture contained therein will not evaporate off, and skin maceration and infection

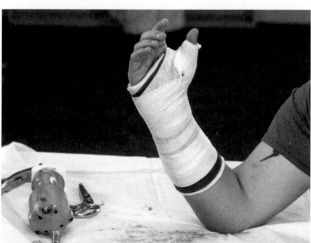
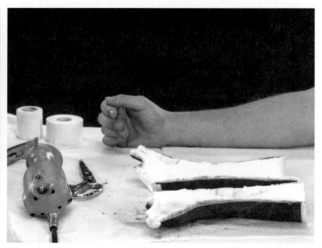

FIGURE 24.12 Bivalve thumb spica cast.

may result.[8] Instruct patients that, when bathing or showering, the best technique for keeping the cast dry (other than avoiding water all together) is to adequately cover the affected body part with a waterproof material[8] and hold it in such a way that water runs away from the cast.

- Avoid scratching or putting objects in the cast.
  - Objects are often unclean and can introduce bacteria to skin in areas that cannot be cleaned.
  - Objects can get stuck in the cast, leading to constant contact that can cause skin breakdown or infection.
  - Scratching could break the skin and cause bleeding. The untreatable wound, created by an unclean object on an uncleanable body part, is at high risk for infection.
- Avoid sliding or shifting the limb inside of the cast to scratch.
- The cast should be removed and replaced if any of the following occur:
  - The interior cast padding gets wet.
  - The cast has an offending odor or significant skin breakdown is observed.
  - Something gets stuck in the cast.
  - The cast loosens and is no longer appropriately stabilizing the fracture. This can be due to a decrease in swelling, settling or compression of padding material, or soft tissue atrophy secondary to prolonged immobilization.
  - The patient experiences pain or symptoms of compartment syndrome.

Special Considerations

When caring for an injured person, the treatment of the injury is just part of what you need to account for in your treatment plan. Patients are often also coping with the financial, social, emotional, and psychological consequences of the injury. Just as treatment of a musculoskeletal injury must include any and all overlapping strategies that will expedite healing (think RICE principles), so too

must your planning when considering the full effect of injury and treatment on a patient's life experience.

Modalities

Scenarios may arise where modalities will need to be applied in conjunction with casting, such as superficial ultrasound, electrical stimulation, or bone stim for healing. If any of these treatments or any other topically applied treatment is required, discuss the treatment with a doctor or whoever will apply or supervise the application of the modality where skin access will be necessary. The modalities can be applied by simply cutting a window in the cast and removing the portion desired. Cut through the padding material and the stockinette to expose the desired area. The modality can then be applied. Once treatment is over, the piece can be put back in place and held with an elastic bandage wrapped around the cast.

Dermatological Considerations

In conjunction with the fracture, a dermal abrasion or laceration may have occurred that will also need care during the immobilization period. Likewise, a patient who has preexisting skin issues, such as ulcers, may need a window in the cast to allow access and treatment. Use generous layers of gauze padding to cover the wound before applying stockinette, padding, and cast material to create a subtle outline of the desired area once the cast material is applied. Then cut a window according to the outline made by the gauze pads. Cut through the padding material and the stockinette to expose the desired area, treat as necessary, then replace the cast piece and hold it firm by wrapping an elastic bandage around the cast. If the lesion is too large and cutting a window of appropriate size would compromise the stability of the cast, you may need to consider a removable brace or a bivalve triple-cut technique as alternative options.[8,12]

Socioeconomic and Cultural Considerations

A cast is a relatively cheap, customizable immobilization modality. As such, it serves as the gold standard of care for most common fracture patterns that are deemed

---

Athletic Training Education Competency

The athletic training education curriculum mandates that all athletic trainers understand the impact of both internal and environmental forces at play when dealing with the complex experience of injury.[18]

- PS 2: Explain the theoretical background of psychological and emotional responses to injury and forced inactivity (e.g., cognitive appraisal model, stress response model).
- PS 3: Describe how psychosocial considerations affect clinical decision making related to return to activity or participation (e.g., motivation, confidence).

appropriate for conservative management. For some stable fracture patterns, removable bracing can also be applied. However, these are often expensive and not covered by insurance in situations where casting is available and considered, at least by the insuring institution, to be a better option.

If the patient has greater financial means or favorable insurance or if your institution is able to supply these materials at little or no cost to recipients, then the array of immobilization techniques at your disposal are more numerous. Conversely, if bracing may prove to be too expensive for some patients because it is not covered by insurance, their insurance plan comes with a high deductible, or they do not have insurance and are self-pay, then a cast will be the most effective and most affordable option, even if it is inconvenient. In environments where services are billable, the reapplication of a cast due to damage, breakdown, or loosening will further cost the patient if the supplies are not covered by insurance.

Also, along these lines, you will have to consider your patient's access to health care. In rural environments, small medical offices may not have resources such as CT, MRI, or even X-ray. The nearest office with such resources may be several hours away by car. Is your patient from out of town? Do you have contact with a practitioner who can more readily follow up with the patient? How can you apply your knowledge, available resources, and techniques to craft a treatment plan that meets the goals of healing while not forcing the patient or her family to incur undue hardship?

You will also need to consider the financial effect of prolonged immobilization on your patient. Applying a cast to a patient who may have managed with a removable brace may render them unable to work based on employer safety standards and significantly affect their quality of life. Your patient's inability to afford repeated copays or serial X-rays may dissuade them from following the standard plan of care for his injury. With careful conversation regarding the risks versus financial benefits, lengthening the time between follow-up visits, although not ideal, may encourage a degree of patient compliance and prevent adverse patient behavior such as not following up at all or attempting to remove the cast at home.

If your patient is an athlete, some sports allow for participation with appropriate padding.[5] However, will participation in the cast expose the athlete to being targeted or open them up to further injury? Work culture, sport culture, familial culture, and socioeconomic implications can all affect casting as a treatment in terms of patient compliance or noncompliance. Although these factors are outside of your control, keeping them in mind can lead you to have more productive and relatable discussion with your patient and can create an opportunity to provide helpful insight that may lead to increased patient compliance, improved outcomes, and overall patient satisfaction. Casting is about more than just treating the problem—as in all of health care, it is about treating the patient.

CLINICAL BOTTOM LINE

- The skill of casting involves more than cast application and removal.
- Effective communication with your patient includes both obvious and subtle insights into her experience, such as planning for weight-bearing considerations, driving, practicing good hygiene in the cast, and managing discomfort in safe and effective ways.
- Identifying and anticipating obstacles to patient compliance are as essential to treatment success as appropriate, pathology-specific application.
- The ability to plan and execute a treatment strategy that accounts for the global influence of injury and immobilization on a patient is what sets athletic trainers apart from technicians in the clinical setting.

 Go to HK*Propel* to complete the activities and case studies for this chapter.

APPENDIX

Standard Medical Terminology and Abbreviations

A	Anterior	AT	Athletic trainer
A:	Assessment	ATC	Certified athletic trainer
Ⓐ	Assistance	Ⓑ	Bilateral
ā	Before	BE	Below elbow
AAROM	Active assistive range of motion	b.i.d.	Twice a day
a.c.	Before meals	BK	Below knee
abd	Abduction	BOS	Base of support
ABG	Arterial blood gases	BP	Blood pressure
AC joint	Acromioclavicular joint	bpm	Beats per minute
ACL	Anterior cruciate ligament	BS	Blood sugar; breath sounds; bowel sounds
add	Adduction	BUN	Blood urea nitrogen
ADL	Activities of daily living	Bx	Biopsy
ad lib.	As desired; at discretion	c̄	With
adm	Admitted; admission	C	Celsius; centigrade
AFO	Ankle foot orthosis	CA	Carcinoma; cancer
AIDS	Acquired immunodeficiency syndrome	C&S	Culture and sensitivity
AE	Above elbow	CABG	Coronary artery bypass graft
AK	Above knee	CAD	Coronary artery disease
A-line	Arterial line	cal	Calories
ALS	Amyotrophic lateral sclerosis	cap	Capsule
AMA	Against medical advice	CAT	Computerized axial tomography
AMB	Ambulation; ambulates; ambulating	CBC	Complete blood count
amt	Amount	cc	Cubic centimeter
ANS	Autonomic nervous system	CC, C/C	Chief complaint
ant	Anterior	CGA	Contact guard assist
AP	Anterior–posterior (anteroposterior)	CHF	Congestive heart failure
ARF	Acute renal failure	CHI	Closed head injury
AROM	Active range of motion	cm	Centimeter
ASA	Aspirin	CNS	Central nervous system
ASAP	As soon as possible	CO2	Carbon dioxide
ASHD	Arteriosclerotic heart disease	c/o	Complains of
ASIS	Anterior superior iliac spine	cont.	Continue

CMC	Carpometacarpal		FBS	Fasting blood sugar
COPD	Chronic obstructive pulmonary disease		FH	Family history
CPAP	Continuous positive airway pressure		flex.	Flexion
CPR	Cardiopulmonary resuscitation		fl oz	Fluid ounce
CSF	Cerebrospinal fluid		FROM	Functional range of motion
CT	Computed tomography		ft	Foot; feet
CTR	Carpal tunnel release		FUO	Fever of unknown origin
cu mm	Cubic millimeter		FWB	Full weight-bearing
CV	Cardiovascular		Fx	Fracture
CVA	Cerebrovascular accident		G	Good muscle strength (grade 4)
CXR	Chest X-ray		GB	Gall bladder
d	Day		GH joint	Glenohumeral joint
Ⓓ	Dependent		GI	Gastrointestinal
DC, D/C	Discharge		gm	Gram
DC	Doctor of chiropractic medicine		g, gr	Grain
DDS	Doctor of dental surgery		GTT	Glucose tolerance test
DIP	Distal interphalangeal (joint)		h	Hour
DJD	Degenerative joint disease		HA, H/A	Headache
DO	Doctor of osteopathic medicine		H&P	History and physical
DOB	Date of birth		HBV	Hepatitis B virus
DOE	Dyspnea on exertion		HCT, Hct	Hematocrit
DM	Diabetes mellitus		HEENT	Head, eyes, ears, nose, throat
dr	Dram		HEP	Home exercise program
Dr.	Doctor		HGB, Hgb	Hemoglobin
DTR	Deep tendon reflexes			
DVT	Deep vein thrombosis		HIPS	History, inspection, palpation, special tests
Dx	Diagnosis		HIV	Human immunodeficiency virus
ECG	Electrocardiogram		HOPS	History, observation, palpation, special tests
ECHO	Echocardiogram		HR	Heart rate
ED	Emergency department		hr.	Hour
EEG	Electroencephalogram		hs	At bedtime
EKG	Electrocardiogram		Ht	Height
EMG	Electromyogram		HTN	Hypertension
ENT	Ear, nose, throat		Hx	History
ER	Emergency room		I&O	Intake and output
ETOH	Ethyl alcohol		Ⓘ	Independent
eval.	Evaluation		ICU	Intensive care unit
ext	Extension		IDDM	Insulin-dependent diabetes mellitus
F	Fahrenheit; fair muscle strength (grade 3)		IM	Intramuscular
f	Female		IMP	Impression
FACP	Fellow of the American College of Physicians		in.	Inches
			IP	Inpatient
FACS	Fellow of the American College of Surgeons		IV	Intravenous

kg.	Kilogram		NPO	Nothing by mouth
KUB	Kidney, ureter, bladder		NSR	Normal sinus rhythm
L	Left; liter		NWB	Non-weight-bearing
Ⓛ	Left		O	Objective; oriented
lat	Lateral		O2	Oxygen
lb	Pound		OA	Osteoarthritis
LBP	Low back pain		OX4	Oriented to time, place, person, situation
LCL	Lateral collateral ligament		OBS	Organic brain syndrome
LE	Lower extremity		OH	Occupational history
LLQ	Left lower quadrant		OP	Outpatient
LOC	Loss of consciousness		OR	Operating room
LP	Lumbar puncture		ORIF	Open reduction, internal fixation
LTG	Long-term goal		OT	Occupational therapy; occupational therapist
LUQ	Left upper quadrant		oz	Ounce
m	Murmur; meter; male		p̄	After
max	Maximum		P	Plan; posterior; pulse; poor muscle strength (grade 2)
MCL	Medial collateral ligament			
med	Medial		PA	Posterior–anterior (posteroanterior); physician assistant
meds	Medications			
MFT	Muscle function test		pc	After meals
MD	Muscular dystrophy; medical doctor		PCL	Posterior cruciate ligament
mg	Milligram		PE	Physical examination
MI	Myocardial infarction		per	By
ml	Milliliter		PET	Positron emission tomography
min	Minutes; minimum		PFT	Pulmonary function test
mm	Millimeter		PID	Pelvic inflammatory disease
MMT	Manual muscle test		PIP	Proximal interphalangeal
mo	Month		PM, p.m.	Afternoon
mod	Moderate		PMH	Past medical history
MP, MCP	Metacarpophalangeal		PNF	Proprioceptive neuromuscular facilitation
MRI	Magnetic resonance imaging		PNI	Peripheral nerve injury
MS	Musculoskeletal; multiple sclerosis		PNS	Peripheral nervous system
MVA	Motor vehicle accident		p.o.	By mouth
MVP	Mitral valve prolapse		pos	Positive
N	Normal muscle strength (grade 5)		poss	Possible
neg	Negative		postop	Postoperation
NG	Nasogastric		PRE	Progressive resistive exercise
NIDDM	Non-insulin-dependent diabetes mellitus		preop	Preoperation
NKA	No known allergy		prn	As needed
NKDA	No known drug allergy		pro	Pronation
nn	Nerve		PROM	Passive range of motion
noc	Night		PSIS	Posterior superior iliac spine

pt	Patient		SI(J)	Sacroiliac (joint)
PT	Physical therapy; physical therapist		Sig	Instruction to patient; directions for use; give as follows
PT/PTT	Prothrombin time; partial thromboplastin time		SLE	Systemic lupus erythematosus
PVD	Peripheral vascular disease		SLR	Straight leg raise
PWB	Partial weight-bearing		SOAP	Subjective, objective, assessment, plan
Px	Physical examination		SOB	Shortness of breath
q	Every		SOC	Start of care
qd	Every day		SpGr	Specific gravity
qh	Every hour		S/P	Status post
q2h	Every 2 hours		sq	Subcutaneous
q.i.d.	Every other day		SR	Systems review
qt	Quart		S/S	Signs and symptoms
®	Right; respiration		STAT	Immediately
R	Right		STD	Sexually transmitted disease
RA	Rheumatoid arthritis		STG	Short-term goal
RBC	Red blood cell count		sup	Supination; superior
RD	Registered dietitian		Sx	Symptoms
re:	Regarding		T	Temperature; trace muscle strength (grade 1)
rehab	Rehabilitation		T&A	Tonsillectomy and adenoidectomy
reps	Repetitions		tab	Tablet
resp	Respiratory; respiration		TB	Tuberculosis
RLQ	Right lower quadrant		TBI	Traumatic brain injury
RN	Registered nurse		tbsp	Tablespoon
R/O	Rule out		TEDS	Thromboembolic disease stockings
ROM	Range of motion		TENS, TNS	Transcutaneous electrical nerve stimulator
ROS	Review of symptoms			
RROM	Resistive range of motion		THR	Total hip replacement
RT	Respiratory therapy; respiratory therapist		TIA	Transient ischemic attack
RTC	Return to clinic		t.i.d.	Three times a day
RTO	Return to office		TKR	Total knee replacement
RUQ	Right upper quadrant		TM(J)	Temporomandibular (joint)
RSD	Reflex sympathetic dystrophy		Tx	Treatment; traction
Rx	Recipe; prescription; therapy; intervention plan		UA	Urinalysis
			UMN	Upper motor neuron
$\bar{s}$	Without		URI	Upper respiratory infection
S	Subjective		US	Ultrasound
SAQ	Short arc quad		UTI	Urinary tract infection
SBA	Standby assistance		UV	Ultraviolet
SCI	Spinal cord injury		VC	Vital capacity
SC joint	Sternoclavicular joint		VD	Venereal disease
SH	Social history		v.o.	Verbal orders

vol	Volume		←	From; regressing backward
VS	Vital signs		→	To; progressing forward, approaching
WBC	White blood cell count; white blood count		1°	Primary
w/c	Wheelchair		2°	Secondary
W/cm2	Watts per square centimeter		~	Approximately; about
WDWN	Well developed, well nourished		@	At
wk	Week		>	Greater than
WFL	Within functional limits		<	Less than
WNL	Within normal limits		=	Equals
wt	Weight		+, (+)	Plus; positive
x	Number of times performed (×2 = twice; ×3 = three times)		−, (−)	Minus; negative
+1 (+2)	Assistance of 1 person (2 persons) required		#	Number (when placed before the number: #1); pound (when placed after the number: 1#)
y.o.	Years old		/	Per
yd	Yard		%	Percent
yr	Year		+, &, et	And
♂	Male		°	Degree
♀	Female		√	Flexion
↓	Down; downward; decrease		/	Extension
↑	Up; upward, increase		±, +/−	Plus or minus
Δ	Change		//	Parallel to
⊥	Perpendicular to		// bars	Parallel bars
↔	To and from			

Reprinted from S.J. Shultz, P.A. Houglum, D.H. Perrin, 2016, *Examination of Musculoskeletal Injuries* 4E (Champaign, IL: Human Kinetics), 28-31.

GLOSSARY

acclimatization—The process or result of becoming accustomed to a new climate or set of conditions; complex series of changes or adaptations that occur in response to heat stress in a controlled environment over the course of 7 to 14 days.

achondroplasia—A hereditary condition signified by short limbs due to ossification of long bone cartilage.

activities of daily living (ADLs)—Tasks that enable people to meet their basic needs. Examples include eating, dressing, hygiene, housecleaning, and shopping.

acute—A condition or injury with a rapid onset and a short course, usually resulting from a single mechanism of injury; not chronic.

acute anterior compartment syndrome—A serious, often limb-threatening, condition where pressure builds up in the anterior compartment of the lower leg. The increasing pressure affects the neurovascular structures in the lower leg. Causes of acute anterior compartment syndrome in the lower leg include a direct blow or fracture.

adenosine triphosphate (ATP)—A molecule that carries energy within cells. It is the main energy currency of the cell.

advocacy—The act of supporting a cause, person, or plan.

aerobic—Relating to, involving, or requiring free oxygen.

agonal breathing—Labored, gasping breaths; the body's final attempt to sustain life.

airborne contact—Occurs when a person inhales infected droplets that have become airborne (i.e., exposure to bacteria or virus through coughing and sneezing).

airway adjuncts—Devices used once an airway has been established to maintain an open airway.

alleviation—Something that lessens the signs and symptoms of a condition or injury.

altered mental status (AMS)—General term used to describe various changes in a patient's mental functioning that can range from slight confusion to coma. These can include signs and symptoms such as confusion, amnesia, disorientation, and unusual or strange behavior.

amino acids—The individual building blocks for protein structure. The type of protein made and its function are determined by the sequence and types of amino acids present in its structure.

anaerobic—Relating to, involving, or requiring an absence of free oxygen.

anaphylaxis—A severe, potentially life-threatening allergic reaction.

anatomical position—The reference position for the body for nomenclature and measurements. The position is the body standing erect, with the arms at the side and the palms facing forward.

anemia—A condition in which one's body lacks enough healthy red blood cells to carry adequate oxygen to the tissues, which can lead to extreme fatigue.

anesthesia—The absence of sensation.

aneurysm—Localized enlargement of an arterial wall.

anosmia—Loss of smell.

antagonist muscle—A muscle with the opposite action of the prime mover.

antalgic gait—Gait in which the patient has pain during the stance phase and so remains on the painful leg for as short a time as possible.

antioxidants—Substances that can prevent or slow damage to cells caused by free radicals.

antithrombic—An agent that reduces the formation of blood clots (thrombi).

apnea—Temporary breathing cessation.

approximation—Bringing tissue edges together for suturing.

arrhythmia—Irregular heartbeat.

arthralgia—Joint pain.

arthrokinematics—Description of the movement of the joint surfaces when a bone moves through a range of motion.

aseptic technique—Practices and procedures to prevent contamination from pathogens.

aspiration—The accidental sucking in of food particles or fluids into the lungs.

assessment—The process by which the patient's condition or injury is appraised or evaluated. It evolves collecting information from the patient's medical history, reported symptoms, and laboratory or diagnostic results.

athletic trainers—Health care professionals who work with active people. Their services include injury and illness prevention, wellness promotion and education, emergent care, examination, clinical diagnosis, therapeutic intervention, and rehabilitation of injuries and medical conditions.

atrophy—A reduction of muscle mass due to injury or immobility.

auscultation—The process of listening to sounds within the body; done with a stethoscope.

autonomic nervous system—A part of the nervous system that controls resting functions, such as heart rate, respiratory rate, and digestion.

avascular necrosis—Without blood supply.

AVPU scale—An acronym for "alert, verbal, pain, unresponsive;" a system to measure and record a patient's level of consciousness.

basal metabolic rate—The minimum daily calories required to maintain normal resting bodily functions; does not include energy for daily activities or exercise.

baseline—Initial values or measurements (e.g., vital signs, ROM) to which subsequent measurements can be compared.

baseline concussion testing—A series of physical and cognitive tests that measure healthy brain function before a sports season starts and prior to an injury occurring. The results of the baseline testing can be compared to test results postinjury to monitor recovery and return to play.

big data—A large set of information that can be analyzed to identify patterns, trends, or human behaviors.

bilateral—Both sides; during examination, the injured or affected area is compared with the noninjured side of the body.

bioavailability—The amount and rate at which a drug dose reaches the action site unchanged. A medication that reaches the action site unchanged has a bioavailability of 100%.

biofeedback—A modality used to measure muscular contractions through visual and auditory signals to assist patients in strengthening and muscular and postural control.

biological value—A measure of the efficiency of the protein in food for the maintenance and growth of bodily tissues.

blepharospasm—Involuntary eyelid closure.

blindisms—Repetitive movements like hand waving, rocking, or finger flicking. There is no inherent harm in displaying blindisms other than the social stigma.

blood-borne pathogens—Pathogenic microorganisms that are present in human blood and can cause disease in humans. These pathogens include, but are not limited to, hepatitis B virus (HBV) and human immunodeficiency virus (HIV).

Board of Certification (BOC)—A credentialing agency that provides certification for athletic trainers and maintains standards for athletic training professional practice and continuing education.

body composition—The proportions of fat and fat-free mass in the body.

body substance isolation (BSI)—An approach to infection control expanding on the original concept of universal precautions. BSI covers all body substances (e.g., blood, urine, feces, tears) of people undergoing medical interventions, especially during out-of-hospital care of those who might be infected with infectious diseases, such as HIV or hepatitis.

bone-building years—Time during which peak bone mass is developed, generally considered to take place in women from the late teen years to the late 20s.

bone stress response—Swelling within the bone as a response to undue stresses.

boosting—Enacting an autonomic dysreflexia (AD) immediately before competition in an attempt to gain a physiological advantage.

boxer fracture—Fracture of the fifth metacarpal neck having apex dorsal angulation.

bradycardia—Heart rate that is slower than normal.

break test—Test for strength completed by having the athletic trainer apply resistance while the patient holds a contraction; typically performed in the mid-range of motion.

budgeting—Creating a planned process to manage the financial resources of the health care setting.

bullying—Unwanted aggressive behaviors toward a young person by another youth or group of youths, not including siblings or current dating partner, that involves an observed or perceived power imbalance and is repeated multiple times or is highly likely to be repeated.

bursitis—Injury resulting in inflammation of a bursa.

capillary refill—The time it takes for color to return to an external capillary bed after pressure is applied to cause blanching; usually less than 2 seconds.

capital equipment—Fixed assets such as equipment or facilities.

carbohydrate loading—A practice that competitive and elite athletes use to supersaturate their muscles with optimal glycogen levels.

cardiorespiratory fitness (CRF)—The ability to perform exercise involving large muscle groups at moderate to high intensities for prolonged periods.

case-control study—Study that identifies patients who have the outcome of interest (cases) and control patients without the same outcome and looks for exposure of interest.

cast index—The ratio of sagittal to coronal width from the inside edges of the cast at the fracture site.

causal-comparative/quasi-experimental—A study that determines a cause-and-effect relationship; similar to experimental design, but without randomization of groups.

catastrophic injury—Fatalities, permanent disability injuries, serious injuries (fractured neck or serious head injury) even though the athlete has a full recovery, temporary or transient paralysis, heat stroke due to exercise, or sudden cardiac arrest.

central nervous system (CNS)—Portion of the nervous system made up of the brain and spinal cord.

cerebrospinal fluid (CSF)—Clear, colorless body fluid found around the brain and spinal cord.

certified specialist in sports dietetics (CSSD)—An RD with additional education and specific knowledge, skills, and expertise for competency in sports dietetics practice.

chain of command—The official hierarchy of authority that dictates who is in charge of whom and of whom permission must be asked.

chief complaint—The main reason the patient is seeing the athletic trainer; the patient's primary complaint.

chronic—A condition or injury with a long duration or slow progression, usually resulting from repetitive stress; the opposite of acute.

cirrhosis—Scarring of the liver.

clinical diagnosis—The use of clinical methods to establish the cause and nature of a patient's condition or injury and the subsequent functional impairment caused by the pathology.

clinical prediction rules—Guidelines that consider that various components of the history, physical examination, and basic laboratory results to inform the diagnosis, prognosis, or treatment or intervention of a patient.

clonus—Rhythmic alternation of muscular contractions caused by hyperactive stretch reflex from an upper motor neuron lesion.

closed kinetic chain (CKC) exercises—Exercises done when an extremity is fixed to an object like the floor or wall.

cognitive appraisal—A person's evaluation of a situation that influences his perception of stress.

cohort study—Identifies two groups (cohorts) of patients (one that received the exposure of interest and one that did not) and follows these cohorts for the outcome of interest.

Commission on Accreditation of Athletic Training Education (CAATE)—Organization that develops, maintains, and oversees academic requirements of programs for athletic trainers, which leads to the process of accrediting academic programs.

commotio cordis—Sudden arrhythmic death caused by an impact to the chest wall. It is mostly seen in athletes between the ages of 8 and 18 who play sports with projectiles, such as baseballs, hockey pucks, or lacrosse balls. The timing and location of the impact are important factors in determining whether or not an athlete will have this condition. Immediate CPR and defibrillation are imperative for preventing death; even with CPR and AED use, survival is rare.

compartment syndrome—Neurovascular compromise in soft tissue resulting from increased pressure in a rigid fascial compartment that prevents adequate muscle perfusion.

competencies—Observable and measurable knowledge and skills applied to a profession.

complex carbohydrates—Long chains of carbohydrates containing more than 10 monosaccharide units. Whole grains, starchy vegetables, and legumes are examples of complex carbohydrates.

compounding—To combine two or more elements (drug components).

computed tomography (CT)—A radiographic study that uses ionizing radiation and the principles of tomography to make a series of three-dimensional cross-sectional images that are stored and reconstructed by a computer.

concentric contraction—A muscle contraction where the fibers shorten as the muscle contracts. The opposite of an eccentric contraction.

concentric muscular contraction—Shortening of a muscle while contracting; critical for power.

confidentiality—An ethical duty of a psychologist to hold information discussed with a client private and not share this information with anyone unless certain circumstances are met concerning public safety.

contact healing—A form of primary healing where the bone is held tightly together.

continuing education—Education beyond certification that promotes continued competence, development of current knowledge and skills, and enhancement of professional skills and judgment.

continuous quality improvement (CQI)—A concept where the health care team members work together to routinely and continually assess how the entity (e.g., department, institution, clinic) is doing and what can be done better.

contraindication—Any symptom or circumstance indicating the inappropriateness of an otherwise advisable treatment, procedure, or exercise.

core temperature—The temperature of the body, specifically in deep structures of the body, in comparison to temperatures of peripheral tissues.

correlational research—A study that assesses relationships between two or more variables.

cortical bone—Also known as compact bone; the dense bone responsible for skeletal mass that is imperative to body structure and weight-bearing.

crepitus—A grating or crackling sound and sensation created during movement due to irregularities between structures; occurs from the ends of a bone fracture rubbing or when there is air present in spaces where it should not be (e.g., pleural space).

critical appraisal—Authors evaluate and synopsize individual research studies.

cryotherapy—The application of cold.

cyanosis—Bluish or purplish discoloration of the skin or mucous membranes due to the tissues near the skin surface having low oxygen saturation.

Deaf—People with hearing loss who share the same social structures, cultural views, and history and use American Sign Language (ASL) as their primary mode of communication.

debride—To remove dead, contaminated, or adherent tissue or foreign material from a wound.

decerebrate—Abnormal body posture that involves holding the arms and legs straight out, plantarflexing the feet, and arching the head and neck backward. The muscles are tightened and held rigidly.

decorticate—Abnormal posturing in which a person is stiff with flexed arms, clenched fists, and legs held out straight. The arms are flexed in toward the body and the wrists and fingers are bent and held on the chest.

dehydration—Excessive loss of body water.

density—The weight of a product as compared to its size. Typically, products that boast higher density offer greater protection and are more resistant to deformation and impact.

depersonalization—Detachment from one's thoughts and feelings. Chronic depersonalization refers to depersonalization-derealization disorder and can be found in the DSM-5 under dissociative disorders.

derealization—A feeling that one's surroundings are not real.

dermatomes—A delineated area of the skin innervated by a single nerve root. Each cord segment has a represented skin area.

descriptive research—A systematic collection of information through description to describe a phenomenon.

diagnostic medical sonography (DMS)—An imaging and therapeutic modality that images or treats deep structures of the body by measuring and recording the reflection of high-frequency sound waves.

diagnostic overshadowing—Attributing all symptoms to the primary condition or disability and overlooking other medical issues.

diaphoresis—Unusual degree of sweating.

diaphoretic—Excessive sweating for no apparent reason.

diaphragmatic breathing—A style of breathing that uses slowed abdominal breaths to stimulate the vagus nerve and lower the body's stress response.

diaphysis—The shaft of long bone.

diastolic—Minimum arterial pressure during relaxation and dilatation of the ventricles of the heart when the ventricles fill with blood.

diathermy—A therapeutic modality used particularly when a heating effect in the tissues is desired without motor or sensory stimulation.

dietary supplements—A product taken orally that contains one or more ingredients (such as vitamins or amino acids) that are intended to supplement one's diet and are not considered food.

differential diagnosis—Identification of a condition or injury by comparison of the symptoms of two or more similar conditions or injuries.

direct contact—Passing of an infectious substance from one person to another—for example, when infected blood from one coworker splashes into the eye of another coworker or when someone directly touches body fluids of an infected person (i.e., percutaneous or mucosal contact).

disability—An umbrella term for impairments, activity limitations, and participation restrictions.

disablement model—A structure for assessing patient health status that describes the effect of injury or disease on patient function.

displaced fracture—Translation, angulation, rotation, or shortening occurring between two opposing segments of a fractured bone.

docosahexaenoic acid (DHA)—An omega-3 fatty acid that is a primary structural component of the human brain, cerebral cortex, skin, and retina.

dose–response relationship—The relationship between the quantity of a substance or exposure (i.e., amount of exercise) and its overall effect on the body.

drug—A chemical that causes a physiological effect when introduced into the body.

drug absorption—The movement of a drug or medication through the body systems from the point of introduction (site of administration) to the bloodstream.

drug distribution—The movement of a drug to and from the bloodstream and other tissues in the body.

dual-energy X-ray absorptiometry (DEXA)—The use of low-dose X-rays to measure bone mineral density and body composition.

dyspnea—Difficulty breathing; shortness of breath.

dysrhythmia—Abnormal physiological rhythm.

eccentric contraction—A muscle contraction where the fibers lengthen as the muscle contracts. The opposite of a concentric contraction.

eccentric muscular contraction—Elongation of muscle while contracting to an opposing force (deceleration).

ecchymosis—Skin discoloration; often black and blue that later changes to green and yellow.

effectiveness—When a prevention program works under real-world conditions.

efficacious—When a prevention program works under ideal conditions.

effleurage—Massage technique of stroking an identified body area.

eicosapentaenoic acid (EPA)—An omega-3 fatty acid found in the flesh of cold-water fish.

electrocardiogram—A test that measures the electrical activity of the heartbeat.

electrolyte—Micronutrients that separate into ions in solution, thus acquiring the capacity to conduct electricity. The main electrolytes that are mandatory for optimal cellular hydration and functions are sodium, potassium, chloride, calcium, magnesium, and phosphate.

electromagnetic energy modalities—A high energy source that is transmitted by the movement of photons.

electrotherapy—A passive form of treatment where many different forms of electrical stimulation are initiated; used primarily for pain and spasm reduction in addition to increased tissue healing.

emergency medical services (EMS)—A system that represents the combined efforts of several professionals and agencies to provide prehospital emergency care to the sick and injured.

emergency medical technician (EMT)—Someone trained in basic life support, including AED use, airway adjuncts, and assisting patients with certain medications.

emesis—Vomiting.

emotional intelligence—A conglomeration of social skills that involve a person's ability to manage interpersonal relationships with empathy through awareness, control, and emotional expression.

emotive—Being demonstrative; expressing emotions.

empathy—The ability to understand a patient's perspective.

empiric—Anticipated or likely.

end feel—Quality of the sensation felt when stressing a joint at the end range of motion.

endemic transmission—Transmission at a predictable rate.

endotracheal intubation—Procedure by which a tube is inserted through the mouth into the trachea to maintain the patient's airway.

engineering controls—Means controls (e.g., sharps disposal containers, self-sheathing needles, or safer medical devices, such as sharps with engineered injury protections and needleless systems) that isolate or remove the bloodborne pathogens hazard from the workplace.

epidemiology—The study of the distribution and determinants of health-related states or events (including disease), and the application of this study to the control of diseases and other health problems.

epiphora—Excessive eye watering.

epiphyseal plate—Also known as the growth plate; a hyaline cartilage plate found in the metaphysis that remains open during bone-growing years.

epiphysiolysis—A medical injury or condition where the epiphysis loosens or separates from the bone shaft.

epiphysis—The end portion of long bone.

ergogenic aid—Training technique, mechanical device, nutritional ingredient or practice, pharmacological method, or psychological technique that can improve exercise performance capacity or enhance training adaptations.

ergonomics—The science concerned with fitting a job to a person's anatomical, physiological, and psychological characteristics to enhance human efficiency and well-being.

erythema—Superficial reddening of the skin.

ethnicity—A group of people with a distinct shared ancestry and cultural identity.

etiology—In medicine, the cause, set of causes, or attributes that contribute to disease, illness, or injury.

euhydration—Normal state of body water content; absence of absolute or relative hydration or dehydration.

evaluation—The systematic process that allows the athletic trainer to make a clinical judgment or diagnosis.

evidence-based practice—The use of the best available evidence from research to guide decision making in patient treatment and care.

examination—The act or process of inspecting the body to determine the presence or absence of an injury or pathology.

expendable—Disposable services or items that are replaced routinely

expense—The amount paid for an item or service.

experimental research—Also known as true experiment, this study determines cause-and-effect relationships through random assignment to control and experimental groups.

exposure—The time at risk for developing a condition.

exposure control plan (ECP)—Written plan that eliminates or minimizes employee exposure as defined by the Occupational Safety and Health Administration.

exposure determination—Who is at risk based on job classification where exposure to blood or OPIMs may occur without regard to the use of PPE.

facility planning—The process of managing, designing, and facilitating the function and use of a space.

fatty acids—Molecules that are long chains of lipid-carboxylic acid found in fats and oils.

female athlete triad—Condition related to low energy availability and variations and degrees of physiological changes associated with menstrual cycle disruption; ultimately, may cause bone mineral losses, stress fractures, or osteoporosis.

fibroblastic proliferation—The haphazard laying down of collagen tissue during the repair process following soft tissue injury.

flexibility—The ability of a joint to move through a full range of motion.

formulary—An entity that maintains a list of drugs that are available as part of a service or insurance provision.

fracture reduction—Correction of a displaced fracture using slight exaggeration of the deformity, traction, and then reversal of the deformity to reestablish anatomical alignment.

free radicals—Unstable molecules the body produces as a reaction to environmental and other pressures.

gap healing—A form of secondary healing where bone must form across an injured area that is not approximated.

gastric emptying—The time it takes for food and fluids to leave the stomach.

Glasgow Coma Scale (GCS)—Common scoring system used to describe the level of consciousness in a person following a traumatic brain injury. Summation of scores for eye, verbal, and motor responses.

glucose—A simple sugar that is an important energy source in living organisms; a component of many carbohydrates.

glycogen—A long chain of glucose molecules linked together; the main form from which energy is derived in working muscles.

goal setting—A method of deciding what you want to accomplish and systematically devising a plan to accomplish the results that you desire based on short-term, step-by-step, realistic, measurable, and recorded standards.

gold standard—Considered the best method of measurement, based on validity and reliability.

goniometer—Apparatus used to measure range of motion and joint angles. Different sizes and types of goniometers are available to measure different joints.

handwashing facility—A facility providing an adequate supply of running potable water, soap, and single-use towels or air-drying machines.

hard of hearing—People who have a milder form of hearing loss but can still communicate efficiently with the hearing community.

head-tilt/chin-lift maneuver—Procedure used to prevent the tongue from obstructing the airway. The maneuver is performed by tilting the patient's head backward by applying pressure to the forehead and the chin. It is the preferred method of opening the airway.

health—A state of complete physical, mental, and social well-being; not merely the absence of disease or infirmity.

health care administration—The planning, direction, and coordination of medical and health services.

health care team—A group of health care professionals who work together to provide patient-centered care.

health disparities—Health differences that are linked with social, economic, or environmental disadvantage that increase the vulnerability of marginalized groups.

health equity—All people have same opportunity to attain health.

hearing loss—A general term that describes people who are hard of hearing or deaf.

hematochezia—Vomiting of blood.

hemoglobin A1c—Glycosylated hemoglobin; a measure of the average blood glucose level over the lifetime of a red blood cell, approximately 2 to 3 months.

hemolytic—Destruction of red blood cells.

hemorrhage—Abnormal and severe internal or external bleeding.

hepatitis—Inflammation of the liver.

hesitation—Inability to start urine stream.

heterotopic ossification—Benign process characterized by heterotopic ossification, or bone formation, within large muscles.

human immunodeficiency virus (HIV)—A retrovirus that is the etiologic agent of acquired immunodeficiency syndrome (AIDS).

hydration—The process of replacing water in the body.

hydrodensitometry—Also known as underwater weighing; uses water displacement to measure body volume and thus body composition.

hydroxyapatite—A mineral that is the main inorganic constituent of bone.

hyperandrogenism—Condition of high levels of androgen in women.

hyperesthesia—Heightened or increased sensation.

hyperglycemia—High blood sugar.

hyperhydration—Excessive water in the body.

hypermobility—Excessive joint play (movement) that permits increased mobility.

hypertension—Also known as high blood pressure, it causes the heart to contract against higher levels of pressure in the blood vessels. Diagnosed as resting blood pressure above 130/80.

hyperthermia—Elevated core temperature.

hypertonia—An abnormally high muscle tone or tension.

hypertrophy—Increase in bulk.

hypoesthesia—Decreased sensation.

hypoglycemia—Low blood sugar.

hypomobility—Restricted joint movement (play) that limits normal range of motion; the opposite of hypermobility.

hyponatremia—Low blood sodium levels.

hypoperfusion—Inadequate delivery of vital oxygen and nutrients to body tissues.

hyposmia—Reduced ability to smell.

hypotension—Low blood pressure.

hypothermia—Core temperature below 35°C (95°F).

hypovolemic—State of decreased blood volume or diminished body fluid.

hypoxia—Deficiency in the amount of oxygen that reaches the tissues of the body.

ICD-10—A medical classifications system created by the World Health Organization. ICD-10 stands for International Statistical Classification of Diseases and Related Health Problems, 10th edition.

impedance—A measure of the amount of opposition to the flow of a current in the body; used during bioelectrical impedance to estimate body fat.

implicit bias—Unconscious judgment and behavior toward members of a group.

incidence—The proportion of members of a population who develop new cases of a condition during a specified period of time.

indirect calorimetry—Measurement of oxygen consumption and carbon dioxide production to determine substrate use and caloric burn.

indirect contact—When a person touches an object that contains the blood or OPIM of an infected person, and that fluid then enters his body at a correct entry site (i.e., sharing items such as razors and toothbrushes).

instability—The lack of ability to maintain alignment of bony segments, usually due to a torn or lax ligament and weak muscles.

instructional self-talk—Does not have an influence on motivation; is meant to help improve focus on technical aspects of a movement.

insulin resistance—The body's response to insulin is impaired, resulting in elevated levels of glucose in the blood.

insurance (medical)—An arrangement with an agency (government or company) to provide guaranteed compensation to providers for medical services in return for payment.

interprofessional practice (IPP)—When two or more professions learn with, about, and from each other to promote effective collaboration and improve health outcomes.

intersectionality—Overlapping of racial, ethnic, or cultural identities.

intrinsic plus position—MCP joints flexed to as close to 70 to 90 degrees as is comfortably achievable with the PIP and DIP joints extended.

isokinetic—Contraction similar to isotonic (concentric and eccentric) but done at constant speed.

isokinetic contraction—Similar to an isotonic contraction in that the muscle fibers change length, but the speed of the movement remains constant during the movement.

isometric—Strengthening where joint angle and muscular length do not change.

isometric contraction—Muscle contraction in a fixed position with no shortening or lengthening of the muscle fibers.

isotonic—Muscle contraction that occurs with constant tension as the muscle changes length.

isotonic contraction—Muscle contraction with shortening or lengthening of the muscle fibers while the tension or load remains the same throughout. Concentric and eccentric contractions are isotonic contractions.

jaundice—Condition in which the skin, whites of the eyes, and mucous membranes turn yellow because of a high level of bilirubin.

jaw-thrust technique—Procedure used to prevent the tongue from obstructing the airway. The jaw-thrust maneuver is used on patients with a suspected cervical spine injury because it allows for the athletic trainer to clear the tongue from the airway with minimal neck movement. It is performed by placing the fingers under the lower jaw to physically push it upwards to open the mouth.

jugular vein distention—Bulging of the neck veins caused by increased pressure in the superior vena cava.

key indicators—A measurable factor that identifies the success of an organization, employee, or project based on specific desired outcomes.

Koplik's spots—Clustered, white oral lesions.

laxity—Increased joint movement.

leadership—Influence over others or the art of motivating others to achieve a common goal.

lifestyle disease—Diseases caused by unhealthy lifestyle habits, such as inactivity, poor sleep, smoking, and poor nutrition.

likelihood ratio—Indicates how many times a patient with an injury or disease will have a certain diagnostic result compared to patients without the injury or disease.

low energy availability—The state of lacking enough calories (energy) for both the body's requirements and exercise.

macronutrients—A type of food (e.g. fat, protein, carbohydrate) required in large amounts in the diet.

magnetic resonance imaging (MRI)—An imaging technique that uses a strong magnetic field and radio waves to produce cross-sectional images of the body.

malaise—Feeling of general discomfort, uneasiness, weakness, or pain; often the first sign of an infection or other condition.

mallet finger—Rupture of one or more of the distal extensor tendons of the hand or an avulsion of the extensor tendon from the distal phalanx of the thumb or finger.

management—A process of directing, supervising, or overseeing people.

manual muscle test (MMT)—A technique for estimating the relative strength of a specific muscle.

marginalization—Making assumptions and prejudging cultural or ethnic groups.

massage—The manipulation of the body's soft tissues through techniques that bring about specific responses, including stroking, rubbing, kneading, compressing, applying percussion and vibration.

mass casualty incident—Any emergency situation where the number of patients outnumbers the resources (e.g., personnel, equipment) available.

mechanical energy modalities—Modalities that use an object to provide a force to soft-tissue structures that creates a therapeutic effect.

mechanism of injury (MOI)—Manner by which the injury occurred.

medical control—Usually a physician at a local hospital who directs medical care or decisions for EMS providers; this direction can be done in real time over the radio or cell phone during a call, but also includes preestablished protocols that EMS personnel must follow.

medical emergency—Emergencies that are not caused by an outside force, illness, or condition.

meditation—A practice consisting of relaxation training (e.g., diaphragmatic breathing and mental imagery) that emphasizes remaining in the present moment with an attitude of acceptance and nonjudgment; helps patients tolerate the pain of their injury during rehabilitation.

mental health services—Inpatient or outpatient treatment or counseling or use of prescription medication for problems with emotions, nerves, or mental health.

mental imagery—Cognitive representations of real or imagined actions without actual stimuli from the present environment.

meta-analysis—A systematic review that uses quantitative methods to summarize the results.

metabolic equivalent—MET, where 1 MET is the energy expenditure of sitting.

metabolism—Entirety of all chemical processes that convert the essential nutrients we consume in our food to energy in our bodies.

metaphysis—Narrow portion of long bone that separates the epiphysis from the diaphysis.

microassaults—Most closely aligned with old-fashioned isms like sexism or racism. Assaults can be verbal, nonverbal, implicit, or explicit (i.e., intentional) discriminatory behavior.

microinsult—Insensitive or rude remarks that convey contempt for the target.

microinvalidations—Dismissive of the feelings or experiences of a member of a group or denying one's own biases toward a social group; these behaviors can be unconscious.

micronutrients—Vitamins and minerals that must be obtained from our food in order to maintain optimal health.

microorganisms—Organisms of microscopic or submicroscopic size.

minerals—A chemical element required as an essential nutrient by organisms to perform functions necessary for life.

mission—A statement of an organization's definition and philosophy.

mood disorder—Also known as an affective disorder; type of psychological disorder characterized by an elevation or lowering of a person's emotional state that severely affects function (e.g., depression or bipolar).

mortality—Relating to death, specifically the risk of death attributable to a disease.

muscular dystrophy—Hereditary condition marked by progressive wasting of muscles.

muscular fitness—A composite of muscular strength, endurance and power.

myalgia—Muscle pain.

myasthenia gravis—Rare, chronic autoimmune disease marked by muscular weakness without atrophy.

myelinated—Nerve fiber enclosed in a sheath that improves impulse conduction.

myoclonus—Sudden, involuntary jerking of a muscle or group of muscles.

myotome—Muscle or muscle group innervated by a single nerve root.

National Athletic Trainers' Association (NATA)—Membership organization of athletic trainers.

nature of illness (NOI)—For nontraumatic or nonorthopedic conditions, the manner by which the condition or illness developed.

negative predictive value (NPV)—The proportion of patients with a negative diagnostic test who do not have an injury or disease.

negative self-talk—Typically negatively influences performance, increases anxiety, and destroys confidence.

neuromotor—Training that incorporates motor skills, such as balance, coordination, and proprioceptive exercises.

nuclear medicine—A discipline that uses radioactive isotopes in the diagnosis and treatment of disease, including many types of cancers; heart disease; gastrointestinal, endocrine, and neurological disorders; and other abnormalities within the body.

nutrient density—Food that is high in nutrients but relatively low in calories. Nutrient-dense foods contain vitamins, minerals, complex carbohydrate, lean protein, and healthy fat.

nutrition—Act or process of nourishing or being nourished; specifically, the sum of the processes by which a person takes in and uses food substances that are necessary for human function.

occupational exposure—Reasonably anticipated contact of the skin, eye, or mucous membrane with blood or OPIMs that may result from the performance of the employee's duties.

opacification—Process of becoming cloudy or opaque.

open kinetic chain (OKC) exercises—Exercises where an extremity (e.g., arm or leg) is free to move in space and not fixed to an object.

operational plan—Detailed account and plans for individual departments and organizational teams to achieve an organization's strategic plan goals.

oppression—Unjust treatment with regard to status.

ossification—Natural process of bone formation.

osteoblast—Cell that secretes the matrix necessary for bone formation.

osteoclast—Cell that absorbs bone tissue during bone growth and healing.

osteocytes—Cell formed when an osteoblast becomes embedded in the matrix it has secreted.

osteokinematics—Movement of long bones that produces motion.

osteopenia—Mild thinning of bone mass; a precursor to osteoporosis.

osteoporosis—Medical condition in which bones become brittle and fragile due to loss of tissue; typically results from deficiency in calcium or vitamin D or hormonal changes.

otalgia—Ear pain.

other potentially infectious materials (OPIMs)—Other bodily fluids or tissues that have been infected with pathogens, including semen, vaginal secretions, cerebrospinal fluid, synovial fluid, pleural fluid, saliva, and other bodily fluids.

otorrhea—Ear discharge.

outcome goals—Goals focused on the desired end result (e.g., "Finish 1st in the race.").

outcome measures—The instrument used to study the end result of health care services; these measures take patient's experiences, preferences, and values into account and help integrate evidence-based practice into athletic trainers' clinical practice.

over the counter (OTC)—A drug that is sold retail without a prescription.

overload—A gradual increased stress (i.e., exercise) must be applied to the body to continue adaptations.

palliation—Something that reduces or relieves the pain or other symptoms without curing the condition.

paramedic—Someone who has extensive training in advanced life support, including intubation, emergency pharmacology, cardiac monitoring, and other advanced assessment and treatment skills.

parenteral—Contact with blood, semen, or another body fluid from an infected patient.

paresthesia—Abnormal sensations such as tingling, prickling, and numbness.

parotitis—Swollen parotid glands.

pathologic fractures—Fracture caused by disease rather than trauma.

pathological reflexes—An abnormal automatic response from the nervous system that may have primitive origins and indicate a loss of cortical inhibition.

pathophysiology—The disordered physiological processes associated with disease or injury.

patient advocacy—When health care providers assist patients with communication regarding their health needs and obtain information pertinent to their health so that they can make informed decisions.

patient-centered care (PCC)—Collaboration of a cohesive team of health care providers to focus on a patient's needs.

performance goals—Goals focused on a specific performance standard (e.g., "Run it in 12.2 seconds.").

perfusion—The passage of fluid through the circulatory system to organs or tissues, usually referring to the delivery of blood to an area.

peripheral nervous system (PNS)—Portion of the nervous system outside the brain and spinal cord.

peristalsis—Involuntary contraction and relaxation of the smooth muscle of the intestines.

personal protective equipment (PPE)—Protective clothing, goggles, gloves, and equipment that protect the athletic trainer from exposure to infection or disease from contact with a patient.

person-first terminology—Statements that identify the person first and then the disability.

petrissage—Massage technique of kneading an identified body area.

pharmacodynamics—The study of how a drug affects the body, which includes time, intensity, and adverse effects.

pharmacokinetics—How the body processes a drug, which includes metabolism, absorption distribution, and elimination.

pharmacology—The science of drug action, effect, and uses.

pharmacy—An entity that sells, dispenses, and prepares medications.

phonophobia—Fear of loud sounds.

photophobia—Sensitivity to light.

phytonutrients—A substance found in certain plants that is believed to be beneficial to human health and help prevent various diseases.

pitting edema—Swelling, usually in the extremities, that when pressed will maintain the depression created for some time.

placebo effect—A beneficial effect produced by a placebo drug or treatment that cannot be attributed to the properties of the placebo itself and must therefore be due to the patient's belief in that treatment.

plethysmography—A body composition technique using air displacement for measurement of body volume and thus body composition; typically conducted with the BodPod.

point tenderness—Localized sore spot identified during palpation.

poliomyelitis or polio—A viral infection that affects motor cells of the spinal cord.

polymerize—Combination of single molecules into poly-molecular chains.

polyopia—Perception of more than one image of a single object.

position of function—Placing the body so that the ankle is in neutral dorsiflexion (no equinus), there is 30 degrees of wrist extension, and the thumb is opposed to midway between maximal radial and palmar abduction.

positive predictive value (PPV)—The proportion of patients with a positive diagnostic test who have an injury or disease.

positive self-talk—A cognitive behavioral strategy used in sport to help an athlete redirect attention toward a task, boost motivation and effort, and improve attitude.

postprofessional education—Formal education in athletic training beyond the professional master's degree; can occur through doctoral education or a residency program.

power distance—The level of comfort that group members have with power, influence, and wealth inequalities.

preparticipation physical examination—Physical examination to help assess and maintain the health and safety of athletes; sports physicals.

prevalence—The proportion of members of a population affected by a condition at any given time.

prevention—The action taken to decrease the chance of getting a disease, condition, or injury.

primary data—Raw data collected by the researcher.

primary healing—Wound or tissue healing where scar tissue does not have to fill a gap in the injured tissue.

process goals—Goals focused on "the how," or the small goals you need to focus on to get to the end result (e.g., "Give maximum effort and have a great attitude today.").

product liability—The responsibility of the manufacturer, distributor, and seller of a product to deliver products free of defects that could cause harm and to compensate for any injury caused by defective merchandise.

professional education—Formal education for entry into the athletic training profession that occurs at the graduate level.

professional ethics—A standard to ensure that the highest standards of integrity, conduct, and care are maintained and employed.

progression—A systematic increase in workload (duration or intensity) to increase fitness levels.

progressive muscle relaxation—An exercise that systematically tenses and relaxes individual muscle groups through directing conscious attention, active contraction, and relaxation.

progressive strengthening (progressive resistance) exercises—When strengthening concepts are used across the phases of rehabilitation; application is based on tissue healing, patient feedback, and safety.

prophylactic procedures—Various techniques used to guard or protect a body part from injury or reinjury.

proprioception—Also known as kinesthesia; the ability to identify a body's position in space.

proprioceptive neuromuscular facilitation (PNF)—A rehabilitation technique primarily used to increase both active and passive range of motion through neuromuscular engagement by relying on reflexive stretching.

protective equipment—Various items worn to help reduce the risk of injury from sport or activity.

proton pump inhibitors (PPIs)—These medications block stomach acid, irreversibly binding to and inhibiting hydrogen-potassium pump.

provocation—Something that increases or aggravates the signs and symptoms of a condition or injury.

psychological skills training—A deliberate, structured training program of psychological strategies and methods that improve physical performance through training aspects involved in the mental aspects of competition.

public health—The science of promoting the health of people and their communities.

qualitative—The use of descriptive characteristics that are observable but not numerically measurable; provides input about relationship systems. Examples include focus groups or independent observations.

quality assurance—Also known as quality improvement; a systematic continuous evaluation of health care services to ensure patient safety and beneficial health care outcomes.

quantitative—The use of numbers as measurable data that can be statistically analyzed. Examples include percentages, frequencies, and specific medical values such as laboratory results.

race—A societal category that is not grounded in biology.

radiographic image—Also called a radiograph or X-ray; an image obtained through the use of ionizing radiation (X-rays) in combination with an image receptor (either film or digital).

radiologist—A physician specifically trained to supervise and interpret radiology examinations.

randomized controlled trials—Includes a randomized group of patients in an experimental group and a control group.

referral—The practice of sending a patient to another health care provider for consultation or care; delegation of care.

reflex—An involuntary response to a stimulus. Reflexes are specific and predictable; in this case, they are caused by stimulation of tendons.

registered dietitian (RD)—Food and nutrition experts who have met the criteria from the Commission on Dietetic Registration (CDR) to earn the RD credential.

relative energy deficiency in sport (RED-S)—Impaired physiological functioning caused by relative energy deficiency; includes, but is not limited to, impairments of metabolic rate, menstrual function, bone health, immunity, protein synthesis, and cardiovascular health.

relative humidity—The amount of water vapor present in air; expressed as a percentage of the amount needed for saturation at the same temperature.

relaxation techniques—A variety of methods used to reduce tension, stress, and anxiety in the body.

release of information (ROI)—A statement signed by a patient that releases confidential information to specified designees.

resistance training—Also known as strength training or weight-lifting, it is exercise intended to improve muscular strength and endurance.

resonance—Sound quality that is either deep or full and reverberating.

revenue—Income or earning of an organization.

rigidity—Also known as stiffness; the amount of bending or compression that occurs in response to a measured amount of applied stress.

risk—The probability that an adverse event or consequence will occur.

risk factor—Elements that increase the probability that an adverse event or consequence will occur.

Russel's sign—Calluses on the back of hand or knuckles from self-induced vomiting.

Salter-Harris fracture—Fracture involving the epiphyseal plate.

Schwann cells—Myelin-secreting glial cells that form the myelin sheath around the axon.

secondary data—Data already collected by primary sources that is accessible to researchers, such as the government census or organizational records.

secondary healing—Wound or tissue healing where the wound edges cannot be approximated and granulation tissue must fill the gap in the wound.

self-talk—A person's internal dialogue that can be used to influence her sense of confidence, self-worth, and perception of the world.

sensitivity—The proportion of patients with the injury or disease who have a positive test or result. The higher the sensitivity, the more correctly the test has identified patients with that injury or disease.

sepsis—Life-threatening organ dysfunction as a host responds to an infection.

shivering—Involuntary response to decreased core temperature in an effort to generate heat through muscle contractions.

shock—Critical condition that is brought on by a sudden drop in blood flow through the body. The circulatory system fails to maintain adequate blood flow, decreasing the delivery of oxygen and nutrients to vital organs.

shrinkers—Elastic compression socks that are pulled over a residual amputated limb.

signs—Objective evidence or manifestation of a condition or injury.

simple carbohydrates—Formed from 10 or fewer monosaccharides. Dairy products, fruit, and sucrose are examples of simple carbohydrates.

skinfolding—A technique that estimates body fat percentage from several thickness folds of skin and subcutaneous fat across the body.

soft-tissue mobilization (STM)—A form of manual therapy intended to address soft-tissue injury that uses instruments and hands-on techniques to enhance healing, reduce pain, and increase range of motion.

special population—For the purposes of athletic training, this term includes people in a population subset based on job duties, age, gender identity, and disability.

specificity—Adaptations of the body to exercise are specific to the type of training undertaken.

specificity—The proportion of patients without the injury or disease who have a negative result. The higher the specificity, the more correctly the test has identified patients without the injury or disease.

spina bifida—A congenital spinal cord injury in which the neural tube does not close completely during the first 4 to 6 weeks of fetal development.

spinal cord injury (SCI)—An injury that results in complete or partial loss of motor and sensory function below the lesion.

spinal motion restriction (SMR)—Attempting to maintain the spine in anatomic alignment (spinal neutral) and minimizing gross movement irrespective of adjuncts or devices.

splenomegaly—Enlarged spleen.

sports-relaxed concussion (SRC)—A traumatic brain injury induced by biomechanical forces with several common features that may be used in clinically defining the nature of the injury.

standard precautions (SP)—Combines major features of universal precautions (UP) and body substance isolation (BSI) and are based on the principle that all blood, body fluids, secretions, excretions except for sweat, nonintact skin, and mucous membranes may contain transmissible infectious agents.

state anxiety—The psychological and physiological transient reactions directly related to adverse situations in a specific moment.

stereotype—A belief regarding characteristics of a social group; these are preconceived generalizations.

stigma—When people are shamed because they are different from a social standard.

stoicism—Not showing emotion after painful or pleasurable experiences.

strategic planning—A process of creating a future plan based on definition objectives and outcomes for the organization.

stress fracture—A fracture of bone caused by repeated mechanical stresses.

stress syndrome—Inflammatory process of bone caused by repeated mechanical stresses; often precedes stress fracture.

stress tolerance—The ability to withstand stress without breaking.

subchondral—Layer of bone found just below the cartilage that acts as a shock absorber in weight-bearing joints.

surveillance—The systematic, ongoing collection, analysis, and dissemination of data in order to prevent and control injuries and illnesses.

symptoms—Any perceived subjective change related to the condition or injury reported by the patient.

syncope—Temporary loss of consciousness.

systematic review—Authors have systematically searched for, appraised, and summarized all of the medical literature for a specific topic.

systolic—Pressure in the arteries during the contraction of the ventricles.

tachycardia—Heart rate is faster than normal.

tachypnea—Rapid respirations.

tactical athletes—People in service professions (e.g., military, firefighters, law enforcement, and emergency responders).

tapotement—Massage technique of percussing an identified body area.

tendinopathy—Injury to a tendon; for example, tendinitis, tendinosis, and tenosynovitis.

tenesmus—Straining to defecate or urinate.

tensile strength—Measurement of how much tensile force a material can withstand before it fails. This is often reported as pounds per square inch.

therapeutic exercise—A component of rehabilitation that addresses the return of injured patients to pain-free function or activity.

therapeutic modality—The application of an implement or device that causes physiological changes that improve or facilitate normal function.

thermal energies—Heat and cold therapies that transfer thermal energy through conduction, convection, radiation, and conversion.

thermal gradient—The difference between the temperature of the environment and the temperature of the body.

thermoregulation—The body's ability to maintain a normal core temperature, which is rigorously maintained at approximately 37°C (99°F).

thermotherapy—The application of heat.

thready pulse—A scarcely perceptible, often rapid pulse that feels like a fine mobile thread under a palpating finger.

trabecular bone—Also known as spongy bone; porous bone containing red bone marrow found at the ends of long bones.

trait anxiety—The stable tendency to attend to, experience, and report negative emotions, such as fears, worries, and anxiety, across many situations.

triage—The process of sorting patients based on the severity of the injury and medical need to establish treatment and transportation priorities.

trigger point—An area in the muscle or fascia that when stimulated will cause pain that typically radiates; there may be a palpable nodule present. Trigger points are not caused by acute trauma.

triglycerides—The major form of fat stored by the body. Triglycerides serve as the backbone for many types of lipids (fats). Triglycerides come from the food we eat and are also produced by the body.

type 2 diabetes—A chronic medical condition where the body does not produce enough insulin, resulting in elevated blood sugar levels.

ultrasound—A deep-heating modality that is inaudible to the human ear.

universal precautions—Approach to infection control. According to the concept of universal precautions, all human blood and certain human body fluids are treated as if known to be infectious for HIV, HBV, and other blood-borne pathogens.

urinalysis—Tests to detect or measure certain substance in the urine.

$\dot{V}O_2$max—A measure of the maximal volume of oxygen the lungs can take in and the working muscles can distribute and use.

vector-borne contact—Transmitted by an animal (i.e., exposure to infected animals such as dogs, raccoons, insects, and bats).

viscoelastic—Exhibiting both viscous and elastic components when deformed.

vision—An aspirational declaration of an organization's future.

vitamins—Organic compounds that are needed in small quantities to sustain life and help the body grow and develop normally.

Wallerian degeneration—Degeneration of nerve fiber that occurs distal to the site of injury when the nerve fiber is cut or crushed.

Wolff's law—A law that states that tissue, particularly bone, will adapt to the loads under which it is placed.

work practice controls—Controls that reduce the likelihood of exposure by altering the manner in which a task is performed (e.g., prohibiting recapping of needles by a two-handed technique).

REFERENCES

Chapter 1

1. Athletic Training. National Athletic Trainers' Association. https://www.nata.org/about/athletic-training. Accessed August 13, 2020.

2. Strategic implementation team defines profession. *NATA News.* December, 2007:14.

3. Athletic training. The National Athletic Trainers' Association website. www.nata.org/about/athletic-training. Accessed May 2, 2019.

4. Job settings. The National Athletic Trainers' Association website. www.nata.org/about/athletic-training/job-settings. Accessed April 10, 2019.

5. Board of Certification. Practice analysis, 7th ed. Board of Certification website. https://bocatc.org/system/document_versions/versions/24/original/boc-pa7-content-outline-20170612.pdf?1497279231. Published 2015. Accessed November 29, 2016.

6. Prentice W. *Principles of Athletic Training: A Competency-Based Approach.* New York: McGraw-Hill; 2011.

7. Webber M. *Dropping the Bucket and Sponge.* Prescott, AZ: Athletic Training History; 2011.

8. Delforge GD, Behnke RS. The history and evolution of athletic training education in the United States. *J Athl Train.* 1999;34(1):53-61.

9. Commission on Accreditation and Administration of Athletic Training Education Directory. Archived from the original on 2011-05-21. https://caate.net/archived-actions/. Accessed August 13, 2020.

10. Breitbach AP, Richardson R. Interprofessional education and practice in athletic training. *Athl Train Educ J.* 2015;10(2):170-182.

11. Standards of Professional Practice Board of Certification website. https://www.bocatc.org/system/document_versions/versions/154/original/boc-standards-of-professional-practice-2018-20180619.pdf?1529433022. Accessed August 13, 2020.

12. Code of Ethics. https://www.nata.org/membership/about-membership/member-resources/code-of-ethics. Accessed August 13, 2020.

13. Health sciences. Whitworth University website. http://catalog.whitworth.edu/undergraduate/healthsciences/. Accessed August 13, 2020.

14. About CAATE. Commission on Accreditation and Administration of Athletic Training Education website. https://caate.net/. Accessed August 13, 2020.

15. World Health Organization, Framework for Action on Interprofessional Education & Collaborative Practice, 2010 Interprofessional Education Collaborative Expert Panel. *Core Competencies for Interprofessional Collaborative Practice: Report of an Expert Panel.* Washington, DC: Interprofessional Education Collaborative; 2011.

16. Interprofessional Education Collaborative Expert Panel. *Core Competencies for Interprofessional Collaborative Practice: 2016 Update.* https://nebula.wsimg.com/2f68a39520b03336b41038c370497473?AccessKeyId=DC06780E69ED19E2B3A5&disposition=0&alloworigin=1.

17. Athletic training accredited programs. https://caate.net/search-for-accredited-program/. Accessed August 13, 2020.

18. Board of Certification. https://www.bocatc.org/. Accessed August 13, 2020.

19. NATA. Accessed May 10, 2012.

20. Ebel RG. *Far Beyond the Shoe Box: Fifty Years of the National Athletic Trainers' Association.* New York: Forbes; 1999.

21. Lisher SM. *A Descriptive History of the Discipline of Athletic Training Education* [master's thesis]. Glassboro; NJ: Rowan University; 2002.

22. Professional education programs. National Athletic Trainers' Association website. http://nata.org/ProfessionalEduPrgmsNATA. Accessed August 1, 2008.

Chapter 2

1. National Athletic Trainers' Association. *Athletic Training Educational Competencies.* 5th ed. 2011.

2. Akobeng AK. Principles of evidence-based medicine. *Arch Dis Child.* 2005;90(8):837-840.

3. Bernardo WM, Nobre MRC, Jatene FB. Evidence based clinical practice: part II-searching evidence databases. *Rev Bras Reumatol.* 2004;44(6):403-409.

4. Bhandari M, Giannoudis PV. Evidence-based medicine: what it is and what it is not. *Injury.* 2006;37(4):302-306.

5. Davies P. What is evidence-based education? *Br J Educ Stud.* 1999;47(2):108-121.

6. Fineout-Overholt E, Melnyk BM, Stillwell SB, Williamson KM. Evidence-based practice step by step: critical appraisal of the evidence: part I. *Am J Nurs.* 2010;110(7):47-52.

7. Kreder HJ. Evidence-based surgical practice: what is it and do we need it? *World J Surg.* 1999;23(12):1232-1235.

8. Martinoff R, Kreder H. Finding evidence: evidence-based practice. *Hand clinics.* 2009;25(1):15-27.

9. Melnyk BM, Fineout-Overholt E, Stillwell SB, Williamson KM. Evidence-based practice: step by step: the seven steps of evidence-based practice. *Am J Nurs.* 2010;110(1):51-53.

10. Sackett DL, Rosenberg WM, Gray JM, Haynes RB, Richardson WS. Evidence-based medicine: what it is and what it isn't. 1996. *Clin Orthop Relat Res.* 2007;455:3-5.

11. Steves R, Hootman JM. Evidence-based medicine: what is it and how does it apply to athletic training? *J Athl Train.* 2004;39(1):83.

12. Stillwell SB, Fineout-Overholt E, Melnyk BM, Williamson KM. Evidence-based practice, step by step: asking the clinical question: a key step in evidence-based practice. *Am J Nurs.* 2010;110(3):58-61.

13. Devereaux P, Bhandari M, Clarke M, et al. Need for expertise based randomised controlled trials. *BMJ.* 2005;330(7482):88.

14. Bartunek JM, Seo MG. Qualitative research can add new meanings to quantitative research. *J Organ Behav.* 2002;23(2):237-242.

15. Creswell JW, Creswell JD. *Research Design: Qualitative, Quantitative, and Mixed Methods Approaches.* Thousand Oaks, CA: Sage; 2017.

16. Denzin NK, Lincoln YS. *The Sage Handbook of Qualitative Research.* Thousand Oaks, CA: Sage; 2005.

17. Given LM. *The Sage Encyclopedia of Qualitative Research Methods.* Thousand Oaks, CA: Sage; 2008.

18. Glesne C. *Becoming Qualitative Researchers: An Introduction.* Upper Saddle River, NJ: Pearson; 2015.

19. Lougen C. Sources: The Sage Encyclopedia of Qualitative Research Methods. *Ref User Serv Q.* 2011;49(1):101-102.

20. Mack N, Woodsong C, MacQueen KM, Guest G, Namey E. *Qualitative Research Methods: A Data Collectors Field Guide.* Research Triangle Park, NC: Family Health International; 2005.

21. Marshall C, Rossman GB. *Designing Qualitative Research.* Thousand Oaks, CA: Sage; 2014.

22. Savin-Baden M, Major CH. *Qualitative Research: The Essential Guide to Theory and Practice.* Routledge; 2013.

23. Strauss A. *The Discovery of Grounded Theory: Strategies for Qualitative Research.* Chicago, IL: Aldine; 1967.

24. Taylor SJ, Bogdan R. *Introduction to Qualitative Research Methods: The Search for Meaning.* Hoboken, NJ: Wiley; 1984.

25. Thomas R. Five ways of doing qualitative analysis: Phenomenological psychology, grounded theory, discourse analysis, narrative research, and intuitive inquiry by F.J. Weitz, K. Charmaz, L.M. McMullen, R. Josselson, R. Anderson and E. McSpadden. Book review. Wiley Online Library website. https://onlinelibrary.wiley.com/doi/abs/10.1111/j.2044-8295.2012.02104.x. Published April 16, 2012.

26. Foley G, Timonen V. Using grounded theory method to capture and analyze health care experiences. *Health Serv Res.* 2015;50(4):1195-1210.

27. Goertzen MJ. Introduction to quantitative research and data. *Libr Technol Rep.* 2017;53(4):12.

28. Hill A, Spittlehouse C. *What is critical appraisal? Volume 3, number 2.* http://citeseerx.ist.psu.edu/viewdoc/download?doi=10.1.1.524.2610&rep=rep1&type=pdf. Hayward Medical Communications; 2001.

29. Critical appraisal tools to make sense of evidence. McMaster University website. www.nccmt.ca/knowledge-repositories/search/87. Accessed October 10, 2017.

30. Greenhalgh T. *How to Read a Paper: The Basics of Evidence-Based Medicine.* Chichester, England: John Wiley & Sons; 2014.

31. Haynes B. Of studies, syntheses, synopses, summaries, and systems: the "5S" evolution of information services for evidence-based healthcare decisions. *Evid Based Nurs.* 2007;10(1):6-7.

32. Hollands H, Kertes PJ. Measuring the size of a treatment effect: relative risk reduction, absolute risk reduction, and number needed to treat. *Evid Based Ophthalmol.* 2008;9(2):72-76.

33. *International Classification of Functioning, Disability and Health. Agenda item 13.9 of the Fifty-Fourth World Health Assembly.* World Health Organization website. https://apps.who.int/gb/archive/pdf_files/WHA54/ea54r21.pdf?ua=1. Published May 22, 2001.

34. International Classification of Functioning, Disability and Health (ICF). World Health Organization website. www.who.int/classifications/icf/en. Accessed December 7, 2017.

35. Sharma S. Levels of evidence. *Evid Based Ophthalmol.* 2002;3(1):5-6.

36. Bhandari M, Montori VM, Devereaux PJ, et al. Doubling the impact: publication of systematic review articles in orthopaedic journals. *JBJS.* 2004;86(5):1012-1016.

37. Parsons JT, Valovich McLeod TC, Snyder AR, Sauers EL. Change is hard: adopting a disablement model for athletic training. *J Athl Train.* 2008;43(4):446-448.

38. Snyder AR, Parsons JT, Valovich McLeod TC, Curtis Bay R, Michener LA, Sauers EL. Using disablement models and clinical outcomes assessment to enable evidence-based athletic training practice, part I: disablement models. *J Athl Train.* 2008;43(4):428-436.

39. Valovich McLeod TC, Snyder AR, Parsons JT, Curtis Bay R, Michener LA, Sauers EL. Using disablement models and clinical outcomes assessment to enable evidence-based athletic training practice, part II: clinical outcomes assessment. *J Athl Train.* 2008;43(4):437-445.

40. Nagi SZ. Some conceptual issues in disability and rehabilitation. In Sussman MB, ed. *Sociology and Rehabilitation.* Washington, D.C.: American Sociological Association; 1965.

41. Whiteneck G. Conceptual models of disability: past, present, and future. Paper presented at: Workshop on disability in America: A new look; September 10, 2006; Washington, DC.

42. Baldini A, Morel-Journel N, Paparel P, Ruffion A, Terrier JE. Patient-reported long-term sexual outcomes following plication surgery for penile curvature: A retrospective 58-patient study. *Prog Urol.* 2017;27(1):10-16.

43. Stone PW. Popping the (PICO) question in research and evidence-based practice. *Appl Nurs Res.* 2002;15(3):197-198.

44. Santos CMdC, Pimenta CAdM, Nobre MRC. The PICO strategy for the research question construction and evidence search. *Rev Lat Am Enfermagem.* 2007;15(3):508-511.

45. Akobeng AK. Understanding diagnostic tests 2: likelihood ratios, pre-and post-test probabilities and their use in clinical practice. *Acta Paediatr.* 2007;96(4):487-491.

46. Banning M. A review of clinical decision making: models and current research. *J Clin Nurs.* 2008;17(2):187-195.

47. Huang X, Lin J, Demner-Fushman D. Evaluation of PICO as a knowledge representation for clinical questions. *AMIA Annu Symp Proc.* 2006;2006:359-363.

48. O'Sullivan D, Wilk S, Michalowski W, Farion K. Using PICO to align medical evidence with MDs decision making models. *Stud Health Technol Inform.* 2013;192:1057.

49. Stevens KR. Systematic reviews: the heart of evidence-based practice. *AACN Clin Issues* 2001;12(4):529-538.

50. Hertel J. Research training for clinicians: the crucial link between evidence-based practice and third-party reimbursement. *J Athl Train.* 2005;40(2):69.

51. Akobeng AK. Understanding diagnostic tests 1: sensitivity, specificity and predictive values. *Acta Paediatr.* 2007;96(3):338-341.

52. Deeks JJ, Altman DG. Diagnostic tests 4: likelihood ratios. *Br Med J.* 2004;329(7458):168-169.

53. Wales NS. Moving beyond sensitivity and specificity: using likelihood ratios to help interpret diagnostic tests. *Aust Prescr.* 2003;26(5).

54. Steurer J, Fischer JE, Bachmann LM, Koller M, ter Riet G. Communicating accuracy of tests to general practitioners: a controlled study. *Br Med J.* 2002;324(7341):824-826.

55. Denegar CR, Fraser M. How useful are physical examination procedures? Understanding and applying likelihood ratios. *J Athl Train.* 2006;41(2):201.

56. Knowles SB, Marshall SW, Guskiewicz KM. Issues in estimating risks and rates in sports injury research. *J Athl Train.* 2006;41(2):207.

57. Loong T-W. Understanding sensitivity and specificity with the right side of the brain. *Br Med J.* 2003;327(7417):716-719.

58. Resnick, DB. What is Ethics in research and why is it important? List adapted from Shamoo A and Resnik D. 2015. Responsible Conduct of Research, 3rd ed. New York: Oxford University Press; 2015.

59. Resnik DB, Konecny B, Kissling GE. Conflict of interest and funding disclosure policies of environmental, occupational, and public health journals. *J Occup Environ Med.* 2017;59(1):28-33.

60. Shamoo AE, Resnik DB. *Responsible Conduct of Research.* Oxford, England: Oxford University Press; 2009.

61. WMA declaration of Helsinki—Ethical principles for medical research involving human subjects. World Medical Association website. www.wma.net/policies-post/wma-declaration-of-helsinki-ethical-principles-for-medical-research-involving-human-subjects. Updated October, 2013.

62. The National Commission for the Protection of Human Subjects of Biomedical and Behavioral Research. *The Belmont Report. Ethical Principles and Guidelines for the Protection of Human Subjects of Research.* Washington, D.C.: U.S. Government Printing Office; 1979. https://videocast.nih.gov/pdf/ohrp_appendix_belmont_report_vol_2.pdf.

63. Protection of Human Subjects. 45 C.F.R. §46.101. 2009.

64. Compliance and reporting. Department of Health and Human Services website. www.hhs.gov/ohrp/compliance-and-reporting/index.html. Accessed October 10, 2017.

65. Guidance for Institutional Review Boards and Clinical Investigators. U.S. Food and Drug Administration website. www.fda.gov/RegulatoryInformation/Guidances/ucm126420.htm. Accessed October 10, 2017.

66. U.S. Department of Health and Human Services. *Institutional Review Board (IRB) Written Procedures: Guidance for Institutions and IRBs.* www.fda.gov/downloads/regulatoryinformation/guidances/ucm512761.pdf. Published May 2018.

Chapter 3

1. World Health Organization Constitution. Accessed August 12, 2019. https://www.who.int/about/who-we-are/constitution

2. CDC - Public Health System and the 10 Essential Public Health Services - OSTLTS. Accessed August 12, 2019. https://www.cdc.gov/publichealthgateway/publichealthservices/essentialhealthservices.html

3. Fineberg HV. Public health and medicine where: the twain shall meet. *Am J Prev Med.* 2011;41(4 Suppl 3):S149-151. doi:10.1016/j.amepre.2011.07.013

4. White F. Primary health care and public health: foundations of universal health systems. *Med Princ Pract.* 2015;24(2):103-116. doi:10.1159/000370197

5. Obtain Certification. NATA. Published March 19, 2015. Accessed May 1, 2020. https://www.nata.org/about/athletic-training/obtain-certification

6. Lam KC, Valier ARS, Anderson BE, McLeod TCV. Athletic Training Services During Daily Patient Encounters: A Report From the Athletic Training Practice-Based Research Network. *J Athl Train.* 2016;51(6):435-441. doi:10.4085/1062-6050-51.8.03

7. Hoffman M, Bovbjerg V, Hannigan K, et al. Athletic Training and Public Health Summit. *J Athl Train.* 2016;51(7):576-580. doi:10.4085/1062-6050-51.6.01

8. van Mechelen W, Hlobil H, Kemper HC. Incidence, severity, aetiology and prevention of sports injuries. A review of concepts. *Sports Med.* 1992;14(2):82-99. doi:10.2165/00007256-199214020-00002

9. Thacker SB. Public health surveillance and the prevention of injuries in sports: what gets measured gets done. *J Athl Train.* 2007;42(2):171-172.

10. Thacker SB, Berkelman RL. Public health surveillance in the United States. *Epidemiol Rev.* 1988;10:164-190. doi:10.1093/oxfordjournals.epirev.a036021

11. Thacker SB, Qualters JR, Lee LM, Centers for Disease Control and Prevention. Public health surveillance in the United States: evolution and challenges. *MMWR supplements*. 2012;61(3):3-9.

12. Lee LM, Thacker SB, Centers for Disease Control and Prevention (CDC). The cornerstone of public health practice: public health surveillance, 1961--2011. *MMWR supplements*. 2011;60(4):15-21.

13. WHO | Epidemiology. Accessed August 15, 2019. https://www.who.int/topics/epidemiology/en/

14. Kerr ZY, Dompier TP, Snook EM, et al. National collegiate athletic association injury surveillance system: review of methods for 2004-2005 through 2013-2014 data collection. *J Athl Train*. 2014;49(4):552-560. doi:10.4085/1062-6050-49.3.58

15. Orchard JW, Meeuwisse W, Derman W, et al. Sport Medicine Diagnostic Coding System (SMDCS) and the Orchard Sports Injury and Illness Classification System (OSIICS): revised 2020 consensus versions. *Br J Sports Med*. 2020;54(7):397-401. doi:10.1136/bjsports-2019-101921

16. Bahr R, Clarsen B, Derman W, et al. International Olympic Committee consensus statement: methods for recording and reporting of epidemiological data on injury and illness in sport 2020 (including STROBE Extension for Sport Injury and Illness Surveillance (STROBE-SIIS)). *Br J Sports Med*. 2020;54(7):372-389. doi:10.1136/bjsports-2019-101969

17. Lohmander LS, Englund PM, Dahl LL, Roos EM. The long-term consequence of anterior cruciate ligament and meniscus injuries: osteoarthritis. *Am J Sports Med*. 2007;35(10):1756-1769. doi:10.1177/0363546507307396

18. Covassin T, Beidler E, Ostrowski J, Wallace J. Psychosocial aspects of rehabilitation in sports. *Clin Sports Med*. 2015;34(2):199-212. doi:10.1016/j.csm.2014.12.004

19. Bahr R, Clarsen B, Ekstrand J. Why we should focus on the burden of injuries and illnesses, not just their incidence. *Br J Sports Med*. 2018;52(16):1018. doi:10.1136/bjsports-2017-098160

20. Finch C. A new framework for research leading to sports injury prevention. *J Sci Med Sport*. 2006;9(1-2):3-9; discussion 10. doi:10.1016/j.jsams.2006.02.009

21. Bahr R. No injuries, but plenty of pain? On the methodology for recording overuse symptoms in sports. *Br J Sports Med*. 2009;43(13):966. doi:10.1136/bjsm.2009.066936

22. Padua DA, DiStefano LJ, Hewett TE, et al. National Athletic Trainers' Association Position Statement: Prevention of Anterior Cruciate Ligament Injury. *J Athl Train*. 2018;53(1):5-19. doi:10.4085/1062-6050-99-16

23. Bahr R, Holme I. Risk factors for sports injuries--a methodological approach. *Br J Sports Med*. 2003;37(5):384-392. doi:10.1136/bjsm.37.5.384

24. Meeuwisse WH. Assessing Causation in Sport Injury: A Multifactorial Model. *Clin J Sport Med*. 1994;4(3):166-170.

25. Braveman P, Gottlieb L. The social determinants of health: it's time to consider the causes of the causes. *Public Health Rep*. 2014;129 Suppl 2:19-31. doi:10.1177/00333549141291S206

26. Disparities | Healthy People 2020. Accessed August 22, 2019. https://www.healthypeople.gov/2020/about/foundation-health-measures/Disparities#6

27. Braveman P. What are health disparities and health equity? We need to be clear. *Public Health Rep*. 2014;129 Suppl 2:5-8. doi:10.1177/00333549141291S203

28. Bauer UE, Briss PA, Goodman RA, Bowman BA. Prevention of chronic disease in the 21st century: elimination of the leading preventable causes of premature death and disability in the USA. *Lancet*. 2014;384(9937):45-52. doi:10.1016/S0140-6736(14)60648-6

29. Determinants of Health | Healthy People 2020. Accessed August 29, 2019. https://www.healthypeople.gov/2020/about/foundation-health-measures/Determinants-of-Health

30. Hafeez H, Zeshan M, Tahir MA, Jahan N, Naveed S. Health Care Disparities Among Lesbian, Gay, Bisexual, and Transgender Youth: A Literature Review. *Cureus*. 9(4). doi:10.7759/cureus.1184

31. Zahran HS, Bailey CM, Damon SA, Garbe PL, Breysse PN. Vital Signs: Asthma in Children - United States, 2001-2016. *MMWR Morb Mortal Wkly Rep*. 2018;67(5):149-155. doi:10.15585/mmwr.mm6705e1

32. Volerman A, Chin MH, Press VG. Solutions for Asthma Disparities. *Pediatrics*. 2017;139(3). doi:10.1542/peds.2016-2546

33. Sullivan K, Thakur N. Structural and Social Determinants of Health in Asthma in Developed Economies: a Scoping Review of Literature Published Between 2014 and 2019. *Curr Allergy Asthma Rep*. 2020;20(2):5. doi:10.1007/s11882-020-0899-6

34. Flay BR. Efficacy and effectiveness trials (and other phases of research) in the development of health promotion programs. *Prev Med*. 1986;15(5):451-474.

35. McLeroy KR, Bibeau D, Steckler A, Glanz K. An ecological perspective on health promotion programs. *Health Educ Q*. 1988;15(4):351-377.

36. Norcross MF, Johnson ST, Bovbjerg VE, Koester MC, Hoffman MA. Factors influencing high school coaches' adoption of injury prevention programs. *J Sci Med Sport*. 2016;19(4):299-304. doi:10.1016/j.jsams.2015.03.009

37. Joy EA, Taylor JR, Novak MA, Chen M, Fink BP, Porucznik CA. Factors influencing the implementation of anterior cruciate ligament injury prevention strategies by girls soccer coaches. *J Strength Cond Res*. 2013;27(8):2263-2269. doi:10.1519/JSC.0b013e31827ef12e

Chapter 4

1. Peer KS, Schlabach GA. The professional values of program directors and head athletic trainers: the impact of the hidden curriculum. *Athl Train Educ J (National Athletic Trainers' Association)*. 2011;6(4):194-201.

2. Volberding J. Relationship between cultural competence and athletic training students' confidence in providing

culturally competent care. *Athl Train Sports Health Care.* 2014;6(1):31-36. doi:10.3928/19425864-20140103-02

3. Jeffreys MR, Dogan E. Evaluating cultural competence in the clinical practicum. *Nurs Educ Perspect.* 2013;34(2):88-94. doi:10.1097/00024776-201303000-00005

4. Perera-Diltz DM, Greenidge WL. Mindfulness techniques to promote culturally appropriate engagement. *J Creativ Ment Health.* 2018;13(4):490-504. doi:10.1080/1540138 3.2018.1459215

5. Long TB. Overview of teaching strategies for cultural competence in nursing students. *J Cult Divers.* 2012;19(3):102-108.

6. Abrums ME, Leppa C. Beyond cultural competence: teaching about race, gender, class, and sexual orientation. *J Nurs Educ.* 2001;40(6):270-275.

7. Miller LR, Peck BM. Patient-centered care: An examination of provider–patient communication over time. *Health Serv Res Manag Epidemiol.* 2019;6:1-7.

8. Ratka A, Pharm D. Empathy and the development of affective skills. *Am J Pharm Educ.* 2018;82(10):1140-1143.

9. Dekker ABE, Keulen M, Vagner G, et al. Physician self-assessed empathy does not correlate with patient perceptions of physician empathy. *Orthop J Harv Med Sch.* 2019;20:18-22.

10. Crocker AF, Smith SN. Person-first language: Are we practicing what we preach? *J Multidiscip Healthc.* 2019;12:125-129.

11. Guide to reporting on persons with an impairment. International Paralympic Committee website. www.paralympic.org/sites/default/files/document/141027103527844_2014 _10_31+Guide+to+reporting+on+persons+with+an+impairment.pdf. Updated October 2014. Accessed May 5, 2020.

12. Hudon C, Fortin M, Haggerty JL, Lambert M, Poitras M-E. Measuring patients' perceptions of patient-centered care: a systematic review of tools for family medicine. *Ann Fam Med.* 2011;9(2):155-164. doi:10.1370/afm.1226

13. Liddell DL. JDSC Supplemental guide for bias-free writing. *J Coll Stud Dev.* 2018;59(1):1-2.

14. Taylor P, Lopez MH, Martinez J, Velasco G. When labels don't fit: Hispanics and their views of identity. Pew Research Center website. April 4, 2012. www.pewresearch.org/hispanic/2012/04/04/when-labels-dont-fit-hispanics-and-their-views-of-identity.

15. Fernandez R. What's in a label? Not enough. *Hartford Courant.* March 2, 2001:A13.

16. Diversity research: NCAA race and gender demographics database. National Collegiate Athletic Association website. www.ncaa.org/about/resources/research/diversity-research. Updated 2019. Accessed May 5, 2020.

17. Quick facts: United States. United States Census Bureau website. www.census.gov/quickfacts/fact/table/US/PST045218. Updated 2019. Accessed May 5, 2020.

18. Bozo J, Revels-Macalinao M, Huynh V. Examining skin color and discrimination among ethnic minority adoles-

cents. *Race Soc Probl.* 2018;10(4):320-331. doi:10.1007/s12552-018-9250-4

19. Garcia JA, Sanchez GR, Sanchez-Youngman S, Vargas ED, Ybarra VD. Race as lived experience. *Du Bois Rev: Soc Sci Res Race.* 2015;12(2):349-373.

20. Vargas ED, Winston NC, Garcia JA, Sanchez GR. Latina/o or Mexicana/o? The relationship between socially assigned race and experiences with discrimination. *Sociol Race Ethn.* 2016;2(4):498-515.

21. Livermore DA. *Leading With Cultural Intelligence: The Real Secret to Success.* New York, NY: Amacom; 2015.

22. Dovidio JF, Hewstone M, Glick P, Esses VM. Prejudice, stereotyping and discrimination: theoretical and empirical overview. In Dovidio JF, Hewstone M, Glick P, Esses VM, eds. *The SAGE Handbook of Prejudice, Stereotyping and Discrimination.* London: SAGE; 2010:3-28. doi:10.4135/9781446200919.n1

23. Tocar SD. Comparative analysis of some cultural dimensions systems: a qualitative value-based approach. *Int J Cross Cult Manag.* 2019; I(1):21-34.

24. Hoffmann DE, Tarzian AJ. The girl who cried pain: a bias against women in the treatment of pain. *J Law Med Ethics.* 2001;29(1):13-27.

25. Jarrett C. Ouch! The different ways people experience pain. *The Psychologist.* 2011 June;24:416-420. https://thepsychologist.bps.org.uk/volume-24/edition-6/ouch-different-ways-people-experience-pain.

26. Waters J. Just why do women face a fight for equal health? *Community Practitioner.* 2019;92(9):36-41.

27. Thiederman S. Stoic or shouter, the pain is real. *RN.* 1989;52(6):49-51.

28. Campbell CM, Edwards RR. Ethnic differences in pain and pain management. *Pain Manag.* 2012;2(3):219-230. doi:10.2217/pmt.12.7

29. Briggs E. Cultural perspectives on pain management. *J Perioper Pract.* November 2008;18(11):468-471.

30. Kim HJ, Greenspan JD, Ohrbach R, et al. Racial/ethnic differences in experimental pain sensitivity and associated factors—cardiovascular responsiveness and psychological status. *PLoS One.* 2019;14(4):1-22.

31. Tung W-C, Li Z. Pain beliefs and behaviors among Chinese. *Home Health Care Manag Pract.* 2014;27(2):95-97. doi:10.1177/1084822314547962

32. Booker SQ. African Americans' perceptions of pain and pain management. *J Transcult Nurs.* 2016;27(1):73-80.

33. Shavers VL, Bakos A, Sheppard VB. Race, ethnicity and pain among the US population. *J Health Care Poor Underserved. 2010;21(1):177-220.*

34. Arimura T, Hosoi M, Tsukiyama Y, et al. Pain questionnaire development focusing on cross-cultural equivalence to the original questionnaire: The Japanese version of the short-form McGill Pain Questionnaire. *Pain Med.* 2012;13(4):541-551. doi:10.1111/j.1526-4637.2012.01333.x

35. The National CLAS Standards. Office of Minority Health. U.S. Department of Health and Human Services website. https://minorityhealth.hhs.gov/omh/browse.aspx?lvl=2&lvlid=53. Accessed July 17, 2020.

36. Treating the non-English speaking patient. *Dental Assistant*. March/April 2005;74(2):20-21.

37. Race: The Power of an Illusion. Ask the Experts. Public Broadcasting System website. www.pbs.org/race/000_About/002_04-experts-01-10.htm. Updated 2003. Accessed May 6, 2020.

38. Garcia JD. Race and ethnicity. In Brown N, González LT, McIlwraith T, eds. *Perspectives: An Open Invitation to Cultural Anthropology*. Arlington, VA: American Anthropological Association; 2017:211-212.

39. Mukhopadhyay C, Henze RC. How real is race? Using anthropology to make sense of human diversity. *Phi Delta Kappan*. 2003;84(9):669-678.

40. Freeman, Lauren. Confronting diminished epistemic privilege and epistemic injustice in pregnancy by challenging a "panoptics of the womb". *J Med Philos*. 2014;40(1):44-68.

41. Ratts MJ. Charting the center and the margins: addressing identity, marginalization, and privilege in counseling. *J Ment Health Couns*. 2017;39(2):87-103. doi:10.17744/mehc.39.2.01

42. Chapman EN, Kaatz A, Carnes M. Physicians and implicit bias: how doctors may unwittingly perpetuate health care disparities. *J Gen Intern Med*. 2013;28(11):1504-1510. doi:10.1007/s11606-013-2441-1

43. Operario D, Fiske ST. Racism equals power plus prejudice: a social psychological equation for racial oppression. In Eberhardt JL, Fiske ST, eds. *Confronting Racism: The Problem and the Response*. Thousand Oaks CA: Sage; 1998: 33–54.

44. Crisp RJ, Nicel JK. Disconfirming intergroup evaluations: asymmetric effects for in-groups and out-groups. *J Soc Psychol* 2004;144(3):247-271. doi:10.3200/socp.144.3.247-271

45. Cohrs JC, Duckitt J. Prejudice, types and origins of. *The Encyclopedia of Peace Psychology*. November 13, 2011. doi:10.1002/9780470672532.wbepp218

46. Implicit bias in health care. *Quick Safety*. April 2016;23:1-4. www.jointcommission.org/resources/news-and-multimedia/newsletters/newsletters/quick-safety/quick-safety-issue-23-implicit-bias-in-health-care. Accessed May 6, 2020.

47. Project Implicit website. https://implicit.harvard.edu/implicit. Accessed May 21, 2020.

48. Lang KR, Dupree CY, Kon AA, Duzinski DM. Calling out implicit racial bias as a harm in pediatric care: *Camb Q Healthcare Ethics*. 2016;25(3):540-552.

49. Nelson S. Race, racism, and health disparities: What can I do about it? *Creat Nurs*. 2016;22(3):161-165.

50. Fitzgerald C, Hurst S. Implicit bias in healthcare professionals: a systematic review. *BMC Med Ethics*. 2017;18(1).19. doi:10.1186/s12910-017-0179-8

51. Bekker S, Ahmed OH, Bakare U, et al. We need to talk about manels: the problem of implicit gender bias in sport and exercise medicine. *Brit J Sport Med*. 2018;52(20):1287-1289. doi:10.1136/bjsports-2018-099084

52. Hall WJ, Chapman MV, Lee KM, et al. Implicit racial/ethnic bias among health care professionals and its influence on health care outcomes: a systematic review. *Am J Public Health*. 2015;105(12):E60-E76.

53. Cuevas AG, O'Brien K, Saha S. What is the key to culturally competent care: reducing bias or cultural tailoring? *Psychol Health*. 2017;32(4):493-507. doi:10.1080/08870446.2017.1284221

54. Cramer DN, McElveen JS. Undoing racism in social work practice. *Race, Gender & Class*. 2003;10(2):41.

55. Goodman D. Oppression and privilege: two sides of the same coin. *J Intercult Commun Res*. 2015;(18):1-14.

56. Kaplin D. Microaggressions and macroaggressions in religiously diverse communities. *NY Psychologist*. 2017;XXIX(3):16-24.

57. Hodge DR. Spiritual microaggressions: Understanding the subtle messages that foster religious discrimination. *J Ethn Cult Divers Soc Work*. 2019:1-17. doi:10.1080/15313204.2018.1555501

58. Mcintosh P. *On Privilege, Fraudulence, and Teaching as Learning*. New York, NY: Routledge; 2020

59. Mcintosh P. Extending the knapsack: using the White privilege analysis to examine conferred advantage and disadvantage. *Women & Therapy*. 2015;38(3-4):232-245. doi:10.1080/02703149.2015.1059195

60. Berk RA. Microaggressions trilogy: Part 1. Why do microaggressions matter? *J Fac Dev*. 2017;31(1):63-73.

61. Berk RA. Microaggressions trilogy: Part 2. Microaggressions in the academic workplace. *J Fac Dev*. 2017;31(2):69-83.

62. Hunn V, Harley D, Elliott W, Canfield JP. Microaggression and the mitigation of psychological harm: Four social workers' exposition for care of clients, students, and faculty who suffer "a thousand little cuts." *J Pan Afr Stud (Online)*. 2015;7(9):41-54.

63. Rini R. How to take offense: responding to microaggression. *J Am Philos Assoc*. 2018;4(3):332-351. doi:10.1017/apa.2018.23

64. Nadal KL, Griffin KE, Wong Y, Hamit S, Rasmus M. The impact of racial microaggressions on mental health: counseling implications for clients of color. *J Couns Dev*. 2014;92(1):57-66. doi:10.1002/j.1556-6676.2014.00130.x

65. Huynh VW. Ethnic microaggressions and the depressive and somatic symptoms of Latino and Asian American adolescents. *J Youth Adolesc*. 2012;41(7):831-846. doi:10.1007/s10964-012-9756-9

66. Schultz RA. Embodied nonverbal microaggressions from the perspective of dance/movement therapists: interpretative phenomenological analysis. *Am J Dance Ther*. 2018;40:224-239. doi:10.1007/s10465-018-9282-8

67. Berk RA. Microaggressions trilogy: Part 3. Microaggressions in the classroom. *J Fac Dev.* 2017;31(3):95-110.

68. Swann G, Minshew R, Newcomb ME, Mustanski B. Validation of the sexual orientation microaggression inventory in two diverse samples of LGBTQ youth. *Arch Sex Behav.* 2016;45(6):1289-1298.

69. Darvin J. Becoming a more culturally responsive teacher by identifying and reducing microaggressions in classrooms and school communities. *J Multicult Educ.* 2018;12(1):2-9.

70. Rethorn ZD, Cook C, Reneker JC. Social determinants of health: if you are not measuring them, you aren't seeing the big picture. *J Orthop Sports Phy Ther.* 2019;49(12):872-874. doi:10.2519Zjospt.2019.0613

71. Palmer RT, Maramba DC. Racial microaggressions among Asian American and Latino/a students at a historically Black university. *J Coll Stud Dev.* 2015;56(7):705-722. doi:10.1353/csd.2015.0076

72. Sue DW, Capodilupo CM, Torino GC, et al. Racial microaggressions in everyday life: implications for clinical practice. *Am Psychol.* 2007;62(4):271-286.

73. Sue DW, Nadal KL, Capodilupo CM, Lin AI, Torino GC, Rivera DP. Racial microaggressions against Black Americans: implications for counseling. *J Couns Dev.* 2008;86(3):330-338.

74. Pappas E, Zampeli F, Xergia SA, Georgoulis AD. Lessons learned from the last 20 years of ACL-related in vivo-biomechanics research of the knee joint. *Knee Surgery, Sports Traumatology, Arthroscopy.* 2013;21(4):755-66.

75. Byrd CM. Microaggressions self-defense: A role-playing workshop for responding to microaggressions. *Soc Sci.* 2018;7(96):1-11. doi:10.3390/socsci7060096

76. Kaskan ER, Ho IK. Microaggressions and female athletes. *Sex Roles.* 2014;74(7-8):275-287. doi:10.1007/s11199-014-0425-1

77. Sue DW, Alsaidi S, Awad MN, Glaeser E, Calle CZ, Mendez N. Disarming racial microaggressions: Microintervention strategies for targets, White allies, and bystanders. *Am Psychol.* 2019;74(1):128.

78. Wong G, Derthick AO, David EJR, Saw A, Okazaki S. The what, the why, and the how: A review of racial microaggressions research in psychology. *Race Soc Probl.* 2014;6(2):181-200.

79. Jacob G, Meta van dH, Jama N, Moore AM, Ford-Jones L, Wong PD. Adverse childhood experiences: basics for the paediatrician. *Paed Child Healt Can.* 2019;24(1):30-37.

80. Bryan RH. Getting to why: adverse childhood experiences' impact on adult health. *JNP.* 2019;15(2):153-157.e1.

81. Ortiz R. Building resilience against the sequelae of adverse childhood experiences: rise up, change your life, and reform health care. *Am J Lifestyle Med.* 2019;13(5):470-479. doi:10.1177/1559827619839997

82. Chaby L, Cavigelli S, White A, Wang K, Braithwaite V. Long-term changes in cognitive bias and coping response as a result of chronic unpredictable stress during adolescence. *Front Hum Neurosci.* July 2013;7:1-11.

83. Burke-Harris N, Renschler T. ACE-Q materials. Center for Youth Wellness website. https://centerforyouthwellness.org/aceq-pdf. Updated 2015. Accessed May 6, 2020.

84. Naik P. When trauma-informed pedagogy is not enough: the need for increased school-based mental health services in public schools. https://ksr.hkspublications.org/2019/10/08/when-trauma-informed-pedagogy-is-not-enough-the-need-for-increased-school-based-mental-health-services-in-public-schools. Updated October 8, 2019. Accessed May 6, 2020.

85. Tebb KP, Gingi P, Lauren T, Diaz A, Brindis CD. Innovative approaches to address social determinants of health among adolescents and young adults. *Health Equity.* 2018;2(1):321-328.

86. Friedman C. The social determinants of health index. *Rehabil Psychol.* Feb 2020;65(1):11-21. doi:10.1037/rep0000298

87. Dykes DC, White AA. Getting to equal: strategies to understand and eliminate general and orthopaedic healthcare disparities. *Clin Orthop Relat Res.* 2009;467(10):2598-2605. doi:10.1007/s11999-009-0993-5

88. Fortier MA, Anderson CT, Kain ZN. Ethnicity matters in the assessment and treatment of children's pain. *Pediatrics.* 2009;124(1):378-380.

89. Taenzer AH, Clark C, Curry CS. Gender affects report of pain and function after arthroscopic anterior cruciate ligament reconstruction. *Anesthesiology.* 2000;93(3):670-675.

90. Shavers VL, Bakos A, Sheppard VB. Race, ethnicity and pain among the US population. *J Health Care Poor Underserved. 2010;21(1):177-220.*

91. Jarrett C. Ouch! The different ways people experience pain. *Psychologist.* Jun 2011;24(6):416-420.

92. Blendon R et al. Disparities in physician care: experiences and perceptions of a multi-ethnic America. *Health Affairs.* 2008;27:507-517.

93. Palit S, Kerr KL, Kuhn BL, et al. Exploring pain processing differences in Native Americans. *Health Psychology. 2013;32(11):1127-1136.*

94. Sidani S. Effects of patient-centered care on patient outcomes: an evaluation. *Res Ther Nurs Pract.* 2008;22(1):24-37. doi:10.1891/1541-6577.22.1.24

95. Braveman P. Health disparities and health equity: concepts and measurement. *Annu Rev Public Health.* 2006;27(1):167-194. doi:10.1146/annu rev.publhealth.27.021405.102103

96. Ibrahim SA, O'Connor MI. Movement is life. www.movementislifecaucus.com/wp-content/uploads/Movement-Is-Life-A-Catalyst-For-Change-Proceedings-Report.pdf. Accessed May 6, 2020.

97. Edwards I, Delany CM, Townsend AF, Swisher LL. New perspectives on Queens University at Kingston, International. https://quic.queensu.ca/php/toolsForSuccess/part_1_thinking_about_culture/part_1_thinking_about_culture4.html. Accessed May 20, 2020.

98. Hsieh N, Ruther M. Sexual minority health and health risk factors: Intersection effects of gender, race, and sexual identity. *Am J Prev Med.* 2016;50(6):746-755.

99. Lord B, Khalsa S. Influence of patient race on administration of analgesia by student paramedics. *BMC Emerg Med.* 2019;19(1):32.

100. Kharat AA, Borrego ME, Raisch DW, Roberts MH, Blanchette CM, Petersen H. Assessing disparities in the receipt of inhaled corticosteroid prescriptions for asthma by Hispanic and non-Hispanic white patients. *Ann Am Thorac Soc.* 2015 Feb;12(2):174-183.

101. Okunseri C, Okunseri E, Chilmaza CA, Harunani S, Xiang Q, Szabo A. Racial and ethnic variations in waiting times for emergency department visits related to nontraumatic dental conditions in the United States. *J Am Dent Assoc.* 2013;144(7):828-836.

102. Woodley LK. Reducing health disparities in pediatric asthma. *Pediatric Nursing.* Jul/Aug 2019;45(4):191-198.

103. Kozhimannil KB, Henning-Smith C. Racism and health in rural America. *Johns Hopkins University Press.* 2018;29(1):35-43.

104. Krahn GL, Klein Walker D, Correa-De-Araujo R. Persons with disabilities as a unique health disparity population. *Am J Public Health.* Apr 2015;105(S2):S198-206.

105. Campinha-Bacote J. Delivering patient-centered care in the midst of a cultural conflict: The role of cultural competence. *Online J Issues Nurs.* 2011;16(2):1-8.

106. Marra J, Covassin T, Shingles RR, Canady RB, Mackowiak T. Assessment of certified athletic trainers' levels of cultural competence in the delivery of health care. *JAT.* 2010;45(4):380-385. doi:10.4085/1062-6050-45.4.380

107. Paparella-Pitzel S, Eubanks R, Kaplan SL. Comparison of teaching strategies for cultural humility in physical therapy. *J Allied Health.* 2016;45(2):139-146.

108. Hughes M. Cultural safety requires cultural intelligence. *Kai Tiaki New Zealand.* July 2018;24-25.

109. Tervalon M, Murray-García J. Cultural humility versus cultural competence: a critical distinction in defining physician training outcomes in multicultural education. *J Health Care Poor Underserved.* 1998;9(2):117-125. doi:10.1353/hpu.2010.0233

110. Greene-Moton E, Minkler M. Cultural competence or cultural humility? Moving beyond the debate. *Health Promotion Practice.* 2019;21(1):142-145. doi:10.1177/1524839919884912

111. Berlin EA, Fowkes WC, Jr. A teaching framework for cross- cultural health care. *West J Med.* 1983;139(6):934-938.

112. Mostow C, Crosson J, Gordon S, et al. Treating and precepting with RESPECT: a relational model addressing race, ethnicity, and culture in medical training. *J Gen Intern Med.* Nov 2010;25(11):1257.

113. Mostow C, Crosson J, Gordon S, et al. Treating and precepting with RESPECT: a relational model addressing race, ethnicity, and culture in medical training. *J Gen Intern Med.* May 2010; 25(Suppl 2):146-154.

114. Campinha-Bacote J. The process of cultural competence in the delivery of healthcare services: A model of care. *J Transcult Nurs.* 2002;13(3):181-184.

115. Leape LL. Full disclosure and apology: an idea whose time has come. *Physician Exec.* 2006;32(2):16-18.

116. Byju AS, Mayo K. Medical error in the care of the unrepresented: disclosure and apology for a vulnerable patient population. *J Med Ethics.* 2019;45(12):821-823. doi:10.1136/medethics-2019-105633

117. Koehn D. Why saying "I'm sorry" isn't good enough: the ethics of corporate apologies. *Business Ethics Quarterly.* 2013;23(2):239-268. doi:10.5840/beq201323216

118. National Athletic Trainers' Association. *Ethnicity demographic data: 2012.* http://members.nata.org/members1/documents/membstats/2012-02.htm. Accessed September 20, 2012.

Chapter 5

1. Taylor MK, Gebremichael MD, Wagner CE. Mapping the literature of health care management. *J Med Libr Assoc.* 2007;95(2):e58-65.

2. Goldsmith SB. *Understanding Health Care Management.* Salsbury, MA: Jones & Bartlett; 2012.

3. Thompson JM. Health services administration. In Chisholm S, ed. *The Health Professions: Trends and Opportunities in U.S. Healthcare.* Salsbury, MA: Jones & Bartlett; 2007;357-372.

4. Cadarette SM, Wong L. An introduction to health care administrative data. *Can J Hosp Pharm.* 2015;68(3):232-237.

5. Cowie MR, Blomster JI, Curtis LH, et al. Electronic health records to facilitate clinical research. *Clin Res Cardiol.* 2017;106(1):1-9.

6. Ray R, Konin J. *Management Strategies in Athletic Training.* 4th ed. Champaign, IL: Human Kinetics; 2011.

7. Hughes RG. *Patient Safety and Quality: An Evidence-Based Handbook for Nurses.* Rockville, MD: Agency for Healthcare Research and Quality; 2008.

8. Occupational outlook handbook, 2016-2017. U.S. Bureau of Labor Statistics website. www.bls.gov/ooh/management/medical-and-health-services-managers.htm. Accessed April 30, 2017.

9. Carnevale AP, Smith N, Gulish, A, Beach BH. *Healthcare.* Washington, D.C.: Georgetown University; 2012. https://cew.georgetown.edu/wp-content/uploads/2014/11/Healthcare.FullReport.090712.pdf.

10. Lombardi DM, Schermerhorn, JR. *Healthcare Management.* Hoboken, NJ: Wiley and Sons; 2007.

11. Katz RL. Skills of an effective administrator. *Harv Bus Rev.* 1974;52:90-102.

12. Kubica AJ. Transitioning middle managers. How executives can ensure their success. *Healthc Exec.* 2008;23(2):58, 60.

13. Love DB, Ayadi MF. Redefining the core competencies of future healthcare executives under healthcare reform. *Admin Issues J.* 2015;5(2):3-16.

14. Nieva V, Sorra J. Safety culture assessment: a tool for improving patient safety in healthcare organizations. *Qual Saf Health Care*. 2003;12(suppl 2):ii17-ii23.

15. Ali N, Tretiakov A, Whiddett D, Hunter I. Knowledge management systems success in healthcare: Leadership matters. *Int J Med Inform*. 2017;97:331-340.

16. Health insurance coverage of the total population, 2016. Kaiser Family Foundation website. www.kff.org/other/state-indicator/total-population/?currentTime-frame=0&sortModel=%7B%22colId%22:%22Loca-tion%22,%22sort%22:%22asc%22%7D. Accessed April 30, 2017.

17. Cubanski J, Swoope C, Boccuti C, et al. A primer on Medicare: Key facts about the Medicare program and the people it covers. Kaiser Family Foundation website. www.kff.org/report-section/a-primer-on-medicare-what-is-medicare. Published March 20, 2015. Accessed May 30, 2017.

18. The Medicare part D prescription drug benefit. Kaiser Family Foundation website. www.kff.org/medicare/fact-sheet/the-medicare-prescription-drug-benefit-fact-sheet. Accessed May 17, 2017.

19. Barr DA. *An Introduction to U.S. Health Policy*. Baltimore, MD: Johns Hopkins University; 2010.

20. Peer KS, Rakich JS. Accreditation and continuous quality improvement in athletic training education. *J Athl Train*. 2000;35(2):188.

21. NQC Quality Academy: Useful quality improvement tools. National Quality Center website. http://nationalqualitycenter.org/resources/nqc-quality-academy-useful-quality-improvement-tools. Updated 2009. Accessed May 30, 2017.

22. Health Security Act. U.S. Congress 1994.

23. Health Security Act. U.S. Congress 1994.

24. Clinton's health care plan laid to rest. CQ Almanac website. https://library.cqpress.com/xsite/static.php?source=cqalmanac&type=public&page=expired. Accessed May 30, 2017.

25. HIPAA Privacy Rule 164.502. HIPAA Survival Guide website. www.hipaasurvivalguide.com/hipaa-regulations/164-502.php. Updated August 14, 2002. Accessed May 17, 2017.

26. HIPAA titles: Health Insurance Portability and Accountability Act of 1996. Highmark website. www.highmark.com/hmk2/hipaa/titles.shtml. Accessed May 27, 2017.

27. Labor and Employment Practice. HIPAA/HITECH enforcement action alert. *The National Law Review*. March 22, 2012. www.natlawreview.com/article/hipaahitech-enforcement-action-alert. Accessed September 19, 2017.

28. Tovino SA. The HIPAA privacy rule and the EU GDPR: illustrative comparisons. *Seton Hall L Rev*. 2017;47:973-1103.

29. Health Information Technology for Economic and Clinical Health Act. U.S. Congress 2009.

30. California Confidentiality of Medical Information Act. California civil code section 56.

31. Title 22, California Code of Regulations, Sections 70749, 70751, 71527, and 71549.

32. American Recovery and Reinvestment Act. U.S. Congress 2009.

33. Business Records Exception, Federal Evidence 803(6). Pub. L. 93–595, §1, Jan. 2, 1975.

34. Medicare Conditions of Participation, 42 CFR Sections 482.24. June 17, 1986.

35. National health expenditures: 2014 highlights. Centers for Medicare and Medicaid Services website. www.cms.gov/Research-Statistics-Data-and-Systems/Statistics-Trends-and-Reports/NationalHealthExpendData/downloads/highlights.pdf. Accessed May 30, 2017.

36. Jones, N. Health care in America: Follow the money. *National Public Radio*. March 19, 2012. www.npr.org/sections/health-shots/2012/03/19/148932689/health-care-in-america-follow-the-money?t=1592375437295

37. Atchinson BK, Fox DM. The politics of the Health Insurance Portability and Accountability Act. *Health Aff (Millwood)*. 1997;16(3):146-150.

38. Patient Protection and Affordable Care Act. U.S. Congress 2010.

39. The Privacy Act , 5 U.S.C. § 552a, U.S. Congress 19744.

40. Health Insurance Portability and Accountability Act (HIPAA). U.S. Congress 1996. 45 CFR 160, and 164.

41. Patient Protection and Affordable Care Act of 2009: Health insurance exchanges. National Association of Insurance Commissioners website. www.naic.org/documents/committees_b_Exchanges.pdf. Accessed May 30, 2017.

42. Institute of Medicine of the National Academies. *Performance Measurement: Accelerating Improvement*. Washington D.C.: National Academies Press; 2006.

43. U.S. Department of Health and Human Services. *Quality Improvement*. Washington, D.C.: Author: 2011. www.hrsa.gov/quality/toolbox/508pdfs/qualityimprovement.pdf. Accessed September 15, 2017.

44. Field RI. Why Is health care regulation so complex? *P T*. 2008;33(10):607-608.

45. Steinhoff M, Hoffman A. How do international laws and regulations intersect with HIPAA and other U.S. laws and regulations? Presentation at: Academic Medical Center Conference; June 13, 2017; Chapel Hill, NC.https://nchica.org/wp-content/uploads/2017/06/Hoffman-Steinhoff.pdf. Accessed September 19, 2017.

46. Tipton SJ, Forkey S, Choi YB. Toward proper authentication methods in electronic medical record access compliant to HIPAA and CIA triangle. *J Med Syst*. 2016;40(4):100.

47. Groves P, Kayyali B, Knott D, van Kuiken S. The big data revolution in healthcare: Accelerating value and innovation. *McKinsey and Company*. April 1, 2013. www.mckinsey.com/industries/healthcare-systems-and-services/our-insights/the-big-data-revolution-in-us-health-care.

48. Dulin M, Lovin C, Wright J. Bringing big data to the forefront of healthcare delivery: the experience of Carolina's

healthcare system. *Front Health Serv Manage.* 2017;33(1):1.

49. Gandomi A, Haider M. Beyond the hype: Big data concepts, methods, and analytics. *Int J Inf Manage.* 2015;35(2):137-144.

50. Murdoch TB, Detsky AS. The inevitable application of big data to health care. *JAMA.* 2013;309(13):1351-1352.

51. Sivarajah U, Kamal MM, Irani Z, Weerakkody V. Critical analysis of big data challenges and analytical methods. *J Bus Res.* 2017;70:263-286.

52. Blumenthal D, Tavenner M. The "meaningful use" regulation for electronic health records. *N Engl J Med.* 2010;363(6):501-504.

53. Appari A, Eric Johnson M, Anthony DL. Meaningful use of electronic health record systems and process quality of care: Evidence from a panel data analysis of US acute-care hospitals. *Health Serv Res.* 2013;48(2):354-375.

54. Billing 101. National Athletic Trainers Association website. www.nata.org/practice-patient-care/revenue-reimbursement/general-revenue-reimbursement/billing-101. Accessed May 6, 2017.

55. Reed LS. Private health insurance in the United States: an overview. *Soc Secur Bull.* 1965;28(Dec):3-48. www.ssa.gov/policy/docs/ssb/v28n12/v28n12p3.pdf. Accessed September 15, 2017.

56. Blumberg A, Davidson A. Accidents of history created U.S. health system. *All Things Considered.* October 22, 2009. www.npr.org/templates/story/story.php?storyId=114045132. Accessed May 30, 2017.

57. Meaningful Use. HealthIT.gov website. www.healthit.gov/topic/meaningful-use-and-macra/meaningful-use. Updated October 22, 2019. Accessed July 27, 2020.

Chapter 6

1. Andersen J, Courson RW, Kleiner DM, McLoda TA. National Athletic Trainers' Association position statement: emergency planning in athletics. *J Athl Train.* 2002;37(1):99.

2. Ferreira J, Mueller J, Papa A. (Strategic knowledge management: theory, practice and future challenges. *J Knowl Manage.* 2018;24(2):121-126. doi:10.1108/JKM-07-2018-0461

3. Hersey P, Blanchard KH, Johnson DE. *Management of Organizational Behavior.* Upper Saddle River, NJ: Prentice Hall; 2007.

4. Papanek ML. Kurt Lewin and his contributions to modern management theory. *Acad Manage Proceed.* 1973;1973(1).

5. Hoffman M, Tadelis S. People management skills, employee attrition, and manager rewards: An empirical analysis. *Natl Bureau of Econ Rsch.* 2018; No. w24360.

6. Müller O, Fay M, vom Brocke J. The effect of big data and analytics on firm performance: An econometric analysis considering industry characteristics. *J Manage Info Sys.* 2018;35(2):488-509.

7. Bytheway A, *Investing in Information: The Information Management Body of Knowledge.* Geneva, Switzerland: Springer; 2015.

8. Cyert RM, March JG. A behavioral theory of organizational objectives. In: Haire M; ed. *Modern Organization Theory.* New York, NY: Wiley; 1959; 76-90.

9. Scott Morton MS. *The Corporation of the 1990s: Information Technology and Organizational Transformation.* Oxford, England: Oxford University Press; 1991.

10. Senge PM. *The Fifth Discipline.* New York, NY: Doubleday; 1990.

11. Earl MJ. *Management Strategies for Information Technology.* Upper Saddle River, NJ Prentice-Hall; 1989.

12. Degner LF, Sloan JA, Venkatesh P. The control preferences scale. *Can J Nurse Res.* 1997;29(3):21-43.

13. Von Halle B, Goldberg L. *The Decision Model.* Boca Raton, FL: Taylor & Francis: 2010.

14. Konin JG, Ray R. *Management Strategies in Athletic Training.* 5th ed. Champaign, IL: Human Kinetics; 2018.

15. Burns JM. *Leadership.* 1st ed. New York, NY: Harper and Row; 1978.

16. Konin JG, Ray R. *Management Strategies in Athletic Training.* 5th ed. Champaign, IL: Human Kinetics; 2018.

17. Rost JC. *Leadership for the Twenty-First Century.* 1st ed. New York, NY: Praeger; 1991.

18. Nellis SM. Leadership and management: techniques and principles for athletic training. *J Athl Train.* 1994;29(4):328.

19. Kutz MR. Leadership in athletic training: implications for practice and education in allied health care. *J Allied Health.* 2010;39(4):265-279.

20. Laurent TG, Bradney DA. Leadership behaviors of athletic training leaders compared with leaders in other fields. *J Athl Train.* 2007;42(1):120.

21. Kutz MR, Scialli J. Leadership content important in athletic training education with implications for allied health care. *J Allied Health.* 2008;37(4):203-213.

22. Calfee DL. Get your mission statement working! *Manage Rev.* 1993;82:54-57.

23. Lammers T. The effective and indispensable mission statement. *Inc.* 1992;14:75-77.

24. Block MK, Rhodes WM. *The Impact of the Federal Sentencing Guidelines.* Washington, D.C.: US Department of Justice, National Institute of Justice; 1987.

25. National Collegiate Athletic Association. 2017-18 NCAA sports sponsorship and participation rates report. NCAA Publications website. www.ncaapublications.com/p-4368-2013-14-ncaa-sports-sponsorship-and-participation-rates-report.aspx. Updated 2014. Accessed August 5, 2018.

26. Carpman JR, Grant MA. *Design That Cares: Planning Health Facilities for Patients and Visitors.* 3rd ed. San Francisco, CA: Jossey-Bass; 2016.

27. Aparicio S, Welch Bacon CE, Parsons JT, et al. Staffing levels at National Collegiate Athletic Association foot-

ball bowl subdivision-level institutions. *J Athl Train.* 2015;50(12):12771285.

28. Our three divisions. National Collegiate Athletic Association website. www.ncaa.org/about/resources/media-center/ncaa-101/our-three-divisions. Updated 2016. Accessed August 5, 2018.

29. Flynn RB. *Facility Planning for Physical Education, Recreation, and Athletics.* Reston, VA: American Alliance for Health, Physical Education, Recreation and Dance; 1993.

30. Bayer C, Gamble M, Gentry R, Joshi S. *AIA Guide to Building Life Cycle Assessment in Practice.* Washington, D.C.: American Institute of Architects; 2010.

31. Prentice W, Arnheim D. *Principles of Athletic Training: A Competency-Based Approach.* 15th ed. New York, NY: McGraw-Hill Education; 2014.

32. Secor MR. Designing athletic training facilities or "where do you want the outlets?" *Athl Train.* 1985;19(1):19-21.

33. Sabo J. Design & construction of an athletic training facility. *NATA News.* 2001(May);5(1):10-22.

34. Peterson E. Insult to injury: feeling understaffed, underequipped and undervalued, athletic trainers say a minimum of space and equipment will yield extensive benefits. *Athl Bus.* 1999;23(9):57-60.

35. Terranova AB, Henning JM. National Collegiate Athletic Association division and primary job title of athletic trainers and their job satisfaction or intention to leave athletic training. *J Athl Train.* 2011;46(3):312-318.

36. Judge LW, Petersen JC, Bellar DM, Craig BW, Cottingham MP, Gilreath EL. The current state of NCAA Division I collegiate strength facilities: size, equipment, budget, staffing, and football status. *J Strength Cond Res.* 2014;28(8):2253-2261.

37. Petersen JC. High school indoor athletic facility space planning guidelines. *J Facility Plann Des Manage.* 2013;1(1):1-15.

38. Judge LW, Petersen JC, Bellar DM, Craig BW, Gilreath EL. CSCS certification and school enrollment impacts upon high school strength facilities, equipment, and safety. *J Strength Cond Res.* 2013;27(9):2626-2633.

39. Smith M, Ourand J. Five issues for the next NCAA president. *Street Smith Sports Business J.* 2009;12(32):1-25.

40. Recommendations and guidelines for appropriate medical coverage of intercollegiate athletics. National Athletic Trainers' Association website. www.nata.org/sites/default/files/amciarecsandguides.pdf. Updated 2007. Accessed August 5, 2018.

41. Mazerolle SM, Pitney WA, Casa DJ, Pagnotta KD. Assessing strategies to manage work and life balance of athletic trainers working in the National Collegiate Athletic Association Division I setting. *J Athl Train.* 2011;46(2):194-205.

42. Mazerolle SM, Bruening JE, Casa DJ, Burton LJ. Work-family conflict, part II: job and life satisfaction in National Collegiate Athletic Association Division IA certified athletic trainers. *J Athl Train.* 2008;43(5):513-522.

43. Petersen J. An analysis of indoor physical education facilities in Indiana high schools. *Indiana AHPERD J.* 2007;36(2):30-35.

44. Petersen JC. *Indoor Activity Space and Ancillary Space Analysis for New Mexico High Schools* [dissertation]. Albuquerque, NM: University of New Mexico; 1997.

45. Gallucci AR, Petersen JC. The size and scope of collegiate athletic training facilities and staffing. *J Athl Train.* 2017;52(8):785-794.

46. Benson HR. An introduction to benchmarking in healthcare. *Radiol Manage.* 1994(Fall);16(4):35-39.

47. Ettorchi-Tardy A, Levif M, Michel P. Benchmarking: A Method for Continuous Quality Improvement in Health. *Healthcare Policy.* 2012;7(4):e101-e119.

48. Hanney SR, Gonzalez-Block MA, Buxton MJ, Kogan M. The utilization of health research in policy-making: concepts, examples and methods of assessment. *Health Res Policy Syst.* 2003;1:2. doi:10.1186/1478-4505-1-2

49. National Collegiate Athletic Association. 2013-14 NCAA sports sponsorship and participation rates report. NCAA Publications website. www.ncaapublications.com/p-4368-2013-14-ncaa-sports-sponsorship-and-participation-rates-report.aspx. Updated 2014. Accessed January 10, 2016.

50. Petersen JC. High school indoor athletic facility space planning guidelines. *Facility Plann Des Manage.* 2013;1(1):1-15.

51. BOC facility principles. Board of Certification website. www.bocatc.org/system/document_versions/versions/42/original/boc-facility-principles-20170615.pdf?1497543426. Published 2013. Accessed August 1, 2018.

52. McLeod TCV, Bliven KCH, Lam KC, Bay RC, Valier ARS, Parsons JT. The national sports safety in secondary schools benchmark (N4SB) study: defining athletic training practice characteristics. *J Athl Train.* 2013;48(4):483-492.

53. Wham GS, Saunders R, Mensch J. Key factors for providing appropriate medical care in secondary school athletics: athletic training services and budget. *J Athl Train.* 2010;45(1):75-86.

54. Badgeley MA, McIlvain NM, Yard EE, Fields SK, Comstock RD. Epidemiology of 10,000 high school football injuries: patterns of injury by position played. *J Phys Act Health.* 2013;10(2):160-169.

55. Mayer M. Patient advocacy in research: merely an afterthought? *Patient.* 2011;4(2):69-71. doi:10.2165/11590710-000000000-00000

56. Advocacy. National Athletic Trainers' Association website. www.nata.org/advocacy. Accessed April 22, 2019.

57. Reiger PT. Professional organizations and their role in advocacy. *Semin Oncol Nurs.* 2002;18(4):276-289.

58. Sheldon, MR. Policy-making theory as an analytical framework in policy analysis: implications for research design and professional advocacy. *Phys Ther.* 2016;96(1):101-110.

59. Carleton BC. From professional advocacy to patient advocacy: a gambit for pharmacists. *J Am Pharm Assoc.* 2001;41(1);17-18.

60. Walter G. How to be an advocate for your profession and your practice park. *Clin Gast Hep.* 2017;15(10):1489-1491.

Chapter 7

1. Needlestick Safety and Prevention Act. U.S. Government Publishing Office website. www.gpo.gov/fdsys/pkg/PLAW-106publ430/html/PLAW-106publ430.htm. Published November 6, 2000. Accessed September 22, 2019.

2. Bloodborne pathogens. United States Department of Labor: Occupational Safety and Health Administration website. www.osha.gov/pls/oshaweb/owadisp.show_document?p_table=STANDARDS&p_id=10051#1910.1030(b). Published December 6, 1991. Updated April 3, 2012. Accessed May 20, 2020.

3. Exposure to blood: what healthcare personnel need to know. Centers for Disease Control and Prevention website. www.cdc.gov/HAI/pdfs/bbp/Exp_to_Blood.pdf. Updated July 2003. Accessed September 21, 2017.

4. Hepatitis B: FAQ for the public. Centers for Disease Control and Prevention website. www.cdc.gov/hepatitis/hbv/bfaq.htm#overview. Published May 2013. Accessed September 21, 2017.

5. HIV basic statistics. Centers for Disease Control and Prevention website. www.cdc.gov/hiv/basics/statistics.html. Published June 6, 2017. Updated September 6, 2017. Accessed September 21, 2017.

6. Standard precautions for all patient care. Centers for Disease Control and Prevention website. www.cdc.gov/infectioncontrol/basics/standard-precautions.html. Published January 26, 2017. Accessed September 21, 2017.

7. Siegel JD, Rhinehart E, Jackson M, Chiarello L, Health Care Infection Control Practices Advisory Committee. 2007 Guideline for isolation precautions: preventing transmission of infectious agents in health care settings. *Am J Infect Control.* 2007 Dec;35(10 Suppl 2):S65-164.

8. National Learning Consortium. Continuous quality improvement (CQI) strategies to optimize your practice. www.healthit.gov/sites/default/files/tools/nlc_continuousqualityimprovementprimer.pdf. Published April 30, 2013. Accessed September 15, 2017.

9. Occupational safety and health standards for shipyard employment. U.S. Department of Labor, Occupational Safety and Health Administration website. www.osha.gov/pls/oshaweb/owadisp.show_document?p_table=STANDARDS&p_id=202. Published May 2, 2011. Accessed September 21, 2017.

10. Eye safety. The National Institute for Occupational Safety and Health website. www.cdc.gov/niosh/topics/eye/eye-infectious.html. Published June 29, 2013. Accessed September 21, 2017.

11. Latex allergy: A prevention guideline. The National Institute for Occupational Safety and Health website. www.cdc.gov/niosh/docs/98-113/pdfs/98-113.pdf. Accessed September 15, 2017.

12. Paal P, Ellerton J, Sumann G, Demetz F, Mair P, Brugger H, International Commission for Mountain Emergency Medicine (ICAR MEDCOM). Basic life support ventilation in mountain rescue. Official recommendations of the International Commission for Mountain Emergency Medicine (ICAR MEDCOM). *High Alt Med Biol.* 2007;8(2):147-154.

13. Centers for Disease Control and Prevention. Guideline for hand hygiene in health-care settings: recommendations of the Healthcare Infection Control Practices Advisory Committee and the HICPAC/SHEA/APIC/IDSA Hand Hygiene Task Force. *MMWR Morb Mortal Wkly Rep.* 2002;51(RR-16):1-45.

14. Jumaa PA. Hand hygiene: simple and complex. *Int J Infect Dis.* 2005 Jan;9(1):3-14.

15. WHO guidelines on hand hygiene in health care. World Health Organization website. http://whqlibdoc.who.int/publications/2009/9789241597906_eng.pdf. Published 2009. Accessed September 15, 2017.

16. Kampf G, Kramer A. Epidemiologic background of hand hygiene and evaluation of the most important agents for scrubs and rubs. *Clin Microbiol Rev.* 2004;17(4):863-893.

17. Todd EC, Michaels BS, Holah J, Smith D, Greig JD, Bartleson CA. Outbreaks where food workers have been implicated in the spread of foodborne disease. Part 10. Alcohol-based antiseptics for hand disinfection and a comparison of their effectiveness with soaps. *J Food Prot.* 2010;73(11):2128-2140.

18. Show me the science: when and how to use hand sanitizer. Centers for Disease Control and Prevention website. www.cdc.gov/handwashing/show-me-the-science-hand-sanitizer.html. Published July 13, 2017. Accessed September 21, 2017.

19. Zinder SM, Basler RSW, Foley J, Scarlata C, Vasily DB. National Athletic Trainers' Association position statement: skin diseases. *J Athl Train.* 2010;45(4):411-428.

20. Beam JW, Buckley B, Holcomb WR, Ciocca M. National Athletic Trainers' Association position statement: management of acute skin trauma. *J Athl Train* 2016;51(12):1053-1070.

21. Katch RK, Berry DC. Effectiveness of four-decontamination techniques on bacterial growth on CPR manikins after use in a CPR course. *Int J First Aid Educ.* 2017;1(1):29.

22. Bloodborne pathogen exposure incidents. U.S. Department of Health, Occupational Safety and Health Administration website. www.osha.gov/OshDoc/data_BloodborneFacts/bbfact04.pdf. Published January 2011. Accessed September 21, 2017.

Chapter 8

1. Henderson JP. *The 2015 Athletic Trainer Practice Analysis Study.* Omaha, NE: Board of Certification; 2015.

2. Bernhardt DT, Roberts WO, eds. *PPE: Preparticipation Physical Evaluation.* 5th ed. American Academy of Family

Physicians, American Academy of Pediatrics, American College of Sports Medicine, American Medical Society for Sports Medicine, American Orthopaedic Society for Sports Medicine, American Osteopathic Academy of Sports Medicine; 2019.

3. Miller DJ, Blum AB, Levine WN, Ahmad CS, Popkin CA. Preparticipation evaluation of the young athlete: what an orthopaedic surgeon needs to know. *Am J Sports Med.* 2015;44(6):1605-1615. doi:10.1177/0363546515598994

4. Walsh Flanagan K, Cuppett M. *Medical Conditions in the Athlete.* 3rd ed. Champaign, IL: Human Kinetics; 2017.

5. Conley KM, Bolin DJ, Carek PJ, Konin JG, Neal TL, Violette D. National Athletic Trainers' Association position statement: preparticipation physical examinations and disqualifying conditions. *J Athl Train.* 2014;49(1):102-120. doi:10.4085/1062-6050-48.6.05

6. Lehman PJ, Carl RL. The preparticipation physical evaluation. *Pediatr Ann.* 2017;46(3):e85-e92. doi:10.3928/19382359-20170222-01

7. Caswell SV, Cortes N, Chabolla M, Ambegaonkar JP, Caswell AM, Brenner JS. State-specific differences in school sports preparticipation physical evaluation policies. *Pediatrics.* 2015;135(1):26-32. doi:10.1542/peds.2014-1451

8. Ljungqvist A, Jenoure P, Engebretsen L, et al. The International Olympic Committee (IOC) consensus statement on periodic health evaluation of elite athletes. *Int Sport J.* 2009;10(3):124-144. doi:10.1136/bjsm.2009.064394

9. O'Connor DP, Knoblauch MA. Electrocardiogram testing during athletic preparticipation physical examinations. *J Athl Train.* 2010;45(3):265-272. doi:10.4085/1062-6050-45.3.265

10. Washington R. Electrocardiograms during preparticipation athletic evaluations: is the selective use a compromise to mass screening? *J Pediatr.* 2015;167(4):789-790. doi:10.1016/j.jpeds.2015.07.040

11. O'Connor FG, Kugler JP, Oriscello RG. Sudden death in young athletes: screening for the needle in a haystack. *Am Fam Physician.* 1998;57(11):2763-2770. www.aafp.org/afp/1998/0601/p2763.html. Accessed April 10, 2019.

12. Bonci CM, Bonci LJ, Granger LR, et al. National Athletic Trainers' Association position statement: preventing, detecting, and managing disordered eating in athletes. *J Athl Train.* 2008;43(1):80-108. http://natajournals.org/doi/pdf/10.4085/1062-6050-43.1.80. Accessed June 25, 2018.

13. Mirabelli MH, Devine MJ, Singh J, Mendoza M. The preparticipation sports evaluation. *Am Fam Physician.* 2015;92(5):371-376. doi:10.1542/pir.32-5-e53

14. Parsons JT. *2014-15 NCAA Sports Medicine Handbook.* 2014. www.ncaapublications.com/productdownloads/MD15.pdf. Accessed June 10, 2017.

15. Meehan WP, D'Hemecourt P, Collins CL, Taylor AM, Comstock RD. Computerized neurocognitive testing for the management of sport-related concussions. *Pediatrics.* 2012;129(1):38-44. www.ncbi.nlm.nih.gov/pmc/articles/PMC3255470/pdf/peds.2011-1972.pdf. Accessed July 12, 2018.

16. McCrory P, Meeuwisse W, Dvorak J, et al. Consensus statement on concussion in sport—the 5th international conference on concussion in sport held in Berlin, October 2016. *Br J Sports Med.* 2017:bjsports-2017-097699. doi:10.1136/bjsports-2017-097699

17. Dorrel B, Long T, Shaffer S, Myer GD. The functional movement screen as a predictor of injury in National Collegiate Athletic Association Division II athletes. *J Athl Train.* 2018;53(1):29-34. doi:10.4085/1062-6050-528-15

18. Whittaker JL, Booysen N, De La Motte S, et al. Predicting sport and occupational lower extremity injury risk through movement quality screening: a systematic review. *Br J Sports Med.* 2017;51(7):580-585. doi:10.1136/bjsports-2016-096760

19. Letafatkar A, Hadadnezhad M, Shojaedin S, Mohamadi E. Relationship between functional movement screening score and history of injury. *Int J Sports Phys Ther.* 2014;9(1):21-27. www.ncbi.nlm.nih.gov/pmc/articles/PMC3924605/pdf/ijspt-02-021.pdf. Accessed July 11, 2018.

20. Havenith G. Interaction of clothing and thermoregulation. *Exog Dermatology.* 2002;1(5):221-230. doi:10.1159/000068802

21. Sawka MN, Young AJ, Francesconi RP, Muza SR, Pandolf KB. Thermoregulatory and blood responses during exercise at graded hypohydration levels. *J Appl Physiol.* 1985;59(5):1394-1401. doi:10.1152/jappl.1985.59.5.1394

22. Kenney WL, Tankersley CG, Newswanger DL, Hyde DE, Puhl SM, Turner NL. Age and hypohydration independently influence peripheral vascular response to heat stress. *J Appl Physiol.* 1990;68(5):1902-1908.

23. Adams JD, Sekigucho Y, Suh HG, et al. Dehydration impairs cycling performance, independently of thirst: a blinded study. *Med Sci Sports Exerc.* 2018;50(8):1697-1703.

24. Mora-Rodriguez R, Del Coso J, Hamouti N, Estevez E, Ortega JF. Aerobically trained individuals have greater increases in rectal temperature than untrained ones during exercise in the heat at similar relative intensities. *Eur J Appl Physiol.* 2010;109:973-981. doi:10.1007/s00421-010-1436-4

25. Sawka MN, Coyle EF. Influence of body water and blood volume on thermoregulation and exercise performance in the heat. *Exerc Sport Sci Rev.* 1999;27(1):167-218.

26. Périard JD, Racinais S, Sawka MN. Adaptations and mechanisms of human heat acclimation: applications for competitive athletes and sports. *Scand J Med Sci Sport.* 2015;25(S1):20-38. doi:10.1111/sms.12408

27. Salamunes ACC, Stadnik AMW, Neves EB. The effect of body fat percentage and body fat distribution on skin surface temperature with infrared thermography. *J Therm Biol.* 2017;66(November 2016):1-9. doi:10.1016/j.jtherbio.2017.03.006

28. Casa DJ, Guskiewicz KM, Anderson SA, et al. National Athletic Trainers' Association position statement: preventing sudden death in sports. *J Athl Train.* 2012;47(1):96-118.

www.guideline.gov/summaries/summary/38461/national-athletic-trainers-association-position-statement-preventing-sudden-death-in-sports.

29. Armstrong LE, Maresh CM. The induction and decay of heat acclimatisation in trained athletes. *Sport Med.* 1991;12(5):302-312.

30. Heat acclimatization. Korey Stringer Institute website. https://ksi.uconn.edu/prevention/heat-acclimatization. Accessed July 4, 2018.

31. Casa DJ, DeMartini JK, Bergeron MF, et al. National Athletic Trainers' Association position statement: exertional heat illnesses. *J Athl Train.* 2015;50(9):986-1000. doi:10.4085/1062-6050-50.9.07

32. Wet bulb globe temperature monitoring. Korey Stringer Institute website. https://ksi.uconn.edu/prevention/wet-bulb-globe-temperature-monitoring. Accessed July 9, 2018.

33. Activity guidelines and rest break guidelines. Georgia High School Association website. www.ghsa.net/sites/default/files/documents/sports-medicine/HeatPolicy2018.pdf. Accessed July 9, 2018.

34. Inter-Association Task Force on exertional heat illnesses consensus statement. National Athletic Trainers' Association website. www.nata.org/sites/default/files/inter-association-task-force-exertional-heat-illness.pdf. Accessed February 13, 2018.

35. McDermott BP, Anderson SA, Armstrong LE, et al. National Athletic Trainers' Association position statement: fluid replacement for the physically active. *J Athl Train.* 2017;52(9):877-895. doi:10.4085/1062-6050-52.9.02

36. Heat stroke prevention. Korey Stringer Institute website. https://ksi.uconn.edu/emergency-conditions/heat-illnesses/exertional-heat-stroke/heat-stroke-prevention. Updated August 5, 2019. Accessed August 27, 2019.

37. Torii M. Maximal sweating rate in humans. *J Hum Ergol (Tokyo).* 1995;24(2):137-152. doi:10.11183/jhe1972.24.137

38. Volpe SL, Poule KA, Bland EG. Estimation of prepractice hydration status of National Collegiate Athletic Association Division I athletes. *J Athl Train.* 2009;44(6):624-629.

39. Maughan RJ, Shirreffs SM. Dehydration and rehydration in competitive sport. *Scand J Med Sci Sports.* 2010;20(Suppl 3):40-47. doi:10.1111/j.1600-0838.2010.01207.x

40. Nuccio RP, Barnes KA, Carter JM, Baker LB. Fluid balance in team sport athletes and the effect of hypohydration on cognitive, technical, and physical performance. *Sport Med.* 2017;47(10):1951-1982. doi:10.1007/s40279-017-0738-7

41. Baker LB, Lang JA, Kenney WL. Change in body mass accurately and reliably predicts change in body water after endurance exercise. *Eur J Appl Physiol.* 2009;105:959-967. doi:10.1007/s00421-009-0982-0

42. Cheuvront SN, Ely BR, Kenefick RW, Sawka MN. Biological variation and diagnostic accuracy of dehydration assessment markers. *Am J Clin Nutr.* 2010;92(3):565-573. doi:10.3945/ajcn.2010.29490.

43. Armstrong LE, Maresh CM, Castellani JW, et al. Urinary indices of hydration status. *Int J Sport Nutr.* 1994;4:265-279.

44. McKenzie AL, Munoz CX, Armstrong LE. Accuracy of urine color to detect equal to or greater than 2% body mass loss in men. *J Athl Train.* 2015;50(12):1306-1309. doi:10.4085/1062-6050-51.1.03

45. Adams JD, Johnson EC, Jansen LT, Mauromoustakos AT, Perrier E, Kavouras SA. Assessment of hydration state by combining urine color and void number. *FASEB J.* 2017;31(1 Suppl).

46. Hew-Butler TD, Rosner MH, Fowkes Godek S, et al. Statement of the 3rd International Exercise-Associated Hyponatremia Consensus Development Conference, Carlsbad, California, 2015. *Br J Sports Med.* 2015;49:1432-1446. doi:10.1136/bjsports-2015-095004

47. Hew-Butler TD. Overhydrating presents health hazards for young football players. The Conversation website. https://theconversation.com/overhydrating-presents-health-hazards-for-young-football-players-100365. Published August 1, 2018.

48. Pollak AN, Barnes L, Ciotola JA, Gulli B, eds. *Emergency Care and Tranportation of the Sick and Injured.* 10th ed. Burlington, MA: Jones & Bartlett Learning; 2011.

49. Cappaert TA, Stone JA, Castellani JW, et al. National Athletic Trainers' Association position statement: environmental cold injuries. *J Athl Train.* 2008;43(6):640-658.

50. McMamara EC, Johe DH, Endly DA, eds. *Outdoor Emergency Care.* 5th ed. Upper Saddle River, NJ: Pearson Education; 2012.

51. Fudge J. Exercise in the cold: preventing and managing hypothermia and frostbite injury. *Sports Health.* 2016;8(2):133-139. doi:10.1177/1941738116630542

52. Baumgartner EA, Belson M, Rubin C, Patel M. Hypothermia and other cold-related morbidity emergency department visits: United States, 1995-2004. *Wilderness Environ Med.* 2008;19(4):233-237. doi:10.1580/07-WEME-OR-104.1

53. Castro RRT, Mendes F, Nobrega ACL. Risk of hypothermia in a new Olympic event: the 10-km marathon swim. *Clinics.* 2009;64(4):351-357. doi:10.1590/S1807-59322009000400014

54. Lightning safety tips and resources. National Weather Service website. www.weather.gov/lightning. Accessed July 18, 2018.

55. Jensenius JS. A detailed analysis of lightning deaths in the United States from 2006 through 2017. National Weather Service website. www.weather.gov/media/safety/06-17lightning_fatality_analysis.pdf. Accessed July 19, 2018.

56. Cherington M, Breed DW, Yarnell PR, Smith WE. Lightning injuries during snowy conditions. *Br J Sports Med.* 1998;32:333-335. www-ncbi-nlm-nih-gov.moravian.idm.oclc.org/pmc/articles/PMC1756127/pdf/v032p00333.pdf.

57. Houser AP, Larson SL, Fast JS. U.S. Army platoon gets struck by lightning, a case series. *Curr Sports Med Rep.* 2018;17(4):126-128.

58. Walsh KM, Cooper MA, Holle RL, Rakov VA, Roeder WP, Ryan M. National Athletic Trainers' Association position statement: lightning safety for athletics and recreation. *J Athl Train*. 2013;48(2):258-270. doi:10.4085/1062-6050-48.2.25

59. Thomson EM, Howard TM. Lightning injuries in sports and recreation. *Curr Sports Med Rep*. 2013;12(2):120-124. doi:10.1249/JSR.0b013e318287728f

60. Kithil R. An overview of lightning detection equipment. National Lightning Safety Institute website. www.lightningsafety.com/nlsi_lhm/overview2002.html. Accessed August 23, 2019.

61. Lightning. Korey Stringer Institute website. https://ksi.uconn.edu/emergency-conditions/lightning. Accessed July 18, 2018.

62. Schilling JF. Educational preparation and experiences in the industrial-occupational setting: a qualitative study of the athletic training graduates' perspective. *Athl Train Educ J*. 2011;6(2):99-106. http://natajournals.org/doi/pdf/10.4085/1947-380X-6.2.99

63. Ergonomics. U.S. Department of Labor, Occupational Safety and Health Administration website. www.osha.gov/SLTC/ergonomics. Accessed August 21, 2018.

64. MacLeod D. Ten principles of ergonomics. www.danmacleod.com/ErgoForYou/10_principles_of_ergonomics.htm. Accessed August 21, 2018.

Chapter 9

1. World Health Organization. *Preamble to the Constitution of the World Health Organization as Adopted by the International Health Conference. New York, 19-22 June, 1946*. Geneva: World Health Organization; 1946.

2. Mandsager K, Harb S, Cremer P, Phelan D, Nissen SE, Jaber W. Association of cardiorespiratory fitness with long-term mortality among adults undergoing exercise treadmill testing. *JAMA Netw Open*. 2018;1(6):e183605-e183605. doi:10.1001/jamanetworkopen.2018.3605

3. Äijö M, Kauppinen M, Kujala UM, Parkatti T. Physical activity, fitness, and all-cause mortality: An 18-year follow-up among old people. *J Sport Health Sci*. 2016;5(4):437-442. doi:10.1016/j.jshs.2015.09.008

4. Saint-Maurice PF, Coughlan D, Kelly SP, et al. Association of leisure-time physical activity across the adult life course with all-cause and cause-specific mortality. *JAMA Netw Open*. 2019;2(3):e190355-e190355. doi:10.1001/jamanetworkopen.2019.0355

5. Simon HB. Exercise and health: dose and response, considering both ends of the curve. *Am J Med*. 2015;128(11):1171-1177. doi:10.1016/j.amjmed.2015.05.012

6. Moore SC, Patel AV, Matthews CE, et al. Leisure time physical activity of moderate to vigorous intensity and mortality: a large pooled cohort analysis. *PLoS Med*. 2012;9(11):e1001335. doi:10.1371/journal.pmed.1001335

7. Shah RV, Murthy VL, Colangelo LA, et al. Association of fitness in young adulthood with survival and cardiovascular risk: the coronary artery risk development in young adults (CARDIA) study. *JAMA Intern Med*. 2016;176(1):87-95. doi:10.1001/jamainternmed.2015.6309

8. Juraschek SP, Blaha MJ, Blumenthal RS, et al. Cardiorespiratory fitness and incident diabetes: the FIT (Henry Ford ExercIse Testing) project. *Diabetes Care*. 2015;38(6):1075-1081. doi:10.2337/dc14-2714

9. Hussain N, Gersh BJ, Gonzalez Carta K, et al. Impact of cardiorespiratory fitness on frequency of atrial fibrillation, stroke, and all-cause mortality. *Am J Cardiol*. 2018;121(1):41-49. doi:10.1016/j.amjcard.2017.09.021

10. Vainshelboim B, Müller J, Lima RM, et al. Cardiorespiratory fitness and cancer incidence in men. *Ann Epidemiol*. 2017;27(7):442-447. doi:10.1016/j.annepidem.2017.06.003

11. Fu Q, Levine BD. Exercise and the autonomic nervous system. *Handb Clin Neurol*. 2013;117:147-160. doi:10.1016/B978-0-444-53491-0.00013-4

12. Davison K, Bircher S, Hill A, Coates AM, Howe PRC, Buckley JD. Relationships between obesity, cardiorespiratory fitness, and cardiovascular function. *J Obes*. 2010;2010:191253. doi:10.1155/2010/191253

13. Murphy M, Nevill A, Neville C, Biddle S, Hardman A. Accumulating brisk walking for fitness, cardiovascular risk, and psychological health. *Med Sci Sports Exerc*. 2002;34(9):1468-1474. doi:10.1097/00005768-200209000-00011

14. Kawano M, Shono N, Yoshimura T, Yamaguchi M, Hirano T, Hisatomi A. Improved cardio-respiratory fitness correlates with changes in the number and size of small dense LDL: randomized controlled trial with exercise training and dietary instruction. *Intern Med*. 2009;48(1):25-32. doi:10.2169/internalmedicine.48.1527

15. König D, Väisänen SB, Bouchard C, et al. Cardiorespiratory fitness modifies the association between dietary fat intake and plasma fatty acids. *Eur J Clin Nutr*. 2003;57(7):810-815. doi:10.1038/sj.ejcn.1601613

16. Kelley GA, Kelley KS, Franklin B. Aerobic exercise and lipids and lipoproteins in patients with cardiovascular disease: a meta-analysis of randomized controlled trials. *J Cardiopulm Rehabil*. 2006;26(3):131-139; quiz 140-141, discussion 142-144.

17. Rajendran P, Chen Y-F, Chen Y-F, et al. The multifaceted link between inflammation and human diseases. *J Cell Physiol*. 2018;233(9):6458-6471. doi:10.1002/jcp.26479

18. Nieman DC, Wentz LM. The compelling link between physical activity and the body's defense system. *J Sport Health Sci*. 2019;8(3):201-217. doi:10.1016/j.jshs.2018.09.009

19. Pedersen BK. Anti-inflammatory effects of exercise: role in diabetes and cardiovascular disease. *Eur J Clin Invest*. 2017;47(8):600-611. doi:10.1111/eci.12781

20. Overweight and obesity. National Heart, Lung, and Blood Institute website. www.nhlbi.nih.gov/health-topics/overweight-and-obesity. Accessed July 9, 2019.

21. NHLBI Obesity Education Initiative Expert Panel on the Identification, Evaluation, and Treatment of Obesity in

Adults (US). *Clinical Guidelines on the Identification, Evaluation, and Treatment of Overweight and Obesity in Adults: The Evidence Report.* Bethesda, MD: National Heart, Lung, and Blood Institute; 1998. www.ncbi.nlm.nih.gov/books/NBK2004.

22. Centers for Disease Control and Prevention. *National Diabetes Statistics Report, 2017.* Atlanta, GA: Centers for Disease Control and Prevention, US Department of Health and Human Services; 2017.

23. Kirwan JP, Sacks J, Nieuwoudt S. The essential role of exercise in the management of type 2 diabetes. *Cleve Clin J Med.* 2017;84(7 Suppl 1):S15-S21. doi:10.3949/ccjm.84.s1.03

24. Schellenberg ES, Dryden DM, Vandermeer B, Ha C, Korownyk C. Lifestyle interventions for patients with and at risk for type 2 diabetes: a systematic review and meta-analysis. *Ann Intern Med.* 2013;159(8):543-551. doi:10.7326/0003-4819-159-8-201310150-00007

25. Colberg SR, Sigal RJ, Yardley JE, et al. Physical activity/exercise and diabetes: a position statement of the American Diabetes Association. *Diabetes Care.* 2016;39(11):2065-2079. doi:10.2337/dc16-1728

26. Zanuso S, Sacchetti M, Sundberg CJ, Orlando G, Benvenuti P, Balducci S. Exercise in type 2 diabetes: genetic, metabolic and neuromuscular adaptations. A review of the evidence. *Br J Sports Med.* 2017;51(21):1533-1538. doi:10.1136/bjsports-2016-096724

27. Church TS, Blair SN, Cocreham S, et al. Effects of aerobic and resistance training on hemoglobin A1c levels in patients with type 2 diabetes: a randomized controlled trial. *JAMA.* 2010;304(20):2253-2262. doi:10.1001/jama.2010.1710

28. Wendell CR, Gunstad J, Waldstein SR, Wright JG, Ferrucci L, Zonderman AB. Cardiorespiratory fitness and accelerated cognitive decline with aging. *J Gerontol A Biol Sci Med Sci.* 2014;69(4):455-462. doi:10.1093/gerona/glt144

29. Zhu N, Jacobs DR, Schreiner PJ, et al. Cardiorespiratory fitness and cognitive function in middle age: the CARDIA study. *Neurology.* 2014;82(15):1339-1346. doi:10.1212/WNL.0000000000000310

30. Farrell SW, Abramowitz AR, Willis BL, et al. The relationship between cardiorespiratory fitness and Montreal cognitive assessment scores in older adults. *Gerontology.* 2018;64(5):440-445. doi:10.1159/000489336

31. Dolezal BA, Neufeld EV, Boland DM, Martin JL, Cooper CB. Interrelationship between sleep and exercise: a systematic review. *Adv Prev Med.* 2017;2017:1364387. doi:10.1155/2017/1364387

32. Dishman RK, Sui X, Church TS, Kline CE, Youngstedt SD, Blair SN. Decline in cardiorespiratory fitness and odds of incident sleep complaints. *Med Sci Sports Exerc.* 2015;47(5):960-966. doi:10.1249/MSS.0000000000000506

33. Papasavvas T, Bonow RO, Alhashemi M, Micklewright D. Depression symptom severity and cardiorespiratory fitness in healthy and depressed adults: a systematic review and meta-analysis. *Sports Med.* 2016;46(2):219-230. doi:10.1007/s40279-015-0409-5

34. Dishman RK, Sui X, Church TS, Hand GA, Trivedi MH, Blair SN. Decline in cardiorespiratory fitness and odds of incident depression. *Am J Prev Med.* 2012;43(4):361-368. doi:10.1016/j.amepre.2012.06.011

35. Berryman JW. Exercise is medicine: a historical perspective. *Curr Sports Med Rep.* 2010;9(4):195. doi:10.1249/JSR.0b013e3181e7d86d

36. Warburton DER, Jamnik V, Bredin SSD, Shephard RJ, Gledhill N. The 2019 Physical Activity Readiness Questionnaire for Everyone (PAR-Q+) and electronic Physical Activity Readiness Medical Examination (ePARmed-X+). *Health Fit J Can.* 2018;11(4):80-83. doi:10.14288/hfjc.v11i4.270

37. Kline GM, Porcari JP, Hintermeister R, et al. Estimation of $\dot{V}O_2$ max from a one-mile track walk, gender, age, and body weight. *Med Sci Sports Exerc.* 1987;19(3):253-259.

38. McSwegin PJ, Plowman SA, Wolff GM, Guttenberg GL. The validity of a one-mile walk test for high school age individuals. *Meas Phys Educ Exerc Sci.* 1998;2(1):47-63. doi:10.1207/s15327841mpee0201_4

39. Cooper KH. A means of assessing maximal oxygen intake. Correlation between field and treadmill testing. *JAMA.* 1968;203(3):201-204.

40. Flouris A, Metsios G, Koutedakis Y. Enhancing the efficacy of the 20 m multistage shuttle run test. *Br J Sports Med.* 2005;39(3):166. doi:10.1136/bjsm.2004.012500

41. Hong AR, Kim SW. Effects of resistance exercise on bone health. *Endocrinol Metab* (Seoul). 2018;33(4):435-444. doi:10.3803/EnM.2018.33.4.435

42. Layne JE, Nelson ME. The effects of progressive resistance training on bone density: a review. *Med Sci Sports Exerc.* 1999;31(1):25-30.

43. Yang J. Enhanced skeletal muscle for effective glucose homeostasis. *Prog Mol Biol Transl Sci.* 2014;121:133-163. doi:10.1016/B978-0-12-800101-1.00005-3

44. Elia M. Organ and tissue contribution to metabolic weight. In: Kinney J, Tucker H, eds. *Energy Metabolism: Tissue Determinants and Cellular Corollaries.* Philadelphia, PA: Raven Press; 1999:61-79.

45. Volaklis KA, Halle M, Meisinger C. Muscular strength as a strong predictor of mortality: A narrative review. *Eur J Intern Med.* 2015;26(5):303-310. doi:10.1016/j.ejim.2015.04.013

46. Volaklis K, Mamadjanov T, Meisinger C, Linseisen J. Association between muscular strength and depressive symptoms : A narrative review. *Wien Klin Wochenschr.* 2019;131(11-12):255-264. doi:10.1007/s00508-019-1491-8

47. Roberts HC, Denison HJ, Martin HJ, et al. A review of the measurement of grip strength in clinical and epidemiological studies: towards a standardised approach. *Age Ageing.* 2011;40(4):423-429. doi:10.1093/ageing/afr051

48. Levinger I, Goodman C, Hare DL, Jerums G, Toia D, Selig S. The reliability of the 1RM strength test for untrained middle-aged individuals. *J Sci Med Sport.* 2009;12(2):310-316. doi:10.1016/j.jsams.2007.10.007

49. Golding LA, Myers CR, Sinning WE. *Y's Way to Physical Fitness: The Complete Guide to Fitness Testing and Instruction*. 3rd ed. Champaign, IL: Human Kinetics; 1989.

50. Clemons JM, Campbell B, Jeansonne C. Validity and reliability of a new test of upper body power. *J Strength Cond Res*. 2010;24(6):1559-1565. doi:10.1519/JSC.0b013e-3181dad222

51. Margaria R, Aghemo P, Rovelli E. Measurement of muscular power (anaerobic) in man. *J Appl Physiol*. 1966;21(5):1662-1664. doi:10.1152/jappl.1966.21.5.1662

52. Rikli RE, Jones CJ. *Senior Fitness Test Manual*. 2nd ed. Champaign, IL: Human Kinetics; 2013.

53. Harris C, Wattles AP, DeBeliso M, Sevene-Adams PG, Berning JM, Adams KJ. The seated medicine ball throw as a test of upper body power in older adults. *J Strength Cond Res*. 2011;25(8):2344. doi:10.1519/JSC.0b013e-3181ecd27b

54. Engin A. The definition and prevalence of obesity and metabolic syndrome. *Adv Exp Med Biol*. 2017;960:1-17. doi:10.1007/978-3-319-48382-5_1

55. Flegal KM, Kruszon-Moran D, Carroll MD, Fryar CD, Ogden CL. Trends in obesity among adults in the United States, 2005 to 2014. *JAMA*. 2016;315(21):2284-2291. doi:10.1001/jama.2016.6458

56. Donnelly JE, Blair SN, Jakicic JM, et al. American College of Sports Medicine position stand. Appropriate physical activity intervention strategies for weight loss and prevention of weight regain for adults. *Med Sci Sports Exerc*. 2009;41(2):459-471. doi:10.1249/MSS.0b013e3181949333

57. Turocy PS, DePalma BF, Horswill CA, et al. National Athletic Trainers' Association position statement: safe weight loss and maintenance practices in sport and exercise. *J Athl Train*. 2011;46(3):322-336. doi:10.4085/1062-6050-46.3.322

58. Yusuf S, Hawken S, Ounpuu S, et al. Obesity and the risk of myocardial infarction in 27,000 participants from 52 countries: a case-control study. *Lancet*. 2005;366(9497):1640-1649. doi:10.1016/S0140-6736(05)67663-5

59. Hayes PA, Sowood PJ, Belyavin A, Cohen JB, Smith FW. Sub-cutaneous fat thickness measured by magnetic resonance imaging, ultrasound, and calipers. *Med Sci Sports Exerc*. 1988;20(3):303-309.

60. Heyward VH, Stolarczyk LM. *Applied Body Composition Assessment*. Champaign, IL: Human Kinetics; 1996.

61. Dempster P, Aitkens S. A new air displacement method for the determination of human body composition. *Med Sci Sports Exerc*. 1995;27(12):1692-1697.

62. Bolanowski M, Nilsson BE. Assessment of human body composition using dual-energy X-ray absorptiometry and bioelectrical impedance analysis. *Med Sci Monit*. 2001;7(5):1029-1033.

63. Damilakis J, Adams JE, Guglielmi G, Link TM. Radiation exposure in X-ray-based imaging techniques used in osteoporosis. *Eur Radiol*. 2010;20(11):2707-2714. doi:10.1007/s00330-010-1845-0

64. Jackson AW, Baker AA. The relationship of the sit and reach test to criterion measures of hamstring and back flexibility in young females. *Res Q Exerc Sport*. 1986;57(3):183-186. doi:10.1080/02701367.1986.10605395

65. Lemmink KAPM, Kemper HCG, Greef MHG, Rispens P, Stevens M. The validity of the sit-and-reach test and the modified sit-and-reach test in middle-aged to older men and women. *Res Q Exerc Sport*. 2003;74(3):331-336. doi:10.1080/02701367.2003.10609099

66. Hancock GE, Hepworth T, Wembridge K. Accuracy and reliability of knee goniometry methods. *J Exp Orthop*. 2018;5:46. doi:10.1186/s40634-018-0161-5

67. Akizuki K, Yamaguchi K, Morita Y, Ohashi Y. The effect of proficiency level on measurement error of range of motion. *J Phys Ther Sci*. 2016;28(9):2644-2651. doi:10.1589/jpts.28.2644

68. Keogh JWL, Cox A, Anderson S, et al. Reliability and validity of clinically accessible smartphone applications to measure joint range of motion: A systematic review. *PLoS ONE*. 2019;14(5):e0215806. doi:10.1371/journal.pone.0215806

69. Milanese S, Gordon S, Buettner P, et al. Reliability and concurrent validity of knee angle measurement: smart phone app versus universal goniometer used by experienced and novice clinicians. *Man Ther*. 2014;19(6):569-574. doi:10.1016/j.math.2014.05.009

70. Kjær IGH, Torstveit MK, Kolle E, Hansen BH, Anderssen SA. Normative values for musculoskeletal- and neuromotor fitness in apparently healthy Norwegian adults and the association with obesity: a cross-sectional study. *BMC Sports Sci Med Rehabil*. 2016;8(1):37. doi:10.1186/s13102-016-0059-4

71. Gibson AL, Dale W, Vivian H. *Advanced Fitness Assessment and Exercise Prescription*. 8th ed. Champaign, IL: Human Kinetics; 2018.

72. Bushman B. Neuromotor exercise training. *ACSMs Health Fit J*. 2012;16(6):4. doi:10.1249/FIT.0b013e31826f7bfa

73. Garber CE, Blissmer B, Deschenes MR, et al. American College of Sports Medicine position stand. Quantity and quality of exercise for developing and maintaining cardiorespiratory, musculoskeletal, and neuromotor fitness in apparently healthy adults: guidance for prescribing exercise. *Med Sci Sports Exerc*. 2011;43(7):1334-1359. doi:10.1249/MSS.0b013e318213fefb

74. Piercy KL, Troiano RP, Ballard RM, et al. The Physical Activity Guidelines for Americans. *JAMA*. 2018;320(19):2020-2028. doi:10.1001/jama.2018.14854

75. Suni JH, Oja P, Laukkanen RT, et al. Health-related fitness test battery for adults: aspects of reliability. *Arch Phys Med Rehabil*. 1996;77(4):399-405.

76. Dingenen B, Malfait B, Nijs S, et al. Postural stability during single-leg stance: a preliminary evaluation of non-contact lower extremity injury risk. *J Orthop Sports Phys Ther*. 2016;46(8):650-657. doi:10.2519/jospt.2016.6278

77. Springer BA, Marin R, Cyhan T, Roberts H, Gill NW. Normative values for the unipedal stance test with eyes open and closed. *J Geriatr Phys Ther.* 2007;30(1):8-15. doi:10.1519/00139143-200704000-00003

78. Duncan PW, Weiner DK, Chandler J, Studenski S. Functional reach: a new clinical measure of balance. *J Gerontol.* 1990;45(6):M192-197.

79. Rogers ME, Page P, Takeshima N. Balance training for the older athlete. *Int J Sports Phys Ther.* 2013;8(4):517-530.

80. Gray GW. *Lower Extremity Functional Profile.* Adrian, MI: Wynn Marketing; 1995.

81. Olmsted LC, Carcia CR, Hertel J, Shultz SJ. Efficacy of the Star Excursion Balance Tests in detecting reach deficits in subjects with chronic ankle instability. *J Athl Train.* 2002;37(4):501-506.

82. Gribble PA, Hertel J, Plisky P. Using the Star Excursion Balance Test to assess dynamic postural-control deficits and outcomes in lower extremity injury: a literature and systematic review. *J Athl Train.* 2012;47(3):339-357. doi:10.4085/1062-6050-47.3.08

83. van Lieshout R, Reijneveld EAE, van den Berg SM, et al. Reproducibility of the Modified Star Excursion Balance Test composite and specific reach direction scores. *Int J Sports Phys Ther.* 2016;11(3):356-365.

84. Coughlan GF, Fullam K, Delahunt E, Gissane C, Caulfield BM, Sci M. A comparison between performance on selected directions of the Star Excursion Balance Test and the Y Balance Test. *J Athl Train.* 2012;47(4):366-371.

85. Lai WC, Wang D, Chen JB, Vail J, Rugg CM, Hame SL. Lower quarter Y-Balance test scores and lower extremity injury in NCAA Division I athletes. *Orthop J Sports Med.* 2017;5(8):2325967117723666. doi:10.1177/2325967117723666

86. Ainsworth BE, Haskell WL, Herrmann SD, et al. 2011 Compendium of Physical Activities: a second update of codes and MET values. *Med Sci Sports Exerc.* 2011;43(8):1575-1581. doi:10.1249/MSS.0b013e31821ece12

87. American College of Sports Medicine. *ACSM Guidelines for Exercise Testing and Prescription.* 10th ed. Philadelphia, PA: Wolters Kluwer Health; 2017.

88. van Teeffelen WM, de Beus MF, Mosterd A, et al. Risk factors for exercise-related acute cardiac events. A case-control study. *Br J Sports Med.* 2009;43(9):722-725. doi:10.1136/bjsm.2009.057307

89. American Thoracic Society, American College of Chest Physicians. ATS/ACCP Statement on cardiopulmonary exercise testing. *Am J Respir Crit Care Med.* 2003;167(2):211-277. doi:10.1164/rccm.167.2.211

90. Gibbons RJ, Balady GJ, Bricker JT, et al. ACC/AHA 2002 guideline update for exercise testing: summary article. A report of the American College of Cardiology/American Heart Association Task Force on Practice Guidelines (Committee to Update the 1997 Exercise Testing Guidelines). *J Am Coll Cardiol.* 2002;40(8):1531-1540. doi:10.1016/s0735-1097(02)02164-2

91. Fletcher GF, Ades PA, Kligfield P, et al. Exercise standards for testing and training. *Circulation.* 2013;128(8):873-934. doi:10.1161/CIR.0b013e31829b5b44

92. Olsen O, Sjøhaug M, van Beekvelt M, Mork PJ. The effect of warm-up and cool-down exercise on delayed onset muscle soreness in the quadriceps muscle: a randomized controlled trial. *J Hum Kinet.* 2012;35:59-68. doi:10.2478/v10078-012-0079-4

93. Law RYW, Herbert RD. Warm-up reduces delayed onset muscle soreness but cool-down does not: a randomised controlled trial. *Aust J Physiother.* 2007;53(2):91-95.

94. Devlin J, Paton B, Poole L, et al. Blood lactate clearance after maximal exercise depends on active recovery intensity. *J Sports Med Phys Fitness.* 2014;54(3):271-278.

95. Menzies P, Menzies C, McIntyre L, Paterson P, Wilson J, Kemi OJ. Blood lactate clearance during active recovery after an intense running bout depends on the intensity of the active recovery. *J Sports Sci.* 2010;28(9):975-982. doi:10.1080/02640414.2010.481721

96. Holick MF. Sunlight, UV-radiation, vitamin D and skin cancer: how much sunlight do we need? *Adv Exp Med Biol.* 2008;624:1-15. doi:10.1007/978-0-387-77574-6_1

97. Moodycliffe AM, Nghiem D, Clydesdale G, Ullrich SE. Immune suppression and skin cancer development: regulation by NKT cells. *Nat Immunol.* 2000;1(6):521-525. doi:10.1038/82782

98. Ambros-Rudolph CM, Hofmann-Wellenhof R, Richtig E, Müller-Fürstner M, Soyer HP, Kerl H. Malignant melanoma in marathon runners. *Arch Dermatol.* 2006;142(11):1471-1474. doi:10.1001/archderm.142.11.1471

99. Lynn J, Urda J, Pierce P. Sun exposure and exercise: the good, the bad, and the behavior change. *ACSMs Health Fit J.* 2016;20(3):11. doi:10.1249/FIT.0000000000000200

100. Wysong A, Gladstone H, Kim D, Lingala B, Copeland J, Tang JY. Sunscreen use in NCAA collegiate athletes: identifying targets for intervention and barriers to use. *Prev Med.* 2012;55(5):493-496. doi:10.1016/j.ypmed.2012.08.020

101. Berko J, Ingram DD, Shubhaya S, Parker JD. Deaths attributed to heat, cold, and other weather events in the United States, 2006-2010. *Natl Health Stat Report.* 2014;76:1-15.

102. Pasqua LA, Damasceno MV, Cruz R, et al. Exercising in air pollution: the cleanest versus dirtiest cities challenge. *Int J Environ Res Public Health.* 2018;15(7):1502. doi:10.3390/ijerph15071502

103. Giorgini P, Rubenfire M, Bard RL, Jackson EA, Ferri C, Brook RD. Air pollution and exercise: a review of the cardiovascular implications for health care professionals. *J Cardiopulm Rehabil Prev.* 2016;36(2):84. doi:10.1097/HCR.0000000000000139

104. An R, Zhang S, Ji M, Guan C. Impact of ambient air pollution on physical activity among adults: a systematic review and meta-analysis. *Perspect Public Health.* 2018;138(2):111-121. doi:10.1177/1757913917726567

Chapter 10

1. Beck KL, Thomson JS, Swift RJ, Von Hurst PR. Role of nutrition in performance enhancement and postexercise recovery. *Open Access J Sport Med.* 2015;2015(6):259-267. doi:10.2147/OAJSM.S33605

2. Schonbrun Z. Next arms race in major sports is at the food table. *The New York Times.* October 6, 2015: SP3.

3. Cuellar C. Nutrition is Iowa's next frontier in college football development's feeding frenzy. *Des Moines Register.* May 12, 2017.

4. Stark R. Food for thought. NCAA Champion Magazine website. www.ncaa.org/static/champion/food-for-thought/#sthash.GEZgYF4J.7RNFZEdT.dpbs. Published 2015. Accessed November 7, 2018.

5. Myerberg P. NCAA schools put money where athletes' mouths are. *USA TODAY Sports.* April 26, 2015.

6. Be a Board Certified Sports Dietitian (CSSD). Eat Right website. www.scandpg.org/sports-nutrition/be-a-board-certified-sports-dietitian-cssd. Updated August 18, 2015. Accessed November 7, 2018.

7. McDermott BP, Anderson SA, Armstrong LE, et al. National Athletic Trainers' Association position statement: fluid replacement for the physically active. *J Athl Train.* 2017;52(9):877-895. doi:10.4085/1062-6050-52.9.02

8. Sammarone Turocy P, DePalma BF, Horswill CA, et al. National Athletic Trainers' Association position statement: safe weight loss and maintenance practices in sport and exercise. *J Athl Train.* 2011;46(3):322-336.

9. Buell JL, Franks R, Ransone J, Powers ME, Laquale KM, Carlson-Phillips A. National Athletic Trainers' Association position statement: evaluation of dietary supplements for performance nutrition. *J Athl Train.* 2013;48(1):124-136. doi:10.4085/1062-6050-48.1.16

10. Bonci CM, Bonci LJ, Granger LR, et al. National Athletic Trainers' Association position statement: preventing, detecting, and managing disordered eating in athletes. *J Athl Train.* 2008;43(1):80-108. http://natajournals.org/doi/pdf/10.4085/1062-6050-43.1.80.

11. Thomas DT, Erdman KA, Burke LM. American College of Sports Medicine position statement: nutrition and athletic performance. *Med Sci Sport Exerc.* 2016;48(3):543-568. doi:10.1249/MSS.0000000000000852

12. U.S. Department of Health and Human Services and U.S. Department of Agriculture. *2015-2020 Dietary Guidelines for Americans.* 8th ed. Washington, D.C.: Author; 2015. https://health.gov/sites/default/files/2019-09/2015-2020_Dietary_Guidelines.pdf.

13. Romijn JA, Coyle EF, Sidossis LS, et al. Regulation of endogenous fat and carbohydrate metabolism in relation to exercise intensity and duration. *Am J Physiol Metab.* 1993;265(3):E380-E391.

14. Maunder E, Plews DJ, Kilding AE. Contextualising maximal fat oxidation during exercise: determinants and normative values. *Front Physiol.* 2018;9:Article 599. doi:10.3389/fphys.2018.00599

15. Burke LM, Hawley JA, Wong SHS, Jeukendrup AE. Carbohydrates for training and competition. *J Sports Sci.* 2011;29(1):S17-S27. doi:10.1080/02640414.2011.585473

16. Kanter M. High-quality carbohydrates and physical performance. *Nutr Today.* 2018;53(1):35-39. doi:10.1097/NT.0000000000000238

17. Bussau VA, Fairchild TJ, Rao A, Steele P, Fournier PA. Carbohydrate loading in human muscle: an improved 1 day protocol. *Eur J Appl Physiol.* 2002;87(3):290-295. doi:10.1007/s00421-002-0621-5

18. Jäger R, Kerksick CM, Campbell BI, et al. International Society of Sports Nutrition position stand: protein and exercise. *J Int Soc Sports Nutr.* 2017;14(20). doi:10.1186/s12970-017-0177-8

19. Thomas DT, Erdman KA, Burke LM. Position of the Academy of Nutrition and Dietetics, Dietitians of Canada, and the American College of Sports Medicine: nutrition and athletic performance. *J Acad Nutr Diet.* 2016;116(3):501-528. doi:10.1016/j.jand.2015.12.006

20. Kerksick CM, Arent S, Schoenfeld BJ, et al. International Society of Sports Nutrition position stand: nutrient timing. *J Int Soc Sports Nutr.* 2017;14:33. doi:10.1186/s12970-017-0189-4

21. Berger C, Goltzman D, Langsetmo L, et al. Peak bone mass from longitudinal data: implications for the prevalence, pathophysiology, and diagnosis of osteoporosis. *J Bone Min Res.* 2010;25(9):1948-1957. doi:10.1002/jbmr.95

22. Dawson-Hughes B, Harris S, Lichtenstein A, Dolnikowski G, Palermo N, Rasmussen H. Dietary fat increases vitamin D-3 absorption. *J Acad Nutr Diet.* 2015;115(2):225-230.

23. Mulligan GB, Licata A. Taking vitamin D with the largest meal improves absorption and results in higher serum levels of 25-hydroxyvitamin D. *J Bone Miner Res.* 2010;25(4):928-930. doi:10.1002/jbmr.67

24. Ross AC, Taylor CL, Yaktine AL, Del Valle HB. DRI: Dietary reference intakes: Calcium Vitamin D Committee to review dietary reference intakes for vitamin d and calcium food and nutrition board. 2011. www.nap.edu. Accessed November 15, 2018.

25. Tovey A. How much vitamin D is needed to achieve optimal levels? Vitamin D Council website. www.vitamindcouncil.org/how-much-vitamin-d-is-needed-to-achieve-optimal-levels/#.XABJiHpKhTY. Accessed November 29, 2018.

26. Kimball SM, Mirhosseini N, Holick MF. Evaluation of vitamin D_3 intakes up to 15,000 international units/day and serum 25-hydroxyvitamin D concentrations up to 300 nmol/L on calcium metabolism in a community setting. *Dermatoendocrinol.* 2017;9. doi:10.1080/19381980.2017.1300213

27. Lunn WR, Pasiakos SM, Colletto MR, et al. Chocolate milk and endurance exercise recovery: protein balance, glycogen, and performance. *Med Sci Sport Exerc.* 2012;44(4):682-691. doi:10.1249/MSS.0b013e3182364162

28. Akil M, Celenk C. Iron metabolism and importance of iron in exercise. *Int J Acad Res.* 2013;5(4):223-230.

29. Reinke S, Von Haehling S, Anker S, et al. Absolute and functional iron deficiency in professional athletes during training and recovery. *Int J Cardiol.* 2012;156(2):186-191.

30. Institute of Medicine (U.S.) Panel on Micronutrients. *Dietary Reference Intakes for Vitamin A, Vitamin K, Arsenic, Boron, Chromium, Copper, Iodine, Iron, Manganese, Molybdenum, Nickel, Silicon, Vanadium, and Zinc.* Washington, D.C.: National Academy Press; 2001.

31. Alaunyte I, Stojceska V, Plunkett A. Iron and the female athlete: a review of dietary treatment methods for improving iron status and exercise performance. *J Int Soc Sport Nutr.* 2015;12(38). doi:10.1186/s12970-015-0099-2

32. Alghannam AF, Gonzalez JT, Betts JA. Restoration of muscle glycogen and functional capacity: role of post-exercise carbohydrate and protein co-ingestion. *Nutrients.* 2018;10(2). doi:10.3390/nu10020253

33. Gonzalez JT, Fuchs CJ, Betts JA, van Loon LJC. Glucose plus fructose ingestion for post-exercise recovery-greater than the sum of its parts? *Nutrients.* 2017;9(4). doi:10.3390/nu9040344

34. Pritchett K, Pritchett R. Chocolate milk: a post-exercise recovery beverage for endurance sports. *Med Sport Sci.* 2012;59:127-134. doi:10.1159/000341954

35. Karp JR, Johnston JD, Tecklenburg S, Mickleborough TD, Fly AD, Stager JM. Chocolate milk as a post-exercise recovery aid. *Int J Sport Nutr Exerc Metab.* 2006;16(1):78-91.

36. Şimşek T, Uzelli Şimşek H, Zafer Cantürk N. Response to trauma and metabolic changes: posttraumatic metabolism. *Ulus Cer Derg.* 2014;30:153-159. doi:10.5152/UCD.2014.2653

37. Aranow C. Vitamin D and the immune system. *J Investig Med.* 2011;59(6):881-886. doi:10.231/JIM.0b013e31821b8755

38. Lin P-H, Sermersheim M, Li H, Lee PHU, Steinberg SM, Ma J. Zinc in wound healing modulation. *Nutrients.* 2018;10(16). doi:10.3390/nu10010016

39. Chow O, Barbul A. Immunonutrition: role in wound healing and tissue regeneration. *Adv Wound Care.* 2014;3(1):46-53. doi:10.1089/wound.2012.0415

40. Guo S, Dipietro LA. Factors affecting wound healing. *J Dent Res.* 2010;89(3):219-229. doi:10.1177/0022034509359125

41. Joy E, De Souza MJ, Nattiv A, et al. 2014 Female Athlete Triad Coalition consensus statement on treatment and return to play of the female athlete triad. *Curr Sports Med Rep.* 2014;13(4):219-232. doi:10.1249/JSR.0000000000000077

42. Mountjoy M, Sundgot-Borgen J, Burke LM, et al. The IOC consensus statement: beyond the female athlete triad-relative energy deficiency in sport (RED-S). *Br J Sport Med.* 2014;48:491-497. doi:10.1136/bjsports-2014-093502

43. Creighton D, Shrier I, Shultz R, Meeuwisse W, Matheson G. Return-to-play in sport: a decision-based model. *Clin J Sport Med.* 2010;20(5):379-385.

44. Kerksick CM, Wilborn CD, Roberts MD, et al. ISSN exercise and sports nutrition review update: research and recommendations. *J Int Soc Sports Nutr.* 2018;15(38). doi:10.1186/s12970-018-0242-y

45. Dietary Supplement Health and Education Act of 1994. National Institutes of Health website. https://ods.od.nih.gov/About/DSHEA_Wording.aspx. Published October 25, 1994. Accessed December 2, 2018.

46. 2018-19 NCAA banned drugs list. NCAA website. www.ncaa.org/2018-19-ncaa-banned-drugs-list. Accessed November 11, 2018.

47. Dietary supplements for exercise and athletic performance. National Institutes of Health website. https://ods.od.nih.gov/factsheets/ExerciseAndAthleticPerformance-Consumer. Updated October 4, 2017.

48. Bérdi M, Köteles F, Hevesi K, Bárdos G, Szabo A. Elite athletes' attitudes towards the use of placebo-induced performance enhancement in sports. *Eur J Sport Sci.* 2015;15(4):315-321. doi:10.1080/17461391.2014.955126

49. Trojian TH, Beedie CJ. Placebo effect and athletes. *Curr Sports Med Rep.* 2008;7(4):214-217. doi:10.1249/JSR.0b013e31817ed050

50. Maughan RJ, Shirreffs SM. Dehydration and rehydration in competitive sport. *Scand J Med Sci Sport.* 2010;20(Suppl 3):40-47. doi:10.1111/j.1600-0838.2010.01207.x

51. Goldstein ER, Ziegenfuss TN, Kalman DS, et al. International society of sports nutrition position stand: caffeine and performance. *J Int Soc Sports Nutr.* 2010;7(5).

52. Mickleborough TD. Omega-3 polyunsaturated fatty acids in physical performance optimization. *Int J Sport Nutr Exerc Metab.* 2013;23:83-96.

53. Shei R-J, Lindley MR, Mickleborough TD. Omega-3 polyunsaturated fatty acids in the optimization of physical performance. *Mil Med.* 2014;179. doi:10.7205/MILMED-D-14-00160

54. Da Boit M, Hunter AM, Gray SR. Fit with good fat? The role of n-3 polyunsaturated fatty acids on exercise performance. *Metabolism.* 2017;66:45-54. doi:10.1016/j.metabol.2016.10.007

55. Nutrition and Allergies EFSA Panel on Dietetic Products. Scientific opinion on the tolerable upper intake level ofeicosapentaenoic acid (EPA), docosahexaenoic acid (DHA) and docosapentaenoic acid (DPA). *EFSA J.* 2012;10(7). doi:10.2903/j.efsa.2012.2815

56. International Society for the Study of Fatty Acids and Lipids. *Recommendations for Intake of Polyunsaturated Fatty Acids in Healthy Adults.* www.issfal.org/assets/issfal 03 pufaintakereccomdfinalreport.pdf. Published June 28, 2004.

57. FAO/WHO. *Interim Summary of Conclusions and Dietary Recommendations on Total Fat & Fatty Acids.* 2008. www.who.int/nutrition/topics/FFA_summary_rec_conclusion.pdf?ua=1. Accessed December 2, 2018.

58. Kumar PR, Essa MM, Al-Adawi S, et al. Omega-3 fatty acids could alleviate the risks of traumatic brain injury—a mini review. *J Tradit Complement Med.* 2014;4(2):89-92. doi:10.4103/2225-4110.130374

59. Dyall S, Michael-Titus A. Neurological benefits of omega-3 fatty acids. *Neuromolecular.* 2008;10(4):219-235.

60. Mills J, Bailes J, Sedney C, Hutchins H, Sears B. Omega-3 fatty acid supplementation and reduction of traumatic axonal injury in a rodent head injury model. *J Neurosurg.* 2011;114(1):77-84.

Chapter 11

1. NFHS rules changes affecting risk (1982-2016). National Federation of State High School Associations (NFHS) website. www.nfhs.org/media/1017463/1982-2016_nfhs_risk_minimization_rules.pdf. Accessed June 5, 2017.

2. Gieck J, McCue III FC. Fitting of protective football equipment. *Am J Sports Med.* 1980;8(3):192-196. http://journals.sagepub.com/doi/pdf/10.1177/036354658000800309. Accessed May 3, 2017.

3. Biasca N, Wirth S, Tegner Y. The avoidability of head and neck injuries in ice hockey: an historical review. *Br J Sport Med.* 2002;36:410-427. http://bjsm.bmj.com/content/bjsports/36/6/410.full.pdf. Accessed June 6, 2017.

4. Swartz EE, Mihalik JP, Beltz NM, Day MA, Decoster LC. Face mask removal is safer than helmet removal for emergent airway access in American football. *Spine J.* 2014;14:996-1004. doi:10.1016/j.spinee.2013.10.032

5. Bonfield CM, Shin SS, Kanter AS. Helmets, head injury and concussion in sport. *Phys Sportsmed.* 2015;43(3):236-246. doi:10.1080/00913847.2015.1039922

6. Stamp J. Leatherhead to radio-head: the evolution of the football helmet. *Smithsonian Magazine.* October 1, 2012. www.smithsonianmag.com/arts-culture/leatherhead-to-radio-head-the-evolution-of-the-football-helmet-56585562.

7. Pfriem SD. Standards-based regulation of athletic protective headgear—policy background, mechanisms and evaluation. *J Law Heal.* 2016;29(1):55-84.

8. About ANSI. American National Standards Institute website. www.ansi.org/about_ansi/overview/overview?menuid=1. Accessed June 5, 2017.

9. Home page. Athletic Equipment Managers Association (AEMA) website. http://equipmentmanagers.org. Published 2013. Accessed June 5, 2017.

10. Introduction. Hockey Equipment Certification Council (HECC) website. http://hecc.net. Published 2017. Accessed June 5, 2017.

11. About OSHA. Occupational Safety and Health Administration website. www.osha.gov/aboutosha. Published 2017. Accessed June 5, 2017.

12. Home page. ASTM International website. www.astm.org. Published 2017. Accessed June 5, 2017.

13. About us. CSA Group website. www.csagroup.org/about-csa-group/. Published 2017. Accessed June 5, 2017.

14. About NOCSAE. National Operating Committee on Standards for Athletic Equipment (NOCSAE) website. nocsae.org/about-nocsae. Published 2011. Accessed June 5, 2017.

15. Home page. Sports and Fitness Industry Association (SFIA) website. www.sfia.org. Published 2017. Accessed June 5, 2017.

16. Gould TE, Piland SG, Caswell SV, et al. National Athletic Trainers' Association position statement: preventing and managing sport-related dental and oral injuries. *J Athl Train.* 2016;51(10):1062-6050-51.8.01. doi:10.4085/1062-6050-51.8.01

17. Casa DJ, DeMartini JK, Bergeron MF, et al. National Athletic Trainers' Association position statement: exertional heat illnesses. *J Athl Train.* 2015;50(9):986-1000. doi:10.4085/1062-6050-50.9.07

18. Broglio SP, Cantu RC, Gioia GA, et al. National Athletic Trainers' Association position statement: management of sport concussion. *J Athl Train.* 2014;49(2):245-265. doi:10.4085/1062-6050-49.1.07

19. Swartz EE, Boden BP, Courson RW, et al. National Athletic Trainers' Association position statement: acute management of the cervical spine—injured athlete. *J Athl Train.* 2009;44(3):306-331. doi:10.4085/1062-6050-44.3.306

20. Casa DJ, Guskiewicz KM, Anderson SA, et al. National Athletic Trainers' Association position statement: preventing sudden death in sports. *J Athl Train.* 2012;47(1):96-118. www.guideline.gov/summaries/summary/38461/national-athletic-trainers-association-position-statement-preventing-sudden-death-in-sports.

21. Andersen JC, Courson RW, Kleiner DM, McLoda TA. National Athletic Trainers' Association position statement: emergency planning in athletics. *J Athl Train.* 2002;37(1):99-104.

22. Lloyd J, Gutmann J, DelRossi G. Do ill-fitting helmets amplify the risk of head injury among youth football? *J Head Trauma Rehabil.* 1986;26(5):437.

23. Valovich McLeod TC. Proper fit and maintenance of ice-hockey helmets. *Athl Ther Today.* 2005;10(6):54-57.

24. Burnett E, White J, Scurr J. The influence of the breast on physical activity participation in females. *J Phys Act Heal.* 2015;12(4):588-594. doi:10.1123/jpah.2013-0236

25. Black AM, Patton DA, Eliason PH, Emery CA. Prevention of sport-related facial injuries. *Clin Sport Med.* 2017;36:257-278. doi:10.1016/j.csm.2016.11.002

26. Pujalte GGA. Eye injuries in sports. *Athl Ther Today.* 2010;15(5):14. http://ezproxy.leedsbeckett.ac.uk/login?url=http://search.ebscohost.com/login.aspx?direct=true&db=edb&AN=54955948&site=eds-live&scope=site.

27. Faure CE, Armstrong A. Examination of football helmet fit and players' helmet air maintenance. *Appl Res Coach.* 2015;30(1):56-84. https://illiad.radford.edu/illiad/illiad.dll?Action=10&Form=75&Value=380174. Accessed April 17, 2017.

28. McGuine TA, Hetzel S, McCrea M, Brooks MA. Protective equipment and player characteristics associated with the incidence of sport-related concussion in high school football players: a multifactorial prospective

study. *Am J Sports Med.* 2014;42(10):2470-2478. doi:10.1177/0363546514541926

29. 2017 NOCSAE reconditioner licensees. National Federation of State High School Associations (NFHS) website. www.nfhs.org/media/1018157/5-2017_nocsae_reconditioners.pdf. Accessed June 5, 2017.

30. Farrington T, Onambele-Pearson G, Taylor RL, Earl P, Winwood K. A review of facial protective equipment use in sport and the impact on injury incidence. *Br J Oral Maxillofac Surg.* 2011;50:233-238. doi:10.1016/j.bjoms.2010.11.020

31. McIntosh AS, Janda DH. Evaluation of cricket helmet performance and comparison with baseball and ice hockey helmets. *Br J Sport Med.* 2003;37(4):325-330. http://bjsm.bmj.com/content/bjsports/37/4/325.full.pdf. Accessed May 24, 2017.

32. Breedlove KM, Breedlove EL, Bowman TG, Nauman EA. Impact attenuation capabilities of football and lacrosse helmets. *J Biomech.* 2016;49:2838-2844. doi:10.1016/j.jbiomech.2016.06.030

33. Trojian TH, Beedie CJ. Placebo effect and athletes. *Curr Sports Med Rep.* 2008;7(4):214-217. doi:10.1249/JSR.0b013e31817ed050

34. Daneshvar DH, Baugh CM, Nowinski CJ, McKee AC, Stern RA, Cantu RC. Helmets and mouth guards: the role of personal equipment in preventing sport-related concussions. *Clin Sport Med.* 2011;30:145-163. doi:10.1016/j.csm.2010.09.006

35. Helmet laboratory testing performance results. NFL Player Health and Safety website. www.playsmartplaysafe.com/resource/helmet-laboratory-testing-performance-results. Published 2017. Accessed June 13, 2017.

36. Swartz EE, Broglio SP, Cook SB, et al. Early results of a helmetless-tackling intervention to decrease head impacts in football players. *J Athl Train.* 2015;50(12):1219-1222. doi:10.4085/1062-6050-51.1.06

37. McCrory P, Meeuwisse W, Dvorak J, et al. Consensus statement on concussion in sport—the 5th international conference on concussion in sport held in Berlin, October 2016. *Br J Sports Med.* 2017;51(11):838-847. doi:10.1136/bjsports-2017-097699

38. Navarro RR. Protective equipment and the prevention of concussion—what is the evidence? *Curr Sports Med Rep.* 2011;10(1):27-31.

39. Rowson S, Duma SM. Development of the STAR evaluation system for football helmets: integrating player head impact exposure and risk of concussion. *Ann Biomed Eng.* 2011;39(8):2130-2140. doi:10.1007/s10439-011-0322-5

40. Fitting instructions and helmet care. Riddell website. http://team.riddell.com/wp-content/uploads/360_web.pdf. Accessed June 6, 2017.

41. Helmet fitting guide. International Federation American Football website. http://ifaf.org/pdf/health_safety/helmet_fitting.pdf. Accessed September 3, 2017.

42. Schutt helmet fitting instructions. Schutt Sports website. https://s3-us-west-2.amazonaws.com/schutt-pdfs/Helmet_Fitting_Guide.pdf. Accessed September 3, 2017.

43. Rowson B, Rowson S, Duma SM. Hockey STAR: a methodology for assessing the biomechanical performance of hockey helmets. *Ann Biomed Eng.* 2015;43(10):2429-2443. doi:10.1007/s10439-015-1278-7

44. Reid C. Lacrosse helmets 101. Lacrosse.com website. www.lacrosse.com/guide/lacrosse-helmets-101. Published 2015. Accessed June 8, 2017.

45. Policy I: Helmets. USA Cycling website. www.usacycling.org/policy-i-helmets.htm. Published 2013. Accessed June 10, 2017.

46. Ross DS, Ferguson A, Bosha P, Cassas K. Factors that prevent roughstock rodeo athletes from wearing protective equipment. *Curr Sport Med Rep.* 2010;9(6):342-346.

47. Trojian TH, Mohamed N. Demystifying preventive equipment in the competitive athlete. *Curr Sports Med Rep.* 2012;11(6):304-308. https://illiad.radford.edu/illiad/illiad.dll?Action=10&Form=75&Value=380070. Accessed April 13, 2017.

48. Delaney JS, Al-Kashmiri A, Drummond R, Correa JA. The effect of protective headgear on head injuries and concussions in adolescent football (soccer) players. *Br J Sports Med.* 2008;42(2):110-115; discussion 115. doi:10.1136/bjsm.2007.037689

49. Broglio SP, Ju Y-Y, Broglio MD, Sell TC. The efficacy of soccer headgear. *J Athl Train.* 2003;38(3):220-224. www.journalofathletictraining.org. Accessed September 15, 2017.

50. Menger R, Menger A, Nanda A. Rugby headgear and concussion prevention: misconceptions could increase aggressive play. *Neurosurg Focus.* 2016;40(4):1-7. doi:10.3171/2016.1.FOCUS15615

51. Maher ME, Hutchison MG, Cusimano MD, Comper P, Schweizer TA. Concussions and heading in soccer: a review of the evidence of incidence, mechanisms, biomarkers and neurocognitive outcomes. *Brain Inj.* 2014;28(3):271-285. doi:10.3109/02699052.2013.865269

52. Delaney JS, Frankovich R. Head injuries and concussions in soccer. *Clin J Sport Med.* 2005;15(4):214-217. https://illiad.radford.edu/illiad/illiad.dll?Action=10&Form=75&Value=385224. Accessed September 11, 2017.

53. Benson BW, Mohtadi NG, Rose MS, Meeuwisse WH. Head and neck injuries among ice hockey players wearing full face shields vs half face shields. *JAMA.* 2015;282(24):2328-2332. doi:10.1001/jama.282.24.2328

54. Woods SE, Diehl J, Zabat E, Daggy M, Engel A, Okragly R. Is it cost-effective to require recreational ice hockey players to wear face protection? *South Med J.* 2008;1001(10):991-995. https://illiad.radford.edu/illiad/illiad.dll?Action=10&Form=75&Value=381991. Accessed June 7, 2017.

55. Asplund C, Bettcher S, Borchers J. Facial protection and head injuries in ice hockey: a systematic review. *Br J Sports Med.* 2009;43:993-999. doi:10.1136/bjsm.2009.060152

56. Protective eyewear for young athletes. American Academy of Ophthalmology website. www.aao.org/clinical-statement/protective-eyewear-young-athletes. Published April 2013. Accessed May 25, 2017.

57. Micieli JA, Easterbrook M. Eye and orbital injuries in sports. *Clin Sport Med.* 2017;36:299-314. doi:10.1016/j.csm.2016.11.006

58. Vinger PF. A practical guide for sports eye protection. *Phys Sportsmed.* 2000;28(6):49-69. https://illiad.radford.edu/illiad/illiad.dll?Action=10&Form=75&Value=382106. Accessed June 12, 2017.

59. Westerman B, Stringfellow PM, Eccleston JA. EVA mouthguards: how thick should they be? *Dent Traumatol.* 2002;18(1):24-27. doi:10.1034/j.1600-9657.2002.180103.x

60. Pawar PG, Suryawanshi MM, Patil AK, et al. Importance of mouth guards in sports: A review. *J Evol Med Dent Sci.* 2013;2(46):8903-8908. https://jemds.com/data_pdf/priyadarshini (fareedi-6).pdf. Accessed April 24, 2017.

61. Knapik JJ, Marshall SW, Lee RB, et al. Mouthguards in sport activities: history, physical properties and injury prevention effectiveness. *Sport Med.* 2007;37(2):117-144. doi:10.2165/00007256-200737020-00003

62. American Dental Association. The importance of using mouthguards. *JADA.* 2004;135:1061. http://forbestimpressions.com/documents/patient_40.pdf. Accessed May 25, 2017.

63. Mouthguards. American Dental Association website. www.ada.org/en/member-center/oral-health-topics/mouthguards. Published 2016. Accessed May 25, 2017.

64. Stuart MJ, Link AA, Smith AM, Krause DA, Sorenson MC, Larson DR. Skate blade neck lacerations: a survey and case follow-up. *Clin J Sport Med.* 2009;19:494-497. https://illiad.radford.edu/illiad/illiad.dll?Action=10&Form=75&Value=381988. Accessed June 7, 2017.

65. Hansman H. The sorry state of the sports bra industry. *Outside Online.* March 1, 2017. www.outsideonline.com/2157141/lack-support.

66. Mason B, Page K-A, Fallon K. An analysis of movement and discomfort of the female breast during exercise and the effects of breast support in three cases. *J Sci Med.* 1999;2(2):134-144. http://ac.els-cdn.com.lib-proxy.radford.edu/S1440244099801935/1-s2.0-S1440244099801935-main.pdf?_tid=c93f828c-4a5a-11e7-b605-00000aab0f26&acdnat=1496714124_92b189fdd67ec8197f9cd593558d647d. Accessed June 5, 2017.

67. Bowles K-A, Steele JR, Munro BJ. Features of sports bras that deter their use by Australian women. *J Sci Med Sport.* 2011;15:195-200. doi:10.1016/j.jsams.2011.11.248

68. Brown N, White J, Brasher A, Scurr J. An investigation into breast support and sports bra use in female runners of the 2012 London Marathon. *J Sports Sci.* 2014;32(9):801-809. doi:10.1080/02640414.2013.844348

69. Standard test method and performance specification used in evaluating the performance characteristics of chest protectors for commotio cordis. NOCSAE website. https://nocsae.org/standard/standard-test-method-and-performance-specification-used-in-evaluating-the-performance-characteristics-of-chest-protectors-for-commotio-cordis-2. Updated July 2019. Accessed April 2, 2020.

70. Richards D, Ivarsson BJ, Scher I, Hoover R, Rodowicz K, Cripton P. Ice hockey shoulder pad design and the effect on head response during shoulder-to-head impacts. *Sport Biomech.* 2016;15(4):385-396. doi:10.1080/14763141.2016.1163414

71. Protective equipment and clothing guidelines 2015. USA Rugby website. https://assets.usarugby.org/docs/refereeing/protective-equipment-clothing-guidelines.pdf. Accessed October 23, 2017.

72. Bieniek JM, Sumfest JM. Sports-related testicular injuries and the use of protective equipment among young male athletes. *Urology.* 2014;84:1485-1489. doi:10.1016/j.urology.2014.09.007

73. Yang J, Bowling JM, Lewis MA, Marshall SW, Runyan CW, Mueller FO. Use of discretionary protective equipment in high school athletes: prevalence and determinants. *Am J Public Health.* 2005;95(11):1996-2002. doi:10.2105/AJPH.2004.050807

74. Jastifer J, Kent R, Crandall J, et al. Athletic shoe in football: apparel or protective equipment? *Sports Health.* 2017;March/April:126-131.

75. Langone KA. How to evaluate and recommend athletic shoes. *Pod Manag.* 2010;October:107-115. www.aapsm.org/pdf/articles/recommend-athletic-shoes.pdf. Accessed June 14, 2017.

76. Footwear—Running shoe anatomy. AAPSM website. www.aapsm.org/runshoe-running-anatomy.html. Accessed June 15, 2017.

77. NATA. Appropriate prehospital management of the spine-injured athlete: updated from 1998 document. ACBSP website. https://acbsp.com/wp-content/uploads/2018/11/Appropriate-Prehospital-Care-of-the-Spine-Injured-Athlete.pdf. Published 2015.

78. Lenhardt CS, Mihalik JP, Lynall RC, Fraser MA, Petschauer M, Swartz EE. The effect of football shoulder pad removal technique and equipment removal training on cervical spine motion, time to task completion, and perceived task difficulty. *Athl Train Sport Heal Care.* 2015;7(6):1-10. https://illiad.radford.edu/illiad/illiad.dll?Action=10&Form=75&Value=382162. Accessed June 12, 2017.

79. Martinez DC, Bowman TG, Boergers RJ. The role of practice on lacrosse helmet facemask removal time. 2015;20(July):37-43.

80. Endres B, Decoster LC, Swartz EE. Football equipment removal in an exertional heat stroke scenario: time and difficulty. *Athl Train Sport Health Care.* 2014;6(5):213-219. https://illiad.radford.edu/illiad/illiad.dll?Action=10&Form=75&Value=382163. Accessed June 12, 2017.

81. Miller KC, Long BC, Edwards J. Necessity of removing American football uniforms from humans with hyperthermia before cold-water immersion. *J Athl Train.* 2015;50(12):1240-1246. doi:10.4085/1062-6050-51.1.05

82. Heat illnesses. Korey Stringer Institute website. http://ksi.uconn.edu/emergency-conditions/heat-illnesses. Accessed September 21, 2017.

83. Swartz EE, Belmore K, Decoster LC, Armstrong CW. Emergency face-mask removal effectiveness: a comparison of traditional and nontraditional football helmet face-mask attachment systems. *J Athl Train*. 2010;45(6):560-569. doi:10.4085/1062-6050-45.6.560

84. Decoster LC, Shirley CP, Swartz EE. Football face-mask removal with a cordless screwdriver on helmets used for at least one season of play. *J Athl Train*. 2005;40(3):169-173.

85. Bradney DA, Bowman TG. Lacrosse helmet facemask removal. *J Athl Train*. 2013;48(1):47-56. doi:10.4085/1062-6050-48.1.02

86. Riddell Sports. Riddell revolution speed quick release. www.youtube.com/watch?v=CiXH1Jw_naA. Published 2013. Accessed September 11, 2017.

87. Swartz EE, Mihalik JP, Decoster LC, Al-Darraji S, Bric J. Emergent access to the airway and chest in American football players. *J Athl Train*. 2015;50(7):681-687. doi:10.4085/1062-6050-50.4.04

88. Riddell Sports. RipKord shoulder pad removal system. www.youtube.com/watch?v=WbwSFVb_uXY. Published 2011. Accessed September 11, 2017.

89. Commotio cordis. Korey Stringer Institute website. http://ksi.uconn.edu/emergency-conditions/cardiac-conditions/commotio-cordis. Accessed September 4, 2017.

90. Mills BM, Conrick KM, Anderson S, et al. Prehospital care of the spine-injured athlete consensus recommendations on the prehospital care of the injured athlete with a suspected catastrophic cervical spine injury. *J Athl Train*. 2020;55(6):563-572. doi:10.4085/1062-6050-0434.19

91. Courson R, Ellis J, Herring SA, et al. Best practices and current care concepts in prehospital care of the spine-injured athlete in American tackle football. *J Athl Train*. 2020;55(6):545-562. doi:10.4085/1062-6050-430-19

92. Mihalik JP, Lynall RC, Fraser MA, et al. Football equipment removal improves chest compression and ventilation efficacy. *Prehospital Emerg Care*. 2016;20(5):578-585. doi:10.3109/10903127.2016.1149649

Chapter 12

1. Steves R, Hootman JM. Evidence-based medicine: what is it and how does it apply to athletic training? *J Athl Train*. 2004;39(1):83-87.

2. Denegar CR, Hertel J. Editorial: clinical education reform and evidence-based clinical practice guidelines. *J Athl Train*. 2002;37(2):127-128.

3. Sackett D, Rosenburg W, Gray J, Haynes R, Richardson W. Evidence-based medicine: what it is and it isn't. *BMJ*. 1996;312:71-72.

4. National Athletic Trainers' Association. *Athletic Training Education Competencies*. 5th ed. www.nata.org/sites/default/files/competencies_5th_edition.pdf. Published 2011. Accessed April 3, 2020.

5. Perrin DH, McLeod IA. *Athletic Taping, Bracing, and Casting*. 4th ed. Champaign, IL: Human Kinetics; 2019.

6. NFHS rules changes affecting risk (1982-2019). National Federation of State High School Associations (NFHS) website. https://nfhs.org/media/1020416/1982-2019-nfhs-risk-minimization-rules-8-28-19.pdf. Published August 28, 2019. Accessed April 3, 2020.

7. Playing rules. NCAA website. www.ncaa.org/playing-rules. Accessed April 3, 2020.

8. Goodell R. 2019 official playing rules of the National Football League. National Football League (NFL) website. https://operations.nfl.com/media/3831/2019-playing-rules.pdf. Published 2019. Accessed April 3, 2020.

9. Konin JG, Ray R. *Management Strategies in Athletic Training*. 5th ed. Champaign, IL: Human Kinetics; 2019.

10. Callaghan MJ. Role of ankle taping and bracing in the athlete. *Br J Sports Med*. 1997;31(2):102-108. doi:10.1136/bjsm.31.2.102

11. Malina R, Plagenz L, Rarick G. Effect of exercise upon the measurable supporting strength of cloth and tape ankle wraps. *Res Q*. 1963;34(2):158-165.

12. Manfroy PP, Ashton-Miller JA, Wojtys EM. The effect of exercise, prewrap, and athletic tape on the maximal active and passive ankle resistance to ankle inversion. *Am J Sports Med*. 1997;25(2):156-163. doi:10.1177/036354659702500203

13. Keil A. *Strap Taping for Sports and Rehabilitation*. Champaign, IL: Human Kinetics; 2012.

14. Bragg RW, Macmahon J, Overom E, et al. Failure and fatigue characteristics of adhesive athletic tape. *Med Sci Sports Exerc*. 2002;33(3):403-410.

15. Williams S, Whatman C, Hume PA, Sheerin K. Kinesio taping in treatment and prevention of sports injuries. *Sports Med*. 2012;42(2):153-164. doi:10.2165/11594960-000000000-00000

16. Mostafavifar M, Wertz J, Borchers J. A systematic review of the effectiveness of kinesio taping for musculoskeletal injury. *Phys Sportsmed*. 2012;40(4):33-40. doi:10.3810/psm.2012.11.1986

17. Parreira PC, Costa LC, Hespanhol LJ, Lopes A, Costsa L. Current evidence does not support the use of Kinesio Taping in clinical practice: a systematic review. *J Physiother*. 2014;60(1):31-39. doi:10.1016/j.jphys.2013.12.008

18. Bassett K, Lingman S, Ellis R. The use and treatment efficacy of kinaesthetic taping for musculoskeletal conditions: A systematic review. *N Z J Physiother*. 2010;38(2):56-62.

19. Nelson N. Kinesio taping for chronic low back pain: A systematic review. *J Bodyw Mov Ther*. 2016;20(3):672-681. doi:10.1016/j.jbmt.2016.04.018

20. Ghozy S, Dung N, Morra M, et al. Efficacy of kinesio taping in treatment of shoulder pain and disability: a systematic review and meta-analysis of randomised controlled trials. *Physiotherapy*. 2019;107:176-188. doi:10.1016/j.physio.2019.12.001

21. Zhang X, Liu L, Wang B, Liu X, Li P. Evidence for kinesio taping in management of myofascial pain syndrome: a systematic review and meta-analysis. *Clin Rehabil*. 2019;33(5):865-874. doi:10.1177/0269215519826267

22. Kerkhoffs GM, Struijs PA, Marti RK, et al. Different functional treatment strategies for acute lateral ankle ligament injuries in adults. *Cochrane Database Syst Rev.* 2002;(3):CD002938.

23. Lardenoye S, Theunissen E, Cleffken B, Brink PR, de Bie RA, Poeze M. The effect of taping versus semi-rigid bracing on patient outcome and satisfaction in ankle sprains: a prospective, randomized controlled trial. *BMC Musculoskelet Disord.* 2012;13(1):81. doi:10.1186/1471-2474-13-81

24. Kemler E, van de Port I, Backx F, van Dijk CN. A systematic review on the treatment of acute ankle sprain: brace versus other functional treatment types. *Sports Med.* 2011;41(3):185-197. doi:10.2165/11584370-000000000-00000

25. Lin C-WC, Hiller CE, de Bie RA. Evidence-based treatment for ankle injuries: a clinical perspective. *J Man Manip Ther.* 2010;18(1):22-28. doi:10.1179/106698110X12595770849524

26. Fabian E, Gowling T, Jackson R. Walking boot design: A gait analysis study. *Orthopedics.* 1999;22:503-508.

27. Pietrosimone BG, Grindstaff TL, Linens SW, Uczekaj E, Hertel J. A systematic review of prophylactic braces in the prevention of knee ligament injuries in collegiate football players. *J Athl Train.* 2008;43(4):409-415.

28. Salata MJ, Gibbs AE, Sekiya JK. The effectiveness of prophylactic knee bracing in American football. *Sports Health.* 2010;2(5):375-379. doi:10.1177/1941738110378986

29. Leppänen M, Aaltonen S, Parkkari J, Heinonen A, Kujala U. Interventions to prevent sports related injuries: a systematic review and meta-analysis of randomised controlled trials. *Sports Med.* 2014;44(4):473-486. doi:10.1007/s40279-013-0136-8

30. Lowe WR, Warth RJ, Davis EP, Bailey L. Functional bracing after anterior cruciate ligament reconstruction: a systematic review. *JAAOS - J Am Acad Orthop Surg.* 2017;25(3):239-249. doi:10.5435/JAAOS-D-15-00710

31. Yang X, Feng J, He X, Wang F, Hu Y. The effect of knee bracing on the knee function and stability following anterior cruciate ligament reconstruction: A systematic review and meta-analysis of randomized controlled trials. *Orthop Traumatol Surg Res.* 2019;105(6):1107-1114. doi:10.1016/j.otsr.2019.04.015

32. Cleary MA, Walsh Flanagan K. *Acute and Emergency Care in Athletic Training.* Champaign, IL: Human Kinetics; 2020.

Chapter 13

1. Andersen JC, Courson RW, Kleiner DM, McLoda TA. National Athletic Trainers' Association position statement: Emergency planning in athletics. *J Athl Train.* 2002;37(1):99-104.

2. Parsons JT. *2014-15 NCAA Sports Medicine Handbook.* 2014. www.ncaapublications.com/productdownloads/MD15.pdf. Accessed June 10, 2017.

3. The National Federation of State High School Associations (NFHS) website. www.nfhs.org. Accessed June 5, 2017.

4. Drezner JA, Courson RW, Roberts WO, Mosesso VN, Link MS, Maron BJ. Inter-association task force recommendations on emergency preparedness and management of sudden cardiac arrest in high school and college athletic programs: a consensus statement. *J Athl Train.* 2007;42(1):143-158.

5. Casa DJ, Anderson SA, Baker L, et al. The inter-association task force for preventing sudden death in collegiate conditioning sessions: best practices recommendations. *J Athl Train.* 2012;47(4):477-480. doi:10.4085/1062-6050-47.4.08

6. Casa DJ, Almquist J, Anderson SA, et al. The inter-association task force for preventing sudden death in secondary school athletics programs: best-practices recommendations. *J Athl Train.* 2013;48(4):546-553. doi:10.4085/1062-6050-48.4.12

7. Casa DJ, Guskiewicz KM, Anderson SA, et al. National Athletic Trainers' Association position statement: preventing sudden death in sports. *J Athl Train.* 2012;47(1):96-118. www.guideline.gov/summaries/summary/38461/national-athletic-trainers-association-position-statement-preventing-sudden-death-in-sports.

8. Huggins RA, Scarneo SE, Casa DJ, et al. The inter-association task force document on emergency health and safety: best-practice recommendations for youth sports leagues. *J Athl Train.* 2017;52(4):384-400. doi:10.4085/1062-6050-52.2.02

9. Courson RW, Goldenberg M, Adams KG, et al. Inter-association consensus statement on best practices for sports medicine management for secondary schools and colleges. *J Athl Train.* 2014;49(1):128-137. doi:10.4085/1062-6050-49.1.06

10. National Athletic Trainers' Association official statement on athletic heath care provider "time outs" before athletic events. National Athletic Trainers' Association website. www.nata.org/sites/default/files/TimeOut.pdf. Published August 1, 2012.

11. Trauma center levels explained. American Trauma Society website. www.amtrauma.org/?page=traumalevels. Accessed April 7, 2018.

12. Swartz EE, Boden BP, Courson RW, et al. National Athletic Trainers' Association position statement: acute management of the cervical spine– injured athlete. *J Athl Train.* 2009;44(3):306-331. doi:10.4085/1062-6050-44.3.306

13. Singletary EM, Charlton NP, Epstein JL, et al. Part 15: First aid: 2015 American Heart Association and American Red Cross guidelines update for first aid. *Circulation.* 2015;132(18):S574-S589. doi:10.1161/CIR.0000000000000269

14. Goffinett ASW, Pickett JR. Spine boarding in athletic trauma: a paradigm shift. *NATA News.* 2014;(July):30-31.

15. Hoffman JR, Wolfson AB, Todd K, Mower WR. Selective cervical spine radiography in blunt trauma: methodology of the national emergency X-radiography utilization

study (NEXUS). *Ann Emerg Med.* 1998;32(4):461-469. https://ac-els-cdn-com.lib-proxy.radford.edu/S0196064498701763/1-s2.0-S0196064498701763-main.pdf?_tid=2938e3be-ae6e-11e7-9a48-00000aab0f27&acdnat=1507717562_4fd42dd37250b11c55a1f7b65ea1c672. Accessed October 11, 2017.

16. Stiell IG, Wells GA, Vandemheen K, et al. The Canadian C-spine rule for radiography in alert and stable trauma patients. *JAMA.* 2001;286(15):1841-1848. doi:10.1001/jama.286.15.1841

17. Official statement: EMS changes to pre-hospital care of the athlete with acute cervical spine injury. National Athletic Trainers' Association website. www.nata.org/sites/default/files/c-spine-management.pdf. Published 2014.

18. Appropriate prehospital management of the spine-injured athlete: updated from 1998 document. National Athletic Trainers' Association website. www.nata.org/sites/default/files/Executive-Summary-Spine-Injury-updated.pdf. Published August 5, 2015.

19. Walsh KM, Cooper MA, Holle RL, Rakov VA, Roeder WP, Ryan M. National Athletic Trainers' Association position statement: lightning safety for athletics and recreation. *J Athl Train.* 2013;48(2):258-270. doi:10.4085/1062-6050-48.2.25

20. Cappaert TA, Stone JA, Castellani JW, et al. National Athletic Trainers' Association position statement: environmental cold injuries. *J Athl Train.* 2008;43(6):640-658.

21. Casa DJ, DeMartini JK, Bergeron MF, et al. National Athletic Trainers' Association position statement: exertional heat illnesses. *J Athl Train.* 2015;50(9):986-1000. doi:10.4085/1062-6050-50.9.07

22. McDermott BP, Anderson SA, Armstrong LE, et al. National Athletic Trainers' Association position statement: fluid replacement for the physically active. *J Athl Train.* 2017;52(9):877-895. doi:10.4085/1062-6050-52.9.02

23. Casa DJ, Csillan D. Preseason heat-acclimatization guidelines for secondary school athletics. *J Athl Train.* 2009;44(3):332-333. doi:10.4085/1062-6050-44.3.332

24. National Council for Behavioral Health. Mental Health First Aid. www.mentalhealthfirstaid.org. Published 2018. Accessed April 8, 2018.

25. Neal TL, Diamond AB, Goldman S, et al. Inter-association recommendations for developing a plan to recognize and refer student-athletes with psychological concerns at the collegiate level: an executive summary of a consensus statement. *J Athl Train.* 2013;48(5):716-720. doi:10.4085/1062-6050-48.4.13

26. Neal TL, Diamond AB, Goldman S, et al. Interassociation recommendations for developing a plan to recognize and refer student-athletes with psychological concerns at the secondary school level: a consensus statement. *J Athl Train.* 2015;50(3):231-249. doi:10.4085/1062-6050-50.3.03

27. Critical incident stress management—emergency medical services. Virginia Department of Health website. www.vdh.virginia.gov/emergency-medical-services/emergency-operations/cism-critical-incident-stress-management. Accessed April 8, 2018.

28. ATs care. National Athletic Trainers' Association website. www.nata.org/membership/about-membership/member-resources/ats-care. Accessed May 2, 2018.

29. Mihalik JP, Lynall RC, Fraser MA, et al. Football equipment removal improves chest compression and ventilation efficacy. *Prehospital Emerg Care.* 2016;20(5):578-585. doi:10.3109/10903127.2016.1149649

30. Endres B, Decoster LC, Swartz EE. Football equipment removal in an exertional heat stroke scenario: time and difficulty. *Athl Train Sport Heal Care.* 2014;6(5):213-219. https://illiad.radford.edu/illiad/illiad.dll?Action=10&Form=75&Value=382163. Accessed June 12, 2017.

31. Lenhardt CS, Mihalik JP, Lynall RC, Fraser MA, Petschauer M, Swartz EE. The effect of football shoulder pad removal technique and equipment removal training on cervical spine motion, time to task completion, and perceived task difficulty. *Athl Train Sport Heal Care.* 2015;7(6):1-10. https://illiad.radford.edu/illiad/illiad.dll?Action=10&Form=75&Value=382162. Accessed June 12, 2017.

32. Martinez DC, Bowman TG, Boergers RJ. The role of practice on lacrosse helmet facemask removal time. *J Athl Train.* 2014;49(3):S-128.

33. Best practices for NCAA championships competition venue safety and security. NCAA website. www.ncaa.org/sites/default/files/Best_Practices_for_Venue_Safety_and_Security.pdf. Accessed February 27, 2018.

34. Courson R, Ellis J, Herring SA, et al. Best practices and current care concepts in prehospital care of the spine-injured athlete in American tackle football. *J Athl Train.* 2020;55(6):545-562. doi:10.4085/1062-6050-430-19

35. Mills BM, Conrick KM, Anderson S, et al. Prehospital care of the spine-injured athlete consensus recommendations on the prehospital care of the injured athlete with a suspected catastrophic cervical spine injury. *J Athl Train.* 2020;55(6):563-572. doi:10.4085/1062-6050-0434.19

Chapter 14

1. Cleary MA, Walsh Flanagan K. *Acute and Emergency Care in Athletic Training.* Champaign, IL: Human Kinetics; 2020.

2. Teasdale G. Forty years on: Updating the Glasgow Coma Scale. *Nurs Times.* 2014;110(42):12-16. www.nursingtimes.net. Accessed April 9, 2019.

3. McCrory P. Smelling salts. *Br J Sports Med.* 2006;40:659-660. doi:10.1136/bjsm.2006.029710

4. American Heart Association. *Highlights of the 2015 American Heart Association Guidelines Update for CPR and ECC.* 2015. https://eccguidelines.heart.org/wp-content/uploads/2015/10/2015-AHA-Guidelines-Highlights-English.pdf.

5. Casa DJ, Guskiewicz KM, Anderson SA, et al. National Athletic Trainers' Association position statement: Prevent-

ing sudden death in sports. *J Athl Train.* 2012;47(1):96-118. www.guideline.gov/summaries/summary/38461/national-athletic-trainers-association-position-statement-preventing-sudden-death-in-sports.

6. Drezner JA, Courson RW, Roberts WO, Mosesso VN, Link MS, Maron BJ. Inter-Association task force recommendations on emergency preparedness and management of sudden cardiac arrest in high school and college athletic programs: a consensus statement. *J Athl Train.* 2007;42(1):143-158. www.journalofathletictraining.org. Accessed February 13, 2018.

7. Popp JK, Berry DC. Athletic training students demonstrate airway management skill decay, but retain knowledge over 6 months. *Athl Train Educ J.* 2016;11(4):173-180. doi:10.4085/1104173

8. Pollak AN, Barnes L, Ciotola JA, Gulli B, eds. *Emergency Care and Transportation of the Sick and Injured.* 10th ed. Burlington, MA: Jones & Bartlett Learning; 2011.

9. O'Connor FG, Kugler JP, Oriscello RG. Sudden death in young athletes: screening for the needle in a haystack. *Am Fam Physician.* 1998;57(11):2763-2770. www.aafp.org/afp/1998/0601/p2763.html. Accessed April 10, 2019.

10. Lauschke J, Maisch B. Athlete's heart or hypertrophic cardiomyopathy? *Clin Res Caridol.* 2009;98:80-88. doi:10.1016/j.lpm.2012.02.007

11. McCallum L, Higgins D. Measuring body temperature. *Nurs Times [online].* 2012;45:20-22. www.nursing-times.net/clinical-archive/assessment-skills/measuring-body-temperature/5051350.article. Accessed April 15, 2019.

12. Casa DJ, Almquist J, Anderson SA, et al. The Inter-Association Task Force for preventing sudden death in secondary school athletics programs: best-practices recommendations. *J Athl Train.* 2013;48(4):546-553. doi:10.4085/1062-6050-48.4.12

13. Casa DJ, DeMartini JK, Bergeron MF, et al. National Athletic Trainers' Association position statement: exertional heat illnesses. *J Athl Train.* 2015;50(9):986-1000. doi:10.4085/1062-6050-50.9.07

14. *Inter-Association Task Force on Exertional Heat Illnesses Consensus Statement.* 2003. www.nata.org/sites/default/files/inter-association-task-force-exertional-heat-illness.pdf. Accessed February 13, 2018.

15. Cappaert TA, Stone JA, Castellani JW, et al. National Athletic Trainers' Association position statement: environmental cold injuries. *J Athl Train.* 2008;43(6):640-658.

16. Miller KC, Hughes LE, Long BC, Adams WM, Casa DJ. Validity of core temperature measurements at 3 rectal depths during rest, exercise, cold-water immersion, and recovery. *J Athl Train.* 2017;52(4):332-338. doi:10.4085/1062-6050-52.2.10

17. Berry DC, Seitz SR. Educating the educator: use of pulse oximetry in athletic training. *Athl Train Educ J.* 2012;7(2):74-80. doi:10.5608/070274

18. Courson R, Ellis J, Herring SA, et al. Best practices and current care concepts in prehospital care of the spine-injured athlete in American tackle football. *J Athl Train.* 2020;55(6):545-562. doi:10.4085/1062-6050-430-19

19. National Athletic Trainers' Association. *Appropriate Prehospital Management of the Spine-Injured Athlete: Updated from 1998 Document.* 2015.

20. Swartz EE, Boden BP, Courson RW, et al. National Athletic Trainers' Association position statement: acute management of the cervical spine–injured athlete. *J Athl Train.* 2009;44(3):306-331. doi:10.4085/1062-6050-44.3.306

21. Mihalik JP, Lynall RC, Fraser MA, et al. Football equipment removal improves chest compression and ventilation efficacy. *Prehospital Emerg Care.* 2016;20(5):578-585. doi:10.3109/10903127.2016.1149649

22. Endres B, Decoster LC, Swartz EE. Football equipment removal in an exertional heat stroke scenario: time and difficulty. *Athl Train Sport Heal Care.* 2014;6(5):213-219. https://illiad.radford.edu/illiad/illiad.dll?Action=10&Form=75&Value=382163. Accessed June 12, 2017.

23. Andersen JC, Courson RW, Kleiner DM, McLoda TA. National Athletic Trainers' Association position statement: emergency planning in athletics. *J Athl Train.* 2002;37(1):99-104.

24. Mills BM, Conrick KM, Anderson S, et al. Prehospital care of the spine-injured athlete consensus recommendations on the prehospital care of the injured athlete with a suspected catastrophic cervical spine injury. *J Athl Train.* 2020;55(6):563-572. doi:10.4085/1062-6050-0434.19

25. Hazinski MF, Nolan JP, Aickin R, et al. Part 1: Executive summary: 2015 international consensus on cardiopulmonary resuscitation and emergency cardiovascular care science with treatment recommendations. *Circulation.* 2015;132(16 Suppl 1):S2-S39. doi:10.1161/CIR.0000000000000270

26. Board of Certification. *Certification Maintenance Requirements for Certified Athletic Trainers.* Omaha, NE: Author, 2019. www.bocatc.org/system/document_versions/versions/164/original/boc-certification-maintenance-requirements-20180914.pdf?1536935092. Accessed April 10, 2019.

27. Roberts K, Whalley H, Bleetman A. The nasopharyngeal airway: Dispelling myths and establishing the facts. *Emerg Med J.* 2005;22(6):394-396. doi:10.1136/emj.2004.021402

28. Singletary EM, Zideman DA, De Buck EDJ, et al. Part 9: First aid: 2015 international consensus on first aid science with treatment recommendations. *Circulation.* 2015;132(16 Suppl 1);S269-S311. doi:10.1161/CIR.0000000000000278

29. Beam JW, Buckley B, Holcomb WR, Ciocca M. National Athletic Trainers' Association position statement: management of acute skin trauma. *J Athl Train.* 2016;51(12):1053-1070. doi:10.4085/1062-6050-51.7.01

30. Singletary EM, Charlton NP, Epstein JL, et al. Part 15: First aid: 2015 American Heart Association and American Red Cross guidelines update for first aid. *Circulation.* 2015;132(18):S574-S589. doi:10.1161/CIR.0000000000000269

31. Berry DC, Seitz SR, Payne EK. Educating the educator: use of advanced bleeding control mechanisms in athletic training: a shift in the thought process of prehospital care.

Part 1: tourniquets. *Athl Train Educ J.* 2014;9(3):142-151. doi:10.4085/0904193

32. Gutierrez G, Reines HD, Wulf-Gutierrez ME. Clinical review: hemorrhagic shock. *Crit Care.* 2004;8:373-381. doi:10.1186/cc2851

33. Fischer PE, Perina DG, Delbridge TR, et al. Prehospital emergency care spinal motion restriction in the trauma patient—a joint position statement. *Prehospital Emerg Care.* 2018;22(6):659-661. doi:10.1080/10903127.201 8.1481476

34. Conway D, Payne EK, Strapp E, Scifers JR. Spinal immobilization. *Athl Train Sport Heal Care.* 2019;11(2):53-56. doi:10.3928/19425864-20190130-01

35. White IV CC, Domeier RM, Millin MG. Prehospital emergency care EMS spinal precautions and the use of the long backboard-resource document to the position statement of the National Association of EMS Physicians and the American College of Surgeons Committee on Trauma. *Prehospital Emerg Care.* 2014;18(2):306-314. doi:10.31 09/10903127.2014.884197

36. Hoffman JR, Wolfson AB, Todd K, Mower WR. Selective cervical spine radiography in blunt trauma: methodology of the National Emergency X-Radiography Utilization Study (NEXUS). *Ann Emerg Med.* 1998;32(4):461-469. https://ac-els-cdn-com.lib-proxy.radford.edu/S0196064498701763/1-s2.0-S0196064498701763-main.pdf?_tid=2938e3be-ae6e-11e7-9a48-00000aab0f27&acd-nat=1507717562_4fd42dd37250b11c55a1f7b65ea1c672. Accessed October 11, 2017.

37. Stiell IG, Wells GA, Vandemheen K, et al. The Canadian CT Head Rule for patients with minor head injury. *Lancet.* 2001;357(9266):1391-1396. doi:10.1016/S0140-6736(00)04561-X

38. Chang CJ, Weston T, Tedeschi F, White M, Young CC. Inter-association consensus statement: the management of medications by the sports medicine team. *J Athl Train.* 2018;53(11):1103-1112. doi:10.4085/1062-6050-53-11

39. McDermott BP, Anderson SA, Armstrong LE, et al. National Athletic Trainers' Association position statement: fluid replacement for the physically active. *J Athl Train.* 2017;52(9):877-895. doi:10.4085/1062-6050-52.9.02

40. Papa L. Potential blood-based biomarkers for concussion. *Sport Med Arthosc.* 2016;24(3):108-115. doi:10.1097/JSA.0000000000000117

41. O'Connell B, Kelly ÁM, Mockler D, et al. Use of blood biomarkers in the assessment of sports-related concussion—a systematic review in the context of their biological significance. *Clin J Sport Med.* 2018;28(6):561-571. doi:10.1097/JSM.0000000000000478

Chapter 15

1. Doherty C, Delahunt E, Caulfield B, Hertel J, Ryan J, Bleakley C. The incidence and prevalence of ankle sprain injury: A systematic review and meta-analysis of prospective epidemiological studies. *Sports Med.* 2014;44(1):123-140.

2. Waterman BR, Owens BD, Davey S, Zacchilli MA, Belmont PJ. The epidemiology of ankle sprains in the United States. *J Bone Joint Surg Am.* 2010;92(13):2279-2284.

3. Grassi A, Quaglia A, Canata GL, Zaffagnini S. An update on the grading of muscle injuries: A narrative review from clinical to comprehensive systems. *Joints.* 2016;4(1):39-46.

4. Maffulli N, Del Buono A, Oliva F, et al. Muscle injuries: A brief guide to classification and management. *Transl Med UniSa.* 2015;12:14-18.

5. Beiner JM, Jokl P. Muscle contusion injury and myositis ossificans traumatica. *Clin Orthop Rel Res.* 2002,S403:S110-119.

6. Bass E. Tendinopathy: Why the difference between tendinitis and tendinosis matters. *Int J Massage Bodywork.* 2012;5(1):14-17.

7. Kaeding C, Best TM. Tendinosis: Pathophysiology and nonoperative treatment. *Sports Health.* 2009;1(4):284-292.

8. Goel R, Abzug JM. De Quervain's tenosynovitis: A review of the rehabilitative options. *Hand.* 2015;10(1):1-5.

9. Stahl S, Vida D, Meisner C, Stahl AS, Schaller HE, Held M. Work-related etiology of de Quervain's tenosynovitis: A case-control study with prospectively collected data. *BMC Musculoskelet Disord.* 2015;16:126-135.

10. Baoge L, Van Den Steen E, Rimbaut S, et al. Treatment of skeletal muscle injury: A review. *ISRN Orthop.* 2012;2012:689012.

11. Petersen W, Rembiotzki IV, Koppenburg AG, et al. Treatment of acute ankle ligament injuries: A systematic review. *Arch Orthop Trauma Surg.* 2013;133(8):1129-1141.

12. Brosseau L, Casimiro L, Milne S, et al. Deep transverse friction massage for treating tendinitis. *Cochrane Database Syst Rev.* 2002;4.

13. Loew LM, Brosseau L, Tugwell P, et al. Deep transverse friction massage for treating lateral elbow or lateral knee tendinitis. *Cochrane Database Syst Rev.* 2002;8(11).

14. Nurkovic J, Jovasevic L, Konicanin A, et al. Treatment of trochanteric bursitis: Our experience. *J Phys Ther Sci.* 2016;28(7):2078-2081.

15. Andres BM, Murrell GAC. Treatment of tendinopathy: What works, what does not, and what is on the horizon. *Clin Orthop Relat Res.* 2008;466(7):1539-1554.

16. Bley B, Abid W. Imaging of tendinopathy: A physician's perspective. *J Orthop Sports Phys Ther.* 2015;45(11):826-828.

17. Hodgson RJ, O'Connor PJ, Grainger AJ. Tendon and ligament imaging. *Br J Radiol.* 2012;85(1016):1157-1172.

18. Lento PH, Primack S. Advances and utility of diagnostic ultrasound in musculoskeletal medicine. *Curr Rev Musculoskelet Med.* 2008;1(1):24-31.

19. Cauley JA. Defining ethnic and racial differences in osteoporosis and fragility fractures. *Clin Orthop Relat Res.* 2011;469(7):1891-1899.

20. Amin S, Achenbach SJ, Atkinson EJ, Khosla S, Melton LJ. Trends in fracture incidence: A population-based study over 20 years. *J Bone Miner Res.* 2014;29(3):581-589.

21. Peck DM. Apophyseal injuries in the young athlete. *Am Fam Physician.* 1995;51(8):1891-1898.

22. Marsell R, Eihorn TA. The biology of fracture healing. *Injury.* 2012;42(6):551-555.

23. Affshana M, Saveethna J. Healing mechanism in bone fracture. *J Pharm Sci Res.* 2015;7(7):441-442.

24. Della Rocca GJ. The science of ultrasound therapy for fracture healing. *Indian J Orthop.* 2009;43(2):121-126.

25. Tamas N, Scammell BE. Principles of bone and joint injury and their healing. *Surgery.* 2015;33(1):7-14.

26. Rowbotham E, Barron D. Radiology of fracture complications. *Orth Trauma.* 2009;23(1):52-60.

27. Jahagirdar R, Scammell BE. Principles of fracture healing and disorders of bone union. *Surgery.* 2008;27(2):63-69.

28. Chen AT, Vallier HA. Noncontiguous and open fractures of the lower extremity: Epidemiology, complications, and unplanned procedures. *Injury.* 2016;47(3):742-747.

29. Axelrad TW, Einhorn TA. Use of clinical assessment tools in the evaluation of fracture healing. *Injury.* 2011;42(3):301-305.

30. Inaba K, DuBose JJ, Barmparas G, et al. Clinical examination is insufficient to rule out thoracolumbar spine injuries. *J Trauma.* 2011;70(1):174-179.

31. Eyler Y, Sever M, Turgut A, et al. The evaluation of the sensitivity and specificity of wrist examination findings for predicting fractures. *Am J Emerg Med.* 2018;36(3):425-429.

32. Schneiders AG, Sullivan SJ, Hendrick PA, et al. The ability of clinical tests to diagnose stress fractures: A systematic review of meta-analysis. *J Orth Sports Phys Ther.* 2012;42(9):760-771.

33. Joshi N, Lira A, Mehta N, Paladino L, Sinert R. Diagnostic accuracy of history, physical examination, and bedside ultrasound for diagnosis of extremity fractures in the emergency department: A systematic review. *Acad Emer Med.* 2013;20(1):1-34.

34. Moore MB. The use of a tuning fork and stethoscope to identify fractures. *J Athl Train.* 2009;44(3):272-274.

35. Wright AA, Hegedus EJ, Lenchik L, Kuhn KJ, Santiago L, Smoliga JM. Diagnostic accuracy of various imaging modalities for suspected lower extremity stress fractures: A systematic review with evidence-based recommendations for clinical practice. *Am J Sports Med.* 2016;44(1):255-263.

36. Einhorn TA, Gerstenfeld LC. Fracture healing: Mechanisms and interventions. *Nat Rev Rheumatol.* 2015;11(1):45-54.

37. Goldstein C, Sprague S, Petrisor BA. Electrical stimulation for fracture healing: Current evidence. *J Orthop Trauma.* 2010;24(1):S62-65.

38. Jayakumar P, Lau S. Fracture management. *Ann R Surg Engl.* 2006;88(4):419-420.

39. Menorca RMG, Fussell TS, Elfar JC. Peripheral nerve trauma: Mechanisms of injury and recovery. *Hand Clin.* 2013;29(3):317-330.

40. Roganovic, Z. Factors influencing the outcome of nerve repair. *Vojnosanit Pregl.* 1998;55(2):119-131.

41. Li R, Liu Z, Pan Y, Chen L, Zhang Z, Lu L. Peripheral nerve injuries treatment: A systematic review. *Cell Biochem Biophys.* 2014;68(3):449-454.

42. Lewandowski J, O'Brien M, Watts J, Scifers JR. Clinical roundtable: Iontophoresis. *Athl Train Sports Health Care.* 2013;5(3):103-105.

43. Kane NM, Oware A. Nerve conduction and electromyography studies. *J Neurol.* 2012;259(7):1502-1508.

44. Rangavajla G, Mokarram N, Masoodzadehgan N, et al. Non-invasive imaging of peripheral nerves. *Cells Tissues Organs.* 2014;200(1):69-77.

45. Domkundwar S, Autkar G, Khadilkar SV, Virarkar M. Ultrasound and EMG-NCV study (electromyography and nerve conduction velocity) correlation in diagnosis of nerve pathologies. *J Ultrasound.* 2017;20(2):111-122.

46. Zaidman CM, Seelig MJ, Baker JC, et al. Detection of peripheral nerve pathology: Comparison of ultrasound and MRI. *Neurology.* 2013;80(18):1634-1640.

47. National Osteoporosis Foundation website. www.nof.org. Accessed August 10, 2020.

Chapter 16

1. Shultz SJ, Houglum PA, Perrin DH. *Examination of Musculoskeletal Injuries.* 4th ed. Champaign, IL: Human Kinetics; 2016.

2. Lombardi NJ, Tucker B, Freedman KB, et al. Accuracy of athletic trainer and physician diagnoses in sports medicine. *Orthopedics.* 2016;39(5):e944-e949. doi:10.3928/01477447-20160623-10

3. Eberman LE, Finn ME. Enhancing clinical evaluation skills: palpation as the principal skill. *Athl Train Educ J.* 2010;5(4):170-175. http://natajournals.org/doi/pdf/10.4085/1947-380X-5.4.170. Accessed October 9, 2017.

4. Norkin C, White D. Chapter 1: Basic concepts. In: *Measurement of Joint Motion: A Guide to Gonimetry.* Philadephia, PA: F.A. Davis; 2009:3-53. doi:10.1108/S0749-742320160000019022

5. Pescatello LS, ed. *ACSM's Guidelines for Exercise Testing and Prescription.* 9th ed. Philadelphia, PA: Lippincott, Williams, & Wilkins; 2014.

6. Norkin C, White D. Appendix A: Normative range of motion values. In: *Measurement of Joint Motion: A Guide to Gonimetry.* Philadelphia, PA: F.A. Davis; 2009:425-430.

7. Hoppenfeld S. *Physical Examination of the Spine & Extremities.* Norwalk, CT: Appleton & Lange; 1976.

8. Comana F. Functional assessments: Posture, movement, core, balance, and flexibility. In: Bryant CX, Green DJ, eds. *ACE Personal Trainer Manual.* 4th ed. San Diego, CA: American Council on Exercise; 2010:135-170.

9. Hegedus EJ, Cook C, Lewis J, Wright A, Park J-Y. Combining orthopedic special tests to improve diagnosis of shoulder pathology. *Phys Ther Sport*. 2015;16:87-92. doi:10.1016/j.ptsp.2014.08.001

10. Nick JM. Deep tendon reflexes: the what, why, where, and how of tapping. *JOGNN*. 2003;32:297-306. doi:10.1177/0884217503253491

11. McCrory P, Meeuwisse W, Dvorak J, et al. Consensus statement on concussion in sport—the 5th international conference on concussion in sport held in Berlin, October 2016. *Br J Sports Med*. 2017;51(11):838-847. doi:10.1136/bjsports-2017-097699

12. Putukian M. Clinical evaluation of the concussed athlete: a view from the sideline. *J Athl Train*. 2017;52(3):236-244. doi:10.4085/1062-6050-52.1.08

13. Putukian M, Raftery M, Guskiewicz KM, et al. Onfield assessment of concussion in the adult athlete. *Br J Sport Med*. 2013;47:285-288. doi:10.1136/bjsports-2013-092158

14. Sports Concussion Assessment Tool, 5th ed. *Br J Sports Med*. 2017;51(11):851-858. doi:10.1136/bjsports-2017-097506SCAT5

15. Patricios J, Fuller GW, Ellenbogen R, et al. What are the critical elements of sideline screening that can be used to establish the diagnosis of concussion? A systematic review. *Br J Sport Med*. 2017;51(10):888-894. doi:10.1136/bjsports-2016-097441

16. Broglio SP, Cantu RC, Gioia GA, et al. National Athletic Trainers' Association position statement: Management of sport concussion. *J Athl Train*. 2014;49(2):245-265. doi:10.4085/1062-6050-49.1.07

17. Stiell IG, Wells GA, Vandemheen K, et al. The Canadian CT Head Rule for patients with minor head injury. *Lancet*. 2001;357(9266):1391-1396. doi:10.1016/S0140-6736(00)04561-X

18. Mower WR, Hoffman JR, Herbert M, Wolfson AB, Pollack CV, Zucker MI. Developing a decision instrument to guide computed tomographic imaging of blunt head injury patients. *J Trauma*. 2005;59(4):954-959. doi:10.1097/01.ta.0000187813.79047.42

19. Podell K, Presley C, Derman H. Sideline sports concussion assessment. *Neurol Clin*. 2017;35(3):435-450. doi:10.1016/j.ncl.2017.03.003

20. Echemendia RJ. The Sport Concussion Assessment Tool, 5th edition (SCAT5): Background and rationale. *Br J Sport Med*. 2017;51:848-850. https://illiad.radford.edu/illiad/illiad.dll?Action=10&Form=75&Value=389118. Accessed November 1, 2017.

21. Matuszak JM, McVige J, McPherson J, Willer B, Leddy JJ. A practical concussion physical examination toolbox: evidence-based physical examination for concussions. *Sports Health*. 2016;8(3):260-269. http://journals.sagepub.com/doi/pdf/10.1177/1941738116641394. Accessed October 30, 2017.

22. Galetta KM, Morganroth J, Moehringer N, et al. Adding vision to concussion testing: a prospective study of sideline testing in youth and collegiate athletes. *J Neuro-Ophthalmol*. 2015;35:235-241. doi:10.1097/WNO.0000000000000226

23. Seidman DH, Burlingame J, Yousif LR, et al. Evaluation of the King-Devick test as a concussion screening tool in high school football players. *J Neurol Sci*. 2015;356(1-2):97-101. doi:10.1016/j.jns.2015.06.021

24. King D, Clark T, Gissane C. Use of a rapid visual screening tool for the assessment of concussion in amateur rugby league: A pilot study. *J Neurol Sci*. 2012;320(1-2):16-21. doi:10.1016/j.jns.2012.05.049

25. Tjarks BJ, Dorman JC, Valentine VD, et al. Comparison and utility of King-Devick and ImPACT® composite scores in adolescent concussion patients. *J Neurol Sci*. 2013;334:148-153. doi:10.1016/j.jns.2013.08.015

26. Neal TL, Diamond AB, Goldman S, et al. Inter-association recommendations for developing a plan to recognize and refer student-athletes with psychological concerns at the collegiate level: an executive summary of a consensus statement. *J Athl Train*. 2013;48(5):716-720. doi:10.4085/1062-6050-48.4.13

27. Neal TL, Diamond AB, Goldman S, et al. Interassociation recommendations for developing a plan to recognize and refer student-athletes with psychological concerns at the secondary school level: a consensus statement. *J Athl Train*. 2015;50(3):231-249. doi:10.4085/1062-6050-50.3.03

28. McGinn T, Guyatt GH, Wyer PC, Naylor CD, Stiell IG, Richardson WS. Users' guides to the medical literature—XXII: How to use articles about clinical decision rules. *JAMA*. 2000;284(1):79-84. doi:10.1001/jama.284.1.79

29. Beneciuk JM, Bishop MD, George SZ. Clinical prediction rules for physical therapy interventions: a systematic review. *Phys Ther*. 2009;89(2):114-124. doi:ptj.20080239 [pii]\r10.2522/ptj.20080239

30. Keogh C, Wallace E, O'Brien KK, Galvin R, Smith SM, Fahey TP. Developing an international register of clinical prediction rules for use in primary care: a descriptive analysis. *Ann Fam Med*. 2014;12(4):359-366. doi:10.1370/afm.1640.INTRODUCTION

31. Hankemeier DA, Popp JK, Walker SE. Familiarity with and use of clinical prediction rules and patient-rated oucome measures. *Athl Train Sport Heal Care*. 2017;9(3):108-123.

32. Knox GM, Snodgrass SJ, Stanton TR, et al. Physiotherapy students' perceptions and experiences of clinical prediction rules. *Physiotherapy*. 2017;103:296-303. doi:10.1016/j.physio.2016.04.001

33. Stiell IG, Wells GA, Vandemheen K, et al. The Canadian C-spine rule for radiography in alert and stable trauma patients. *JAMA*. 2001;286(15):1841-1848. doi:10.1001/jama.286.15.1841

34. Centor RM, Witherspoon JM, Dalton HP, Brody CE, Link K. The diagnosis of strep throat in adults in the emergency room. *Med Decis Mak*. 1981;1(3):239-246. https://illiad.radford.edu/illiad/illiad.dll?Action=10&Form=75&Value=387184. Accessed October 9, 2017.

35. Hoffman JR, Wolfson AB, Todd K, Mower WR. Selective cervical spine radiography in blunt trauma: methodology of the National Emergency X-Radiography Utilization Study (NEXUS). *Ann Emerg Med.* 1998;32(4):461-469. https://ac-els-cdn-com.lib-proxy.radford.edu/S0196064498701763/1-s2.0-S0196064498701763-main.pdf?_tid=2938e3be-ae6e-11e7-9a48-00000aab0f27&acdnat=1507717562_4fd42dd37250b11c55a1f7b65ea1c672. Accessed October 11, 2017.

36. Stiell IG, Greenberg GH, Mcknight RD, Nair RC, McDowell I, Worthington JR. A study to develop clinical decision rules for the use of radiography in acute ankle injuries. *Ann Emerg Med.* 1992;21(4):384-390. www.annemergmed.com/article/S0196-0644(05)82656-3/pdf. Accessed October 5, 2017.

37. Long AS, Scifers JR. Clinical prediction rules for diagnostic imaging after lower extremity trauma. *Int J Athl Ther Train.* 2011;16(6):38-41.

38. Stiell IG, Greenberg GH, Wells GA, et al. Derivation of a decision rule for the use radiography in acute knee injuries. *Ann Emerg Med.* 1995;26(4):405-413. www.annemergmed.com/article/S0196-0644(95)70106-0/pdf. Accessed October 5, 2017.

39. Seaberg DC, Jackson R. Clinical decision rule for knee radiographs. *Am J Emerg Med.* 1994;12(5):541-543. https://ac-els-cdn-com.lib-proxy.radford.edu/0735675794902747/1-s2.0-0735675794902747-main.pdf?_tid=d6fb9804-ae6c-11e7-a158-00000aacb-35f&acdnat=1507716994_8ba157dca27a154d-1972d540e2bc0bbd. Accessed October 11, 2017.

40. Wells PS, Hirsh J, Anderson DR, et al. A simple clinical model for the diagnosis of deep-vein thrombosis combined with impedance plethysmography: Potential for an improvement in the diagnostic process. *J Intern Med.* 1998;243:15-23. doi:10.1046/j.1365-2796.1998.00249.x

41. Almquist J. Back to basics: is it broken? *Athl Ther Today.* 1999;(January):38-39.

42. Raab S, Wolfe BD, Gould TE, Piland SG. Characterizations of a quality certified athletic trainer. *J Athl Train.* 2011;46(6):672-679. http://natajournals.org/doi/pdf/10.4085/1062-6050-46.6.672. Accessed November 30, 2017.

43. Welch Bacon CE, Eppelheimer BL, Kasamatsu TM, Lam KC, Nottingham SL. Athletic trainers' perceptions of and barriers to patient care documentation: a report from the athletic training practice-based research network. *J Athl Train.* 2017;52(7):667-675. doi:10.4085/1062-6050-52.3.15

44. National Athletic Trainers' Association. *Best Practice Guidelines for Athletic Training Documentation.* NATA. August 2017.

45. Nottingham SL, Lam KC, Kasamatsu TM, Eppelheimer BL, Welch Bacon CE. Athletic trainers' reasons for and mechanics of documenting patient care: a report from the athletic training practice-based research network. *J Athl Train.* 2017;52(7):656-666. doi:10.4085/1062-6050-52.3.14

46. Sleszynski SL, Glonek T. Outpatient osteopathic SOAP note form: preliminary results in osteopathic outcomes-based research. *JAOA.* 2005;105(4):181-205. https://illiad.radford.edu/illiad/illiad.dll?Action=10&-Form=75&Value=383374. Accessed July 20, 2017.

47. Zierler-Brown S, Brown TR, Chen D, Blackburn RW. Clinical documentation for patient care: Models, concepts, and liability considerations for pharmacists. *Am J Heal Pharm.* 2007;64(17):1851-1858. doi:10.2146/ajhp060682

48. Henderson JP. *The 2015 Athletic Trainer Practice Analysis Study.* Omaha, NE: Board of Certification; 2015.

49. Snyder AR, Parsons JT, Valovich McLeod TC, Curtis Bay R, Michener LA, Sauers EL. Using disablement models and clinical outcomes assessment to enable evidence-based athletic training practice, part i: disablement models. *J Athl Train.* 2008;43(4):428-436. http://natajournals.org/doi/pdf/10.4085/1062-6050-43.4.428. Accessed July 24, 2017.

50. Snyder AR, Valovich McLeod TC, Sauers EL. Defining, valuing, and teaching clinical outcomes assessment in professional and post-professional athletic training education programs. *Athl Train Educ J.* 2007;2:31-41. www.nataej.org. Accessed December 3, 2017.

51. Fitzpatrick R, Davey C, Buxton MJ, Jones DR. Evaluating patient-based outcome measures for use in clinical trials. *Health Technol Assess (Rockv).* 1998;2(14). https://illiad.radford.edu/illiad/illiad.dll?Action=10&-Form=75&Value=391637. Accessed December 2, 2017.

52. Snyder Valier AR, Jennings AL, Parsons JT, Vela LI. Benefits of and barriers to using patient-rated outcome measures in athletic training. *J Athl Train.* 2014;49(5):674-683. doi:10.4085/1062-6050-49.3.15

53. Valier AR, Lam KC. Beyond the basics of clinical outcomes assessment: selecting appropriate patient-rated outcomes instruments for patient care. *Athl Train Educ J.* 2015;10(1):91-100. doi:10.4085/100191

54. Tongue JR, Epps HR, Forese LL. Communication skills for patient-centered care. Research-based, easily learned techniques for medical interviews that benefit orthopaedic surgeons and their patients. *J Bone Jt Surg.* 2005;87(3):652-658. www.ejbjs.org/cgi/content/full/87/3/652#responses. Accessed November 27, 2017.

55. Schattner A. The silent dimension: Expressing humanism in each medical encounter. *Arch Intern Med.* 2009;169(12):1095-1099. https://illiad.radford.edu/illiad/illiad.dll?Action=10&Form=75&Value=391151. Accessed December 1, 2017.

56. Levinson W, Roter DL, Mulooly JP, Dull VT, Frankel RM. Physician-patient communication: The relationship with malpractice claims among primary care physicians and surgeons. *JAMA.* 1997;277(2):553-559. https://illiad.radford.edu/illiad/illiad.dll?Action=10&-Form=75&Value=391154. Accessed November 30, 2017.

Chapter 17

1. ACR Appropriateness Criteria. American College of Radiology website. www.acr.org/Clinical-Resources/ACR-Appropriateness-Criteria. Accessed May 23, 2018.

2. Waite S, Grigorian A, Alexander RG, et al. Analysis of perceptual expertise in radiology—Current knowledge and a new perspective. *Front Hum Neurosci*. 2019;13:213. doi:10.3389/fnhum.2019.00213

3. Shelmerdine SC, Langan D, Hutchinson JC, et al. Chest radiographs versus CT for the detection of rib fractures in children (DRIFT): a diagnostic accuracy observational study. *Lancet Child Adolesc Health*. 2018;2(11):802-811.

4. Malgo F, Hamdy NAT, Ticheler CHJM, et al. Value and potential limitations of vertebral fracture assessment (VFA) compared to conventional spine radiography: experience from a fracture liaison service (FLS) and a meta-analysis. *Osteoporos Int*. 2017;28(10):2955-2965.

5. Reidelbach CS, Goerke SM, Leschka SC, et al. Comparing the diagnostic performance of radiation dose-equivalent radiography, multi-detector computed tomography and cone beam computed tomography for finger fractures—A phantom study. *PLoS One*. 2019;14(3):e0213339.

6. Philipsen RH, Sánchez CI, Maduskar P, et al. Automated chest-radiography as a triage for Xpert testing in resource-constrained settings: a prospective study of diagnostic accuracy and costs. *Sci Rep*. 2015;5:12215.

7. Im YG, Lee JS, Park JI, Lim HS, Kim BG, Kim JH. Diagnostic accuracy and reliability of panoramic temporomandibular joint (TMJ) radiography to detect bony lesions in patients with TMJ osteoarthritis. *J Dent Sci*. 2018;13(4):396-404.

8. Gunderman RB. *Essential Radiology: Clinical Presentation, Pathophysiology, Imaging*. 3rd ed. New York, NY: Thieme; 2014.

9. du Plessis A, Broeckhoven C, Guelpa A, le Roux SG. Laboratory X-ray micro-computed tomography: a user guideline for biological samples. *Gigascience*. 2017;6(6):1-11. doi:10.1093/gigascience/gix027

10. McCollough CH, Leng S, Yu L, Fletcher JG. Dual- and multi-energy CT: principles, technical approaches, and clinical applications. *Radiology*. 2015;276(3):637-653. doi:10.1148/radiol.2015142631

11. Stewart BK, Huang HK. Single-exposure dual-energy computed radiography. *Med Phys*. 1990;17(5):866-875.

12. Long BW, Hall Rollins J, Smith BJ. *Merrill's Atlas of Radiographic Positioning & Procedures*. 13th ed. St. Louis, MO: Elsevier/Mosby; 2017.

13. Saied AM, Redant C, El-Batouty M, et al. Accuracy of magnetic resonance studies in the detection of chondral and labral lesions in femoroacetabular impingement: systematic review and meta-analysis. *BMC Musculoskelet Disord*. 2017;18(1):83.

14. Lohrke J, Frenzel T, Endrikat J, et al. 25 Years of contrast-enhanced MRI: developments, current challenges and future perspectives. *Adv Ther*. 2016;33(1):1-28.

15. Craig M. *Essentials of Sonography and Patient Care*. 4th ed. St. Louis, MO: Elsevier/Saunders, 2018.

16. Sorensen B, Hunskaar S. Point-of-care ultrasound in primary care: a systematic review of generalist performed point-of-care ultrasound in unselected populations. *Ultrasound J*. 2019;11(1):31. doi:10.1186/s13089-019-0145-4

17. El-Maghraby TA, Moustafa HM, Pauwels EK. Nuclear medicine methods for evaluation of skeletal infection among other diagnostic modalities. *Q J Nucl Med Mol Imaging*. 2006 Sep;50(3):167-192.

18. Love C, Din AS, Tomas MB, Kalapparambath TP, Palestro CJ. Radionuclide bone imaging: an illustrative review. *Radiographics*. 2003 Mar-Apr;23(2):341-358.

19. Bombardieri E, Aktolun C, Baum RP, et al. Bone scintigraphy: procedure guidelines for tumour imaging. *Eur J Nucl Med Mol Imaging*. 2003;30:BP99-BP106.

20. Segall G, Delbeke D, Stabin MG, et al. SNM practice guideline for sodium 18F-fluoride PET/CT bone scans 1.0. *J Nucl Med*. 2010;51:1813-1820. doi:10.2967/jnumed.110.082263

21. Van den Wyngaert T, Strobel K, Kampen WU, et al. The EANM practice guidelines for bone scintigraphy. *Eur J Nucl Med Mol Imaging*. 2016;43(9):1723-1738. doi:10.1007/s00259-016-3415-4

22. ACR Committee on MR Safety. *ACR Manual on MR Safety*. Version 1.0, published 2020. www.acr.org/-/media/ACR/Files/Radiology-Safety/MR-Safety/Manual-on-MR-Safety.pdf.

Chapter 18

1. Emery MS, Horsby K, Lahr R, et al. American Heart Association preparticipation cardiovascular screening for competitive athletes history elements applied to a diverse international screening program. *J Am Coll Cardiol*. 2017;69(11):378.

2. Starkey C, Brown SD, Ryan J. *Examination of Orthopedic and Athletic Injuries*. 3rd ed. Philadelphia, PA: FA Davis; 2010.

3. Anderson MK, Parr GP. *Foundations of Athletic Training: Prevention. Assessment, and Management*. 5th ed. Philadelphia, PA: Wolters Kluwer; 2013.

4. Walker HK, Hall WD, Hurst JW. *Clinical Methods: The History, Physical, and Laboratory Examinations*. 3rd ed. Boston, MA: Butterworths; 1990.

5. Understanding blood pressure readings. American Heart Association website. www.heart.org/en/health-topics/high-blood-pressure/understanding-blood-pressure-readings. Updated November 30, 2017. Accessed May 15, 2020.

6. Ajam T, Mehdirad AA. Electrocardiography. Medscape website. https://emedicine.medscape.com/article/1894014-overview. Updated March 11, 2019. Accessed May 15, 2020.

7. Herbst MK, O'Rourke MC. *Cardiac Ultrasound*. Treasure Island, FL; StatPearls Publishing; 2020. www.ncbi.nlm.nih.gov/books/NBK470584.

8. Urinalysis. University of North Carolina Medical Center website. www.uncmedicalcenter.org/mclendon-clinical-laboratories/available-tests/urinalysis-general-mi-

croscopic. Updated December 16, 2019. Accessed May 15, 2020.

9. Padilla O. Blood tests: Normal values. Merck Manuals website. www.merckmanuals.com/professional/resources/normal-laboratory-values/blood-tests-normal-values. Updated September 2018. Accessed May 15, 2020.

10. Kane NM, Oware A. Nerve conduction and electromyography. *J Neurol.* 2012;259(7):1502-1508.

11. CDC media statement: Measles cases in the U.S. are highest since measles was eliminated in 2000. Centers for Disease Control and Prevention website. www.cdc.gov/media/releases/2019/s0424-highest-measles-cases-since-elimination.html. Published April 25, 2019. Accessed September 2, 2019.

12. Golwalkar M, Pope B, Stauffer J, Snively A, Clemmons N. Mumps outbreaks at four universities—Indiana, 2016. *Morb Mortal Wkly Rep.* 2018;67(29):793-797.

13. Measles, mumps, and rubella (MMR) vaccination: What everyone should know. Centers for Disease Control and Prevention website. www.cdc.gov/vaccines/vpd/mmr/public/index.html. Updated March 28, 2019. Accessed on September 2nd, 2019.

14. Campos-Outcalt, D. Measles: Why it's still a threat. *J Fam Pract.* 2017;66(7):446-449.

15. Mumps clinical information. Minnesota Department of Health website. www.health.state.mn.us/diseases/mumps/hcp/clinical.html#6. Accessed on September 2nd, 2019.

16. Leung AK, Hon KL, Leong KF. Rubella (German measles) revisited. *Hong Kong Med J.* 2019;25(2):134-141.

17. Mount HR, Boyle SD. Aseptic and bacterial meningitis: Evaluation, treatment and prevention. *Am Fam Physician.* 2017;96(5):314-322.

18. Schwartzkopf J. Infectious mononucleosis. *JAAPA.* 2018;31(11):52-53.

19. Shephard, RJ. Exercise and the athlete with infectious mononucleosis. *Clin Sports Med.* 2017;27(2):168-178.

20. American Academy of Pediatrics. Recommendations for prevention and control of influenza in children, 2017-2018. *J Pediatr.* 2017;140(7):1-20.

21. Dobson J, Whitley RJ, Pocock S, Monto AS. Oseltamivir treatment for influenza in adults: a meta-analysis of randomized controlled trials. *Lancet.* 2015;385(9979):1729-1737.

22. Gershon AA, Breuer J, Cohen JI, et al. Varicella zoster virus infection. *Nat Rev Dis Primers.* 2015;2(1):1-41.

23. Gaieski DF, O'Brien NF, Hernandez R. Emergency neurologic life support: Meningitis and encephalitis. *Neurocrit Care.* 2017;27:S124-S133.

24. Hepatitis types. World Health Organization website. www.who.int/hepatitis/topics/en. Accessed on May 29, 2019.

25. Agumadu VC, Ramphul K. Zika virus: A review of literature. *Cureus.* 2018;10(7):e3025. doi:10.7759/cureus.3025

26. Miller MG, Weiler JM, Baker R, Collins J, D'Alonzo G. National Athletic Trainers' Association position statement: management of asthma in athletes. *J Athl Train.* 2005;40(3):224-245.

27. Molis MA, Molis WE. Exercise-induced bronchospasm. *Sports Health.* 2010;2(4):311-317.

28. Kinkade S, Long NA. Acute bronchitis. *Am Fam Physician.* 2016;94(7):259-265.

29. Mostaghim M, Snelling T, McMullan M, Ewe YH, Bajorek B. Impact of clinical decision support on empirical antibiotic prescribing for children with community-acquired pneumonia. *J Paediatr Child Health.* 2019;55:305-311.

30. To KKW, Yip CCY, Yuen KY. Rhinovirus—From bench to bedside. *J Formos Med Assoc.* 2017;116:496-504.

31. Aring AM, Chan MM. Current concepts in adult acute rhinosinusitis. *Am Fam Physician.* 2016;94(2):97-105.

32. Massoth M, Anderson C, McKinney KA. Asthma and chronic rhinosinusitis: Diagnosis and medical management. *Med Sci.* 2019;7(53):1-15.

33. Chinai B, Hunter K, Roy S. Outpatient management of chronic obstructive pulmonary disease: Physician adherence to 2017 global initiative for chronic obstructive lung disease guidelines and effect on patient outcomes. *J Clin Med Res.* 2019;11(8):556-562.

34. Spruit MA, Burtin C, De Boever P, et al. COPD and exercise: does it make a difference? *Breathe.* 2016;12:1-12.

35. Lahousse L, Seys LJM, Joos GF, et al. Epidemiology and impact of chronic bronchitis in chronic obstructive pulmonary disease. *Eur Respir J.* 2017;50:1602470. https://doi.org/10.1183/ 13993003.02470-2016

36. Iqbal AM, Jamal SF. Essential hypertension. StatPearls [Internet]. www.ncbi.nlm.nih.gov/books/NBK539859. Published April 24, 2019. Accessed September 12, 2019.

37. Sharman JE, La Gerche A, Coombes JS. Exercise and cardiovascular risks in patients. *Am J Hypertens.* 2015;28(2):147-158.

38. Rehman S, Nelson VL. Blood Pressure Measurement. StatPearls [Internet]. www.ncbi.nlm.nih.gov/books/NBK482189. Published June 1, 2019. Accessed September 1, 2019.

39. Marian AJ, Braunwald E. Hypertrophic cardiomyopathy: genetics, pathogenesis, clinical manifestations, diagnosis, and therapy. *Circ Res.* 2017;121(7):749-770.

40. Coates A, Mountjoy M, Barr J. Incidence of iron deficiency and iron deficient anemia in elite runners and triathletes. *Clin J Sports Med.* 2017;27(5):493-498.

41. Connes P, Reid H, Hardy-Dessources MD, Morrison E, Hue O. Physiological responses of sickle cell trait carriers during exercise. *Sports Med.* 2008;38(11):931-946.

42. Mitchell BL. Sickle cell trait and sudden death. *Sports Med Open.* 2018;4(1):19. doi: 10.1186/s40798-018-0131-6

43. Exertional sickling. Korey Stringer Institute website. https://ksi.uconn.edu/emergency-conditions/exertional-sickling. Accessed May 24, 2019.

44. Iwakiri K, Kinoshita Y, Habu Y, et al. Evidence-based clinical practice guidelines for gastroesophageal reflux disease 2015. *J Gastroenterol.* 2016;51:751-767.

45. Madisch A, Anderson V, Erick P, et al. The diagnosis and treatment of functional dyspepsia. *Dtsch Arztebl Int.* 2018;115:222-232.

46. Saha, L. Irritable bowel syndrome: Pathogenesis, diagnosis, treatment and evidence-based medicine. *World J Gastroenterol.* 2014;20(22):6759-6773.

47. Fashner J, Gitu AC. Diagnosis and treatment of peptic ulcer disease and *H. pylori* infection. *Am Fam Physician.* 2015;91(4):236-242.

48. Torres J, Mehandru S, Colombel JF. Crohn's disease. *Lancet.* 2017;389(10080):1741-1755.

49. Florez ID, Al-Khalifah R, Sierra JM, et al. The effectiveness and safety of treatment used for acute diarrhea and acute gastroenteritis in children: protocol for a systematic review and network meta-analysis. *Systematic Reviews.* 2016;5(14):1-9. doi:10.1186/s13643-016-0186-8

50. Adams SM, Bornemann PH. Ulcerative colitis. *Am Fam Phys.* 2013;87(10):699-705.

51. Vercellini P, Buggio L, Frattaruolo MP, et al. Medical treatment of endometriosis related pain. *Best Pract Res Clin Obstet Gynaecol.* 2018;51:68-91.

52. Ahn SH, Monsanto SP, Miller C, Singh SS, Thomas R, Tayade C. Pathophysiology and immune dysfunction in endometriosis. *Biomed Res Int.* 2015;2015:1-12.

53. Ackerman KE, Misra M. Amenorrhoea in adolescent female athlete. *Lancet Child Adolesc Health.* 2018;2(9):677-688.

54. McCartney CR, Marshall JC. Polycystic ovary syndrome. *N Engl J Med.* 2016;375:54-64.

55. Kim JH, Lee SM, Lee J-H, et al. Successful conservative management of ruptured ovarian cysts with hemoperitoneum in healthy women. *PLoS ONE.* 2014;9(3):e91171. doi:10.1371/journal.pone.0091171

56. Wawrysiuk S, Naber K, Rechberger T, et al. Prevention and treatment of uncomplicated lower urinary tract infections in the era of increasing antimicrobial resistance—non-antibiotic approaches: a systemic review. *Arch Gynecol Obstet.* 2019;300(4):821-828. doi:10.1007/s00404-019-05256-z

57. Flores-Mireles AL, Walker JN, Caparon M, et al. Urinary tract infections: epidemiology, mechanisms of infection and treatment options. *Nat Rev Microbiol.* 2015;13(5):269-284.

58. DaJusta D, Granberg CF, Villanueva C. Contemporary review of testicular torsion: New concepts, emerging technologies and potential therapeutics. *J Pediatr Urol.* 2013;9(6):723-730.

59. Banyra O, Shulyak A. Acute epididymo-orchitis: Staging and treatment. *Cent European J Urol.* 2002;65(3):139-143.

60. McCrory P, Meeuwisse W, Dvorak J, et al. Consensus statement on concussion in sport—the 5th international conference on concussion in sport held in Berlin, October 2016. *Br J Sports Med.* 2018;51:838-847.

61. Guskiewicz KM, Bruce SL, Cantu RC. National Athletic Trainers' Association position statement. Management of sport-related concussion. *J Athl Train.* 2004;39(3):280-297.

62. Falco-Walter JJ, Scheffer IE, Fisher RS. The new definition and classification of seizures and epilepsy. *Epilepsy Res.* 2018;139:73-79.

63. Seizure first aid and safety. Epilepsy Foundation website. www.epilepsy.com/learn/seizure-first-aid-and-safety. Updated February 25, 2019. Accessed May 24, 2019.

64. Bruehl S. Complex regional pain syndrome. *BMJ.* 2015;351:1-13.

65. Wolffsohn JS, Davies LN. Presbyopia: Effectiveness of correction strategies. *Prog Retin Eye Res.* 2019;68:124-143.

66. Willmann D, Melanson SW. Corneal Injury. StatPearls [Internet]. www.ncbi.nlm.nih.gov/books/NBK459283. Published February 19, 2019. Accessed September 3, 2019.

67. Wipperman JL, Dorsch JH. Evaluation and management of corneal abrasions. *Am Fam Physician.* 2013;87(2):114-120.

68. Watson S, Cabrera-Aguas M, Khoo P. Common eye infections. *Aust Prescr.* 2018;41(3):67-72.

69. Taqi AA, Hussein AS, Jamal NM. Traumatic hyphema frequency and management evaluation: A retrospective case study. *Health Sci J.* 2017; 11(1). doi:10.21767/1791-809X.1000481

70. Greco A, Rizzo MI, De Virgilio A, et al. Emerging concepts in glaucoma and review of literature. *Am J Med.* 2016;129(9):e7-e13.

71. Taylor DJ, Hobby AE, Binns AM, et al. How does age-related macular degeneration affect real-world visual ability and quality of life? A systematic review. *BMJ Open.* 2016;6(12):e011504. doi: 10.1136/bmjopen-2016-011504.

72. Nizami AA, Gulani AC. Cataract. StatPearls [Internet]. www.ncbi.nlm.nih.gov/books/NBK539699. Published June 3, 2019. Accessed September 9, 2019.

73. Dykewicz KS, Wallace DV, Baroody F, et al. Treatment of seasonal allergic rhinitis: An evidence-based focus 2017 guideline update. *Ann Allergy Asthma Immunol.* 2017;119(6):489-511.

74. Kinkade S, Long N. Acute bronchitis. *Am Fam Physician.* 2016;94(7):560-565.

75. Rao A, Berg B, Quezada T, et al. Diagnosis and antibiotic treatment of group A streptococcal pharyngitis in children in a primary care setting: impact of point-of-care polymerase chain reaction. *BMC Pediatr.* 2019;19(24):1-8.

76. Jaworek AJ, Earsai K, Lyons KM, Daggumati S, Hu Amanda, Sataloff RT. Acute infectious laryngitis: a case series. *Ear Nose Throat J.* 2018;97(9):306-309.

77. Farooqi IF, Akram T, Zaka M. Incidence and empiric use of antibiotics therapy for tonsillitis in children. *Int J Appl Res.* 2017;3(12):323-327.

78. Sogebi OA, Oyewole EA, Mabifah TO. Traumatic tympanic membrane perforations: Characteristics and factors affecting outcome. *Ghana Med J.* 2018;52(1):34-40.

79. Rosenfeld RM, Schwartz SR, Cannon CR, et al. Clinical practice guideline: Acute otitis externa. *Otolaryngol Head Neck Surg.* 2014;150(1S):e21-24.

80. American Academy of Pediatrics and American Academy of Family Physicians. Clinical practice guidelines: diag-

nosis and management of acute otitis media. *Pediatrics.* 2004;113(5):1451-1465.

81. Burrows HL, Blackwood RA, Cooke JM. UMHS Otitis media guidelines. University of Michigan Medicine website. www.med.umich.edu/1info/FHP/practiceguides/om/OM.pdf. Published April 2013. Accessed September 9, 2019.

82. Haik, J. Givol O, Kornhaber R, et al. Cauliflower ear—a minimally invasive treatment method in a wrestling athlete: a case report. *Int Med Case Rep J.* 2018;11:5-7. doi: 10.2147/IMCRJ.S152145

83. Jimenez CC, Corcoran MH, Crawley JT, et al. National Athletic Trainers' Association position statement: management of the athlete with type 1 diabetes mellitus. *J Athl Train.* 2007;42(4):536-545.

84. Luksch JR, Collin PB. Thyroid disorders in athletes. *Curr Sports Med Rep.* 2018;17(2):59-64.

85. Van Dijk SM, Hallensleben NDL, van Santvoort HC, et al. Acute pancreatitis: recent advances through randomized trials. *Gut.* 2017;66:2024-2032.

86. Sexually transmitted disease: Data and statistics. Centers for Disease Control and Prevention website. www.cdc.gov/std/stats/default.htm. Accessed September 2, 2019.

87. Workowski KA. Centers for Disease Control and Prevention sexually transmitted disease treatment guidelines. *Clin Infect Dis.* 2015;61(8):S759-S762.

88. Studer L, Cardoza-Favarato G. Human Papillomavirus. StatPearls [Internet]. www.ncbi.nlm.nih.gov/books/NBK448132. Published October 27, 2019. Accessed September 13, 2019.

89. Zinder SM, Basler RS, Foley J. National Athletic Trainers' Association statement: skin diseases. *J. Athl Train.* 2010;45(4):411-428.

90. Braun T, Kahanov L, Dannelly K, Lauber C. CA-MRSA infection incidence and care in high school and intercollegiate athletics. *Med Sci Sports Exerc.* 2016;48(8):1530-1538.

91. Baggish, A, Drezner, JA, Kim, J, Martinez, M, Prutkin, JM. Resurgence of sport in the wake of COVID-19: Cardiac considerations in competitive athletes. *Br J Sports Med.* 2020;54(19):1130-1131.

92. Barzilay, R, Moore, TM, Greenberg, DM, DiDomenico, GE, Brown, LA, White, LK, . . . Gur, RE. Resilience, COVID-19-related stress, anxiety and depression during the pandemic in a large population enriched for healthcare providers. *Transl Psychiatry.* 2020;10(1):291.

93. Demir, GT, Cicioğlu, Hİ, İlhan, EL. Athlete's anxiety to catch the novel coronavirus (Covid-19) scale (AACNCS): Validity and reliability study. *J. Hum. Sci.* 2020;17(2):458-468.

94. Graupensperger, S, Benson, AJ, Kilmer, JR, Evans, MB. Social (un)distancing: Teammate interactions, athletic identity, and mental health of student-athletes during the COVID-19 pandemic. *J Adolesc Health.* 2020;67(5):662-670.

95. Hagen, J, Stone, JD, Hornsby, WG, Stephenson, M, Mangine, R, Joseph, M, Galster, S. COVID-19 surveillance and competition in sport: Utilizing sport science to protect athletes and staff during and after the pandemic. *J Funct Morphol Kinesiol.* 2020;5(3):69.

96. Hull, JH, Loosemore, M, Schwellnus, M. Respiratory health in athletes: Facing the COVID-19 challenge. *Lancet Respir Med.* 2020;8(6):557-558.

97. Labrague, LJ, De los Santos, J. Fear of Covid-19, psychological distress, work satisfaction and turnover intention among frontline nurses. *J Nurs Manag.* 2020; doi: 10.21203/rs.3.rs-35366/v1

98. Mehrsafar, AH, Gazerani, P, Zadeh, AM, Sánchez, JCJ. Addressing potential impact of COVID-19 pandemic on physical and mental health of elite athletes. *Brain Behav Immun.* 2020;87:147-148.

99. Pappa, S, Ntella, V, Giannakas, T, Giannakoulis, VG, Papoutsi, E, Katsaounou, P. Prevalence of depression, anxiety, and insomnia among healthcare workers during the COVID-19 pandemic: A systematic review and meta-analysis. *Brain Behav Immun.* 2020;88:901-907.

100. Reardon, CL, Bindra, A, Blauwet, C, Budgett, R, Campriani, N, Currie, A, . . . Purcell, R. Mental health management of elite athletes during COVID-19: A narrative review and recommendations. *Br J Sports Med.* 2020; doi: 10.1136/bjsports-2020-102884

101. Sarto, F, Impellizzeri, FM, Spörri, J, Porcelli, S, Olmo, J, Requena, B, . . . Buchheit, M. Impact of potential physiological changes due to COVID-19 home confinement on athlete health protection in elite sports: A call for awareness in sports programming. *Sports Med.* 2020;50(8):1417-1419

102. Twenge, JM, Joiner, TE. US Census Bureau-assessed prevalence of anxiety and depressive symptoms in 2019 and during the 2020 COVID-19 pandemic. *Depress Anxiety.* 2020;37(10):954-956.

103. Yeo, TJ. Sport and exercise during and beyond the COVID-19 pandemic. *Eur J Prev Cardiol.* 2020;27(12):1239-1241.

Chapter 19

1. Sharp M-L, Fear NT, Rona RJ, et al. Stigma as a barrier to seeking health care among military personnel with mental health problems. *Epidemiol Rev.* 2015;37(1):144-162.

2. Mental health by the numbers. National Alliance on Mental Illness website. www.nami.org/Learn-More/Mental-Health-By-the-Numbers. Updated September 2019. Accessed October 1, 2019.

3. Suicide facts at a glance—2015. Centers for Disease Control and Prevention website. www.cdc.gov/violenceprevention/pdf/suicide-datasheet-a.pdf. Accessed August 1, 2018.

4. 10 Leading Causes of Death by Age Group, United States, 2015. Centers for Disease Control and Prevention website. www.cdc.gov/injury/images/lc-charts/leading_causes_of_death_age_group_2015_1050w740h.gif. Accessed August 1, 2018.

5. National Athletic Trainers' Association. 10 for 10 slides: NATA—Mental Health Issues with Student-Athletes at the Collegiate Level. Presentation at: NATA Clinical Symposia and AT Expo; June 26, 2018; New Orleans, LA.

6. Mental illness. National Institute of Mental Health website. www.nimh.nih.gov/health/statistics/mental-illness.shtml. Updated February 2019. Accessed April 1, 2019.

7. Schutte NS, Malouff JM, Thorsteinsson EB, Bhullar N, Rooke SE. A meta-analytic investigation of the relationship between emotional intelligence and health. *Pers Individ Dif.* 2007;42(6):921-933.

8. Mayer JD, Caruso DR, Salovey P. Emotional intelligence meets traditional standards for an intelligence. *Intelligence.* 1999;27:267-298.

9. Hamann DL. An assessment of anxiety in instrumental and vocal performances. *JRes Music Educ.* 1982;30(2):77-90. doi:10.2307/3345040

10. Proctor SL, Boan-Lenzo C. Prevalence of depressive symptoms in male intercollegiate student-athletes and nonathletes. *J Clin Sport Psychol.* 2010;4:204-220. doi:10.1123/jcsp.4.3.204

11. Yang J, Peek-Asa C, Corlette JD, Cheng G, Foster DT, Albright J. Prevalence of and risk factors associated with symptoms of depression in competitive collegiate student athletes. *Clin J Sport Med.* 2007;17:481-487. doi:10.1097/JSM.0b013e31815aed6b

12. Trojian T. Depression is under-recognized in the sport setting: time for primary care sports medicine to be proactive and screen widely for depression symptoms. *Br J Sports Med.* 2016;50:137-139. doi:10.1136/bjsports-2015-095582

13. Wolanin A, Gross M, Hong E. Depression in athletes: prevalence and risk factors. *Curr Sports Med Rep.* 2015;14(1):56-60.

14. Hughes L, Leavvey G. Setting the bar: athletes and vulnerability to mental illness. *Br J Psychiatry.* 2012;200(2):95-96.

15. Gulliver A, Griffiths KM, Christensen H, et al. Internet-based interventions to promote mental health help-seeking in elite athletes: an exploratory randomized controlled trial. *J Med Internet Res.* 2012;14(3):e69.

16. Gulliver A, Griffiths KM, Christensen H, et al. Barriers and facilitators to mental health help-seeking for young elite athletes: a qualitative study. *BMC Psychiatry.* 2012;12(1):157.

17. Bruner MW, Munroe-Chandler KJ, Spink KS. Entry into elite sport: a preliminary investigation into the transition experiences of rookie athletes. *J Appl Sport Psychol.* 2008;20(2):236-252.

18. Hanton S, Fletcher D, Coughlan G. Stress in elite sport performers: a comparative study of competitive and organizational stressors. *J Sports Sci.* 2005;23(10):1129-1141.

19. Noblet AJ, Gifford SM. The sources of stress experiences by professional Australian footballers. *J Appl Sport Psychol.* 2002;14(1):1-13.

20. Daley A. Exercise and depression: a review of reviews. *J Clin Psychol Med Settings.* 2008;15(2):140-147.

21. Peluso M, Andrade L. Physical activity and mental health: the association between exercise and mood. *Clinics.* 2005;60(1):61-70.

22. ADHD foundation. ADHD Childhood website. www.adhdchildhood.com. Accessed August 1, 2018.

23. Bipolar disorder—Frequently asked questions. Brain and Behavior Research Foundation website. www.bbrfoundation.org/faq/frequently-asked-questions-about-bipolar-disorder. Accessed August 1, 2018.

24. Tracey J. The emotional responses to the injury and rehabilitation process. *J Appl Sport Psychol.* 2003;15:279-293.

25. Udry E, Gould D, Bridges D, et al. Down but not out: athlete responses to season ending injuries. *J Sport Exerc Psychol.* 1997;19(3):229-248.

26. Wiese-Bjornstal D, Smith A, Shaffer S, et al. An integrated model of response to sport injury: psychological and sociological dynamics. *J Appl Sport Psychol.* 1998;10(1);49.

27. Mainwaring L. Restoration of self: a model for the psychological response of athletes to severe knee injuries. *Can J Rehabil.* 1999;12(3):145-154.

28. Smith, A. Scott S, O'Fallon W, et al. Emotional responses of athletes to injury. *Mayo Clin Proc.* 1990;65(1):38-50.

29. Walker N, Thather J, Lavallee D. Psychological responses to injury in competitive sport: a critical review. *J R Soc Health.* 2007;127(4):174-180.

30. Wiese-Bjornstal D. Psychology and sociocultural affect injury risk, response, and recovery in high-intensity athletes: a consensus statement. *Scand J Med Sci Sport.* 2010;20(2):103-111.

31. Gulliver A, Griffiths K, Mackinnon A, et al. The mental health of Australian elite athletes. *J Sci Med Sport.* 2015;18(3):255-261.

32. Gouttebare V, Frings-Dresen M, Sluiter J. Mental and psychosocial health among current and former professional footballers. *Occup Med.* 2015;65(3):190-196.

33. Hammond T, Gialloreto C, Kubas H, et al. The prevalence of failure-based depression among elite athletes. *Clin J Sport Med.* 2013;23(4):273-277.

34. Rice S, Purcell R, Silva S, et al. The mental health of elite athletes: A narrative systematic review. *Sports Med.* 2016;46:1333-1353.

35. Haggar M, Chatzisarantis N, Griffin M. Injury representations, coping, emotions, and functional outcomes in athletes with sports-related injuries: a test of self-regulatory theory. *J Appl Soc Psychol.* 2005;35(11):2345-2374.

36. Prochaska JO, DiClemente CC. Transtheoretical therapy: Toward a more integrative model of change. *Psychotherapy.* 1982;19:276-288.

37. Clement D. The transtheoretical model: An exploratory look at its applicability to injury rehabilitation. *J Sport Rehabil.* 2008;17(3):269-282.

38. Tongue J, Epps H, Forese L. Communication skills for patient-centered care research-based, easily learned

techniques for medical interviews. *J Bone Joint Surg.* 2005;87(3):652-658.

39. Larson G, Starkey C, Zaichkowsky L. Psychological aspects of athletic injuries as perceived by athletic trainers. *Sport Psychol.* 1996;10:15-24.

40. Weinberg R, Gould D, eds. *Foundations in Sport and Exercise Psychology.* Champaign, IL: Human Kinetics; 2011.

41. Tilton SR. Review of the state-trait anxiety inventory (STAI). *News Notes.* 2008;48(2):1-3.

42. Leddy M, Lambert M, Ogles B. Psychological consequences of athletic injury among high-level competitors. *Res Q Exerc Sport.* 1994;65:347-354.

43. Cassidy C. Understanding sport-injury anxiety. *Athl Ther Today.* 2006;11:57-58.

44. Erlanger D, Kutner K, Barth J, et al. Neuropsychology of sports-related head injury: dementia pugilistica to post-concussion syndrome. *Clin Neuropsychol.* 1999;13(2):193-209.

45. Hutchison M, Mainwaring L, Comper P, et al. Differential emotional responses of varsity athletes to concussion and musculoskeletal injuries. *Clin J Sport Med.* 2009;19(1):13-19.

46. Mainwaring L, Hutchison M, Bisschop S, et al. Emotional response to sport concussion compared to ACL injury. *Brain Inj.* 2010;24(2):589-597.

47. Grandquist M, Hamson-Utley J, Kenow L, et al. *Psychosocial Strategies for Athletic Training.* Philadelphia, PA: FA Davis; 2014.

48. Chmielewski T, Jones D, Day T, et al. The association of pain and fear of movement/reinjury with function during anterior cruciate ligament reconstruction rehabilitation. *J Orthop Sports Phys Ther.* 2008;38(12):746-753.

49. Kvist J, Sporrstedt K, Good L. Fear of reinjury: a hindrance for returning to sports after anterior cruciate ligament reconstruction. *Knee Surg Sports Traumatol Arthrosc.* 2005;13:393-397.

50. Walker N, Thatcher J, Lavallee D, et al. The emotional response to athletic injury: reinjury anxiety. In: Lavallee D, Thatcher J, Jones M, eds. *Coping and Emotion in Sport.* Hauppauge, NY: Nova Science Publishers; 2004;91-103.

51. Johnston L, Carroll D. The psychological impact of injury: effects of prior sport and exercise involvement. *Br J Sports Med.* 2000;34:436-439.

52. Podlog L, Dimmock J, Miller J. A review of return to sport concerns following injury rehabilitation: practitioner strategies for enhancing recovery outcomes. *Phys Ther Sport.* 2011;12:36-42.

53. Podlog L, Eklund R. The psychosocial aspects of a return to sport following serious injury: a review of the literature from a self-determination perspective. *Psychol Sport Exerc.* 2007;8:535-566.

54. Tongue J, Epps H, Forese L. Communication skills for patient-centered care. Research-based, easily learned techniques for medical interviews. *J Bone Joint Surg.* 2005;87(3):652-658.

55. Wiese-Bjornstal D. Reflections on a quarter century of research in sports medicine psychology. *Rev Psicol Deporte.* 2014;23(2):411-421.

56. Knackstedt P. How coaches factor into student-athlete mental health. *Athletic Business.* 2018;43(3):28-29.

57. Brown GT, Hainline B, Krosus E, et al. *Mind, Body and Sport—Understanding and Supporting Student-Athlete Mental Health.* Indianapolis, IN: National Collegiate Athletic Association; 2014.

58. Covassin T, Beidler E, Ostrowski J, Wallace J. Psychosocial aspects of rehabilitation in sports. *Clin Sports Med.* 2015;34:199-212.

59. Feltz D. The psychology of sports injuries. In: Vinger PE, Hoerner ER, eds. *Sports Injuries: The Unthwarted Epidemic.* 2nd ed. Boston, MA: John Wright; 1986;336-344.

60. Clement D, Granquist M, Arvinen-Barrow M. Psychosocial aspects of athletic injuries as perceived by athletic trainers. *J Athletic Train.* 2013;48(4):512-521.

61. Hardy L, Jones J, Gould D. *Understanding Psychological Preparation for Sport.* Hoboken NJ: John Wiley & Sons; 1996.

62. Etzel E, Watson J, Gardner F. Ethical challenges for psychological consultations in intercollegiate athletics. *J Clin Sport Psychol.* 2007;1(3):304-317. doi:10.1123/jcsp.1.3.304

63. Lopez R, Levy J. Student athletes' perceived barriers to and preferences for seeking counseling. *J Coll Couns.* 2013;16(1):19-31.

64. Etzel E, Pinkney J, Hinkle J. College student-athletes and needs assessment. In: Thomas CC, ed. *Multicultural Needs Assessment for College and University Student Populations.* Springfield, IL: C.C. Thomas; 1994:155-172.

65. Williams J, Andersen M. Psychosocial antecedents of sport injury: review and critique of the stress and injury model. *J Appl Sport Psychol.* 1998;10(1):5-25.

66. Ross M, Berger R, Sage G. Effects of stress inoculation training on athletes' post-surgical pain and rehabilitation after orthopedic injury. *J Consult Clin Psychol.* 1996;64:406-410.

67. Jacobson E. Progressive relaxation. *Am J Psychol.* 1987;100(3-4):522-537.

68. Hanrahan S, Andreson M. *The Routledge Handbook of Applied Sport Psychology.* Abingdon: Routledge, Taylor & Francis; 2010.

69. Holmes, P, Collins, D. The PETTLEP approach to motor imagery: A functional equivalence model for sport psychologists. *J Appl Sport Psychol.* 2001;13:60-83.

70. Ievleva L, Orlick T. Mental links to enhanced healing: an exploratory study. *Sport Psychol.* 1991;5(1):25-40.

71. *Diagnostic and Statistical Manual of Mental Disorders: DSM-5.* Arlington, VA: American Psychiatric Publishing; 2013.

72. Bergland C. Diaphragmatic breathing exercises and your vagus nerve. Psychology Today website. www.psychologytoday.com/us/blog/the-athletes-way/201705/

diaphragmatic-breathing-exercises-and-your-vagus-nerve. Published May 16, 2017. Accessed September 25, 2018.

73. Mack S, Jacobi F, Gerschler A, et al. Self-reported utilization of mental health services in the adult German population–Evidence for unmet needs? Results of the DEGS 1-Mental Health Module (DEGS1-MH). *Int J Meth Psych Res*. 2014;23:289-303.

74. Birnbaum HG, Kessler RC, Kelley D, Ben-Hamadi R, Joish VN, Greenberg PE. Employer burden of mild, moderate, and severe major depressive disorder: mental health services utilization and costs, and work performance. *Depress Anxiety*. 2010;27:1-78.

75. Law YW, Yip PS, Zhang Y, Caine ED. The chronic impact of work on suicide and under-utilization of psychiatric and psychosocial services. *J Affect Disord*. 2014;168:254-261.

76. Kessler RC, Heeringa SG, Stein MB, et al. Thirty-day prevalence of DSM-IV mental disorders among non-deployed soldiers in the U.S. Army: Results from the Army Study to Assess Risk and Resilience in Service members (STARRS). *JAMA Psychiatry*. 2014;71(5):504-513.

77. Hayslip B, Petrie TA, MacIntire MM, Jones GM. The influences of skill level, anxiety, and psychological skills use on amateur golfers' performance. *J Appl Sport Psychol*. 2010;22:123-133. doi:10.1080/10413200903554281

78. Harrison, B. Counseling people in the performing arts. Counseling Today website. https://ct.counseling.org/2018/04/counseling-people-in-the-performing-arts. Published April 10, 2018. Accessed May 18, 2019.

79. McCullough KA, Phelps KD, Spindler KP, et al. Return to high school- and college-level football after anterior cruciate ligament reconstruction: A Multicenter Orthopaedic Outcomes Network (MOON) cohort study. *Am J Sports Med*. 2012;40(11):2523-2529. doi:10.1177/0363546512456836

80. Pattyn E, Verhaeghe M, Bracke P. The gender gap in mental health service use. *Soc Psychiatry Psychiatr Epidemiol*. 2015;50:1089-1095. doi:10.1007/s00127-015-1038-x

81. Na HR, Kang EH, Lee JH, Yu BH. The genetic basis of panic disorder. *J Korean Med Sci*. 2011;26:701-710. doi:10.3346/jkms.2011.26.6.701

82. What is stigma? Why is it a problem? National Alliance on Mental Illness website. www.nami.org/stigma. Accessed May 18, 2019.

83. Gadermann AM, Engle CC, Naifeh JA, et al. Prevalence of DSM-IV major depression among U.S. military personnel: meta-analysis and simulation. *Mil Med*. 2012;177(8):47-59. doi:10.7205/milmed-d-12-00103

84. Attention Deficit Hyperactivity Disorder. National Institute of Mental Health website. www.nimh.nih.gov/health/statistics/attention-deficit-hyperactivity-disorder-adhd.shtml. Updated November 2017. Accessed May 19, 2019

85. Locke E, Latham G. The application of goal setting to sports. *J Sport Psychol*. 1985;7:205-222.

86. Locke E, Shaw K, Saari L, Latham G. Goal setting and task performance: 1969-1980. *Psychol Bull*. 1981;90:125-152.

87. Neal T, Diamond A, Goldman S, et al. Inter-association recommendations for developing a plan to recognize and refer student-athletes with psychological concerns at the collegiate level: an executive summary of a consensus statement. *J Athl Train*. 2013;48(5):716-720. doi:10.4085/1062-6050-48.4.13

88. Neal TL, Diamond AB, Goldman S, et al. Interassociation recommendations for developing a plan to recognize and refer student-athletes with psychological concerns at the secondary school level: a consensus statement. *J Athl Train*. 2015;50(3):231-249.

89. Aghajani Inche Kikanloo A, Jalali K, Asadi Z, Shokrpour N, Amiri M, Bazrafkan L. Emotional intelligence skills: is nurses' stress and professional competence related to their emotional intelligence training? A quasi experimental study. *J Adv Med Educ Prof*. 2019;7(3):138-143. doi:10.30476/JAMP.2019.74922.

90. Ni, Preston. How to increase your emotional intelligence. Six essentials. Psychology Today website. www.psychologytoday.com/us/blog/communication-success/201410/how-increase-your-emotional-intelligence-6-essentials. Published October 2014. Accessed April 16, 2020.

91. Michael Phelps launches new mental health campaign. Olympic Channel website. www.olympicchannel.com/en/stories/news/detail/michael-phelps-launches-new-mental-health-campaign. Published June 2018. Accessed April 19, 2020.

92. Duran, H.B. Michael Phelps dives into mental health advocacy with Talkspace. A List website. www.alistdaily.com/lifestyle/michael-phelps-talkspace-mental-health. Published May 30, 2018. Accessed April 19, 2020.

93. Michael Phelps launches mental health campaign. NBC Sports website. https://olympics.nbcsports.com/2018/05/22/michael-phelps-mental-health. Published May 2018. Accessed April 19, 2020.

94. Salovey P, Mayer J. Emotional intelligence. *Imagin Cogn Pers*. 1990;9(3):185-211. doi:10.2190/DUGG-P24E-52WK-6CDG

95. Van Rooy DL, Viswesvaran C. Emotional intelligence: A meta-analytic investigation of predictive validity and nomological network. *J Vocat Behav*. 2004;65(1):71-95. doi:10.1016/S0001-8791(03)00076-9

96. Stein SJ, Book H. *The EQ Edge: Emotional Intelligence and Your Success*. Toronto, Ontario: Stoddart; 2006.

97. Carmeli A. The relationship between emotional intelligence and work attitudes, behavior and outcomes: An examination among senior managers. *J Manag Psychol*. 2003;18(8):788-813.

98. APA dictionary of psychology. American Psychological Association website. https://dictionary.apa.org/cross-cultural-psychology. Accessed May, 3, 2020.

Chapter 20

1. Taylor DM. Americans With Disabilities: 2014. Household economic studies. *Current Population Reports*. Nov

2018;70-152. www.census.gov/content/dam/Census/library/publications/2018/demo/p70-152.pdf.

2. Conley KM, Bolin DJ, Carek PJ, Konin JG, Neal TL, Violette D. *J Athl Train*. 2014;49(1):102-120.

3. Patel DR, Greydanus DE. Sport participation by physically and cognitively challenged young athletes. *Pediatr Clin North Am*. 2010;57:795-817.

4. Achterstraat, P. *Managing Injured Police*. Sydney, Australia: Audit Office of New South Wales; 2008.

5. Pryor RR, Colburn D, Crill MT, Hostler DP, Suyama J. Fitness characteristics of a suburban special weapons and tactics team. *J Strength Cond Res*. 2012;26:752-757.

6. Boyce RW, Hiatt AR, Jones GR. Workers' compensation claims and physical fitness capacity of police officers. *Health Values*. 1992;16:22-29.

7. Holloway-Beth A, Forst L, Freels S, Brandt-Rauf S, Friedman L. Occupational injury surveillance among law enforcement officers using workers' compensation data, Illinois 1980 to 2008. *J Occup Environ Med*. 2016;58:594-600.

8. Orr R. Optimizing the conditioning of new recruits. Paper presented at the Tactical Strength and Conditioning Conference; 2004; San Diego, California.

9. Booth CK, Probert B, Forbes-Ewan C, Coad RA. Australian army recruits in training display symptoms of overtraining. *Mil Med*. 2006;171(11):1059-1064.

10. Knapik JJ, Grier T, Spiess A, et al. Injury rates and injury risk factors among Federal Bureau of Investigation new agent trainees. *BMC Public Health*. 2011;11(1):920.

11. Knapik JJ, Hauret KG, Jones BH. Primary prevention of injuries in initial entry training. *Recruit Med*. 2006;125-146.

12. Knapik JJ, Reynolds KL, Harman E. Soldier load carriage: historical, physiological, biomechanical, and medical aspects. *Mil Med*. 2004;169(1):45-56.

13. Knapik JJ, Sharp MA, Canham-Chervak M, Hauret K, Patton JF, Jones BH. Risk factors for training-related injuries among men and women in basic combat training. *Med Sci Sports Exerc*. 2001;33(6):946-954.

14. Havenetidis K, Kardaris D, Paxinos T. Profiles of musculoskeletal injuries among Greek Army officer cadets during basic combat training. *Mil Med*. 2011;176(3):297-303.

15. Jones BH, Bovee MW, Harris JM, Cowan DN. Intrinsic risk factors for exercise-related injuries among male and female army trainees. *Am J Sport Med*. 1993;21(5):705-710.

16. Reichard AA, Jackson LL. Occupational injuries among emergency responders. *Am J Ind Med*. 2010;53(1):1-11.

17. Walton SM, Conrad KM, Furner SE, Samo DG. Cause, type, and workers' compensation costs of injury to fire fighters. *Am J Ind Med*. 2003;43(4):454-458.

18. Orr R, Stierli M, Amabile ML, Wilkes B. The impact of a structured reconditioning program on the physical attributes and attitudes of injured police officers: A pilot study. *J Aust Strength Cond*. 2013;21(4):42.

19. Knapik JJ, Sharp MA, Canham-Chervak M, Hauret K, Patton JF, Jones BH. Risk factors for training-related injuries among men and women in basic combat training. *Med Sci Sports Exerc*. 2001;33(6)946-954.

20. Defense Health Services Branch. *Australian Defense Force Health Status Report*. Canberra, Australia: Department of Defense; 2000.

21. Cohen SP, Griffith S, Larkin TM, Villena F, Larkin R. Presentation, diagnoses, mechanisms of injury, and treatment of soldiers injured in Operation Iraqi Freedom: an epidemiological study conducted at two military pain management centers. *Anesth Analg*. 2005;101(4):1098-1103.

22. Kaufman KR, Brodine S, Shaffer R. Military training-related injuries: surveillance, research, and prevention. *Am J Prev Med*. (2000);18(3):54-63.

23. O'Connor F. Injuries during Marine Corps officer basic training. *Mil Med*. 2000;165(7):515-520.

24. Wright VJ, Perricelli BC. Age-related rates of decline in performance among elite senior athletes. *Am J Sports Med*. 2008;36(3):443-450.

25. Roy TC, Knapik JJ, Ritland BM, Murphy N, Sharp MA. Risk factors for musculoskeletal injuries for soldiers deployed to Afghanistan. *Aviat Space Environ Med*. 2012;83(11):1060-1066.

26. Park K, Hur P, Rosengren KS, Horn GP, Hsiao-Wecksler ET. Effect of load carriage on gait due to firefighting air bottle configuration. *Ergonomics*. 2010;53(7):882-891.

27. Park K, Hur P, Rosengren KS, Horn GP, Hsiao-Wecksler ET. Changes in kinetic and kinematic gait parameters due to firefighting air bottle configuration. Paper presented at the North American Congress on Biomechanics; 2008; Ann Arbor, Michigan.

28. Louhevaara V, Tuomi T, Smolander J, et al. Cardiorespiratory strain in jobs that require respiratory protection. *Int Arch Occup Environ Health*. 1985;55:195-206.

29. Richmond VL, Rayson MP, Wilkinson DM, et al. Development of an operational fitness test for the Royal Air Force. *Ergonomics*. 2008;51(6):935-946.

30. von Heimburg ED, Rasmussen AK, Medbø JI. Physiological responses of firefighters and performance predictors during a simulated rescue of hospital patients. *Ergonomics*. 2006;49(2):111-126.

31. Ruby B, Gaskill S, Heil D, Sharkey B, Hansen B, Lanford D. Changes in salivary IgA during arduous wildfire suppression relative to work-shift length. *Med Sci Sports Exerc*. 2002;34:S195.

32. Karter MJ, Molis JL. U.S. firefighter injuries—2010. *NFPA Journal*. November/December 2011.

33. Gavin ML. Dwarfism special needs factsheet. Kids Health website. https://kidshealth.org/en/parents/dwarfism-factsheet.html. Accessed January 17, 2019.

34. Marijon E, Tafflet M, Celermajer DS, et al. Sports-related sudden death in the general population. *Circulation*. 2011;124:672-681.

35. Morrison BN, McKinney J, Isserow S, et al. Assessment of cardiovascular risk and preparticipation screening protocols in masters athletes: the masters athlete screening study (MASS): a cross-sectional study. *BMJ Open Sport Exerc Med.* 2018;4(1):e000370.

36. Valovich McLeod TC, Decoster LC, Loud KJ, et al. National Athletic Trainers' Association position statement: prevention of pediatric overuse injuries. *J Athl Train.* 2011;46(2):206-220.

37. Walsh-Flanagan K, Cuppett M. *Medical Conditions in the Athlete.* 3rd ed. Champaign, IL: Human Kinetics; 2016.

38. Derman W, Schwellnus MP, Jordaan E, et al. Sport, sex and age increase risk of illness at the Rio 2016 Summer Paralympic Games: a prospective cohort study of 51,198 athlete days. *Br J Sports Med.* 2018;52(1):17-23.

39. Derman W, Runciman P, Schwellnus M, et al. High precompetition injury rate dominates the injury profile at the Rio 2016 Summer Paralympic Games: a prospective cohort study of 51,198 athlete days. *Br J Sports Med.* 2018;52(1):24-31.

40. Klenck C, Gebke K. Practical management: common medical problems in disabled athletes. *Clin J Sport Med.* 2007;17:55-60.

41. Silva MPM, Duarte E, Silva AAC, et al. Aspects of sports injuries in athletes with visual impairment. *Revista Brasileira de Medicina do Esporte.* 2011;17(5):319-323.

42. Rovner BW. The Charles Bonnet syndrome: a review of recent research. *Curr Opin Ophthalmol.* 2006;17(3):275-277.

43. Winckler C, Miranda AJ. The athlete with visual impairment. *Aspetar Sports Med J.* 2018;7:138-141.

44. Webster JB, Levy CE, Bryant PR, Prusakowski PE. Sports and recreation for persons with limb deficiency. *Arch Phys Med Rehabil.* 2001;82:S38-S44.

45. Rudolph L, Willick SE. Review of Injury Epidemiology in Paralympic Sports. In *Adaptive Sports Medicine* 2018 (pp. 51-58). Springer.

46. Pepper M, Willick S. Maximizing physical activity in athletes with amputations. *Curr Sports Med Rep.* 2009;8(6):339-44.

47. Dec KL, Sparrow KJ, McKeag DB. 2000. The physically-challenged athlete: medical issues and assessment. *Sport Med.* 2000;29(4):245-258.

48. International Paralympic Committee. Classification explained. https://www.paralympic.org/classification. Accessed October 24, 2020.

49. Crutchfield KE. Managing patients with neurologic disorders who participate in sports activities. *Sports Neurology.* 2014;20(6):1657-1666.

50. Definition of intellectual disability. American Association on Intellectual and Developmental Disabilities website. https://aaidd.org/intellectual-disability/definition. Accessed May 16, 2019.

51. Sefton JM, Burkhardt TA. Introduction to the tactical athlete special issue. *J Athl Train.* 2016;51(11):845.

52. Cheng AS, Hung LK. Randomized controlled trial of workplace-based rehabilitation for work-related rotator cuff disorder. *J Occ Rehab.* 2007;17(3):487-503.

53. Goss DL, Christopher GE, Faulk RT, Moore J. Functional training program bridges rehabilitation and return to duty. *Journal of special operations medicine: a peer reviewed journal for SOF medical professionals.* 2009;9(2):29.

54. Hogshead-Makar N, Sorensen EA. Pregnant and parenting student-athletes: resources and model policies. National College Athletic Association. www.ncaa.org/sites/default/files/PregnancyToolkit.pdf.

55. International Paralympic Committee. WADA publish 2021 prohibited list. https://www.paralympic.org/news/wada-publish-2021-prohibited-list?gclid=CjwKCAjwoc_8BRAcEiwAzJevtXklMRu76FUHZowaJXC0gEsYf34WLkD1KJ4bSLtrfI5I205D6eYKzxoCYS0QAvD_BwE. Accessed October 24, 2020.

56. Karlsson A. Autonomic dysreflexia. *Spinal Cord.* 1999;37(6):383-391.

57. Gee C, West C, Krassioukov A. Boosting in elite athletes with spinal cord injury: a critical review of physiology and testing procedures. *Sports Med.* 2015;45(8):1133-1142.

58. Foley DC, McCutcheon H. Detecting pain in people with an intellectual disability. *Accid Emerg Nurs.* 2004;12(4):196-200.

59. Resources. National Pressure Injury Advisory Panel website. www.npuap.org/resources/educational-and-clinical-resources/npuap-pressure-injury-stages. Accessed October 23, 2020.

60. Classification explained. International Paralympic Committee website. www.paralympic.org/classification. Accessed October 23, 2020.

Chapter 21

1. Boggess BR, Bytomski JR. Medicolegal aspects of sports medicine. *Prim Care.* 2013;40(2):525-535.

2. Prentice WE. *Therapeutic Modalities in Rehabilitation.* McGraw Hill; 2017.

3. Knight KL. *Cryotherapy in Sport Injury Management.* Champaign, IL: Human Kinetics: 1995.

4. Steinagel MC. Cryotherapy in sport injury management. *J Athl Train.* 1996;31(3):277.

5. Escalante G. Sports injuries: should you use heat or cold? Bodybuilding website. www.bodybuilding.com/content/sports-injuries-should-you-use-heat-or-cold.html. Published April 29, 2019.

6. Jutte LS, Hawkins J, Miller KC, Long BC, Knight KL. Skinfold thickness at 8 common cryotherapy sites in various athletic populations. *J Athl Train.* 2012;47(2):170-177.

7. Knight KL, Londeree BR. Comparison of blood flow in the ankle of uninjured subjects during therapeutic applications of heat, cold, and exercise. *Med Sci Sports Exerc.* 1980;12(1):76-80.

8. Peake JM, Roberts LA, Figueiredo VC, et al. The effects of cold water immersion and active recovery on inflam-

mation and cell stress responses in human skeletal muscle after resistance exercise. *J Physiol.* 2017;595(3):695-711.

9. Lehmann A, Ivanovic N, Saxer S. [Superficial heat and cold treatments in backache. Are superficial heat and cold treatments effective in adults with low back pain?]. *Pflege Zeitschrift.* 2014;67(9):556-557.

10. Lehmann JF, Warren CG, Scham SM. Therapeutic heat and cold. *Clin Orthop Relat Res.* 1974;(99):207-245.

11. Price R, Lehmann JF. Influence of muscle cooling on the viscoelastic response of the human ankle to sinusoidal displacements. *Arch Phys Med Rehabil.* 1990;71(10):745-748.

12. Price R, Lehmann JF, Boswell-Bessette S, Burleigh A, deLateur BJ. Influence of cryotherapy on spasticity at the human ankle. *Arch Phys Med Rehab.* 1993;74(3):300-304.

13. McMaster WC. Cryotherapy. *Phys Sportsmed.* 1982;10(11):112-119.

14. Merrick MA, Jutte LS, Smith ME. Cold modalities with different thermodynamic properties produce different surface and intramuscular temperatures. *J Athl Train.* 2003;38(1):28-33.

15. Otte JW, Merrick MA, Ingersoll CD, Cordova ML. Subcutaneous adipose tissue thickness alters cooling time during cryotherapy. *Arch Phys Med Rehabil.* 2002;83(11):1501-1505.

16. Hawkins JR, Miller KC. The importance of target tissue depth in cryotherapy application. *J Athl Enhancement.* 2012;1:2.

17. Selkow NM, Day C, Liu Z, Hart JM, Hertel J, Saliba SA. Microvascular perfusion and intramuscular temperature of the calf during cooling. *Med Sci Sports Exerc.* 2012;44(5):850-856.

18. Hubbard TJ, Denegar CR. Does cryotherapy improve outcomes with soft tissue injury? *J Athl Train.* 2004;39(3):278-279.

19. Crawford C, Boyd C, Paat CF, et al. The impact of massage therapy on function in pain populations—A systematic review and meta-analysis of randomized controlled trials: Part I, patients experiencing pain in the general population. *Pain Med.* 2016;17(7):1353-1375.

20. Isabell WK, Durrant E, Myrer W, Anderson S. The effects of ice massage, ice massage with exercise, and exercise on the prevention and treatment of delayed onset muscle soreness. *J Athl Train.* 1992;27(3):208-217.

21. Hawkins SW, Hawkins JR. Clinical applications of cryotherapy among sports physical therapists. *Int J Sports Phys Ther.* 2016;11(1):141-148.

22. Hunter EJ, Ostrowski J, Donahue M, Crowley C, Herzog V. Effect of salted ice bags on surface and intramuscular tissue cooling and rewarming rates. *J Sport Rehabil.* 2016;25(1):70-76.

23. Ottoson D, Lundeberg T. *Pain Treatment by Tens/Transcutaneous Electrical Nerve Stimulation: A Practical Manual.* Berlin: Springer-Verlag; 1988.

24. Chen C, Tabasam G, Johnson M. Does the pulse frequency of transcutaneous electrical nerve stimulation (TENS) influence hypoanalgesia? A systematic review of studies using experimental pain and healthy human participants. *Physiotherapy.* 2008;94(1):11-20.

25. Chesterton LS, Barlas P, Foster NE, Lundeberg T, Wright CC, Baxter GD. Sensory stimulation (TENS): effects of parameter manipulation on mechanical pain thresholds in healthy human subjects. *Pain.* 2002;99:253-262.

26. Bjordal JM, Johnson MI, Ljunggreen AE. Transcutaneous electrical nerve stimulation (TENS) can reduce postoperative analgesic consumption. A meta-analysis with assessment of optimal treatment parameters for postoperative pain. *Eur J Pain.* 2003;7(2):181-188.

27. Brosseau L, Milne S, Robinson V, et al. Efficacy of the transcutaneous electrical nerve stimulation for the treatment of chronic low back pain: a meta-analysis. *Spine.* 2002;27(6):596-603.

28. Johnson M, Martinson M. Efficacy of electrical nerve stimulation for chronic musculoskeletal pain: a meta-analysis of randomized controlled trials. *Pain.* 2007;130(1-2):157-165.

29. Jin D-m, Xu Y, Geng D-f, Yan T-b. Effect of transcutaneous electrical nerve stimulation on symptomatic diabetic peripheral neuropathy: a meta-analysis of randomized controlled trials. *Diabetes Res Clin Pract.* 2010;89(1):10-15.

30. Vance CG, Dailey DL, Rakel BA, Sluka KA. Using TENS for pain control: the state of the evidence. *Pain Manag.* 2014;4(3):197-209.

31. Schwartz MS, Andrasik F, eds. *Biofeedback: A Practitioner's Guide.* New York, NY: Guilford; 2017.

32. De Pinna S. *Transfer of Energy.* Strongville, OH: Gareth Stevens; 2007.

33. Nadler SF. Complications from therapeutic modalities: results from a national survey of clinicians. *Arch Phys Med Rehabil.* 2003;84(6):849-853.

34. Smith G. *Introduction to Classical Electromagnetic Radiation.* Boston, MA: Cambridge University Press; 1997.

35. Reitz J, Milford F, Christy R. *Foundations of Electromagnetic Theory.* 4th ed. Reading, MA: Addison-Wesley; 2008.

36. Hoffman M. Remodeling the blood coagulation cascade. *J Thromb Thrombolysis.* 2003;16(1-2):17-20.

37. Draper DO, Castro JL, Feland B, Schulthies S, Eggett D. Shortwave diathermy and prolonged stretching increase hamstring flexibility more than prolonged stretching alone. *J Orthop Sports Phys Ther.* 2004;34(1):13-20.

38. Garrett CL, Draper DO, Knight KL. Heat distribution in the lower leg from pulsed short-wave diathermy and ultrasound treatments. *J Athl Train.* 2000;35(1):50-55.

39. Jan M-H, Chai H-M, Wang C-L, Lin Y-F, Tsai L-Y. Effects of repetitive shortwave diathermy for reducing synovitis in patients with knee osteoarthritis: an ultrasonographic study. *Phys Ther.* 2006;86(2):236-244.

40. Peres SE, Draper DO, Knight KL, Ricard MD. Pulsed shortwave diathermy and prolonged long-duration stretching increase dorsiflexion range of motion more than identical stretching without diathermy. *J Athl Train.* 2002;37(1):43-50.

41. Chaves ME, Araújo AR, Piancastelli AC, Pinotti M. Effects of low-power light therapy on wound healing: LASER x LED. *An Bras Dermatol.* 2014;89(4):616-623.

42. Cotler HB, Chow RT, Hamblin MR, Carroll J. The use of low level laser therapy (LLLT) for musculoskeletal pain. *MOJ Orthop Rheumatol.* 2015;2(5):00068.

43. Barolet D. Light-emitting diodes (LEDs) in dermatology. *Semin Cutan Med Surg.* 2008;27(4):227-238.

44. Leal-Junior ECP, Vanin AA, Miranda EF, de Carvalho PdTC, Dal Corso S, Bjordal JM. Effect of phototherapy (low-level laser therapy and light-emitting diode therapy) on exercise performance and markers of exercise recovery: a systematic review with meta-analysis. *Lasers Med Sci.* 2015;30(2):925-939.

45. Vinck EM, Cagnie BJ, Cornelissen MJ, Declercq HA, Cambier DC. Increased fibroblast proliferation induced by light emitting diode and low power laser irradiation. *Lasers Med Sci.* 2003;18(2):95-99.

46. Bjordal JM, Johnson MI, Iversen V, Aimbire F, Lopes-Martins RAB. Low-level laser therapy in acute pain: a systematic review of possible mechanisms of action and clinical effects in randomized placebo-controlled trials. *Photomed Laser Surg.* 2006;24(2):158-168.

47. Fung DT, Ng GY, Leung MC, Tay DK. Therapeutic low energy laser improves the mechanical strength of repairing medial collateral ligament. *Lasers Med Sci.* 2002;31(2):91-96.

48. Lam LKY, Cheing GLY. Effects of 904-nm low-level laser therapy in the management of lateral epicondylitis: a randomized controlled trial. *Photomed Laser Surg.* 2007;25(2):65-71.

49. Ng GY, Fung DT. The combined treatment effects of therapeutic laser and exercise on tendon repair. *Photomed Laser Surg.* 2008;26(2):137-141.

50. Porter RD, Mcarthur FG, inventors; Curaelase Inc, assignee. Therapeutic laser treatment. United States patent US 8,033,284. 2011 Oct 11.

51. Prescott MA, inventor; Prescott, Marvin A., assignee. Method and apparatus for therapeutic laser treatment. United States patent US 5,989,245. 1999 Nov 23.

52. Stergioulas A. Low-level laser treatment can reduce edema in second degree ankle sprains. *J Clin Laser Med Surg.* 2004;22(2):125-128.

53. Tumilty S, McDonough S, Hurley DA, Baxter GD. Clinical effectiveness of low-level laser therapy as an adjunct to eccentric exercise for the treatment of Achilles' tendinopathy: a randomized controlled trial. *Arch Phys Med Rehabil.* 2012;93(5):733-739.

54. Chung H, Dai T, Sharma SK, Huang YY, Carroll JD, Hamblin MR. The nuts and bolts of low-level laser (light) therapy. *Ann Biomed Eng.* 2011;40(2):516-533.

55. Ash C, Dubec M, Donne K, Bashford T. Effect of wavelength and beam width on penetration in light-tissue interaction using computational methods. *Lasers Med Sci.* 2017;32(8):1909-1918.

56. Bisht D, Mehrortra R, Singh PA, Atri SC, Kumar A. Effect of helium-neon laser on wound healing. *Indian J Exp Biol.* 1999;37:187-189.

57. Bjordal JM, Couppe C, Chow RT, Tuner J, Ljunggren EA. A systematic review of low level laser therapy with location-specific doses for pain from chronic joint disorders. *Aust J Physiother.* 2003;49:107-116.

58. Draper DO, Sunderland S. Examination of the law of Grotthus-Draper: does ultrasound penetrate subcutaneous fat in humans? *J Athl Train.* 1993;28:246-250.

59. Balmaseda MT, Fatehi MT, Koozekanani SH. Ultrasound therapy: a comparative study of different coupling medium. *Arch Phys Med Rehabil.* 1986;67:147.

60. Pesek J, Kane E, Perrin D. T-Prep ultrasound gel and ultrasound does not affect local anesthesia. *J Athl Train.* 2001;36(2S):S89-S92.

61. Klucinec B, Scheidler M, Denegar C. Transmission of coupling agents used to deliver acoustic energy over irregular surfaces. *J Orthop Sports Phys Ther.* 2000;30(5):263-269.

62. Mihaloyov MR, Roethemeier JL, Merrick MA. Intramuscular temperature does not differ between direct ultrasound application and application with commercial gel packs. *J Athl Train.* 2000;35(2):S-47.

63. Merrick MA, Mihalyov MR, Roethemeier JL. A comparison of intramuscular temperatures during ultrasound treatments with coupling gel or gel pads. *J Orthop Sports Phys Ther.* 2002;32(5):216-220.

64. Docker MF, Foulkes DJ, Patrick MK. Ultrasound couplants for physiotherapy. *Physiotherapy.* 1982;68(4):124-125.

65. Boone L, Ingersol CD, Cordova ML. Passive hip flexion does not increase during or following ultrasound treatment of the hamstring musculature. *J Athl Train.* 1999;34(2):S-70.

66. Dyson M, Brookes M. Stimulation of bone repair by ultrasound (abstract). *Ultrasound Med Biol.* 1982;8(50):50.

67. Fyfe MC, Chahl LA. The effect of single or repeated applications of "therapeutic" ultrasound on plasma extravasation during silver nitrate induced inflammation of the rat hindpaw ankle joint. *Ultrasound Med Biol.* 1985;11:273-283.

68. Oakley EM. Application of continuous beam ultrasound at therapeutic levels. *Physiotherapy.* 1978;64(6):169-172.

69. Patrick MK. Applications of pulsed therapeutic ultrasound. *Physiotherapy.* 1978;64(4):103-104.

70. Strapp E, Guskiewicz K, Hackney A. The cumulative effects of multiple phonophoresis treatments on dexamethasone and cortisol concentrations in the blood. *J Athl Train.* 2000;35(2):S-47.

71. Starkey C. *Therapeutic Modalities for Athletic Trainers.* Philadelphia, PA: F.A. Davis; 2004.

72. Bly N, McKenzie A, West J, Whitney J. Low dose ultrasound effects on wound healing: a controlled study with Yucatan pigs. *Arch Phys Med Rehabil.* 1992;73:656-664.

73. Johns L, Colloton P. Effects of ultrasound on splenocyte proliferation and lymphokine production. *J Athl Train.* 2002;37(2S):S-42.

74. Holcomb WR, Blank C, Davis C. The effect of superficial pre-heating on the magnitude and duration of temperature elevation with 1 MHz ultrasound. *J Athl Train.* 2000;35(2):S-48.

75. Schandelmaier S, Kaushal A, Lytvyn L, et al. Low intensity pulsed ultrasound for bone healing: systematic review of randomized controlled trials. *BMJ.* 2017;356:j656.

76. Mundi R, Petis S, Kaloty R, Shetty V, Bhandari M. Low-intensity pulsed ultrasound: Fracture healing. *Indian J Orthop.* 2009;43(2):132-140.

77. Leighton R, Watson JT, Giannoudis P, Papakostidis C, Harrison A, Steen RG. Healing of fracture nonunions treated with low-intensity pulsed ultrasound (LIPUS): A systematic review and meta-analysis. *Injury.* 2017;48(7):1339-1347.

78. Khanna A, Nelmes RT, Gougoulias N, Maffulli N, Gray J. The effects of LIPUS on soft-tissue healing: a review of literature. *Br Med Bull.* 2009;89: 169-182.

79. Anderson M, Draper D, Schulthies S. A 1:3 mixture of FlexAll and ultrasound gel is as effective a couplant as 100% ultrasound gel, based upon intramuscular temperature rise (Abstract). *J Athl Train.* 2005;40(2):S89-S90.

80. Draper D, Anderson M. Combining topical analgesics and ultrasound, part 1. *Athl Ther Today.* 2005;10(1):26-27.

81. Myrer J, Measom G, Fellingham G. Intramuscular temperature rises with topical analgesics used as coupling agents during therapeutic ultrasound. *J Athl Train.* 2001;36(1):20-26.

82. Anderson M, Eggett D, Draper D. Combining topical analgesics and ultrasound, Part 2. *Athl Ther Today.* 2005;10(2):45.

83. Ashton DF, Draper DO, Myrer JW. Temperature rise in human muscle during ultrasound treatments using Flex-All as a coupling agent. *J Athl Train.* 1998;33(2):136-140.

84. Davidson CJ, Ganion LR, Gehlsen GM, Verhoestra B, Roepke JE, Sevier TL. Rat tendon morphologic and functional changes resulting from soft tissue mobilization. *Med Sci Sports Exerc.* 1997;29:313-319.

85. Kim J, Sung DJ, Lee J. Therapeutic effectiveness of instrument-assisted soft tissue mobilization for soft tissue injury: mechanisms and practical application. *J Exerc Rehabil.* 2017;13(1):12-22. doi:10.12965/jer.1732824.412

86. Kivlan BR, Carcia CR, Clemente FR, Phelps AL, Martin RL. The effect of Astym® therapy on muscle strength: a blinded, randomized, clinically controlled trial. *BMC Musculoskelet Disord.* 2015;16:325.

87. Sevier TL, Stegink-Jansen CW. Astym treatment vs. eccentric exercise for lateral elbow tendinopathy: a randomized controlled clinical trial. *Peer J.* 2015;3:e967.

88. Baker RT, Nasypany A, Seegmiller JG, et al. Instrument-assisted soft tissue mobilization treatment for tissue extensibility dysfunction. *Int J Athl Ther Training.* 2013;18(5):16-21.

89. Loghmani MT, Warden SJ. Instrument-assisted cross fiber massage increases tissue perfusion and alters microvascular morphology in the vicinity of healing knee ligaments. *BMC Complement Altern Med.* 2013;13:240.

90. Hammer WI. The effect of mechanical load on degenerated soft tissue. *J Bodyw Mov Ther.* 2008;12(3):246-256.

91. Lee JJ, Lee JJ, Kim do H, et al. Inhibitory effects of instrument-assisted neuromobilization on hyperactive gastrocnemius in a hemiparetic stroke patient. *Biomed Mater Eng.* 2014;24(6):2389-2394.

92. Howitt S, Jung S, Hammonds N. Conservative treatment of a tibialis posterior strain in a novice triathlete: a case report. *J Can Chiropr Assoc.* 2009;53:23-31.

93. Miners AL, Bougie TL. Chronic Achilles tendinopathy: a case study of treatment incorporating active and passive tissue warm-up, Graston Technique, ART, eccentric exercise, and cryotherapy. *J Can Chiropr Assoc.* 2011;55:269-279.

94. Schaefer JL, Sandrey MA. Effects of a 4-week dynamic-balance-training program supplemented with Graston instrument-assisted soft-tissue mobilization for chronic ankle instability. *J Sport Rehabil.* 2012;21:313-326.

95. Karmali A, Walizada A, Stuber K. The efficacy of instrument-assisted soft tissue mobilization for musculoskeletal pain: A systematic review. *J Contemp Chiropr.* 2019;2:25-33.

96. Kim J, Sung DJ, Lee J. Therapeutic effectiveness of instrument-assisted soft tissue mobilization for soft tissue injury: mechanisms and practical application. *J Exerc Rehabil.* 2017;13(1):12-22.

97. Sandy Fritz. *Mosby's Fundamentals of Therapeutic Massage.* 6th ed. St. Louis, MO: Elsevier; 2017.

98. Hemmings B, Smith M, Graydon J, Dyson R. Effects of massage on physiological restoration, perceived recovery, and repeated sports performance. *Br J Sports Med.* 2000;34(2):109-114.

99. Hemmings BJ. Physiological, psychological and performance effects of massage therapy in sport: a review of the literature. *Phys Ther Sport.* 2001;2(4):165-170.

100. Suzuki M, Tatsumi A, Otsuka T, et al. Physical and psychological effects of 6-week tactile massage on elderly patients with severe dementia. *Am J Alzheimers Dis Other Demen.* 2010;25(8):680-686.

101. Goats GC. Massage—the scientific basis of an ancient art: Part 2. Physiological and therapeutic effects. *Br J Sports Med.* 1994;28(3):153-156.

102. Cho KS. The effect of a hand massage program on anxiety and immune function in clients with cataract surgery under local anesthesia. *J Korean Acad Nurs.* 1999;29(1):97-106.

103. Weerapong P, Hume PA, Kolt GS. The mechanisms of massage and effects on performance, muscle recovery and injury prevention. *Sport Med.* 2005;35(3):235-256.

104. Chang SO. The conceptual structure of physical touch in caring. *J Adv Nurs.* 2001;33(6):820-827.

105. Best TM, Hunter R, Wilcox A, Haq F. Effectiveness of sports massage for recovery of skeletal muscle from strenuous exercise. *Clin J Sport Med.* 2008;18(5):446-460.

106. Roschel H, Barroso R, Tricoli V, et al. Effects of strength training associated with whole-body vibration training on running economy and vertical stiffness. *J Strength Cond Res.* 2015;29(8):2215-2220.

107. Martínez-Pardo E, Romero-Arenas S, Alcaraz PE. Effects of different amplitudes (high vs. low) of whole-body vibration training in active adults. *J Strength Cond Res.* 2013;27(7):1798-1806.

108. Martínez-Pardo E, Romero-Arenas S, Martínez-Ruiz E, Rubio-Arias JA, Alcaraz PE. Effect of a whole-body vibration training modifying the training frequency of workouts per week in active adults. *J Strength Cond Res.* 2014;28(11):3255-3263.

109. Marín PJ, Rhea MR. Effects of vibration training on muscle power: a meta-analysis. *J Strength Cond Res.* 2010;24(3):871-878.

110. Bautmans I, Hees EV, Lemper J-C, Mets T. The feasibility of whole body vibration in institutionalized elderly persons and its influence on muscle performance, balance and mobility: a randomized controlled trial. *BMC Geriatrics.* 2005;5:17.

111. Machado A, García-López D, González-Gallego J, Garatachea N. Whole-body vibration training increases muscle strength and mass in older women: a randomized-controlled trial. *Scan J Med Sci Sports.* 2010;20(2):200-207.

112. Rees SS, Murphy AJ, Watsford ML. Effects of whole-body vibration exercise on lower extremity muscle strength and power in an older population: a randomized clinical trial. *Phys Ther.* 2008;88:462-470.

113. Roelants M, Delecluse C, Verschueren SM. Whole-body-vibration training increases knee-extension strength and speed of movement in older women. *J Am Geriatr Soc.* 2004;53:901-908.

114. Russo CR, Lauretani F, Bandinelli S, et al. High-frequency vibration training increases muscle power in postmenopausal women. *Arch Phys Med Rehabil.* 2003;84:1854-1857.

115. Verschueren SMP, Bogaerts A, Delecluse C, et al. Vitamin D supplementation on muscle strength, muscle mass, and bone density in institutionalized elderly women: a 6-month randomized, controlled trial. *J Bone Miner Res.* 2011;26:42-49.

116. Von Stengel S, Kemmler W, Engelke K, Kalender WA. Effect of whole-body vibration on neuromuscular performance and body composition for females 65 years and older: a randomized-controlled trial. *Scan J Med Sci Sports.* 2012;22;119-127.

117. Ness LL, Field-Fote EC. Whole-body vibration improves walking function in individuals with spinal cord injury: a pilot study. *Gait Posture.* 2009;30;436-440.

118. Sayenko DG, Masani K, Alizadeh-Meghrazi M, Popovic MR, Craven BC. Acute effects of whole body vibration during passive standing on soleus H-reflex in subjects with and without spinal cord injury. *Neurosci Lett.* 2010;482:66-70.

119. Hong C, Lin J, Bender L, Schaeffer J, Meltzer R, Causin P. Magnetic necklace: its therapeutic effectiveness on neck and shoulder pain. *Arch Phys Med Rehabil.* 1982;63(10):462-466.

120. Cepeda MS, Carr DB, Sarquis T, Miranda N, Garcia RJ, Zarate C. Static magnetic therapy does not decrease pain or opioid requirements: a randomized double-blind trial. *Anesth Analg.* 2007;104(2):290-294.

121. Colbert AP, Cleaver J, Brown KA, et al. Magnets applied to acupuncture points as therapy—a literature review. *Acupunct Med.* 2008;26(3):160-170.

122. Collacott EA, Zimmerman JT, White DW, Rindone JP. Bipolar permanent magnets for the treatment of chronic low back pain: a pilot study. *JAMA.* 2000;283(10):1322-1325.

123. Cao HJ, Han M, Li X, et al. Clinical research evidence of cupping therapy in China: A systematic literature review. *BMC Complement Altern Med.* 2010;10:70.

124. Cao HJ, Zhu CJ, Liu JP. Wet cupping therapy for treatment of herpes zoster: A systematic review of randomized controlled trials. *Altern Ther Health Med.* 2010;16:48-54.

125. Lee MS, Choi TY, Shin BC, Han CH, Ernst E. Cupping for stroke rehabilitation: A systematic review. *J Neurol Sci.* 2010;294:70-73.

126. Lee MS, Kim JI, Ernst E. Is cupping an effective treatment? An overview of systematic reviews. *J Acupunct Meridian Stud.* 2011;4(1):1-4.

127. Chen B, Li M-Y, Liu P-D, Guo Y, Chen Z-L. Alternative medicine: an update on cupping therapy. *QJM.* 2015;108(7):523-525.

128. Corbett M, Rice S, Madurasinghe V, et al. Acupuncture and other physical treatments for the relief of pain due to osteoarthritis of the knee: network meta-analysis. *Osteoarthritis Cartilage.* 2013;21(9):1290-1298.

129. Kim J-I, Lee MS, Lee D-H, Boddy K, Ernst E. Cupping for treating pain: a systematic review. *Evid Based Complement Alternat Med.* 2011;2011:467014.

130. Kim T-H, Kim KH, Choi J-Y, Lee MS. Adverse events related to cupping therapy in studies conducted in Korea: a systematic review. *Euro J Int Med.* 2014;6(4):434-440.

131. Lee MS, Kim J-I, Ernst E. Is cupping an effective treatment? An overview of systematic reviews. *J Acupunct Meridian Stud.* 2011;4(1):1-4.

132. Chow RT, Johnson MI, Lopes-Martins RA, Bjordal JM. Efficacy of low-level laser therapy in the management of neck pain: a systematic review and meta-analysis of

randomised placebo or active-treatment controlled trials. *Lancet*. 2009;374(9705):1897-1908.

133. Tsai SR, Hamblin MR. Biological effects and medical applications of infrared radiation. *J Photochem Photobiol B*. 2017;170:197-207.

134. Hawkins D, Abrahamse H. Effect of multiple exposures of low-level laser therapy on the cellular responses of wounded human skin fibroblasts. *Photomed Laser Surg*. 2006;24(6):705-714.

135. Chung H, Dai T, Sharma SK, Huang YY, Carroll JD, Hamblin MR. The nuts and bolts of low-level laser (light) therapy. *Ann Biomed Eng*. 2012;40(2):516-533.

136. Barolet D, Christiaens F, Hamblin MR. Infrared and skin: Friend or foe. *J Photochem Photobiol B*. 2015;155:78-85.

137. Aker PD, Gross AR, Goldsmith CH, Peloso P. Conservative management of mechanical neck pain: systematic overview and meta-analysis. *BMJ*. 1996;313(7068):1291-1296.

138. Çelik G, Özbek O, Yilmaz M, Duman I, Özbek S, Apiliogullari S. Vapocoolant spray vs lidocaine/prilocaine cream for reducing the pain of venipuncture in hemodialysis patients: a randomized, placebo-controlled, crossover study. *Int J Med Sci*. 2011;8(7):623.

139. Kostopoulos D, Rizopoulos K. Effect of topical aerosol skin refrigerant (spray and stretch technique) on passive and active stretching. *J Bodyw Mov Ther*. 2008;12(2):96-104.

140. Park KW, Boyer MI, Calfee RP, Goldfarb CA, Osei DA. The efficacy of 95-Hz topical vibration in pain reduction for trigger finger injection: a placebo-controlled, prospective, randomized trial. *J Hand Surg*. 2014;39(11):2203-2207.

141. Yoon WY, Chung SP, Lee HS, Park YS. Analgesic pretreatment for antibiotic skin test: vapocoolant spray vs ice cube. *Am J Emerg Med*. 2008;26(1):59-61.

142. Le ADK, Enweze L, DeBaun MR, Dragoo JL. Current clinical recommendations for use of platelet-rich plasma. *Curr Rev Musculoskelet Med*. 2018;11(4):624-634.

143. Winke M, Williamson S. Comparison of a pneumatic compression device to a compression garment during recovery from DOMS. *Int J Exerc Sci*. 2018;11(3):375-383.

144. Stanek J. The effectiveness of compression socks on athletic performance and recovery. *J Sport Rehabil*. 2017;26(1):109-114.

145. Cranston A. *The use of intermittent sequential pneumatic compression for recovery following exercise* (Doctoral dissertation, The University of Waikato).

146. Centner C, Wiegel P, Gollhofer A, König D. Effects of blood flow restriction training on muscular strength and hypertrophy in older individuals: A systematic review and meta-analysis. *Sports Medicine*. 2019 Jan 25;49(1):95-108.

147. Bowman EN, Elshaar R, Milligan H, Jue G, Mohr K, Brown P, Watanabe DM, Limpisvasti O. Upper-extremity blood flow restriction: The proximal, distal, and contralateral effects—a randomized controlled trial. *Journal of Shoulder and Elbow Surgery*. 2020 Jun 1;29(6):1267-1274.

148. da Cunha Nascimento D, Petriz B, da Cunha Oliveira S, Vieira DC, Funghetto SS, Silva AO, Prestes J. Effects of blood flow restriction exercise on hemostasis: A systematic review of randomized and non-randomized trials. *International Journal of General Medicine*. 2019;12:91.

Chapter 22

1. Knapik JJ. The importance of physical fitness for injury prevention: part 1. *J Spec Oper Med*. 2015;15(1):123-127.

2. Knapik JJ. The importance of physical fitness for injury prevention: part 2. *J Spec Oper Med*. 2015;15(2):112-115.

3. Haskell WL, Lee I-M, Pate RR, et al. Physical activity and public health: updated recommendation for adults from the American College of Sports Medicine and the American Heart Association. *Circulation*. 2007;116(9):1081.

4. Hootman JM, Macera CA, Ainsworth BE, Martin M, Addy CL, Blair SN. Association among physical activity level, cardiorespiratory fitness, and risk of musculoskeletal injury. *Am J Epidemiol*. 2001;154(3):251-258.

5. O'Donovan G, Blazevich AJ, Boreham C, et al. The ABC of Physical Activity for Health: a consensus statement from the British Association of Sport and Exercise Sciences. *J Sports Sci*. 2010;28(6):573-591.

6. Twitchett E, Brodrick A, Nevill AM, Koutedakis Y, Angioi M, Wyon M. Does physical fitness affect injury occurrence and time loss due to injury in elite vocational ballet students? *J Dance Med Sci*. 2010;14(1):26-31.

7. Andersen JL, Aagaard P. Myosin heavy chain IIX overshoot in human skeletal muscle. *Muscle Nerve*. 2000;23(7):1095-1104.

8. Prentice WE. *Therapeutic Modalities in Rehabilitation*. New York, NY: McGraw Hill; 2017.

9. O'Sullivan SB, Schmitz TJ. *Physical Rehabilitation, vol. 5*. Philadelphia, PA: FA Davis; 2006.

10. Bogdanis GC. Effects of physical activity and inactivity on muscle fatigue. *Front Physiol*. 2012;3:142.

11. Dideriksen K, Boesen AP, Reitelseder S, et al. Tendon collagen synthesis declines with immobilization in elderly humans: no effect of anti-inflammatory medication. *J Appl Physiol*. 2016;122(2):273-282.

12. Sun S, Henriksen K, Karsdal MA, et al. Collagen type III and VI turnover in response to long-term immobilization. *PLoS One*. 2015;10(12):e0144525.

13. Manske RC, DeWitt J. Ligament healing. In: Manske R, ed. *Fundamental Orthopedic Management for the Physical Therapist Assistant*. Saint Louis, MO: Elsevier; 2016.

14. Hammond MA, Wallace JM. Exercise prevents [beta]-aminopropionitrile-induced morphological changes to type I collagen in murine bone. *Bonekey rep*. 2015;4:645.

15. Bolam KA, Skinner TL, Jenkins DG, Galvão DA, Taaffe DR. The osteogenic effect of impact-loading and resistance

exercise on bone mineral density in middle-aged and older men: A pilot study. *Gerontology.* 2016;62(1):22-32.

16. Kisner C, Colby LA, Borstad J. *Therapeutic Exercise: Foundations and Techniques.* Philadelphia, PA: F.A. Davis; 2017.

17. Teasell R, Dittmer D. Complications of immobilization and bed rest. Part 2: Other complications. *Can Fam Physician.* 1993;39:1440.

18. Hoffman MD. Cardiorespiratory fitness and training in quadriplegics and paraplegics. *Sports Med.* 1986;3(5):312-330.

19. Menke NB, Ward KR, Witten TM, Bonchev DG, Diegelmann RF. Impaired wound healing. *Clinics Derm.* 2007;25(1):19-25.

20. Coudeyre E, Lefevre-Colau M-M, Griffon A, et al. Is there predictive criteria for transfer of patients to a rehabilitation ward after hip and knee total arthroplasty? Elaboration of French clinical practice guidelines. *Ann Readapt Med Phys.* 2007;50(5):327-336; 317-326.

21. Valkenet K, van de Port IG, Dronkers JJ, de Vries WR, Lindeman E, Backx FJ. The effects of preoperative exercise therapy on postoperative outcome: a systematic review. *Clinic Rehab.* 2011;25(2):99-111.

22. Fortin PR, Clarke AE, Joseph L, et al. Outcomes of total hip and knee replacement: preoperative functional status predicts outcomes at six months after surgery. *Arthritis Rheum.* 1999;42(8):1722-1728.

23. Orr R, Raymond J, Fiatarone Singh M. Efficacy of progressive resistance training on balance performance in older adults: a systematic review of randomized controlled trials. *Sports Med.* 2008; 38(4):317-343.

24. Behm DG, Muehlbauer T, Kibele A, Granacher U. Effects of strength training using unstable surfaces on strength, power and balance performance across the lifespan: A systematic review and meta-analysis. *Sports Med.* 2015;1:45(12):1645-1669.

25. Johnson BA, Salzberg CL, Stevenson DA. A systematic review: Plyometric training programs for young children. *Strength Cond Res.* 2011;25(9):2623-2633.

26. Zech A, Hübscher M, Vogt L, Banzer W, Hänsel F, Pfeifer K. Balance training for neuromuscular control and performance enhancement: a systematic review. *J Athl Train.* 2010;45(4):392-403.

27. Liu-Ambrose T, Taunton JE, MacIntyre D, McConkey P, Khan KM. The effects of proprioceptive or strength training on the neuromuscular function of the ACL reconstructed knee: a randomized clinical trial. *Scand J Med Sci Sports.* 2003;13(2):115-123.

28. Risberg MA, Mørk M, Jenssen HK, Holm I. Design and implementation of a neuromuscular training program following anterior cruciate ligament reconstruction. *J Orthop Sports Phys Ther.* 2001;31(11):620-631.

29. Huebscher M, Zech A, Pfeifer K, Haensel F, Vogt L, Banzer W. Neuromuscular training for sports injury prevention: a systematic review. *Med Sci Sports Exerc.* 2010;42(3):413-421.

30. Emery CA, Roy TO, Whittaker JL, Nettel-Aguirre A, Van Mechelen W. Neuromuscular training injury prevention strategies in youth sport: a systematic review and meta-analysis. *Br J Sports Med.* 2015;49(13):865-870.

31. Prins J, Cutner D. Aquatic therapy in the rehabilitation of athletic injuries. *Clin Sports Med.* 1999;18(2):447-461.

32. Thein JM, Brody LT. Aquatic-based rehabilitation and training for the elite athlete. *J Orthop Sports Phys Ther.* 1998;27(1):32-41. doi:10.2519/jospt.1998.27.1.32

33. Tovin BJ, Wolf SL, Greenfield BH, Crouse J, Woodfin BA. Comparison of the effects of exercise in water and on land on the rehabilitation of patients with intra-articular anterior cruciate ligament reconstructions. *Phys Ther.* 1994;74(8):710-719.

34. Hindle KB, Whitcomb TJ, Briggs WO, Hong J. Proprioceptive neuromuscular facilitation (PNF): its mechanisms and effects on range of motion and muscular function. *J Hum Kinet.* 2012;31:105-113.

35. Sharman M, Cresswell A, Riek S. Proprioceptive neuromuscular facilitation stretching: mechanisms and clinical implications. *Sports Med.* 2006;36(11):929-939.

36. Caplan N, Rogers R, Parr MK, Hayes PR. The effect of proprioceptive neuromuscular facilitation and static stretch training on running mechanics. *J Strength Cond Res.* 2009;23(4):1175-1180.

37. Etnyre BR, Abraham LD. H-reflex during static stretching and two variations of proprioceptive neuromuscular facilitation techniques. *Electroencephalogr Clin Neurophysiol.* 1986;63(2):174-179.

38. Etnyre BR, Lee EJ. Chronic and acute flexibility of men and women using three different stretching techniques. *Res Q Exerc Sport.* 1988;59(3):222-228.

39. Feland JB, Myrer JW, Merrill RM. Acute changes in hamstring flexibility: PNF versus static stretch in senior athletes. *Phys Ther Sport.* 2001;2:186-193.

40. Cheng C, Liu X, Fan W, Bai X, Liu Z. Comprehensive rehabilitation training decreases cognitive impairment, anxiety, and depression in poststroke patients: a randomized, controlled study. *J Stroke Cerebrovasc Dis.* 2018;27(10):2613-2622.

41. dos Santos, VA Jr, de Sales Santos M, da Silva Ribeiro NM, Maldonado IL. Combining proprioceptive neuromuscular facilitation and virtual reality for improving sensorimotor function in stroke survivors: a randomized clinical trial. *J Cent Nerve Sys Dis.* 2019:11:1179573519863826.

42. Wyszyᐧski S, Stiler-Wyszyᐧska S. Assessment of the impact of hold-relax and contract-relax techniques on the compression pain threshold in patients with lateral humeral epicondylitis. *Med Sci Pulse.* 2018;12:4;15-21.

43. Kahanov LK, Kato M. Therapeutic effect of joint mobilization: joint mechanoreceptors and nociceptors. *Athl Ther Today.* 2007;12(4):28-31.

44. Do Moon G, Lim JY, Kim DY, Kim TH. Comparison of Maitland and Kaltenborn mobilization techniques for improving shoulder pain and range of motion in frozen

shoulders. *J Phys Ther Sci.* 2015;27(5):1391-1395. doi:10.1589/jpts.27.1391

45. Gautam R. Dhamija K, Puri A. Comparison of Maitland and Mulligan mobilization in improving neck pain, ROM and disability. *Int J Physiother Res.* 2014;2(3):482-487.

46. Maitland GD, Hengeveld E, Banks K. *Maitland's Vertebral Manipulation.* 7th ed. London; England: Butterworths Heinemann; 2006.

47. Wyke BD. Articular neurology and manipulative therapy. In: Glasgow EF, ed. *Aspects of Manipulative Therapy.* 2nd ed. Melbourne, Australia: Churchill Livingstone; 1985:72-77.

48. Hengeveld E, Banks K. *Maitland's Peripheral Manipulation.* 4th ed. London: Butterworth-Heinemann; 2005.

49. Zimmy M. Mechanoreceptors in articular tissues. *Am J Anat.* 1998;182(1):16-32.

50. Simons DG, Mense S. Diagnosis and therapy of myofascial trigger points. *Schmerz.* 2003;17(6):419-424.

51. Healey KC, Hatfield DL, Blanpied P, Dorfman LR, Riebe D. The effects of myofascial release with foam rolling on performance. *J Strength Cond Res.* 2014;28(1):61-68.

52. Okamoto T, Masuhara M, Ikuta K. Acute effects of self-myofascial release using a foam roller on arterial function. *J Strength Cond Res.* 2014;28(1):69-73.

53. Lewit K, Simons DG. Myofascial pain: relief by post-isometric relaxation. *Arch Phys Med Rehabil.* 1984;65(8):452-456.

54. Langevin HM, Huijing PA. Communicating about fascia: history, pitfalls, and recommendations. *Int J Ther Massage Bodywork.* 2009;2(4):3-8.

55. MacDonald GZ, Penney MD, Mullaley ME, et al. An acute bout of self-myofascial release increases range of motion without a subsequent decrease in muscle activation or force. *J Strength Cond Res.* 2013;27(3):812-821.

Chapter 23

1. Adeef A. *Absorption and Drug Development.* Hoboken, NJ: Wikey-Intersciences/J. Wiley; 2003.

2. Welling PG, Tse FLS, Dighe SV. *Pharmaceutical Bioequivalence: Drugs and the Pharmaceutical Sciences.* New York, NY: Marcel Dekker; 1991.

3. Prentice WE. *Principles of Athletic Training.* New York, NY: McGraw Hill; 2017.

4. Rowland M, Tozer TN. *Clinical Pharmacokinetics and Pharmacodynamics: Concepts and Applications.* Philadelphia, PA: Lippincott Williams & Wilkins; 2010.

5. Starkey C. *Therapeutic Modalities.* Philadelphia, PA: F.A. Davis; 2013.

6. Asperheim MK. *Introduction to Pharmacology.* 12th ed. St. Louis, MO: Elsevier Saunders; 2011.

7. Kahanov L, Furst D, Johnson S, Roberts J. Adherence to drug-dispensation and drug-administration laws and guidelines in collegiate athletic training rooms. *J Athl Train.* 2003;38(3):252.

8. Kahanov L, Roberts J, Wughalter EM. Adherence to drug-dispensation and drug-administration laws and guidelines in collegiate athletic training rooms: a 5-year review. *J Athl Train.* 2010;45(3):299-305.

9. National Athletic Trainers' Association Consensus Statement: managing prescription and non-prescription medication in the athletic training facility. *NATA News.* 2009:14-16.

10. Nickell R. Eight principles for managing prescription medications in the athletic training room. *Athl Ther Today.* 2005;10(1):6-9.

11. Mangus BC, Miller MG. *Pharmacology: Application in Athletic Training.* Philadelphia, PA: F.A. Davis; 2005.

12. Huff P. Drug distribution in the training room. *Clin Sports Med.* 1998;17(2):211-228.

13. Price KO, Huff PS, Isetts BJ, Goldwire MA. University-based sports pharmacy program. *Am J Health Syst Pharm.* 1995;52(3):302-309.

14. Federal Food, Drug and Cosmetic Act (FDCA). U.S. Congress 1938.

15. Durham-Humphrey Amendment. U.S. Congress 1951.

16. Federal Anti-Tampering Act. U.S. Congress 1983.

17. OBRA '90 Regulations Federal Register. In Omnibus Budget Reconciliation Act. U.S. Congress 1990.

18. Quality, safety, and efficacy of medicines. World Health Organization website. www.who.int/medicines/areas/quality_safety/en. Accessed April 30, 2018.

19. Medicine and healthcare products: regulatory agency. Gov.UK website. www.gov.uk/government/organisations/medicines-and-healthcare-products-regulatory-agency. Accessed April 30, 2018.

20. Drug product database. Government of Canada website. www.canada.ca/en/health-canada/services/drugs-health-products/drug-products/drug-product-database.html. Accessed April 30, 2018.

21. Akici A, Aydin V, Kiroglu A. Assessment of the association between drug disposal practices and drug use and storage behaviors. *Saudi Pharm J.* 2018;26(1):7-13.

22. Kinrys G, Gold AK, Worthington JJ, Nierenberg AA. Medication disposal practices: increasing patient and clinician education on safe methods. *J Int Med Res.* 2018;46(3):927-939.

23. Secure and Responsible Drug Disposal Act. U.S. Congress 2010.

24. Testing. USADA website. www.usada.org/testing. Accessed August 13, 2020.

25. NCAA drug testing program. NCAA website. www.ncaa.org/sport-science-institute/ncaa-drug-testing-program. Accessed April 2, 2018.

26. Herbert D. NCAA drug distribution study for university athletic programs. *Sports Med Stand Malpract Rep.* 1993;5:5-6.

27. Athletic Training Educational Competencies. 5th ed. National Athletic Trainers' Association website. www.

nata.org/sites/default/files/competencies_5th_edition.pdf. Published 2011.

28. Herbert DL. Dispensing prescription medication to athletes. In: Herbert DL, ed. *The Legal Aspects of Sports Medicine.* Canton, OH: Professional Sports; 1990:215-228.

29. Houglum JE. Asthma medications: basic pharmacology and use in the athlete. *J Athl Train.* 2000;35(2):179.

30. Courson R, Patel H, Navitskis L, Reifsteck F, Ward K. Policies and procedures in athletic training for dispensing medication. *Athl Ther Today.* 2005;10(1):10-14.

31. Goldberg L, Elliot DL, MacKinnon DP, et al. Outcomes of a prospective trial of student-athlete drug testing: the Student Athlete Testing Using Random Notification (SATURN) study. *J Adolesc Health.* 2007;41(5):421-429.

32. Green GA, Uryasz FD, Petr TA, Bray CD. NCAA study of substance use and abuse habits of college student-athletes. *Clin J Sport Med.* 2001;11(1):51-56.

33. Wadler GI, Hainline B. *Drugs and the Athlete.* Philadelphia, PA: F.A. Davis; 1989.

34. Controlled Substance Act. U.S. Congress 1970.

35. Coombs G, Cramer M, Ravanelli N, Morris N, Jay O. Acute acetaminophen ingestion does not alter core temperature or sweating during exercise in hot–humid conditions. *Scand J Med Sci Sports.* 2015;25(S1):96-103.

36. Holgado D, Hopker J, Sanabria D, Zabala M. Analgesics and sport performance: beyond the pain-modulating effects. *PM R.* 2018;10(1):72-82.

37. Jankowski CM, Shea K, Barry DW, et al. Timing of ibuprofen use and musculoskeletal adaptations to exercise training in older adults. *Bone Rep.* 2015;1:1-8.

38. Ziltener J-L, Leal S, Fournier P-E. Non-steroidal anti-inflammatory drugs for athletes: an update. *Ann Phys Rehabil Med.* 2010;53(4):278-288.

39. Chou R, Peterson K. *Drug Class Review: Skeletal Muscle Relaxants: Final Report.* Portland, OR: Oregon Health & Science University; 2005.

40. McFadden E Jr, Gilbert IA. Exercise-induced asthma. *N Engl J Med.* 1994;330(19):1362-1367.

41. Miller MG, Baker FRJ. Asthma. In: Casa DJ, Stearns RL, eds. *Emergency Management for Sport and Physical Activity.* Burlington, MA: Jones & Bartlett Learning; 2015:157-168.

42. Miller MG, Weiler JM, Baker R, Collins J, D'Alonzo G. National Athletic Trainers' Association position statement: management of asthma in athletes. *J Athl Train.* 2005;40(3):224.

43. Ari A, Hess D, Myers T, Rau J. *A Guide to Aerosol Delivery Devices for Respiratory Therapists.* Dallas, TX: American Association for Respiratory Care; 2009.

44. Fanta C, Fletcher S, Wood R, Bochner B, Hollingsworth H. An overview of asthma management. Up to Date website. www.uptodate.com/contents/an-overview-of-asthma-management. Published 2009. Accessed August 13, 2020.

45. Fanta CH, Bochner BS, Hollingsworth H. Treatment of acute exacerbations of asthma in adults. *Methods.* 2014;2(3):5.

46. Morton AR, Fitch KD. Asthmatic drugs and competitive sport. *Sports Med.* 1992;14(4):228-242.

47. Naclerio RM, Hadley JA, Stoloff S, Nelson HS. Patient and physician perspectives on the attributes of nasal allergy medications. *Allergy Asthma Proc.* 2007;28 Suppl 1:S11-S17.

48. Biddington C, Popovich M, Kupczyk N, Roh J. Certified athletic trainers' management of emergencies. *J Sport Rehabil.* 2005;14(2):185-194.

49. Olympia RP, Brady J. Emergency preparedness in high school–based athletics: a review of the literature and recommendations for sport health professionals. *Phys Sportsmed.* 2013;41(2):15-25.

50. Reed TS, Bodine WA. Sideline management of anaphylaxis in an athlete. *Simul Healthc.* 2011;6(2):121-124.

51. Koon G, Atay O, Lapsia S. Gastrointestinal considerations related to youth sports and the young athlete. *Transl Pediatr.* 2017;6(3):129.

52. Swoboda KJ, Saul JP, McKenna CE, Speller NB, Hyland K. Aromatic L-amino acid decarboxylase deficiency: Overview of clinical features and outcomes. *Ann Neurol.* 2003;54(S6):S49-S55.

53. Waterman JJ, Kapur R. Upper gastrointestinal issues in athletes. *Curr Sports Med Rep.* 2012;11(2):99-104.

54. Burstein R, Hourvitz A, Epstein Y, et al. The relationship between short-term antibiotic treatments and fatigue in healthy individuals. *Eur J Appl Physiol Occup Physiol.* 1993;66(4):372-375.

55. Fayock K, Voltz M, Sandella B, Close J, Lunser M, Okon J. Antibiotic precautions in athletes. *Sports Health.* 2014;6(4):321-325.

56. McGrew CA. Acute infections. In: McKeag DB, Moeller JL, eds. *ACSM's Primary Care Sports Medicine.* Philadelphia, PA: Lippincott Williams and Wilkins; 2007:251-260.

57. Antibiotic/antimicrobial resistance. Centers for Disease Control and Prevention (CDC) website. www.cdc.gov/drugresistance/index.html. Published April 1, 2018. Accessed April 30, 2018.

58. National Center for Emerging and Zoonnotic Infections Diseases (NCEZID). Centers for Disease Control and Prevention (CDC) website. www.cdc.gov/drugresistance/index.html. Accessed April 30, 2018.

59. Division of Healthcare Quality Promotion (DHQP). Centers for Disease Control and Prevention (CDC) website. www.cdc.gov/drugresistance/index.html. Accessed April 30, 2018.

60. Be antibiotics aware: smart use, best care. Centers for Disease Control and Prevention (CDC) website. www.cdc.gov/features/antibioticuse/index.html. Accessed April 30, 2018.

61. Moura ML, Boszczowski I, Mortari N, et al. The impact of restricting over-the-counter sales of antimicrobial drugs: preliminary analysis of national data. *Medicine.* 2015;94(38): e1605.

62. Zinder SM, Basler RS, Foley J, Scarlata C, Vasily DB. National Athletic Trainers' Association position statement: skin diseases. *J Athl Train.* 2010;45(4):411-428.

63. Brady KT, McCauley JL, Back SE. Prescription opioid misuse, abuse, and treatment in the United States: an update. *Am J Psychiatry.* 2016;173(1):18-26.

64. Dolovich MB, Ahrens RC, Hess DR, et al. Device selection and outcomes of aerosol therapy: evidence-based guidelines: American College of Chest Physicians/American College of Asthma, Allergy, and Immunology. *Chest.* 2005;127(1):335-371.

65. Birkett D, Brøsen K, Cascorbi, I. Clinical pharmacology in research, teaching and health care: Considerations by IUPHAR, the International Union of Basic and Clinical Pharmacology. *Basic Clin Pharmacol Toxicol.*2010,107(1):531-559.

66. Formulary definition. HealthCare.Gov website. www.healthcare.gov/glossary/formulary. Accessed May 4, 2020.

67. Facility definition under Section 503B of the Federal Food, Drug, and Cosmetic Act. U.S. Food & Drug Administration website. www.fda.gov/downloads/Drugs/Guidance/UCM496288.pdf. Published May, 2018. Accessed May 4, 2020.

68. Paoloni JA, Milne C, Orchard J, et al. Non-steroidal anti-inflammatory drugs in sports medicine: guidelines for practical but sensible use. *British J Sport Med.* 2009;43:863-886.

69. Holgado D, Hopker J, Sanabria D, Zabala M. Analgesics and sport performance: beyond the pain-modulating effects. *PM R.* 2018;10(1):72-82.

70. Pelletier JP, Martel-Pelletier J, Rannou F, Cooper C. Efficacy and safety of oral NSAIDs and analgesics in the management of osteoarthritis: Evidence from real-life setting trials and surveys. *Sem Arthritis Rheum.* 2016;45(4):S22-S27.

71. Jankowski CM, Shea K, Barry DW, et al. Timing of ibuprofen use and musculoskeletal adaptations to exercise training in older adults. *Bone Rep.* 2015;1:1-8.

72. Maron BJ, Zipes DP. Introduction: eligibility recommendations for competitive athletes with cardiovascular abnormalities—general considerations. *J Am Coll Cardiol.* 2005;45:1318-1321.

Chapter 24

1. Boyd AS, Benjamin HJ, Asplund C. Splints and casts: indications and methods. *Am Fam Physician.* 2009;80(5):491-499.

2. Brown, SA, Radja, FE. *Orthopaedic Immobilization Techniques: A Step-by-Step Guide for Casting and Splinting.* Urbana, IL: Sagamore; 2015.

3. Egol KA, Koval KJ, Zuckerman JD. *Handbook of Fractures.* 5th ed. Philadelphia, PA: Wolters Kluwer Health; 2015.

4. Eiff MP, Hatch RL. *Fracture Management for Primary Care.* 3rd ed. Philadelphia, PA: Elsevier Saunders; 2018.

5. Honsik K, Boyd A, Rubin AL. Sideline splinting, bracing, and casting of extremity injuries. *Curr Sports Med Rep.* 2003;(2):147-154.

6. Kamat A, Pierse N, Devane P, Mutimer J, Horne G. Redefining the cast index: the optimum technique to reduce redisplacement in pediatric distal forearm fractures. *J Pediatr Orthop.* 2012;32(8);787-791. doi:10.1097/BPO.0b013e318272474d

7. King JC, Nettrour JF, Beckenbagh RD. Traction reduction and cast immobilization for the treatment of boxer's fractures. *Tech Hand Up Extrem Surg.* 1999;3(3):174-180.

8. Nguyen S, McDowell M, Schlechter J. Casting: pearls and pitfalls learned while caring for children's fractures. *World J Orthop.* 2016;7(9):539-545.

9. Perrin DH, McLeod IA. *Athletic Taping, Bracing, and Casting.* 4th ed. Champaign, IL: Human Kinetics; 2019.

10. Prentice, WE. *Arnheim's Principles of Athletic Training: A Competency-Based Approach.* 12th ed. New York, NY: McGraw-Hill; 2006.

11. Thompson SR, Zlotolow DA. *Handbook of Splinting and Casting: Mobile Medicine Series.* Philadelphia, PA: Elsevier Health Sciences; 2012.

12. Zaino CJ, Patel MR, Arief MS, Pivec R. The effectiveness of bivalving, cast spreading, and Webril cutting to reduce cast pressure in a fiberglass short arm cast. *J Bone Joint Surg Am.* 2015;97(5):374-380. doi:10.2106/jbjs.n.00579

13. BSN Medical. *Ortho-Glass: Splinting Course Manual.* Charlotte, NC: Author; 2004.

14. Ootes, D, Lambers KT, Ring, DC. The epidemiology of upper extremity injuries presenting to the emergency department in the United States. *Hand (NY).* 2012;7(1):18-22. doi:10.1007/s11552-011-9383-z

15. Shuler FD, Grisafi FN. Cast-saw burns: evaluation of skin, cast, and blade temperatures generated during cast removal. *J Bone Joint Surg Am.* 2008;90:2626-2630. doi:10.2106/JBJS.H.00119.

16. Roberts A, Shaw KA, Boosman SE, Cameron CD. Effect of casting material on the cast pressure after sequential cast splitting. *J Pediatr Orthop.* 2017; 37(1):74-77. doi:10.1097/BPO.0000000000000574.

17. Stroncek JD, Reichert WM. Overview of wound healing in different tissue types. In: Reichert WM, ed. *Indwelling Neural Implants: Strategies for Contending with the In Vivo Environment.* Boca Raton, FL: CRC Press/Taylor & Francis; 2008:3-40.

18. Fincher L, Carr D, Coursen R, et al. NATA Athletic Training Education Competencies. National Athletic Trainers' Association website. www.nata.org/sites/default/files/competencies_5th_edition.pdf. Accessed June 28, 2020.

INDEX

Note: The italicized *f* and *t* following page numbers refer to figures and tables, respectively.

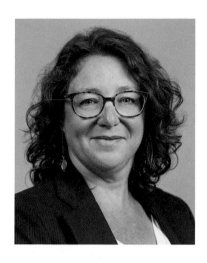

Leamor Kahanov, EdD, ATC, LAT, is the provost of SUNY Oneonta. She previously served as dean of the College of Health Sciences and Education at Misericordia University. Kahanov has also served as the assistant dean of interprofessional education at Indiana State University and as the graduate and undergraduate athletic training program director at San José State University.

Kahanov earned a bachelor's degree in exercise science and athletic training from Indiana University; a master's degree in exercise and sports sciences from the University of Arizona; and a doctorate in education, curriculum, and instruction from the University of San Francisco. She has authored or coauthored more than 80 articles published in peer-reviewed journals as well as 120 professional presentations.

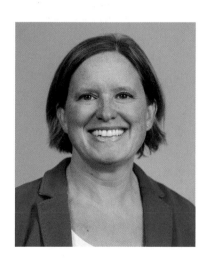

Ellen K. Payne, PhD, LAT, ATC, EMT, is an assistant professor at Moravian College, teaching in the doctor of athletic training program, the master of science in athletic training program, and the undergraduate rehabilitation sciences program. Her previous experience includes teaching athletic training at Radford University and serving as the clinical education coordinator at Marywood University. Prior to becoming an educator, Payne spent six years teaching high school and practicing as an athletic trainer in the San Francisco Bay Area.

Clinically, she has worked with all levels of athletes, from youth sports to professional soccer. In the winter of 2019 she traveled to Spain with the U.S. Paralympic Alpine Ski Team to serve as their athletic trainer during World Cup racing. Payne is also an EMT with Bethlehem Township EMS and a member of the National Ski Patrol. Ellen's research interests include prehospital emergency care, athletic training education, and concussion education. She has authored more than 50 articles and presentations. She currently serves as an assistant editor for the *Athletic Training Education Journal* and is the Eastern Athletic Trainers' Association (EATA) secretary.

CONTRIBUTORS

David C. Berry, PhD, MHA, AT, ATC
Department of Kinesiology
Saginaw Valley State University

Tim Braun, PhD, LAT, ATC, CSCS
School of Health Sciences
Chatham University

Jennifer Doane, MS, RDN, CSSD, LDN, ATC
President, Advantage Nutrition & Wellness LLC

Bryce B. Gaines, LAT, ATC
St. Luke's University Health Network

Marsha Grant-Ford, ATC, PhD
Exercise Science and Physical Education Department
Montclair State University

Angela Hillman, PhD
Applied Health Sciences and Wellness, Division of
Exercise Physiology
College of Health Sciences and Professions
Ohio University

Samuel Johnson, PhD, ATC, CSCS
School of Biological and Population Health Sciences
College of Public Health and Human Sciences
Oregon State University

Paul Knackstedt, MS, Psy D, CMPC
Division of Student Affairs, Cook Counseling Center &
Department of Athletics
Virginia Tech

Monique Mokha, PhD, LAT, ATC, CSCS
Exercise and Sport Science
Nova Southeastern University

James R. Scifers, DScPT, PT, LAT, ATC
Chair, Department of Rehabilitation Sciences
Moravian College

Mitchell Wasik, MS, ATC, LAT
Orthopedics and Sports Medicine
Geisinger/Misericordia University

David A. Wilkenfeld, EdD, LAT, ATC
Department of Rehabilitation Sciences
Moravian College

Loraine Zelna, MS, RT (R)(MR)
Medical Imaging Department
Misericordia University

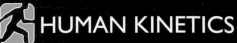

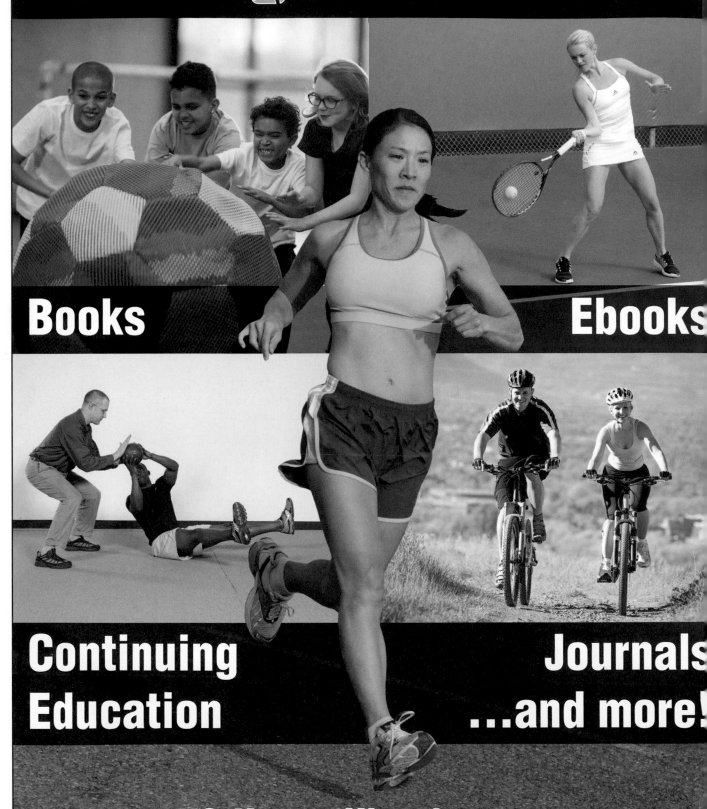

Books

Ebooks

Continuing Education

Journals ...and more!

US.HumanKinetics.com
Canada.HumanKinetics.com